T0332009

John Hughlings Jackson

John Hughlings Jackson

*Clinical Neurology, Evolution, and
Victorian Brain Science*

SAMUEL H. GREENBLATT

*Department of Neurosurgery, Warren Alpert Medical School,
Brown University, Providence, Rhode Island, USA*

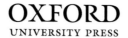

OXFORD
UNIVERSITY PRESS

OXFORD
UNIVERSITY PRESS

Great Clarendon Street, Oxford, OX2 6DP,
United Kingdom

Oxford University Press is a department of the University of Oxford.
It furthers the University's objective of excellence in research, scholarship,
and education by publishing worldwide. Oxford is a registered trade mark of
Oxford University Press in the UK and in certain other countries

First Edition published in 2022

Impression: 1

Published in the United States of America by Oxford University Press
198 Madison Avenue, New York, NY 10016, United States of America

British Library Cataloguing in Publication Data
Data available

Library of Congress Control Number: 2021935484

ISBN 978–0–19–289764–0

DOI: 10.1093/med/9780192897640.001.0001

Printed and bound by
CPI Group (UK) Ltd, Croydon, CR0 4YY

To my wife

Judy

the love of my youth

I offer these

first fruits of my old age

Foreword

Given the exhaustive complexity of modern neuroscience, it is difficult to comprehend the intellectually primordial environment under which the Victorian pioneers of this discipline began to untangle the mysteries of the human brain. Although early Greek physicians, like Hippocrates and Galen, had recognized that certain behavioral functions could be related to cerebral structure, these concepts were lost to supranatural and superstitious beliefs during the middle-ages, and set back decades by the pseudoscience of phrenology that was popular at the turn of the 19th century. By mid-century, however, a number of particularly observant physicians in England, France, Germany, and elsewhere in Europe, began to utilize the scientific method to derive principles of structure-function relationships that might begin to elucidate the mind-body conundrum.

John Hughlings Jackson (1835-1911) was sufficiently prominent among these physicians to be considered, by some, the father of neurology, at least in the English speaking world, and certainly the father of epileptology. He is most noted for recognizing that focal seizures are epilepsy, that they originate in the cortical grey matter of the brain, and that cortical functions can be discretely localized by corelating ictal semiology with pathology at autopsy. This work had practical clinical utility as it initiated the modern era of surgical treatment for epilepsy, but it was much more important for establishing a rigorous scientific approach to the study of brain and behavior. As Greenblatt simply says about Jackson's legacy at the end of this biography he found, "new ways of thinking about old problems."

This highly detailed biography of Jackson is richly researched and referenced, including novel primary source material. The degree of attention paid to Jackson's life and career is not merely of interest because of Jackson's contributions; there were several others who were arguably as, or maybe even more, important, perhaps less recognized, but the place and time of his lifelong dedication to the study of the brain has permitted an extraordinary opportunity to be witness to the birth of modern neuroscience. We are told that Jackson was conservative at base, but highly insightful. He was concerned with human cognition and highly influenced by the philosopher Herbert Spencer. It is particularly instructive to learn about his interactions with other prominent neurologists, neurosurgeons, and proto-neurophysiologists who stimulated the brains of animals to confirm his theories of localization of function. This book presents a vividly descriptive account, as the mind of Jackson attempts to understand the secrets of the mind, together with other prominent intellectuals of the time, in the setting of Victorian England,

Jerome Engel, Jr.
Los Angeles
August 2021

Acknowledgments

These Acknowledgments will be unavoidably autobiographical, because I have been working on Hughlings Jackson intermittently over my entire adult lifetime—now a span of six decades. From those earliest stages I owe deep debts of gratitude to many people, most now departed, beginning when I was an undergraduate at Cornell (B.A. 1961). In the spring of 1960 I was introduced to Jackson's concepts of brain organization by neuroanatomist Marcus Singer. Jackson thus became the subject of my undergraduate honors thesis in history, under the guidance of historians Henry Guerlac and L. Pearce Williams. At the Johns Hopkins Institute of the History of Medicine my mentor for my M.A. (1964) thesis on Jackson was Professor Owsei Temkin (see Greenblatt 2007). At the Cornell University Medical College (M.D. 1966) I was a student with neurologist Fred Plum, and I spent an exciting year (1967–1968) in neurology residency at the Boston VA Hospital, with Norman Geschwind and D. Frank Benson.

In neurosurgery my teachers at the Dartmouth-Hitchcock Medical Center (1970–1974) were Ernest Sachs Jr. (chief), Richard L. Saunders, and Donald H. Wilson. I also enjoyed a brief stint (September–November 1972) with Murray Falconer at the Neurosurgical Unit of Guy's, Maudsley, and King's College Hospitals in London. From that visit I gained my enduring friendship with Charles Polkey (King's College Hospital), who helped greatly in my efforts to grasp something of the ever-changing nosology of epilepsy.

Because this book is based on Jackson's publications, having copies of every item in his bibliography was essential. In the summer of 1992 Christopher C. Taylor obtained those copies, as listed in Jackson's *Selected Writings* (vol. 2, 1932). He was supported by an Undergraduate Teaching and Research Assistantship from the Dean of the College at Brown. In 2006 Jackson's bibliography was expanded and thoroughly reformatted by my fellow Jacksonophiles, George K. York (1951–2021) and David A. Steinberg. They graciously gave me an electronic copy of their *Catalogue Raisonné* of Jackson's writings before its publication. Without their efforts I would have spent at least an additional year doing that bibliographic work. My early work was also advanced when Anne A.J. Andermann (see Andermann 1997) graciously gave me copies of the *Testimonials* for Jackson's appointment at the London Hospital (Jackson 1863b).

In 1995 an eclectic group of neurohistorians was convened in Montreal by Stanley Finger and Harry Whitaker, to found the International Society for the History of the Neurosciences (ISHN). I am indebted to all of the members of this collegial group for many discussions over many years. It would be inequitable to try to name all of them—the list would be nearly synonymous with the Society's membership list. Many of those not specifically mentioned here will find their names in the General Bibliography. However, I will specifically evoke the memory of C.U.M. (Chris) Smith, a fellow founder of the ISHN. We will all miss his critique of this book, which would have been fair, superbly well informed, and incisive.

In 1996 I received a gift of unrestricted funds for my research from MBNA Bank of Delaware, in memory of a patient. By relieving some clinical pressure, that generous donation allowed me to teach a course on the history of neuroscience in Brown's Department of Neuroscience, where Carlos Vargas-Irwin was one of the several students. To all of them I owe thanks for many discussions.

Unfortunately, my scholarly compulsiveness in writing this book did not extend to keeping thorough records of the numerous people who helped along the way, so these Acknowledgments are regrettably incomplete. Doubtless I owe apologies for the omissions of many names. Among the missing would be numerous archivists and librarians, but I can be specific about some of them.

In the summer of 1963 I spent 2 months in Britain searching for Jacksonian material, with support from the American Philosophical Society, Grant No. 3219—Penrose Fund (1962) (see Greenblatt 1965a). For scholarly purposes, my hosts in London were the very accommodating staff at the Wellcome Historical Medical Library. At the York Medical Society, the Secretary, the late Margaret Barnet, was especially helpful. Much more recently, David Pring, the honorary curator of the York Medical Society, has also provided valuable assistance. At the Medical Society of London, Betty Smallwood, the Deputy Registrar, has been helping for more than three decades. At the Brown University Libraries, my late friend, Frank Kellerman, has been sorely missed. Since my arrival at Brown in 1989, I have been peppering the interlibrary loan service with numerous requests. They are always handled promptly and patiently, under the supervision of Bart Hollingsworth. Some other notes in my files include thanks to Edward Brown for information about Philippe Pinel, to Christopher Boes about William Gowers, and to Hugh Buckingham about phoneme analysis in the 1880s.

The lifetime of this project extends back in time to before the present computer age, which has made word processing efficient, enabling, and at times out of whack—hence the need for computer consultants. For several years Christopher DeBlois calmly provided that service, and in more recent years the cheerful expertise of Sherie Simino has been much appreciated. Also in more recent years the skill and conscientiousness of Keith Brough, my editorial assistant, has been essential to the completion of the project. In recent years, the illustrator's skill of Kendall Lane has enhanced the quality of the illustrations immeasurably.

For several weeks in the spring of 2015 Marjorie Perlman Lorch (Birkbeck, University of London) held a Visiting Senior Research Fellowship in Brown's Cogut Center for the Humanities. During that tenure she was able to read and critique all of the available chapters to that point, and we discussed them extensively. Later, with partial support from a research fund at Brown (see MBNA Bank above) Marjorie was able to return to continue our discussions for a week and a half in February–March 2018. By voluntarily identifying so closely with my work, she has put her own professional standing on the line, while enhancing mine. For her courage in that I am most grateful. My connection to Oxford University Press (OUP) was facilitated by Stanley Finger (see ISHN above). At the OUP, my editor, Peter Stevenson, has guided me cheerfully and patiently through myriad problems; and his assistant, Rachel Goldsworthy, has been an unfailing source of advice and assistance.

Also recently, it has occurred to me that generic but sincere thanks are due to the many physicians, surgeons, dentists, and other health professionals, whose skills in the application of modern scientific medicine have kept me alive, functioning well, and comfortable into my ninth decade—and thus able to complete this difficult book.

Finally, and most important, the love and support of my entire family cannot be fully expressed in writing. In particular, the interest and advice of my brother Matt has been much appreciated. The Dedication to my wife speaks for itself.

Contents

Detailed Chapter Contents

List of Illustrations

List of Abbreviations

ALS	amyotrophic lateral sclerosis
BA	British Association for the Advancement of Science
BMA	British Medical Association
BMJ	*British Medical Journal*
EEG	electroencephalography
EOM	extra-ocular movements
F.R.S.	Fellowship of the Royal Society
ICP	intracranial pressure
ILAE	International League Against Epilepsy
ISHN	International Society for the History of the Neurosciences
L.L.D.	Doctor of Laws
L.S.A.	Licentiate of the Society of Apothecaries
M.R.C.S.	Membership of the Royal College of Surgeons
MPC	*Medical Press and Circular*
MTG	*Medical Times and Gazette*
OED	*Oxford English Dictionary*
RCP	Royal College of Physicians
RLOHR	Royal London Ophthalmic Hospital Reports
RMCS	Royal Medical and Chirurgical Society
RSM	Royal Society of Medicine
SW	*Selected Writings (1931–1932)*
TB	tuberculosis
TLE	temporal lobe epilepsy

1

Introduction

Historiography and Practicalities

Who was Hughlings Jackson?

John Hughlings Jackson (1835–1911) was a British neurologist who 'flourished' in the second half of the nineteenth century. He is often called the 'father of English neurology'.[1] More than any other individual in the English-speaking world, Jackson established the methodology for clinical neurology, even to the present day. That is, when a neurologist initially encounters a patient, s/he immediately begins to analyze the patient's problem within a conceptual framework that is quite uniform throughout Western medicine. The essence of the method is the precept that we still teach medical students: first localize the lesion—a single lesion as much as possible—then decide the pathology. Jackson's contemporary, Jean-Martin Charcot (1825–1893), was also working to establish a similar approach.[2] Both men began their work in the 1860s. Thousands of others contributed to it, but mainly beginning in the 1870s. There is one full-length biography of Jackson, which is useful but not really satisfactory.[3]

As a biographical subject, Jackson's primary attraction is the life of his mind, whose growth I will present in this book. His intellectual development is particularly interesting because of his early adherence to the principles of the English philosophical tradition of 'associationism' ('the associationist psychology'). Within this tradition, he was indebted to the Scottish philosopher Alexander Bain (1818–1903) and especially to the Victorian philosopher of evolution, Herbert Spencer (1820–1903). Although Jackson employed Spencer's version of evolutionary theory extensively, he almost never mentioned Charles Darwin (1809–1882) by name in his writings.[4]

Jackson as an Historiographic Problem

Jackson was a distinguished member of the medical establishment in London during its halcyon decades in the middle and later Victorian period, roughly 1860–1900. That standing made him a member of the British intellectual community. Although he was little known to the general public, among British neurologists he was recognized as the most penetrating

---

[1] Critchley and Critchley 1998; often referred to as 'the Critchleys 1998' in this book.

[2] See Goetz et al., 1995, pp.65–72.

[3] The Critchleys 1998. This biography of Jackson is hagiographic in places and not generally analytical. It is valuable for many details, but there are also factual errors, some of which have been found since I wrote my review (Greenblatt 2000).

[4] In 1884 Jackson (J84-02, p.591) used the term 'Darwinism'. Jacyna notes that Jackson also referred to 'the *Origin of Species*' in 1889 (Jacyna 2011, p.3122, citing p.395 in J89-04, but it was actually on p.356). In 1893, concerning a technical anatomical point, Jackson (J93-01, p.129) said, 'Everybody knows of Darwin's researches on the action of the orbicularis palpebrarum during crying, etc.' There is little else.

intellect among a large group of outstanding clinicians. In the decades after his death in 1911, he might have been the subject of a biography by one of the leading neurologists whom he had taught, but there were two problems: (1) no one could find his personal papers,[5] and (2) his voluminous publications are not easy to read.

In 1963 I obtained a copy of Jackson's will and thus 'solved' the first problem by establishing that it is insolvable. He instructed his executor to 'destroy with his own hands all my letters and diaries and all my case books and all correspondence relating thereto'.[6] It appears that he had a faithful executor, because no large cache of Jackson's personal papers has ever been found.[7] Thus, if Jackson's definitive biography were to be written it would have to be done from other sources, mainly his published writings, and therein lies the second rub. Jackson's writing was, as one commentator put it, 'very untidy'.[8] This understatement applies to both style and organization. When he was young, Jackson's style was fairly straightforward. As his theories advanced his prose became increasingly convoluted. Of course, it is the content of his writing, reflecting his thought, that is of primary importance. About this, a perceptive statement of the problems was given by a neurologist-historian who said, from first-hand experience:

> Most of Jackson's numerous papers were written in prose that is not particularly easy to follow. To some extent the difficulty lies in his extreme carefulness with language and in the unfamiliarity of the ideas he attempted to formulate.... Jackson tended to repeat the same idea at more than one place in the same paper, or in different papers, and each time clothed the concept in different words.... Unfortunately, this policy ... sometimes leaves the reader uncertain whether there had been a subtle change in his thought. As well, some of Jackson's interpretations changed as time passed and new data became available, but he tended to let superceded concepts fade from view rather than openly abandon them. Unfortunately for posterity, he never drew all of his ideas together into a definitive statement of his final intellectual position.[9]

A major objective of this book is to identify and understand those subtle changes. As Jackson's theories developed they usually grew in small increments, so each individual change can be hard to appreciate, and yet the sum total of such increments over the years can be a distinctly different position. And finally, in 1885 an editorial writer pointed out that in order to understand Jackson's mature theories—and their changes—it was necessary to have followed and understood their *sequential* development.[10]

---

[5] Jackson's friend, Jonathan Hutchinson (1911, p.1552), remarked on Jackson's 'depredations' of books and recorded Jackson's explanation: 'I did not want the book', he would say, 'I wanted only the information that was in it.' Thus his library in its ultimate condition must have been of very little value.

[6] Jackson 1911a, p.3. I noted this finding, albeit obscurely, in Greenblatt 1965a, p.522. The Critchleys (1998, p.188) cite the same passage from Jackson's will. Swash and Evans 2006, p.666, cite Taylor's 'Biographical memoir' in Jackson 1925, pp.1–27, as their source for the same information about the destruction of Jackson's papers, but no such statement is found in Taylor's memoir.

[7] The executors were Jackson's cousins, Charles Samuel Jackson and 'George William Jackson of Exeter Solicitor'; Charles was specifically directed to destroy Jackson's papers. The Critchleys (1998, p.188) say, without elaboration, that 'a few letters escaped destruction and were given, much later, to a cousin of Jackson's in the United States'.

[8] Walshe 1961, p.28. See Critchley and Critchley 1998, pp.47–51, for other commentaries on this subject; they also remark on the difficulties of Jackson's handwriting.

[9] Eadie 2007c, p.1970. Walshe 1961, p.130, registers essentially the same judgement. A much younger colleague (Leslie Paton, in Chance 1937, p.253) said that, in composing his papers, Jackson 'wrote and rewrote them page by page, four, five or even six times, omitting nothing practical bearing on the subject, believing, as he insisted, that "what might prove of utility to anyone working later on should be included; one never can know what might prove of use in days to come"'.

[10] Jackson 1885i.

Hence the only way to get on with a biography of Jackson's mind is to read all of the 537 items in his bibliography[11] in chronological order. As an *entrée* to Jackson's thought, the utility of his published papers derives partly from the nature of medical publishing in his time. In the nineteenth century the narratives were not sterilized, as they are now. Peer-review as we practice it did not exist, except in the person of a journal's editor. Most articles were single-authored, and the first person singular was commonly employed. Thus, it is potentially feasible to reconstruct the development of Jackson's ideas from his published writings in a way that would be impossible for a twenty-first-century author.

In Jackson's case, the unvarnished honesty of his difficult style is also an advantage. He was not trying to be disingenuous, so penetrating his style potentially leads to a genuine grasp of what he was thinking. An important conduit to his incomplete thoughts was his practice of putting his most recent ideas into long footnotes, which can sometimes seem more impenetrable than the text they were meant to clarify. Nonetheless, his footnotes often provide insights into the ongoing development of his thought, because they show his hesitations and rethinkings. Frequently one finds that Jackson has forecast in a footnote something that he will develop further in a subsequent paper. Despite these problems, Jackson's standing as a seminal figure in neurology has continued to rise, while the earlier prominence of many of his contemporaries has faded.[12] About this phenomenon, there are two caveats, concerning (1) Jackson's biographical sources, and (2) his *Selected Writings* (1931–1932).

The most authoritative biographical sources were published just after Jackson's death by colleagues who knew him to varying degrees. The most important of these were written by Jackson's lifelong friend, Sir Jonathan Hutchinson (1828–1913).[13] Also, in 1946 Hutchinson's son, Herbert, published a *Life and Letters* of his father, which contains many remarks about Jackson.[14] Since Hutchinson was Jackson's only obituarist who knew him well when he was a young adult, we have to rely on Hutchinson's authority about Jackson's early life. This is an important point, because many of the other memoirs of Jackson were written by his admiring junior colleagues.[15] They are generally accurate as of the time when they were written, but their statements about his early years must always be checked against Hutchinson if possible.

In 1931–1932 the publication of the two volumes of *Selected Writings of John Hughlings Jackson* contributed significantly to neurologists' knowledge of Jackson's contributions and thereby to his belatedly rising reputation. The reprinting of the two volumes in 1958 added further to this effect.[16] The editor was Jackson's younger colleague, James Taylor (1859–1946), who chose to arrange the two volumes by subject. Volume One contains Jackson's

---

[11] This number is given by York and Steinberg 2006, p.31. It is inflated because many of his lectures were issued as installments and/or they were published in more than one journal.

[12] See Temkin 1971, p.304; also Eadie 2007c, p.1968.

[13] In addition to a short contribution in Jackson's multi-authored obituary in the *British Medical Journal* (*BMJ*) of October 14, 1911 (Jackson 1911, p.952), Hutchinson wrote 'The late Dr. Hughlings Jackson: Recollections of a lifelong friendship' in the *BMJ* of December 9, 1911 (Hutchinson 1911), which is the best source about Jackson's early life.

[14] H. Hutchinson 1946. Since Herbert Hutchinson had access to his father's papers, the question arises concerning their current location or existence. Beginning in 1872, the Hutchinson family home was in Haslemere, Surrey (Hutchinson 1946, pp.120–127). Despite the extensive efforts of Ms. Greta Turner of the Haslemere Educational Museum in 2003, the main cache of Hutchinson's papers has not been located. For a useful biographical article on Hutchinson see Wales 1963. The ophthalmologist Burton Chance (1868–1965) had access to Jonathan Hutchinson's papers before Herbert Hutchinson wrote his biography of his father; see Chance 1937, pp.254, 285. Chance corresponded with Jackson around 1900; see Chance 1937, p.284.

[15] See e.g. S.A. Kinnier Wilson in 1906 (Martin 1975), Charles Mercier in 1912 (Mercier 1912), and James Taylor in 1925 (Taylor 1925). Taylor probably wrote the first, unsigned part of Jackson's obituary in the *BMJ* of October 14, 1911 ([Jackson] 1911).

[16] The reprinting by Arts & Boeve in 1996 was a limited run.

writings 'On epilepsy and epileptiform convulsions,' and Volume Two is for 'Evolution and dissolution of the nervous system, speech, various papers, addresses and lectures'. Taylor was not interested in the evolution of Jackson's thought, so this arrangement made sense.[17] In my view, however, Jackson's theories developed in close relationship to each other, so the partitioning of subjects in the *Selected Writings* tends to substantiate the false idea that his interwoven theories can actually be separated without losing anything.

Another bedeviling problem with the *Selected Writings* involves Jackson's footnotes. Taylor omitted some footnotes and removed paragraphs from others. He gave general notice of these omissions in his Preface to Volume Two,[18] but readers cannot easily tell where something has gone missing. These omissions are indicated in my footnotes where relevant.

My Approach to Jackson's Historiography

Since I have worked on Hughlings Jackson intermittently throughout my adult life, I come to this self-assigned task with some premises already formulated.

Chronological Analysis

My plan has been to read and analyze all of Jackson's published writings *in chronological order*. As exemplified by the *Selected Writings*, previous historical analyses of his theories have generally dealt with them by subject—aphasia, epilepsy, etc. Historically, his ideas about different subjects evolved in close relationship to each other, especially when he was young. For example, in Chapter 3 we will see that analyzing Jackson's papers on aphasia in 1864, without considering his other papers of the same year, would not produce a comprehensive view of how he was thinking. Sometimes the puzzling inconsistencies in his rapidly evolving theories can seem worse if they are treated separately. I submit that the chronological approach is the only valid way to analyze the continuous development of his thoughts.[19]

A Unified Neurological Pathophysiology

Also in Chapter 3, we will see that from the beginning, as early as 1862, Jackson saw the need to bring together all neurological diseases in a unified pathophysiology. In this regard, Spencer offered generalities about brain function that Jackson could translate into larger conceptualizations, using the data of disease in his ingenious way. The theme of an evolutionary outlook thus contributed greatly to Jackson's effort to create a unified pathophysiology, which is his most important contribution to neurological thought.

---

[17] In 1915 Taylor (p.391) said, 'Jackson's writings are best considered in groups'. Eadie 2013, p.362, offers the same rationale for Taylor's editorial decision.

[18] Jackson 1932, p.vi.

[19] Turner (1993, p.38) complains that 'we too often continue to view and treat Victorian intellectuals as historical figures who did not themselves develop historically'. He implicates the role of authors' collected writings in the ahistorical treatment of Victorian intellectuals (Turner, pp.41–42)—the same charge that I have leveled against Jackson's *Selected Writings*.

The Inadequacies of Premodern Neuroscience, *circa* 1860

When Jackson began he immediately encountered the problem of inadequate knowledge about the central nervous system. That is, in order to have a unified pathophysiology it was necessary to have a unified physiology. This is not to say that nothing was known about it. The British textbooks of the mid-nineteenth century contain a wealth of information about neuroanatomy, neurophysiology, and clinical neurology. Much of it is 'correct' as far as it goes, but that statement applies mainly to the peripheral nervous system and to some of the cranial nerves. There was some conception of the organization and function of the lower brainstem and the spinal cord, but there was little that we would find agreeable about the cerebrum or about the central nervous system as an integrative organ.

Working Out the Normal Neuroscience

It follows that Jackson had to work out an understanding of normal brain organization for his own purposes. However, there is no evidence that he started with any conscious intention to investigate the normal (he called it the 'healthy') nervous system. He simply needed the information to get on with his study of neurological disease. As early as 1863 he implied some recognition of this necessity.[20] In a lecture of 1869 he said that by the 'careful' study of disease we should be able to 'reach a knowledge of the fundamental plan of structure of the nervous system, and thus find out what is the general principle of localisation throughout the nervous system'.[21] In 1873 he said explicitly, 'For some years I have studied cases of disease of the brain, not only for direct clinical, but for anatomical and physiological purposes. Cases of paralysis and convulsion may be looked upon as the results of experiments made by disease on particular parts of the nervous system of man'.[22]

Charcot and Jackson as Co-founders of Modern Neurology

Needless to say, the French consider Charcot to be the founder of modern neurology (Fig. 1.1), while the British accord the same honor to Jackson. I consider them to be co-founders of neurology's basic clinical method, because: (1) they both started in the early 1860s, a decade before anyone else made similar efforts; (2) they had the same objective of a unifying pathophysiology; (3) they both encountered the problem of inadequate neuroscience and used clinical methods to compensate for it; (4) their interests in localization were largely complementary rather than competitive; and (5) each recognized that the other was doing fundamental work.

Although Charcot was senior to Jackson by a decade, his neurological career really began when he was appointed chief of the medical service at the Salpêtrière in Paris in 1862, the same year when Jackson received a junior appointment at Queen Square in London. Charcot overcame the inadequacies of his contemporary neuroscience colleagues by applying his clinico-pathological method to the central lower nervous system.[23] Using the patterns of

---

[20] See Jackson 1863a (discussed below); also Jackson 1864h, pp.1–2.
[21] Jackson 1869a, p.307.
[22] Jackson 1873a, p.84. Jackson 1865f, p.301, used 'experiments of disease'.
[23] See Chapters 2 and 3.

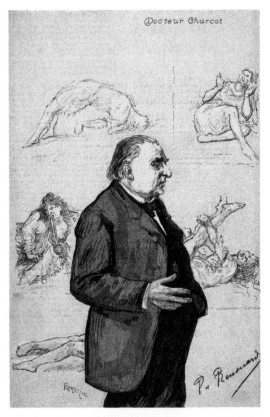

Fig. 1.1 Jean-Martin Charcot. From the 'Front cover of *Revue Illustrée*, a popular tabloid, showing the image that Charcot attained in the general society'.
(Reproduced from La Revue illustrée, 1887. HUMANITIES & SOCIAL SCIENCES LIBRARY / NEW YORK PUBLIC LIBRARY / SCIENCE PHOTO LIBRARY.)

degenerative 'system diseases', he was able to define functional pathways in the spinal cord and brainstem. At the other end of the neuraxis, Jackson used disease patterns to understand the functions of the cerebrum and the principles of its organization.

Some Bibliographic and Other Details

Since Jackson's ideas permeated into many parts of neuroscience and beyond, I hope that the audience for this book will be multidisciplinary. This expectation should lead to a mode of writing that avoids too many technicalities. However, simplification of Jackson's neurological technicalities is impossible, because they are the underpinnings of his theories. I have been particularly concerned to accommodate readers who have some knowledge of clinical and/or basic neuroscience, but not enough to feel comfortable. It was from this concern that I hit upon the idea of using 'Definition Sections', which are located mainly in Chapters 3, 4, and 5. Although my original purpose in creating them was to assist the partially initiated, I like to think that they also serve to clarify my arguments by specifying technical usages. The

Definition Sections are placed in the text where they are immediately relevant, so the only glossary at the end of the book is the Index.

Bibliographies and Formatting

Bibliographies

There are two bibliographies: (1) the Published Writings of John Hughlings Jackson, and (2) the General Bibliography, which contains everything else. The former is based largely on York and Steinberg's *Catalogue Raisonné* of Jackson's publications.[24] Their identification number for each item is given in square brackets at the end of each item's listing. For the items that York and Steinberg missed, each one is noted to be 'Not in York and Steinberg' in my list of Jackson's Published Writings. Doubtless there are still more out there.

In addition to their listing of Jackson's published papers, York and Steinberg's *Catalogue* has two appended lists of privately printed 'pamphlets' (their Appendix 1) and other 'unpublished' material (Appendix 2), which are in the Rockefeller Medical Library, Institute of Neurology, University College London, Queen Square. Those appendices are not reproduced here. A few items in their Appendix 1 are occasionally cited in my footnotes, with references to the *Catalogue*. When there is no clear proof of Jackson's authorship for unsigned items that I attribute to him, or no other identifiable author (e.g., obituaries), his name will be surrounded by square brackets ('[Jackson, J.H.]').

Most of Jackson's papers were originally given at meetings of medical organizations. The chronological listing in his Published Writings is always based on the publication date, but sometimes I will discuss his papers as of the dates of their public delivery, if the date is available. This leads to the question of whether he got to edit and/or enlarge his papers before their publication, and clearly he did in many instances, especially for major lectures.

Italics and underlining

Jackson and his contemporaries liked to use italics. In their hand-written manuscripts they indicated the presence of italics for the type compositor by <u>underlining</u> the words to be italicized. For this reason, underlining was not used in their publications. On the other hand, modern word processors make it easy to underline text, and I have found that option to be an effective way to draw attention to short passages in larger quotations. In all such instances I have indicated the true state of the original by saying 'my underlining' in the footnotes.

Quotations

The main purpose of quotations is evidential—to let historical subjects speak for themselves. In Jackson's case, I hope another advantage to committed readers is the opportunity to learn to read the Jacksonian dialect of Victorian medical English.

Square brackets in footnotes

The footnotes are numbered sequentially in each chapter. In Jackson's Publications *his* footnotes are sometimes numbered sequentially on each page or even in each column. Therefore,

---

[24] York and Steinberg 2006.

the numbers for my footnotes at the ends of indented quotations are surrounded by super-script square brackets (e.g., [99]) to show that they are not part of the original text.

Square brackets around names in bibliographies
In the bibliographies, square brackets around cited names are used when there is no clear author's byline—the name is known or inferred from outside evidence, or the name is actually from the subject of the citation. This is not to be confused with my square brackets at the ends of citations containing York and Steinberg's (2006) numbers for each of their citations. Parentheses are used when only the author's surname is known, but the Christian name is determined from other sources.

Dates
Current European practice is to give dates logically, in day/month/year format, whereas Americans still use month/day/year. In Jackson's time, however, the general British practice was month/day/year. I have used the latter because it is historically accurate for Jackson.

Birth–death years
For the names of deceased individuals who had any importance to Jackson's story, I have given the birth and death dates in the first instance when the name is mentioned in my main text or sometimes in footnotes. Therefore, looking for the first listing of the name in the Index will lead to the dates.

Limited use of honorific titles: Sir, Lord, etc.
Many of the (male) people in Jackson's circle received royal titles in later life. In historical writing there is a sometime practice of forecasting this achievement by inserting 'later' in parentheses before the title, e.g., '(later Sir) Jonathan Hutchinson'. I have eschewed this conceit because I think it predicts a prominence that the individual did not necessarily enjoy before he was honored. However, if the person held the title at the historical time when his actions are being discussed, I have acknowledged the honor. Hutchinson was knighted in 1908, so he was 'Sir Jonathan' when he wrote his biographical memoirs of Jackson in 1911.

2

Prologue to Originality

Jackson's Life, Education, and Environment, 1835–1863

Birth and Family

John Hughlings Jackson was born on April 4, 1835, at Providence Green, Green Hammerton, Yorkshire, in the North of England, about 10 miles northwest of the ancient city of York. He was the youngest of the five children of Samuel Jackson (1805–1858), a native Yorkshireman, and his Welsh wife, Sarah Hughlings (1807?–1836).[1] According to English folklore, Yorkshiremen are supposed to be 'energetic, courageous, cautious in drawing conclusions'[2] and also independent-minded and taciturn—rather like some Americans' characterizations of 'Old Vermonters'. It has been said of Jackson that 'He had a reputation for a Yorkshireman's plain speaking'.[3] But this is not to say that Yorkshire was illiberal. The Yorkshire Philosophical Society (founded in 1821) was the 'mother-society' of the British Association for the Advancement of Science (founded in 1831).[4] Jackson always retained a deep affection for Yorkshire—he made a yearly pilgrimage to his birthplace.[5]

Independence of mind was characteristic of Jackson's family and his environment. He and his siblings were baptized by his great uncle, the Reverend James Jackson, who was a Dissenting Minister.[6] Dissenters were Protestants who dissented from the established Church of England. In the nineteenth century, physical persecution of dissenters was rare or nonexistent, but at the beginning of the century full access to the 'ancient' universities (Cambridge and Oxford) was available only to Anglicans.[7] In York, theological dissension had a long history—many forms of non-Anglican Protestantism were flourishing there.[8] Jackson himself was neither a dissenter nor a believer. When he died in 1911, Hutchinson said: 'I do not believe that Jackson ever made any change in his religious faith. It was one of the simplest kind of agnosticism, and into it he appears to have been born.'[9] Now it's hard to

---

[1] The genealogies of both families have been thoroughly researched by the Critchleys 1998, which is my source for the birth and death dates of Jackson's parents.

[2] T. Buzzard in Jackson 1911b (Obituary) p.952. It was said of another Yorkshireman and physician, Sir William Broadbent (1835–1907), that he had 'a Yorkshireman's sturdiness of mind, amounting almost to stubbornness, which made him cling to his opinion once he had formed it, in face of all differences' (Brown 1955, p.170).

[3] Critchley and Critchley 1998, p.165.

[4] Howarth 1931, p.15. It is now the British Science Association (BSA) or simply 'British Association' (BA).

[5] Taylor 1925, p.2.

[6] Critchley and Critchley 1998, p.7.

[7] This restriction was gradually loosened. By 1900, it had largely disappeared.

[8] Royle 1981, pp.212–218. Dissenters were also called 'nonconformists' or 'free churchmen'. About 'Yorkshire's influence on the foundation of British neurology', see Pearce and Lees 2013. Ackerknecht (1979, pp.89–92) attributes a connection between dissenters and medicine, science, and commerce to the fact that those occupations gradually became open to dissenters in the nineteenth century; see also Birken 1995, about earlier medical dissenters.

[9] Hutchinson 1911, p.1553. Jackson's teacher, Thomas Laycock (see section 'Early Life and Education' in this chapter), was also a Yorkshire native from a dissenting family background. Jacyna (1981, p.116) states that Laycock's variety of dissension included 'the heresy of 'mortalism'. This denied that human beings were composed of spiritual and material elements and that the former left the latter at death to begin a separate

conceive of an agnostic infant, so Hutchinson is implying either that Jackson's family was agnostic and/or that Jackson was agnostic in his later youth.

Jackson's mother died when he was only 1 year old, and his father did not remarry. Jackson and his siblings were raised by their father and his female servants. Samuel Jackson (1805–1858) was a farmer and brewer who had significant substance. He apparently lost a lot of money in the railroad speculation of the 1840s,[10] but he seems to have recovered, and there is evidence that he remained connected to his son's life until his death.[11]

Early Life and Education

We know little about Jackson's primary and secondary education.[12] He finished his secondary education in 1850,[13] at the age of 15, when the ordinary age for leaving school was 14. Later in life he expressed a poor opinion of these schools, and he sometimes attributed his success to the fact that he had not been over-educated.[14] The Critchleys suggest that Jackson's criticism of his early teachers may have been unfair,[15] and I agree. He was not at any disadvantage when he entered and completed medical school. He passed his medical qualifying (licensing) examinations on his first attempts, and his later career certainly bespeaks a well-honed mind. In addition to the basics, he is said to have acquired a 'sound knowledge of Latin and of French' in the course of his schooling.[16]

1850 was a very good year for Jackson. He acquired a substantial inheritance from his maternal grandfather, John Hughlings, who left £2,000 to each of the children of his deceased daughter, Sarah, Jackson's mother. We can infer from this that he too remained connected to his grandchildren's lives in some measure. In any case, this 'handsome sum of money' smoothed the path for Jackson's subsequent education.[17] In the same year Jackson was apprenticed to Dr. William Charles Anderson and his son, Dr. Tempest Anderson, who were

---

existence … the spirit was held to be intrinsic to the body and to perish with it.' I don't know if Jackson's background included this heresy.

[10] Critchley and Critchley 1998, p.8.

[11] Critchley and Critchley 1998, pp.29–31, discovered an affectionate letter from Samuel Jackson to his son, dated March 17, 1854. In a publication of 1864, Hughlings Jackson recalled being 'lodged in a house' during 'a visit at the sea-side' when he was very young (J64-10, p.440). Presumably this was before the speculative railroad bust of the 1840s.

[12] Critchley and Critchley 1998, pp.23–24.

[13] According to Brown 1955, p.16, Jackson 'was educated at Tadcaster and at Nailsworth, Gloucestershire'. There is still in Yorkshire the residential Tadcaster Grammar School, founded in 1557 (http://web.tgsbec.com/prospectus/history-and-heritage/, accessed March 25, 2015), but there is no evidence that he attended there. It seems strange that he would have been sent 220 miles south of York to Nailsworth, east of Bristol, but his mother's family were Welsh, and some lived in Herefordshire, in adjacent England (Critchley and Critchley 1998, pp.15–22). Reynolds and Andrew (2007) have established that Jackson attended the Longfield School, at Halifax, but we don't know when. It was operated by a family named Greenwoods.

[14] Taylor 1925, p.2. Hutchinson 1911, p.1553, makes a similar statement.

[15] Critchley and Critchley 1998, pp.24–25.

[16] Jackson 1911b, p.950. When Jackson obtained his M.D. by examination at St. Andrews (see 'Major Hospital Appointments 1862–1863' in this chapter), one of the requirements was translation of a Latin passage to English (see 'Medical examination papers of the University of St. Andrews. December 1860.' The Lancet 1:149–150, 1861; with thanks to M. Lorch). That he could not read German was a frustration to Jackson; see Mercier 1912, p.86. At an international congress in London in 1881, Jackson regretted that his 'ignorance of foreign languages' impeded his ability to follow some of the papers; see J81-24, p.21. Colleagues who were potential German translators for Jackson included Hutchinson, J.A. Lockhart Clarke (1817–1880) and Thomas Buzzard (1831–1919).

[17] Critchley and Critchley 1998, p.22. According to www.MeasuringWorth.com (accessed January 20, 2017), £2,000 in 1850 was worth £192,900 in 2015.

general practitioners in York. We have no records of Jackson's experience in this capacity, but the Critchleys have used other sources to describe the rigors of the apprenticeship at the same time and place.[18] However, it does not follow automatically that Jackson's life was especially difficult during this period. It may have been quite ordinary, because there is no record that he commented on it in later life.

In 1852, at age 17, Jackson entered the now long-defunct York Medical School,[19] where Dr. Anderson was a lecturer. At this point, we can begin to see some impact of identifiable individuals on Jackson's development. Hutchinson had been a student at York some years before Jackson (1846–1850). In his obituary of Jackson, Hutchinson remarked on the intimacy of their medical school experience—there were only ten or twelve students in the entire school—and on their mutual admiration for a particular instructor:

> ... I believe Chemistry was Dr. Jackson's first love. This was perhaps first awakened at the York School of Medicine, where, in the person of the late Dr. William Proctor, both he and I in succession came under the influence of a most able and attractive teacher ... [we] owed very much to our close intercourse with Dr. Proctor, who taught us chemistry and natural philosophy with enthusiasm, but in almost conversational methods.[20]

So probably it was Proctor who aroused Jackson's first thoughts about scientific method. Aside from this speculation, we can identify at least four areas of study that were important in Jackson's later career, and we know most of his instructors for those subjects.

At the York Medical School, anatomy, physiology, and pathology ('morbid anatomy') were all taught together.[21] 'Demonstrations and Dissections' was a separate course, though taught by the same instructors. Later in life Jackson recalled with gratitude the names of Dr. George Shann and Mr. Samuel W. North as his teachers in this fundamental subject.[22] Clinico-pathological correlation was the central methodological premise of scientific medicine in the nineteenth century.[23] It seeks to correlate the patient's complaints and findings in life with the pathological findings at autopsy. One could argue that this method remains central to our thinking—with imaging often substituting for autopsies. It entered the mainstream of medicine early in the nineteenth century, primarily through the influence of the Parisian school of medicine.[24]

The centrality of clinico-pathological correlation was also emphasized by the most prominent member of the York faculty, Thomas Laycock (1812–1876), a native Yorkshireman, who was Lecturer in Clinical Medicine from 1846 to 1855 (Fig. 2.1). Jackson completed his course in 1855, when Laycock left York to take the prestigious Chair of the Practice of Physic at Edinburgh.[25] Laycock had studied at the Medical School of London University (now University College London) from 1833 to 1835. During the period 1833–1836, he

---

[18] Critchley and Critchley 1998, pp.25–26.

[19] On the history of the School see Wetherill 1961.

[20] Hutchinson 1911, p.1553. In the 1850s, 'natural philosophy' meant 'physics'.

[21] Wetherill 1961; Greenblatt 1965b, p.347.

[22] Jackson 1882d, p.306.

[23] The 'clinico-pathological method' is also known by other names, e.g., 'anatomical diagnosis', 'clinico-anatomical diagnosis'. For reasons that are explained in Chapter 3, I will use 'clinico-pathological' method as the only generic term for this process.

[24] The classical study of 'Paris medicine' is Ackerknecht 1967. Among many other historical analyses are Porter 1997, pp.306–320, and Hannaway and La Berge 1998.

[25] Barfoot 1995. The biographical details in this paragraph are taken from Barfoot's Introduction, pp.1–52, and from Greenblatt 1965b, pp.348–349.

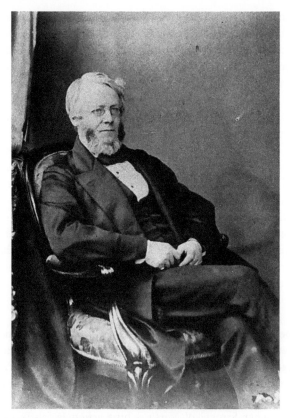

Fig. 2.1 Portrait of Thomas Laycock.
(Reproduced from Barfoot, M. 1995. "To ask the Suffrages of the Patrons": Thomas Laycock and the Edinburgh Chair of Medicine, 1855. Medical History, Suppl.15. Wellcome Trust.)

also studied in Paris. In 1839 he acquired an M.D. *summa cum laude* at the University of Göttingen in Germany. Thus, the York Medical School gave its graduates a solid introduction to the leading medical science of the day. Later in life Jackson told Hutchinson that he did not regret having escaped university training.[26]

In addition to methodological issues, Laycock had a strong interest in the relationship between the nervous system and mental phenomena, but I will defer exploration of his views in relation to Jackson's to Chapter 4.[27] In fact, the subject of psychiatric illness had been in the air at York since the eighteenth century. The York Lunatic Asylum opened in 1777, and there were many other similar institutions by Jackson's time.[28] In 1796, the Quakers, led by William Tuke, opened their famous The Retreat for Persons afflicted with Disorders of the Mind.[29] From the beginning, William Tuke felt that 'it was possible to treat mental affliction with kindliness and humane methods'.[30] William Tuke's great grandson, Daniel Hack Tuke

---

[26] Hutchinson 1911, p.1553.

[27] On Laycock's contributions to the professional discussions of British psychiatrists with regard to mind and brain see Jacyna 1982; and Leff 1991.

[28] See Greenblatt 1965b, p.351; Parsons 2002, p.41; and Rollin and Reynolds 2018.

[29] Sessions and Sessions 1987, p.62.

[30] Sessions and Sessions 1987, p.66. See also Parsons 2002, p.44. Although the famous story about Pinel's unchaining the psychiatric inmates of the Bicêtre in 1798 has been debunked (Weiner 1994), the Enlightenment-driven, humane treatment of the insane was clearly an idea whose time was at hand.

(1827–1895), became a visiting physician to The Retreat in 1853. He was also Lecturer in Psychological Medicine at the York Medical School until he left York in 1859.[31] Hack Tuke conducted an outpatient psychiatry clinic at the Dispensary in York. He also took students to The Retreat,[32] presumably including Jackson, though we have only indirect information about this.[33] We do know that Jackson had an abiding interest in mental illness throughout his career.

Finally, York had an Institute for Diseases of the Eye, founded in 1831. Students saw patients there,[34] so again we can presume that Jackson had that experience. It seems very likely, because he took an early interest in ophthalmology and ophthalmoscopy.[35] One of his first hospital appointments in London, in 1859 or early 1860, was at the Royal London Ophthalmic Hospital, commonly known as 'Moorfields Eye Hospital' or just 'Moorfields'.[36] Jackson's accomplishments in ophthalmology were significant contributions to the growth of the field, especially with regard to the ophthalmoscope, which had been invented by Hermann von Helmholtz (1821–1894) in 1850.[37] The study of ophthalmology was important to Jackson's comprehensive effort to understand neurological disease.

Medical Training: London 1855–1856 and York 1856–1859

In the mid-nineteenth century it was customary for English students who had completed their training at provincial medical schools to proceed to further study in one of London's teaching hospitals. In addition to education, their route to qualifying was through London, by examination of (1) the Worshipful Society of Apothecaries, (2) the Royal College of Surgeons, or (3) the Royal College of Physicians.[38] In 1855, Jackson went to St. Bartholomew's Hospital, which was the largest of London's teaching hospitals. 'Barts' prided itself on its practical bedside teaching.[39] We know very little about Jackson's experience there, with one exception.

---

[31] The exact date of Hack Tuke's appointment to the York Medical School is not well established; see Greenblatt 1965b, p.352; also Wetherill 1961, p.267.

[32] Critchley and Critchley 1998, p.28.

[33] See Jackson 1862b, pp.222–223, where Jackson described a patient who had been 'Under the care of Dr. Shann and Dr. Tuke' at the York County Hospital in August 1855.

[34] Wetherill 1961, p.262.

[35] Chance (1937, p.267) says: 'In a letter ... to the editor of the *British Medical Journal* in 1867 Jackson stated that he had been induced by Dr. John W. Ogle [of St. George's Hospital, London] to employ the ophthalmoscope as a part of his routine of examination'. However, what Jackson actually said was more generic: 'Some years ago, Dr. John W. Ogle pointed out the great value of this instrument to the physician' (Jackson 1867d), so in regard to the priority of Ogle's influence on Jackson, Jackson's statement is ambiguous. In 1862 (Jackson 1862h, p.600), Jackson referred to 'a paper in the *Medical and Chirurgical Transactions*' by J. W. Ogle, but without further citation. We don't know if the eye institute in York had an ophthalmoscope, but the instrument was exciting 'increasing interest' at Moorfields in the 1850s (Collins 1929, p.110).

[36] Greenblatt 1965b, pp.355–356. In 1889 (Jackson 1889h, p.837) Jackson said that ophthalmology was 'the first subject I specially worked at after my student life'. Presumably this refers to his early years in London and his appointment at Moorfields, where Hutchinson was appointed surgeon in 1862 (Collins 1929, p.218). In 1885 Jackson (Jackson 1885f, p.945) acknowledged Hutchinson for his 'earliest instruction in ophthalmology'.

[37] Albert and Edwards 1996, pp.191–192. For a survey of Jackson's work and publications in ophthalmology see Chance 1937.

[38] Medical degrees from the universities of Cambridge and Oxford conferred automatic qualification.

[39] Bonner 1995, pp.170–171. There is no official record of Jackson's attendance at Barts, apparently because he did not sign the student signature book (personal communication [email] from Ms. Katie Ormerod, Assistant Archivist, St. Bartholomew's Hospital, May 19, 2005). This early evasion of bureaucratic formality presaged one of Jackson's lifelong behaviors.

James Paget (1814–1899) was a prominent surgeon and pathologist whose name was later (1874) associated with Paget's Disease of the nipple and (in 1877) Paget's Disease of bone (osteitis deformans). While he was at Barts, Jackson was befriended by Paget.[40] Paget was a direct scion of the clinico-pathological tradition in its English version, which can be traced back at least to John Hunter (1728–1793). Hence, the effect of Paget's teaching would have been to reinforce the importance of the clinico-pathological method that Jackson had already learned at York. We know that, as a student, Jackson made a lasting impression on Paget, because Paget said so four decades later, when he recalled of Jackson,

> I remember you well … You sat regularly at my lectures; you were one of those attentive and watchful students who make lecturers careful, and compel them as far as possible to keep their work up to a level which shall be better than that of their pupils and yet intelligible to them. I well remember you to have been a constant help and guide and promoter of one's best work.[41]

Jackson spent less than a full year in London in 1855–1856. In April 1856 he passed the Apothecaries' examination, thereby becoming a Licentiate of the Society of Apothecaries (L.S.A.).[42] That gave him a license to practice. Shortly thereafter he also passed the examination for Membership of the Royal College of Surgeons (M.R.C.S), which was another form of qualification.[43] Thus doubly armed, he returned to York and took up the position of Resident Medical Officer at the York Dispensary in mid-1856 (Fig. 2.2).[44] His three years in this capacity can be seen as his 'residency' training in general medicine. We know that he saw all manner of cases, because he often referred to his experiences at the York Dispensary in his later writings.[45]

During those years of clinical grooming in York, Jackson began to give some hints of an interest in diseases of the nervous system. In January 1858 he was elected to membership in the York Medical Society. His attendance there was spotty, but he did deliver one paper on a neurological subject at the meeting of January 8, 1859. He also proposed three books for purchase by the Society's library, including one work on the brain.[46] More fundamentally, he began the serious pursuit of clinico-pathological correlation. According to the Critchleys, Jackson was 'an enthusiastic member of the newly-formed Post-Mortem Club, where clinicians and pathologists met periodically to discuss cases informally, especially those of patients who had been admitted on an emergency basis.'[47]

---

[40] Greenblatt 1965b, p.349; Critchley and Critchley 1998, p.31. Paget advocated the establishment of special housing for students at Barts. In 1843 he became Warden of College Hall and a mentor to its students. Whether Jackson benefitted from this arrangement is not known, but it appears that Paget's wardenship lasted only to 1851; see Paget 1902, pp.122–128, and Bonner 1995, p.227.

[41] Paget 1895, p.861.

[42] See Greenblatt 1965b, p.347, footnote 3.

[43] Critchley 1960e, p.614; Greenblatt 1965b, p.350. For further details see Harris 1935, p.131. The Critchleys (1998, p.32) state that Jackson took the Conjoint Examination of the Royal College of Surgeons and the Royal College of Medicine in 1859, rather than the single examination for M.R.C.S. However, this assertion contradicts Critchley 1960e. Although the Conjoint Examination was proposed in 1859, it was decades later before it actually came into being; see Cooke 1972, pp.844–872.

[44] Jackson's official title and exact date of return to York are not clear; see Greenblatt 1965, p.350, footnote 17; and p.351, footnote 22.

[45] See e.g. Jackson 1864j, pp.422, 455; see also Greenblatt 1965b, p.350, footnote 18.

[46] See Greenblatt 1965b, pp.350–351.

[47] Critchley and Critchley 1998, p.32, but they give no source for this statement. In 1882, while urging the importance of such groups, Jackson (Jackson 1882d, pp.305–306) said: 'Many years ago, at York, a club of this sort was formed … Some of the cases we had to deal with were 'coroners' cases'; some of them were cases of sudden or of rapid death.'

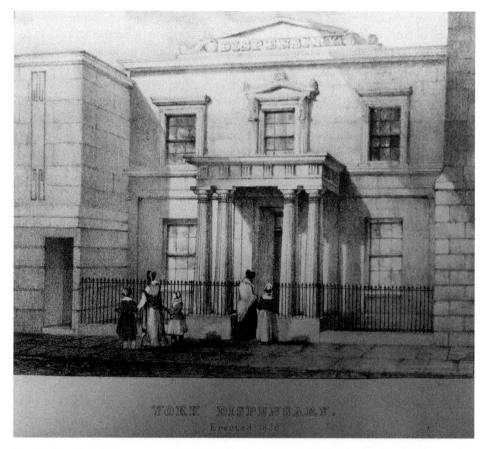

Fig. 2.2 The York Dispensary, erected 1828, where Jackson was Resident Medical Officer 1856–1859.
(Reproduced by kind permission of York Medical Society, David Pring, FRCOG, curator.)

It is important to note that Jackson took his initial qualifying examinations and served most of his 'residency' just before Britain's Medical Act of 1858 was passed by Parliament. The Act did not fully control 'quackery', as its proponents had hoped, but it did leave regulation of the profession to its own good offices. In actuality, brotherly power struggles were legion.

The "medical profession" in 1858 was a hybrid agglomeration of learned, university-educated physicians, surgeons in transition from an old craft to a new "science," and apothecaries who claimed the practical skills of physic and surgery while drug sales wedded them to trade ... The untrained and unlicensed "quack" continued to be an accepted source of health care. Victorian society in 1858 had limited confidence in the power of medical "science" and serious reservations about medical men's social authority and prestige.[48]

The effect of the Act was to create a three-tiered hierarchy by recognizing the large middle group of practitioners who, like Jackson, had some education and training but no university

[48] Peterson 1978, p.38. See also Cherry 1996, pp.27–34, and Roberts 2009.

degrees or equivalent imprimaturs. The quacks were tolerated, but at the bottom they had no access to the newly created *Medical Register*, which recognized general practitioners *and* the higher-level 'physicians'. The latter, as 'consultants', held most of the prestigious positions in the large city hospitals.[49] Thus, when Jackson started his career in the mid-century he was entering a profession that had yet to gain the societal status which it had earned by the time he retired in the early twentieth century. However, this is not to imply that medicine in the mid-century held no enticing prospects. Bright and ambitious youth have always been drawn to the centers of their civilizations. In 1859, age 24, Jackson left York and took up permanent residence in London, just when the entire country was experiencing major changes.

British Society and Culture in the 1850s

The Industrial Revolution began in the late eighteenth century in the Midlands of England—north of London and largely just south of York. For practical reasons of improving efficiency, thermodynamics—*the Science of Energy*[50]—became a crucial concern for many people who were otherwise quite indifferent to the niceties of theoretical physics. Hermann von Helmholtz had published his essay on the conservation of energy in 1847, and its consequences for thermodynamics were the subject of widespread debate and research in Britain in the 1850s and beyond.[51] All of this was directly relevant to the neurosciences in the mid-nineteenth century, because a general conception of 'force' (now called 'energy'[52]) pervaded thinking about the nervous system, including Jackson's analysis of seizures and epilepsy.[53]

Despite the excruciating downsides of the Industrial Revolution, the idea of progress was thriving in the mid-century. Britain had emerged victorious from its Napoleonic wars, and the domestic threat of the revolutionary mob had been largely assuaged without tearing the country apart. In 1859, Queen Victoria (1819–1901) was only 22 years into her long reign (1837–1901). Writing about the period 1850–1870, David Newsome called it Victorian England's

> ... phase of nearly twenty years that has been labelled 'the age of equipoise' ... people came suddenly to realize that their country led the world, not only in its maintenance of political stability while governments were crashing all over Europe [in the revolutions of 1848], but also in its commercial and industrial supremacy and – what affected the population generally and most immediately – in its unrivalled [*sic*] prosperity. So it was that G.M. Young could declare that 'of all decades in our history, a wise man would choose the eighteen-fifties to be young in'.[54]

---

[49] In the *Medical Register* of 1863 Jackson is listed as having registered on January 1, 1859, with a residence (with the Hutchinsons) at 4 Finsbury Circus, London EC. His L.S.A. and M.R.C.S. are noted from 1856, as well as his M.D. of 1860 and M.R.C.P. of 1861. See www.ancestry.co.uk, accessed February 22, 2014.

[50] C. Smith 1998.

[51] See C. Smith 1998, Chapters 7 and 8.

[52] See Youmans 1869. William Thomson (Lord Kelvin) actually introduced the term 'energy' as preferable to 'force' in 1849; see C. Smith 1998, p.13.

[53] In 1881 (Jackson 1881b, pp.449–450) Jackson said, 'I do not use the term force as synonymous either with momentum or energy; it is difficult for me to use the term force without misgivings, since ... it is a term used differently by different people'. See especially Lazar 2015.

[54] Newsome 1997, p.50; my square brackets.

The year of Jackson's migration to London (1859) also coincided with the publication of Darwin's *On the Origin of Species*. Since Spencer's version of evolutionary theory had a prominent role in Jackson's thinking, one might assume that in his youth Jackson's interest would have been aroused by all the tumult that followed Darwin's proclamation. Perhaps, but there is no direct evidence to support such an inference. In fact, the height of the controversy was not reached until the 1870s.[55] Realistically, we can assume that Jackson was aware of the tumult, because it would have been inescapable in his milieu. But it is one thing to know about a controversy and quite another to get involved in it. Jackson had an inherent dislike of controversy, coupled with an explicit preference to remain neutral in contentious situations.

What made Darwin's theory so powerful and so unsettling was the randomness of natural selection. Carried to its logical conclusion, natural selection leaves no role for God and no place for progressivism. With or without God, the basic premise of progressivism is the teleological idea that developments in the natural world are somehow designed to lead to a higher, better order of existence. Some of Darwin's staunchest supporters were troubled by this part of his theory. They tended to endorse evolution while soft-pedaling natural selection.[56] Since Spencer's evolutionism lacked natural selection, it did not suffer this uncomfortable denial of progress. There is no evidence that Jackson read Spencer before 1864, but other versions of evolution were circulating in British culture before Spencer and Darwin appeared.

During most of the nineteenth century before Darwin, the 'development hypothesis' was a sometime topic of discussion in British scientific circles and literary salons. Since it had a rather unstable existence, it meant different things to different people, so it may be best defined by what it is not. The opposite of the development hypothesis is the idea of the fixity of species, which has a biblical origin. That is, God created the species that we have now, so their existence is fixed and immutable. With the development of modern geology in the early nineteenth century there was increasing evidence against the fixity of species. Much of this evidence was marshalled unevenly in a book that was published anonymously in 1844, *Vestiges of the Natural History of Creation*. Its author was Robert Chambers (1802–1871), a journalist and publisher in Edinburgh. He remained tenaciously unidentified as the author until 1884, despite the immutable fact of his death in 1871.[57] *Vestiges* was read widely by literate people in the 1840s and beyond. Thus, before Darwin the development hypothesis was the theory of evolution in a variety of forms and without the crucial mechanism of natural selection.

Evolution was only one factor in a larger trend that was transforming European culture. Historian Owen Chadwick called it *The Secularization of the European Mind in the Nineteenth Century*.[58] One of the most important cultural differences between 1800 and 1900 was the diminished centrality of religion in people's thought processes by the end of the century. In 1800 even avowed atheists could not avoid thinking in theological terms—it was culturally conditioned. One of the 'triumphs' of nineteenth-century science is the fact that our minds are secularized. To think and write in theological terms now requires a conscious choice. This process accelerated in the last third of the nineteenth century, propelled partly by the controversy about evolution.[59]

---

[55] See Bowler 1988, pp.47–71.

[56] See Bowler 1988, pp.2–14; Bowler 2005; and Ruse 2005. See also the foreword by David Hull to Ellegård 1990 (p.2).

[57] See Secord 2000, p.497.

[58] Chadwick 1975.

[59] See e.g. Turner 1978, p.357.

Until Darwin, the British intellectual community generally accepted the premises of 'natural theology'. This was the idea that the works of God can be found in nature, so investigating the natural world is a way of advancing theology. This notion was distinctly British.[60] However, the acrimony of the Darwinian debates strained the earlier truce between theology and science, resulting in what historian Robert Young (1935–2019) called 'the fragmentation of a common context'.[61] By 1880 science was ascendant and the knowledge claims of theology were narrowing.[62] Another way to understand this is through the concept of 'cultural authority'.[63] That is, knowledge claims are considered to be valid only in a society that accepts the authority of their authors. In Chapters 8 and 9 we will see that Jackson claimed that status for medical science in the 1870s.

Now all of this may seem to be at a remove from the history of neuroscience, but it's not. Secularization is relevant to neuroscience because of the mind-brain problem.[64] For practical purposes in our daily work most of us unconsciously adopt a materialist presumption. We blithely assume that brain states cause, or are equivalent to, mental states. In 1800 deliberate expression of that notion would have been tantamount to professional suicide, and it would have been inconsistent with the science of the day. Little was then known about the functions of the cerebral hemispheres. Moreover, until well into the nineteenth century 'mind' and 'soul' were commonly conflated, which put significant theological constraints on neuroscience.

The process of disengaging the mind from the soul, and the mind-soul from the brain, was arguably started by John Locke and his circle in the seventeenth century,[65] but it had not changed cultural patterns to any great extent in 1800. For the scientifically inclined, by 1900 the materialist assumption was pervasive. Jackson's work in the 1860s to the 1890s was a major part of neurology's effort to deal with the methodological problem inherent in the mind-brain dilemma. He agonized over this issue for decades, but in the end it was Jackson's generation who secularized the cerebral hemispheres.

Jackson's Early Career in London, 1859–1863

When Jackson got to London in 1859 (Fig. 2.3) he was apparently thinking deep thoughts, but not about the nervous system. He was thinking about his career and its prospects. We have some access to his internal deliberations at this time because Hutchinson has told us about them. Hutchinson was 7 years' Jackson's senior (Fig. 2.4), so they had not known each other in their separate times at the York Medical School. Jackson arrived in London with a letter of introduction to Hutchinson from Samuel North, their mutual teacher at York, and Jackson lived with the Hutchinson family until 1864.[66] In his obituary for Jackson, Hutchinson recalled:

---

[60] Owsei Temkin (1947, p.307) called it 'a deism which took itself seriously'. Briefly, 'deism' is belief in the existence of a Deity based on reason and reason's reflections on nature, rather than on belief based on pure faith and divine revelation. See also Mayr 1982, pp.371–373.

[61] Young 1985, pp.126–163.

[62] For a review of the historiography of the 'warfare of science with theology' in the nineteenth century see F. Gregory in D. Cahan 2003, pp.329–358. See also Chadwick 1970 and Young 1970a.

[63] Turner 1993.

[64] See the essays in Smith and Whitaker 2014. When we say 'mind-body' we generally mean 'mind-brain', and surely that's what Jackson meant. Therefore, I have used 'mind-brain' rather than 'mind-body', except in direct quotations or in other circumstances where the specification of 'body' as 'brain' is not so clear.

[65] Martensen 2004, p.192.

[66] Hutchinson, H. 1947; Greenblatt 1965b, pp.353–354; Ellis 1993.

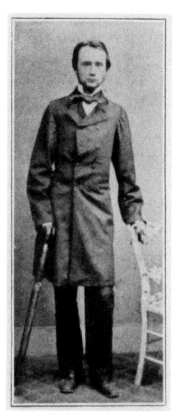

Fig. 2.3 John Hughlings Jackson, *circa* 1860.
(Reproduced with permission from JAMA Ophthalmology. 1937.17(2):244. Copyright© (1937) American Medical Association. All rights reserved.)

… When Dr. Jackson and myself first made acquaintance he had been some two or three years in the profession, and, in the belief that it did not afford attractive scope for mental powers of which he was not unconscious, he was on the point of abandoning it, intending to engage in a literary life. From this I was successful in dissuading him, and for many years I plumed myself upon this as the most successful achievement of my long life. Of late, however, I have had my misgivings, and have doubted whether – great as had been the gain to medicine – it might not have been yet a greater gain to the world at large if Hughlings Jackson had been left to devote his mind to philosophy.[67]

To most of the commentators on Jackson's career, this passage has been canonical. However, Hutchinson tells us what he actually meant in another essay 2 months later.[68] Accordingly, York and Steinberg pointed out that the key to understanding Hutchinson's statement is to emphasize 'engage in a literary life' rather than 'philosophy'.[69] It would have been futile for Jackson to have attempted a purely academic career in the English university system at the time. He had no university degree. On the other hand, a small number of authors did make their livings by

[67] Hutchinson in [Jackson] Obituary 1911b, p.952.
[68] Hutchinson 1911.
[69] York and Steinberg 2002; see also Greenblatt 1965b, p.355.

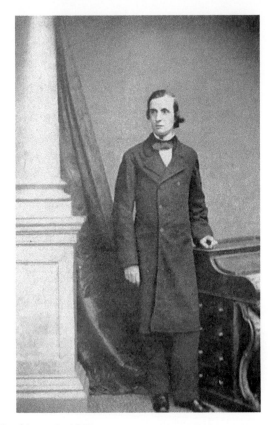

Fig. 2.4 Jonathan Hutchinson in 1862.
(Reproduced from Hutchinson, H. (1946). Jonathan Hutchinson: life and letters. London, UK: Heinemann.)

engaging in the 'literary life'. In his 'Recollections' of Jackson, Hutchinson (Fig. 2.5) spoke of some of the most successful authors who had attracted Jackson: 'In early life he had been much influenced by Carlyle's writings, but subsequently he had found those of Emerson more to his taste'. So Jackson's early literary exemplar probably was Thomas Carlyle.[70] Hutchinson may have been especially sensitive to Jackson's literary tastes, because there is evidence that Jackson 'early aroused in Hutchinson a more philosophic attitude and guided his thoughts and reading into wider circles than those in which Hutchinson had previously moved'.[71]

In addition to Carlyle and Emerson, Hutchinson states that Jackson's favorite authors were Jane Austen and Anthony Trollope, followed possibly by Dickens and Thackeray.[72] In any case, dear reader, *nota bene*! There is no mention of Herbert Spencer in any of this. Because Spencer was such a pervasive presence in Jackson's writings, some of his biographers have assumed that Spencer was Jackson's early muse, but Hutchinson says nothing to that effect. Spencer would enter Jackson's thoughts soon enough, in 1864, but there is no evidence that he was Jackson's motivation to become an author in 1859.

---

[70] Hutchinson 1911, p.1553. This idea leads to the question of which of Carlyle's writings Jackson had read. We don't know, but *Heroes and Hero-Worship* (first published in 1841) was popular at the time.

[71] Chance 1937, p.242; to the same effect, see H. Hutchinson 1946, p.58.

[72] Hutchinson 1911, p.1552. For brief intellectual diversion, Jackson 'devoured' Victorian 'yellowback' novels (Hutchinson 1911, p.1552), but we know nothing of their authors.

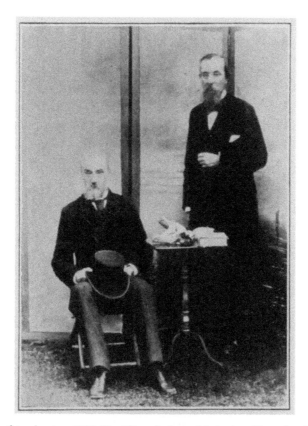

Fig. 2.5 Lifelong friends, *circa* 1888. Hughlings Jackson (sitting) and Jonathan Hutchinson (standing). Taken by Roger Hutchinson at Haslemere, Surrey. It was 'characteristic of Jackson, who hated being photographed'.
(Reproduced with permission from JAMA Ophthalmology. 1937.17(2):244. Copyright© (1937) American Medical Association. All rights reserved.)

Hutchinson actually did help Jackson to start his career in a quasi-literary way. He invited Jackson to join him in his editorial work for the New Sydenham Society[73] and in his duties as a medical reporter for the *Medical Times and Gazette* (*MTG*). The latter was a weekly publication that rivaled *The Lancet* at the time.[74] Hutchinson had been largely supporting himself by this work since 1855. By 1859 he was beginning to make part of his income from practice, which probably made him amenable to sharing the literary work with his new friend. Conveniently for us, Hutchinson's son described his father's journalistic duties:

... He had to attend as reporter all the most important cases and operations in the London Hospitals, and attend meetings of the medical societies, and report on the

---

[73] Hutchinson, H. 1947, pp.58, 73–74. On the New Sydenham Society see E. Gaskell, in Poynter 1968, pp.298–299. On *The Two Sydenham Societies* see Meynell 1985.

[74] *The Lancet* had been founded in 1823 by Thomas Wakley (1795–1862), a crusading reformist (see Bartrip 1990, pp.8–12). Wakley's sons took it over after his death in 1862, and Jackson's first publications in *The Lancet* appeared in 1864–1865 (see York and Steinberg 2006, pp.45–46). In general, the *MTG* provided the medical news with much less commentary. It 'survived until 1885, up to which time it provided *The Lancet* and the *BMJ* with some of their main competition' (Bartrip 1990, p.10).

cases brought up ... The work was of immense educational value, not only in introducing him to all the leading doctors in the Metropolis, and to all the most interesting
work being done, but making him a ready and easy writer, ready with thought and
expression. He learnt to collect and arrange statistics, and to form judgements on a
broad basis.[75]

It is reasonable to assume that the duties and benefits of journalism were essentially the same
for Jackson, especially since they worked together for a time. Jonathan Hutchinson later said
of Jackson's reporting duties, 'In connexion with this kind of work he became well known to
the members of the staff of most of the large London institutions'.76

Although the column in the *MTG* carried only Hutchinson's name until early in 1861,
there are reports that bear the imprint of Jackson's interests starting on October 27, 1860.77
When clear identification of Jackson's authorship is made, it turns out that the subjects of
Jackson's reports were generally about neurological disease.78 Only a limited number of case
reports about other body systems are attributable to Jackson. Thus, by late 1860, at the latest,
Jackson had already begun to exhibit his lifelong interest. This conclusion is consistent with
another important statement by Hutchinson:

> Although I claim the credit of having retained Hughlings Jackson for medicine, I did not
> specialize him. At one period it was proposed that we should work together ... and pub-
> lish our results conjointly. My friend, however, fell, soon after he joined me in London
> life, under the influence of Dr. Brown-Séquard, who told him strongly that it was foolish
> to waste his effort in wide observation of disease in general, and that if he wished to at-
> tain anything he must keep to the nervous system. This advice was opposed to that which
> I offered to him, but as Dr. Brown-Séquard ... was able to offer many attractions, it was
> clearly Dr. Jackson's interest to avail himself of his help.[79]

Since this was the episode that 'specialized' Jackson, it likely occurred before 1861, because
Jackson was in contact with Brown-Séquard in 1860.80 We have seen that Jackson showed
some attraction to the nervous system when he was still in York, so Brown-Séquard was
probably tapping into a preexisting vein of interest. Jackson's contact with Brown-Séquard
at this early stage in his career was particularly important, because English experimental

---

75 Hutchinson, H. 1947, p.38.

76 Hutchinson, J. 1911, p.1552. Despite Jackson's personal connections to Barts and the London Hospital,
Hutchinson said that Jackson 'retained a special attachment to Guy's [Hospital]'. At Guy's, Jackson knew the gen-
eration of prominent physicians after the 'Great Men of Guy's', including William Gull, Walter Moxon, and Samuel
Wilks; see Greenblatt 1965b, p.359; and Eadie 2007b, p.2013.

77 This was a report from the Hospital for the Epileptic and Paralyzed, which appeared for the first time in
the *MTG* on October 27, 1860 (pp.406–407). It consisted of case reports from Brown-Séquard's practice. On
November 3 (pp.432–434) there are long 'Notes of a clinical lecture delivered by Dr. Brown-Séquard, October
22, 1860'. Further reports on November 17 (p.480), December 1 (pp.532–533), December 22 (pp.612–613), and
December 29 (pp.635–636) describe cases of both Brown-Séquard and Ramskill. Before October 27, 1860, most of
Hutchinson's reports involved surgical cases, syphilis, or public health issues.

78 See Greenblatt 1965b, pp.374–375; York and Steinberg 2006, pp.37–42.

79 Hutchinson, J. 1911, p.1551.

80 According to the records of the National Hospital, as reproduced in Gooddy 1964, Brown-Séquard was active
at the Hospital by April 1860, which would have been 'soon', as Hutchinson says, after he and Jackson met. Jackson's
report of Brown-Séquard's lecture in October 1860 shows that Jackson was in contact with Brown-Séquard no later
than that date.

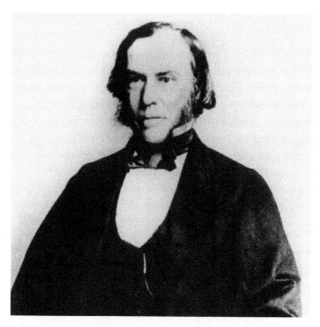

Fig. 2.6 Charles-Edouard Brown-Séquard, at age *circa* 40.

physiology was falling behind its competitors in France and Germany,[81] but Brown-Séquard was in the thick of it.

Charles Edouard Brown-Séquard (1817–1894) (Fig. 2.6) has been described as an 'unhappy wanderer'.[82] He finally stopped wandering when he was appointed to the chair of medicine at the Collège de France in 1878, succeeding the preeminent physiologist Claude Bernard (1813–1878). However, when he met and befriended Jackson in 1860, he was still in his peripatetic mode. Despite his wanderings, Brown-Séquard had been a productive experimental physiologist since the mid-1840s, especially with regard to the sensory pathways in the spinal cord.[83] We still use the eponym 'Brown-Séquard syndrome' to refer to the clinical findings in a patient who has suffered an injury to one half (right or left) of the spinal cord.[84] He had also published on some experimental aspects of epilepsy since 1850.[85] Of particular interest to our story about Jackson in 1859–1860 is Brown-Séquard's active contact with his old friend James Paget. Along with many others, Paget was urging Brown-Séquard to accept an appointment to a new specialty hospital in London.[86] Brown-Séquard agreed and arrived in the spring of 1860.

---

[81] See Geison 1972; Geison 1978, Chapter 2; and Tansey 1992.

[82] Aminoff 1993, p.66; see also papers in Aminoff 1996.

[83] Aminoff 1993, pp.117–130; and Aminoff 2011, pp.46–48, 213–220.

[84] In the *Brown-Séquard syndrome*, 'Paralysis and disturbed proprioception [position sense] are found ipsilateral to the lesion, whereas diminished pain and temperature appreciation, starting one or two levels below the lesion, are found contralaterally' (Koehler and Aminoff, in Koehler et al. 2000, p.200).

[85] Aminoff 2011, pp.183–193.

[86] Aminoff 2011, pp.106–109. There is no evidence that it was Paget who introduced Jackson to Brown-Séquard, though it is possible.

Major Hospital Appointments, 1862–1863

The leading neurological institution that we now refer to as the 'National Hospital' or 'Queen Square' was originally founded in November 1859 as the Hospital for the Relief and Cure of the Paralyzed and Epileptic (now the National Hospital for Neurology and Neurosurgery) (Fig. 2.7).[87] It has always been in Queen Square, which is part of the Bloomsbury district of London. The British Museum and University College London are part of the same area, which was, and still is, vital to the intellectual life of the city.[88] Since the National Hospital was soon to become a major factor in Jackson's life, and he became a uniquely bright star in its galaxy, it is important to understand the hospital's origins and how it got to be what it is.[89]

In the mid-nineteenth century, private specialty hospitals were sprouting up throughout Britain, despite strong opposition, which was partly due to a feeling within the profession that all physicians should be generalists.[90] Moreover, the philanthropic claims of many of them were suspect, because they amounted to private clinics for individual specialists.[91] Such was not the case with the National Hospital. Indeed, 'The hospital's foundation was warmly welcomed by Victorian society'.[92] It was established by two sincere and effective sisters, Johanna and Louisa Chandler, who had cared for their grandmother after her stroke. They saw the need for organized care of such people and resolved to do something about it. Among their advisers was the Lord Mayor of London, Alderman David Wire. He persuaded them to establish an institution for active treatment rather than just another chronic care facility.[93] The first physician appointed to the staff was Jabez Spence Ramskill (1824–1897), and the second was Brown-Séquard. Ramskill was instrumental in the early organization of the hospital, because he had been 'Miss Chandler's' medical attendant,[94] and Brown-Séquard brought his international reputation.

There will be more to say about Jackson's appointment to the National Hospital forthwith, but here I will skip ahead historically to explain the place that it acquired in medical London. The staffing pattern that developed quite rapidly at Queen Square brought a unique opportunity for concentration of instructive cases. Each of the staff physicians naturally had strong neurological interests. In addition, almost all of them had appointments at other, larger teaching hospitals.[95] Thus, they brought their most interesting cases to the National Hospital, or at the least they brought knowledge and discussion thereof. This pattern produced an unparalleled concentration of neurological case material and talent in what was then the world's largest city.[96]

---

[87] Not to be confused with the London Infirmary for Epilepsy and Paralysis, which was founded in 1867 in Marylebone. From 1873 to 1903 it was located in Regent's Park and then in Maida Vale, so in the twentieth century it was generally known as the Maida Vale Hospital for Nervous Diseases. It was merged with Queen Square in 1947 and closed in 1983. See Feiling 1958; and Powell and Kitchen 2007, p.1982.

[88] See Ashton 2012, pp.1–24, 105–130; many other health care entities were established in Queen Square before and after the founding of the National Hospital.

[89] The extensive history of Queen Square by Shorvon and Compston (2019) appeared when my book was nearing completion. I have used its details as much as possible.

[90] See Casper 2014, Introduction, etc.; also Koehler 1999 for international comparisons.

[91] See Peterson 1978, pp.262–263; also Rivett 1986, pp.43–49; Granshaw 1989, pp.205–212; Lorch 2004a, p.125; Weisz 2006, pp.26–43. Despite the opposition to specialist hospitals, the existence of Queen Square was partly defended by the fact that the large general hospitals did not admit epileptics; see Granshaw, p.208; and Casper 2014, p.23.

[92] Lekka 2015, p.40.

[93] Holmes 1954, pp.8–16; see also Rawlings 1913, pp.1–25; Critchley 1960b; and Critchley 1960c.

[94] Lorch 2004a.

[95] This pattern persisted until at least the mid-twentieth century; see Holmes 1954, p.7.

[96] Newsome 1997, p.22.

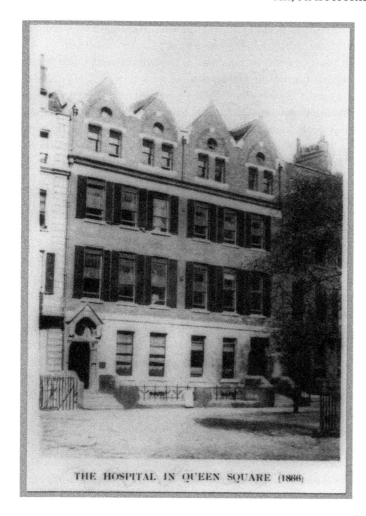

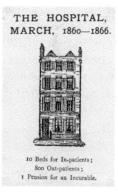

THE HOSPITAL,
MARCH, 1860—1866.

10 Beds for In-patients;
800 Out-patients;
1 Pension for an Incurable.

Fig. 2.7 The National Hospital, Queen Square, in 1866 (left) and 1860–1866 (right).
(Image courtesy of the Queen Square Archives.)

To get back to an exact chronology of Jackson's first years in London is impossible, because he did so many things at once. With regard to hospital positions, he was not officially appointed to the staff of the National Hospital until 1862, at the behest of Brown-Séquard. Before that, in 1859–1860, he quickly acquired appointments to the Royal Ophthalmic Hospital ('Moorfields') and the Metropolitan Free Hospital. Ramskill was on the staff of the latter, and Hutchinson was at both. In addition, Jackson was appointed to the Islington Dispensary, but we have little information about those details. A few years later, when the direction of his professional trajectory was better defined, Jackson resigned all three appointments, but they were important to his early endeavors.[97]

In 1860 and 1861, Jackson sat for examinations to gain advanced qualifications, which shows that he was consciously career-oriented. He wanted to be a consulting Physician, rather than a general practitioner. Until 1860, he had no academic degree, which would have put some constraints on his advancement in London's highly competitive environment. Accordingly, in September 1860, he acquired the M.D. by examination at the University of St. Andrews in Scotland. Over the preceding 140 years there had been some criticism of St. Andrews as a diploma mill, because it had no real faculty of medicine. By the mid-century, the examination apparently had some rigor. The regulations for the medical doctorate were tightened in 1862, so Jackson was among the last external students to be admitted to this examination.[98] In the next year, he also passed the examination of the Royal College of Physicians. He was admitted to its membership on September 30, 1861, gaining the title of M.R.C.P.[99] These credentials were significant factors in his acquisition of the two hospital appointments that he would keep for the rest of his working life.

The National Hospital was a success from the outset, so the need for another staff physician arose in 1861. However, the Board of Management shelved the idea. It was brought up again by Ramskill in April 1862. On May 7, 1862, on the nomination of Brown-Séquard, Jackson was 'elected Assistant Physician on the understanding that he should visit the Hospital twice a day and see the out-patients at their homes for which extra services he will be allowed the Remuneration of fifty pounds per an'.[100] If this sounds burdensome, Jackson thought so too. On July 16, he offered his resignation. The hospital managers decided that he would 'lose his salary of fifty pounds per annum, but not his functions as assistant physician'.[101] When Brown-Séquard resigned his position as Physician on July 15, 1863, to return to America,[102] Jackson was among the four candidates for the post. Two others were appointed, and Jackson did not become a full Physician to the National Hospital until 1867.[103] Critchley speculates that Jackson's youth may have been a factor in his delayed promotion— in 1863 he was only 28.[104]

Jackson's other major hospital appointment was acquired through the good offices of Hutchinson, who had been appointed Assistant Surgeon to the London Hospital in 1859 and Surgeon in 1863.[105] The London is still on the site where Hutchinson and Jackson knew

---

[97]   See Greenblatt 1965b, pp.355–356; and Lorch 2004a, pp.124–125. An incomplete list of Jackson's hospital and teaching appointments is in Greenblatt 1964, pp.160–161.

[98]   Critchley 1960e, p.61, states (without citing his source) that of the 44 examinees, Jackson was one of 36 successful candidates. The Critchleys (1998, p.33) say that Jackson submitted a thesis on an unknown subject, but I think this is an error. In his brief history of medical education at St. Andrews, Shepherd (1972) says nothing about a thesis requirement for the M.D. In his history of the University of St Andrews, Cant (1970, p.111) states that a Commission of 1858 allowed continued granting of the external medical degree 'by examination only', but the M.D.s 'were rationed to ten a year and restricted to practitioners over forty years of age'. Jackson was 25 in 1860, so there are some conflicting details here. In going to St Andrews, Jackson may have been following the example of his friend Lockhart Clarke, who obtained his M.D. there in 1869 ([Clarke] 1880b; on Clarke, see Chapter 6).

[99]   See Greenblatt 1965b, p.358.

[100]   Andermann 1997, pp.474–475.

[101]   Taylor 1925, p.4.

[102]   Aminoff 1993, p.49.

[103]   Greenblatt 1965, pp.363–364.

[104]   Critchley 1960e, p.616.

[105]   Hutchinson, H. 1947, p.76.

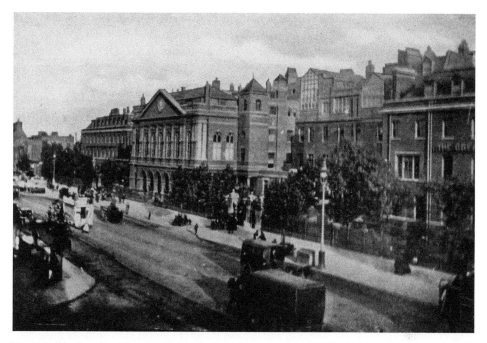

Fig. 2.8 The London Hospital (now the Royal London Hospital) in 1908, when vehicles in the busy street were still horse-drawn.

(By permission of the Antiqua Print Gallery/Alamy Stock Photo.)

it, in London's East End (Fig. 2.8). The words that come to mind to describe this district are 'teeming' and 'Dickensian'. It was, and still is, a place of recent immigrants. It had been this way since the London was founded in 1740. Even then it 'stood in the heart of a notoriously unsavoury area'.[106] Such places are often fertile locations for teaching hospitals. By the mid-nineteenth century, the London was one of the largest 'voluntary' (privately incorporated) hospitals in the city. It had a distinguished medical staff and a medical school that had been founded in 1785. The latter had gained splendid new quarters in 1854.[107]

Jackson was appointed Lecturer on Pathology at the London Hospital Medical College in 1859. We have no information about the details of his appointment, except to point toward the usual suspect, Hutchinson. Jackson was also appointed Lecturer on Physiology in 1863, but we have no information about his activities in either of these offices in the period 1859–1863.[108] Since Jackson had no specific qualifications in physiology, we may wonder how he got such an appointment. Geison has shown that the period 1840–1870 was one of 'stagnancy of English physiology' due to the utilitarian outlook of the London medical schools,[109] so the position in physiology probably was not accorded much importance. On the other

[106] Clark-Kennedy 1979, p.27.

[107] These dates are taken from Clark-Kennedy 1962–1963, Clark-Kennedy 1979, and Morris 1910.

[108] Jackson held teaching appointments with various titles through at least 1870; the best available but still incomplete information on Jackson's dates of appointment is in Greenblatt 1964, p.161. Ellis 1986, pp.13–14, 43, states that in the late eighteenth century student lecture fees at the London Hospital Medical College were paid to the faculty group, which paid the lecturers. This unusual arrangement was apparently still in place in the 1860s. In most schools the fees were paid directly 'to the individual teacher who could charge whatever he could get'.

[109] Geison 1972, p.42; 1978, pp.26–27; see also Butler 1988.

hand, Hutchinson's role in Jackson's appointment as Assistant Physician to the London in 1863 was described by Hutchinson himself in his obituary of Jackson:

> The writer of the obituary in the [London] *Times* suggested that I was probably concerned in his [Jackson's] election to the medical staff of the London. It curiously happened that I was concerned in a manner not exactly that which was intended ... His election as Assistant Physician was a foregone conclusion, for his competitor had retired. Jackson, who had a strong contempt for everything of the nature of red tape and formality, knowing that it was settled, forgot to attend on the day of the election, and I had to persuade an obliging secretary to keep the quorum whilst I ... hunted him up.[110]

The point to notice is that Jackson knew that his competitor had withdrawn. Had he known otherwise, probably he would have been where he was supposed to be. He didn't like red tape, but he craved substance, and he knew that he had to abide some minimum of the former in order to get at the latter. This proposition is substantiated in the privately printed *Testimonials of Dr. J. Hughlings Jackson M.D., Member of the Royal College of Physicians of London*.[111] It consists of 19 letters of recommendation written by many prominent physicians to support Jackson's application for the post at the London. The names included such worthies as Lionel Beale (1828–1906), William Bowman (1816–1892), Brown-Séquard, William Gull (1816–1890), Hutchinson, William Jenner (1815–1898), Laycock, and Samuel Wilks (1824–1911).[112] Some of these men were writing from a distance—testifying to Jackson's reputation in the medical community—but many letters were based on real knowledge of the person. The most telling one came from 'Andrew Clark [(1826–1893)], M.D., F.R.C.P., Assistant Physician to the London Hospital, (late) Professor of Physiology to the London Hospital Medical College'.

> Dr. Hughlings Jackson has been known to me for some years, through frequent conversations and the perusal of his contributions to medical literature.
>
> Able and original, yet peculiarly painstaking and modest; free from affectation and finesse; seeking duty before recompense, and truth before success; versed in the medicine of to-day, and penetrated by the spirit which is shaping the science of the future; already experienced in the practice of his art, and ambitious of increasing its resources and exalting its functions; I consider Dr. Hughlings Jackson to be in every way admirably qualified for the appointment of Assistant Physician to the London Hospital.[113]

This was not just polite hyperbole. Dr. Clark knew his man, because he highlighted the particular characteristics of Jackson that were recognized and admired by his colleagues throughout his life. Along with the other testimonials, it shows that Jackson was already gaining a reputation in the higher circles of medical London. In the next chapters we will see that most of his early recognition started with his work on language disorders, which began in 1864. To understand where Jackson started, however, we need to know something about knowledge of the nervous system and its disorders *circa* 1860.

---

[110] Hutchinson 1911, p.1552; my square brackets.

[111] Jackson 1863b. See also Andermann 1997. I am indebted to Ms. Andermann for long ago sending me a copy of the *Testimonials*.

[112] After Sir Charles Locock introduced potassium bromide in 1857 as the first effective treatment for epilepsy (see Eadie 2012), it was Wilks who popularized it, beginning in 1861 (see Temkin 1971, p.299; Pearce 2002a; and Pearce 2009b). Jackson would have used it early on, because Brown-Séquard was an enthusiast (see Aminoff 2011, p.109). At Queen Square, bromide was also used by Charles Bland Radcliffe (1822–1889) and Ramskill (Scott 1993, p.45).

[113] Clark, A., in Jackson 1863b, p.8, dated 'June 20, 1863'.

3

Laying the Foundations, Starting a Career, 1861–1864

The Situation of Scientific Medicine, *circa* 1860

From antiquity, Western medical theory was based on the humoral physiology of Galen of Pergamon (*circa* 130–200 CE).[1] In the sixteenth century Andreas Vesalius and others began to question Galen, and William Harvey's elucidation of the circulation of the blood in 1628 was a direct contradiction. Nonetheless, many aspects of Galenic medicine (e.g., bloodletting) persisted into the nineteenth century. It was only around 1870 that modern medicine 'was firmly launched on its new scientific course, which gave it the intellectual unity it had lost after the downfall of Galenism . . .'.[2] This change toward the experimental method was led by Claude Bernard (1813–1878) in France and the school of Johannes Müller (1801–1858) in the German-speaking universities.[3] For Western medicine as a whole the decade of the 1860s was transitional.[4] Thus, when Jackson began his medical career in the early 1860s it was just when the transition to modern scientific medicine had been set in motion but not yet consolidated.

The Situation of Clinical Neurology, *circa* 1860

In the early decades of the nineteenth century the Parisian clinico-pathological method was most successful in cardiology and pulmonology, at least in the realm of diagnosis. But the nervous system is far more complex than the heart or the lungs. Good microscopy is required to see neural tracts and cell masses, especially in the spinal cord and brainstem. Because of these constraints the development of clinical neurology lagged behind other specialties until the last third of the nineteenth century. Brown-Séquard expressed this frustration in 1861.

It would be of the utmost importance to find out what part of the brain is altered when there is … paralysis indicating a loss of function in some part of that organ. If the anatomy and the physiology of the brain were better understood it would be possible to know at once where to locate the alteration. But unfortunately we know less about the anatomy and physiology of the brain than about any other organ.[5]

---

[1] Temkin 1973, pp.1–7.
[2] Temkin 1973, p.191.
[3] See Bynum et al. 2006, pp.113–120.
[4] See Poynter 1968, pp.1–43; and Geison 1972, pp.13–47.
[5] Brown-Séquard 1861, p.29.

A few years later, in 1864, Jackson expressed the same thought more succinctly: 'It is the anatomy that is difficult.'[6] When Charcot and Jackson began their neurological careers in the early 1860s, they both found that existing knowledge of normal anatomy and physiology was woefully inadequate, but neither was an experimentalist. Their investigational tool was the clinico-pathological method. To apprehend the normal, they had to 'reverse' the direction of thinking in the clinico-pathological method. That is, they had to reason from the dysfunctions of disease to conclusions about normal function. Charcot considered his 'anatomo-clinical method' ('*méthod anatomo-pathologique*') to be an advanced form of Laennec's 'anatomo-pathological method'.[7] He developed his own method with the aim of creating a more accurate, anatomically based neurological nosology, and one of its major by-products was improved knowledge of functional systems in the spinal cord.[8] Henceforth I will use 'clinico-pathological method' as a generic term, restricting 'anatomo-pathological method' to Charcot's usage. I would not claim that either Charcot or Jackson saw his situation as clearly as I've just stated it. They both had to start from the neuroscience of their day.

Some Aspects of Brain Science, *circa* 1860

The following anatomical definitions will be used in this book.

Definition Section 1—Neuroanatomy

Brain—the entire contents of the skull; i.e., the entire neuraxis[9] above the spinal cord. Dalton (1859, p.321) defined *encephalon* synonymously. The whole brain has three parts. Starting from the top they are the

    (1) **Cerebrum**—all of the contents of the skull above the tentorium;[10] i.e., all of the brain except the two parts in the posterior fossa,[11] which are the

    (2) **Cerebellum**—the small brain that is behind and attached to the

    (3) **Brainstem**—the lowest part of the brain. It connects the cerebrum and cerebellum to the spinal cord. From higher to lower, it consists of the midbrain (*mesencephalon*), pons (*pons Varolii* or *pons cerebelli*), and medulla (*medulla oblongata*), which connects to the spinal cord.

Basal ganglia—masses of brain cells (now called *neurons*), deep in the cerebrum. The term *ganglia* (singular: *ganglion*) now generally refers to the cell masses of the sympathetic chain.[12] We commonly use the term *nucleus* (plural: *nuclei*) to refer to distinct cell masses in the brain and spinal cord, but the term *basal ganglia* has survived to refer to these specific nuclei. The main basal ganglia are the *corpus striatum* (plural: *corpora striata*) and the *thalamus* (plural: *thalami*; nineteenth-century term: *optic thalamus*), one

---

[6] Jackson 1864h, p.147.

[7] See Goetz et al. 1995, p.66.

[8] The classic example of this phenomenon is Charcot's work on amyotrophic lateral sclerosis (ALS); see Goetz et al. 1995, pp.100–108.

[9] Brain and spinal cord; largely synonymous with 'central nervous system'.

[10] Properly addressed as the *tentorium cerebelli*. It is the tough leaf of parchment-like dura (*dura mater*) that separates the cerebrum from the cerebellum inside the back of the skull.

[11] The chamber in the back of the skull below the tentorium, which contains the cerebellum and most of the brainstem. Above the tentorium are multiple *fossae* (spaces) containing the lobes of the brain. The *midbrain* sits in a small, notch-like opening in the tentorium (called the *incisura*) between the two spaces.

[12] A long narrow leash of nerves and their connecting points that lie in the back of the thoracic and abdominal cavities, outside the skull and spinal canal.

on each side. In our current usage, '*the striatum*' refers to the corpus striatum, singular or plural, and '*the thalamus*' is used similarly. Jackson always used 'corpus striatum'.

Cerebral hemisphere (often written as *hemisphere(s)* without the adjective)—the large outcroppings of brain mass that are largely (not entirely) symmetrical on each side. The main divisions of the hemispheres are called *lobes*; they are the *frontal, parietal, occipital,* and *temporal* lobes.

Cortex (plural: *cortices*)—thick sheets of *gray matter* (nerve cell bodies), which connect to other brain areas through *white matter*, which consists of tracts of nerve fibers (*axons*[13]). We now generally use the term *gyrus* (plural: *gyri*) to refer to the individual foldings of the cortical sheets, but the common nineteenth-century term was *convolution*.

In general, our current definitions are the same as they were *circa* 1860, but not entirely.[14] And there is another historical caveat: use of our terms (1) *neuron* and (2) *axon* is anachronistic before 1891, when the neuron theory was instantiated by Santiago Ramón y Cajal (1852–1934), Wilhelm Waldeyer (1836–1921), and others.[15] Signals flow unidirectionally through the web-like *dendrites* of the cell body into the cell body and then out through the (usually) single axon to connect with the dendrites of other neurons. In the mid-nineteenth century, microscopy had identified (1) nerve *cells*, also called *vesicles* or *globules*, and (2) nerve *fibers* (Fig. 3.1),[16] but the exact relationships between these two types of structures were not known. It was assumed that they functioned together to generate and carry signals.

Historically, opinions have swung back and forth between two different ideas about the internal workings of the brain. *Localization* is the idea that some definable functions are carried out, at least to some extent, in one part of the brain. The opposite view is *holism*, which claims that all parts of the brain are equipotential, i.e., not differentiated for specific functions in specific locations. By the 1860s localization was recognized in the brainstem, although it was not labelled 'localization'. Separation of motor and sensory functions in the basal ganglia was also accepted, more or less, but the cortices were the province of the 'mind' or the 'will'.

It would be wrong to assert that nobody knew anything worthwhile about the brain in 1860. A large amount of human anatomy, comparative anatomy, and physiology was available. For the sake of brevity, I will trip lightly through seventeen centuries of prior work, before we look more closely at the situation when Jackson started. Since his ultimate contributions were largely related to the brain, rather than the spinal cord or the peripheral nervous system, we will look mainly at some aspects of how the brain was understood, but the reader will understand that a large body of knowledge and theory is being ignored.[17]

---

[13] The long (sometimes 1–2 m) processes of nerve cells (neurons) that carry signals away from the cell bodies toward other neurons or toward muscles.

[14] See e.g. the definitions in Dunglison 1860; also Swanson 2000. On the other hand, William B. Carpenter (1813–1885), a very influential physiologist, reverted to an older usage and defined the *medulla oblongata* as the entire neuraxis from the corpora striata down to the rostral (upper) end of the spinal cord; see Carpenter 1855, pp.455–456.

[15] See Shepherd 1991, especially pp.177–193.

[16] Todd and Bowman 1857, pp.197–200, used 'vesicles', 'cells', and 'globules'. Dalton 1859, pp.307–315, wrote about 'nerve cells'. When Jackson (Jackson 1865f, p.298) gave a brief review of basic neuroanatomy in 1865, his definitions were essentially the same; see Clarke and Jacyna 1987, pp.58–100. On Todd see Binder et al. 2011; and Binder and Reynolds 2017.

[17] See the extensive descriptions of functional neuroanatomy and neurophysiology in Carpenter 1855, and in Todd and Bowman 1857. Much of this knowledge and theory is analyzed in Clarke and Jacyna 1987, which covers mainly the first two-thirds of the nineteenth century.

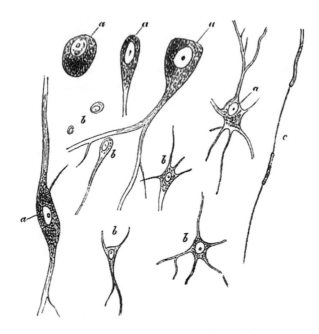

Fig. 3.1 Drawings of large and small 'Nerve-cells' (*a* and *b*) and 'Nerve-fibres' (*c*) in Harley and Brown 1866, fig. 132, p.148, magnified ×350. On p.150 they specifically recommended 'Mr. Lockhart Clarke's method of making preparations of nerve structure . . '. On Lockhart Clarke see Chapter 6.

(Reproduced from Harley, G., Brown, G.T. (1866). Histological Demonstrations: A Guide to the Microscopical Examination of the Animal Tissues in Health and Disease. London: Longmans, Green, and Co.)

Brief History of Cerebral Neuroscience to 1860

Toward the end of classical antiquity, Galen systematized the ancients' theories about all of medical science, including the brain as the organ of mind. His humoral theory of physiological function stated that the brain's role was to distill the 'psychic pneuma' out of the blood, so it could be the carrier of commands to the rest of the body.[18] Some parts of Galen's neurophysiological system persisted into the nineteenth century, but it met its first real challenge in the seventeenth, in the work of Thomas Willis (1621–1675) and his 'Oxford group' of investigators.[19] Willis put the mind in the solid parts of the brain, particularly the cerebral hemispheres, but the cerebrum remained largely the 'chapel of the Deity'.[20]

In the 1790s, Franz Joseph Gall (1758–1828) began to investigate the possibility that different areas of the cerebral cortices might serve different intellectual functions. He called the areas 'organs', so he named his theory 'organology'. This was a form of cortical localization. Organology included the idea that an organ in the brain might cause a prominence ('bump')

[18] 'Humoral' theories of physiological function assume that the site of the changes that drive function is in the liquid (humoral) parts of the body, as contrasted to our 'solidist' point of view. Almost all ancient physiological theories were humoral. Rocca 2003 translates the Greek as 'psychic pneuma'; Singer 1957 uses 'natural spirit'.

[19] See Martensen 2004, p.26 and throughout the volume.

[20] Martensen 2004, pp.98, 139. Willis named the corpora striata and assigned motor and sensory functions to them; see Finger 1994, pp.214–216.

of the overlying skull if the organ were enlarged. It was Gall's sometime associate, Johann Christoph (later Gaspar) Spurzheim (1776–1832), who was associated with the term 'phrenology', though he did not invent the word.[21] Spurzheim emphasized the bumps and thereby brought the whole enterprise into scientific disrepute.[22]

Gall's work was eventually rejected by the biomedical community of Paris, where he lived for his last two decades. It is usually said that the final blow in phrenology's *dénouement* was delivered in a small treatise by the French physiologist Pierre Flourens (1794–1867) in 1842.[23] Flourens' cerebral ablation experiments were carried out largely on pigeons, so he concluded that the hemispheres of the brain are equipotential. Thus, in the scientific community the baby idea of cerebral localization was largely washed away with the bathwater of phrenology. In the European political-social realm, phrenology was accused of being materialistic and therefore anti-Christian, a charge that was not entirely unfounded.[24] The extent of this censure varied geographically. Britain and America were somewhat more tolerant than the continent.

The Functions of the Cerebral Hemispheres, *circa* 1860

In the medical and scientific communities, from the 1840s to the 1860s, localization was generally conflated with phrenology and accordingly besmirched. Nonetheless, Gall's ideas persisted, even if sometimes *sub rosa*. Discussions that opposed phrenology were frequent and acceptable.[25] The existence of this negative attention implies that Gall's arguments were still given enough credence to require such explicit opposition. Interestingly, scholars of literary and social history are now finding evidence of how deeply phrenology penetrated into the culture of the mid-nineteenth century, especially in Britain and the United States.[26]

Regarding Jackson *circa* 1860, we don't have anything to tell us explicitly what he knew about the brain. However, we do know which textbooks were widely used at the time, and we know who he quoted in print in the years immediately after 1860. Carpenter wrote several treatises on human and comparative physiology. His *Principles of Human Physiology* saw its first edition in 1842 and its eighth in 1876.[27] Another standard work was *The Physiological Anatomy and Physiology of Man* (1856) by Robert B. Todd (1809–1860) and William Bowman (1816–1892).[28] Jackson cited Carpenter and Todd frequently, though not always those specific titles. A reference that he did cite directly was the standard American physiology text of the time, *A Treatise on Human Physiology* by John C. Dalton (1825–1889).[29] I will first consider these authors' views of the cerebral cortices and then go on to their

[21] 'The term 'phrenology' was coined in 1815 by the English naturalist and physician Thomas Ignatius Maria Forster (1789–1860); it came into general use in the 1820s. See van Wyhe 2004, p.17, footnote 69; also Noel and Carlson 1970; and Cooter 1984, p.59.

[22] See Greenblatt 1995.

[23] See Ackerknecht and Vallois 1956, especially pp.35–36.

[24] For discussions of these charges and their merits see Temkin 1947, pp.283, 300–307 (reprinted in Temkin 2002, pp.92–93, 105–111); and Ackerknecht and Vallois 1956, pp.18–19.

[25] See e.g. Carpenter 1855, pp.517–522; Brown-Séquard 1861, pp.515–516; and Dalton 1859, pp.368–370.

[26] See e.g. Cooter 1984; Rylance 2000; Tomlinson 2005.

[27] I have used the American edition of 1855, apparently from the fourth British edition of 1853, which would have been available when Jackson was in medical school. For a discussion of Carpenter's books in the science of their time see Winter 1997, pp.35–43.

[28] Todd and Bowman 1857.

[29] Dalton 1859. For a brief biography see [Dalton] 1968.

statements about the basal ganglia *circa* 1860. Brown-Séquard's positions will be considered at the end of this section.

Carpenter, Todd and Bowman, and Dalton all agreed that the hemispheres above the basal ganglia are the province of the mind or the 'will'. Carpenter's description of the physiologically exalted position of the cerebrum is lyrical. He said of the brain: 'its position at the summit of the whole apparatus ... clearly mark it out as the highest in its functional relations, and as ministering, so far as any material instrument may do, to the exercise of those psychical powers, which, in Man, exhibit so remarkable a predominance over the mere animal instincts.'[30] This indicates Carpenter's strong preference to avoid unmitigated materialism.[31] Like Carpenter, Todd and Bowman cited the evidence of comparative anatomy. They said: 'The convolutions of the brain are the centres of intellectual actions, and are intimately associated with the mental phenomena of attention, association, and memory.'[32] Dalton agreed, but he was ambiguous about the physiological meaning of this assertion.[33]

It is important to note that none of those authorities was ascribing any motor function to the cortices. Like Gall, they were locating only intellectual and affective functions in the brain's most prominent structures. With regard to the role of the corpora striata and thalami, there was more disagreement. Clarity is again served by first explaining our modern knowledge of the motor and sensory tracts, whose basics have been well established since the late nineteenth century.[34]

Definition Section 2—Motor and Sensory Tracts

On the motor side, the *corticospinal (pyramidal) tract* was first demonstrated by Flechsig in 1876.[35] It is largely a nonstop pathway. There are some relays in the corpora striata, but the majority of the axons in the tract proceed straight through to the spinal cord on the other (contralateral) side, because the axons of each side cross to the other side in the lower medulla.

As they descend deeply into the hemispheres, axons from the motor cortices come together in a tightly packed area called the *internal capsule*, where they are surrounded by the gray matter of the striata. Lesions in this region commonly cause contralateral hemiplegia (see Definition Section 3) because they interrupt the corticospinal tract. Hemorrhages, strokes, tumors, and other lesions also damage gray matter, which led to the erroneous idea that the damaged gray matter in the striatum is responsible for the associated hemiplegia.

On the sensory side, the situation in the spinal cord and brainstem is more complex, because there are multiple pathways carrying incoming information upward through many relays with different crossing patterns. For practical purposes, (1) all of the sensory pathways cross in the spinal cord or brainstem, and (2) no signals from lower centers get up to the sensory cortex without a relay in the thalamus.

---

[30] Carpenter 1855, p.530.
[31] Carpenter's conservatism and his ultimate success in overcoming charges of materialism are described by Winter 1997, pp.35–43.
[32] Todd and Bowman 1857, p.330.
[33] See Dalton 1859, p.365.
[34] See Finger 1994, Parts II and III.
[35] See Temkin 1971, pp.315–316; also Clarke and O'Malley 1996, p.287.

> So the situation is asymmetrical—there are few relays in the (descending) motor tract
> but many relays on the (ascending) sensory side. In the mid-nineteenth century, this
> asymmetry was not known. It was generally assumed that the arrangement is symmet-
> rical in the two systems.

Unlike some of their contemporaries, Carpenter, and Todd and Bowman agreed that the
majority of the motor and sensory connections of the cortices are made through relays in the
basal ganglia.[36] On the motor side, their idea was that the fibers that descend to the spinal
cord to produce muscular movements originate in the corpora striata. That is, the instructions of the will ('volition') originate in the cortices. They are conveyed from the cortices
to the gray matter of corpora striata and thence downward to the spinal cord. On the sensory side, they said, the fibers carrying incoming sensory information ascend to the 'optic
thalami'. From there the information is relayed to the cortices. Dalton adhered to the older
view that the fibers to and from the cortices mainly pass through the basal ganglia without
connections at that level.[37]

Brown-Séquard shared the conception of the cortices as the province of the will. However,
he was primarily interested in the spinal cord, including its relationships with the brainstem
and the cerebellum. In a lecture published in 1860, he said, 'We pass now to the transmission
of the orders of the will to muscles through the spinal cord',[38] and 'pass' is exactly what he did.
Nothing more was said about the will or its putative location. In 1861 he delivered a series of
*Lectures on the diagnosis and treatment of the various forms of paralytic, convulsive, and mental
affections*.[39] They were given at the Royal College of Physicians of London and at the National
Hospital, so presumably Jackson was in the audience. Here Brown-Séquard expounded on
his reflex theories of neural pathophysiology. To us they are mostly historical curiosities, but
they were part of the debate at the time, and they certainly influenced Jackson's thinking.
Brown-Séquard specifically opposed 'the views of Dr. R. B. Todd, concerning the relations of
these two parts of the encephalon [the corpora striata and thalami], one with voluntary movements and the other with sensibility, [which] are in opposition to many clinical facts'.[40] In
other words, Brown-Séquard sided with Dalton and those who stated that there are no relays
of the motor tract in the basal ganglia. I have emphasized the relationship of the basal ganglia
to the cortices, because it is immediately relevant to Jackson's early efforts to analyze common
neurological phenomena, especially hemiplegia and epileptic seizures.

> Definition Section 3—Some Unilateral Clinical Phenomena
>
> **Hemiplegia**—literally means paralysis of one side of the body, because *plegia* means par-
> alysis, versus *paresis*, which means weakness. However, common usage in Jackson's
> time and ours is to say 'hemiplegia' to refer to any unilateral paralysis, complete or
> incomplete. Hemiplegia is generally the result of a one-sided (almost always contra-
> lateral) lesion of the brain or (rarely) ipsilateral (same-sided) lesion of the spinal cord.

---

[36] Carpenter 1855, pp.489–490; Todd and Bowman 1857, pp.308–311.
[37] Dalton 1859, pp.324–327.
[38] Brown-Séquard 1860, p.45.
[39] Brown-Séquard 1861.
[40] Brown-Séquard 1861, p.199; my square brackets.

Unilateral motor seizures—jerking, repetitive, involuntary movements of one side of the body, which may or may not progress to involve the other side and/or loss of consciousness. Jackson showed that they are usually due to a lesion in the opposite hemisphere. Later he and others realized that seizures that do not necessarily involve motor movements can also come from unilateral brain lesions, but he did not understand that in the 1860s.

Epilepsy—succinctly defined as the 'tendency to epileptic seizures'.[41]

Hemichorea—*chorea* means involuntary jerking and flailing movements of the face and/or extremities and/or trunk, seemingly purposeless and often with a twisting (athetoid) quality. It can be unilateral (hence *hemi*), which implies a contralateral lesion, thought to be in the basal ganglia, but the real localization of the problem remains obscure even now. A variety that was common in Jackson's time was *Sydenham's* or *rheumatic* chorea, which is associated with streptococcal infection and rheumatic fever.

Aphasia—disorder of language due to a brain lesion which is usually unilateral. See Definition Section 4 in this chapter.

Early Neurological Interests and a 'Discarded' Theory, 1861–1863

If we look for common themes in Jackson's reporter's columns in 1861–1862, they are not far to seek. They reflect the interests of his most important colleagues at the time, Hutchinson and Brown-Séquard. The most prominent topic in 1861 was 'syphilitic affections of the nervous system', which showed Hutchinson's influence, because syphilis was one of Hutchinson's specialities. In 1862, there were many 'cases of disease of the cerebellum' *à la* Brown-Séquard.[42] In addition to these topics, Jackson reported on many cases of paralysis of various kinds. His general pattern was to describe a number of cases of the entity under review and then comment on the relevant physiology and pathology. To formulate his comments, he drew on many sources, including the physiological texts that are discussed above.

Jackson and the Situation of Epilepsy in the Early 1860s

Looking back, we can see that many of the themes in Jackson's reporter's columns turned out to be his persisting interests. This was particularly true for the diverse manifestations of epilepsy. It is hard to say that seizures and epilepsy were the special province of any one person in Jackson's circle. They were interesting to every one because they were so common. Treatment of epilepsy was a primary focus of J.S. Ramskill, so Queen Square had an abundance of seizure patients.[43]

From the outset, Jackson took a particular interest in seizures that were not thought to represent 'genuine' epilepsy.[44] He seemed to sense that they were trying to tell him something.

---

[41] Aminoff 1993, p.148. For further definitions see Definition Section 5 in Chapter 4.

[42] Jackson's first two original contributions to the medical literature were both concerned with ophthalmology. They were published outside of his reporter's columns in November 1861 (Jackson 1861f) and December 1862 (Jackson 1862f).

[43] Lorch 2004, pp.125–126.

[44] The other term for 'genuine epilepsy' was 'epilepsy proper'. Jackson used those terms interchangeably, and I will do likewise.

His introductory remarks to his first column on the subject of 'Cases of epilepsy associated with syphilis' (June 22, 1861) included a disclaimer: 'In most of the following cases the convulsions were limited to one side, and in one of them the epileptic fit was not complete, there being no loss of consciousness. It might perhaps … be more correct to call them cases of epileptiform convulsions; but the name of Epilepsy is retained as being more common.'[45]

When Jackson began his career, 'genuine' (grand mal) epilepsy was thought to be a specific disease, whereas convulsions that did not entail the full syndrome of genuine epilepsy, especially those without loss of consciousness, were thought to be symptomatic of some other disease. In truth, none of this was so clear, because the underlying causes were not understood. Temkin summarized the various etiological speculations about epilepsy *circa* 1860:

> If we … focus upon the concepts dominating the pathology of epilepsy around 1860, we find: reflex action, cerebral angiospasm, and changes in the molecular state of the brain through malnutrition or poisoning … several parts of the central nervous system were believed to be affected, either simultaneously or in succession; in none of them was the cause of epilepsy attributed to definite structural changes of a definite organ.[46]

Jackson's First *Suggestions* to Improve Neurological Pathophysiology, 1862–1863

By late 1862, at the latest, Jackson recognized the unsatisfactory state of neurological pathophysiology, and he understood the need for better knowledge of normal function: 'In studying the Natural History of Diseases of the Nervous System, I have experienced great difficulty, not only in arranging notes of cases, but also in thinking of the disease as a lesion of a certain physiological system.' This is the first sentence in a small book that Jackson had published for private circulation in early 1863, *Suggestions for Studying Diseases of the Nervous System on Professor Owens' Vertebral Theory*.[47] Since the Preface is dated 'January 5, 1863', and it was written after the main text, we can conclude that Jackson wrote the 50-page piece in the latter part of 1862. When he wrote the Preface, he had already realized that his basic idea would not solve the problem.

> My motive for writing this pamphlet is to place before myself and my friends, certain vague ideas as to the arrangement of the symptoms of disease on a natural … system. I take Professor Owen's vertebral theory as a basis. I do not pretend to any further originality … than to adapt what is known in physiology to the study of disease. I am not aware that any one has yet attempted to complete [Owen's] Vertebral scheme by allotting viscera, nerves, and arteries, to each vertebral segment … Although I have long had the general idea in my mind … I care very little about the details of the scheme, and will willingly sacrifice all of them, if I can make a better arrangement. I shall begin at once to study over again the whole subject, and … shall try to get aid from Pathology, as well as from Physiology.[48]

---

[45] Jackson 1861b, p.648. In Dunglison 1860, epileptiform is not listed, but 'epileptoid' is. In Dunglison 1874, 'epileptiform' is listed as meaning epileptoid. See also Temkin 1971, p.311.

[46] Temkin 1971, pp.284–285; 'organ' is used here in Gall's localizing sense of the term.

[47] Jackson 1863a.

[48] Jackson 1863a, pp.iii–iv; my square brackets.

Most of Jackson's scheme died an early and merciful death, but embryonic forms of some of his most insightful ideas can be found in these small pages.[49] 'Professor Owen' was Richard Owen (1804–1892), the most prominent comparative anatomist in Britain at the time.[50] He was Thomas Henry Huxley's (1825–1895) main scientific opponent—on the conservative side in the early debates about evolution.[51] In 1846 Owen had proposed the fundamental distinction between 'homologous' and 'analogous' parts in animals, with particular attention to the vertebrate skeleton.[52] He accepted and expanded an older theory, now discredited, which held that the bones of the skull are metamorphosed vertebrae.[53] Those ideas were widely circulated, and Jackson was well aware of them.[54] He thought he could organize his understanding of normal and abnormal neurological functions by thinking about them within the anatomical territories assigned to each of the four separate 'vertebrae' in the human skull.

By the time Jackson wrote his Preface, he knew that his vertebral divisions were not real. On the other hand, in the *Suggestions* he said he was beginning to see large numbers of cases of neurological problems, especially at Queen Square.[55] Half-way through his little treatise he included a section titled 'Ordinary Hemiplegia due to disease of the corpus striatum, or optic thalamus, which are centres for the muscles of the limbs'.[56] Here he said about hemiplegia:

> ...I mean here the ordinary form of that disease, depending...on lesion of the corpus striatum, or thalamus opticus. We get paralysis of the face...and of the arm and leg, but paralysis of motion only...there is very little paralysis of the face...All the sensitive [sensory] nerves escape. I think we find only paralysis of the muscles of the limbs...Is this another way of saying that those muscles less under the control of the will escape, and hence that the corpus striatum and thalamus opticus are able to direct (voluntarily) the limbs only?[57]

The speculation in the last sentence of this passage was important for Jackson's later analysis of seizure patterns and other neurological conundrums. However, in 1863 his analysis of seizures was focused on a theory that he had inherited from Brown-Séquard.

Further on Epilepsy in the *Suggestions*, 1863

In 1852 Brown-Séquard published the results of experiments in which he stimulated the cranial end of cut cervical sympathetic chains of animals. He observed vasoconstriction in the ipsilateral face and ear. In contrast, simply cutting the nerve had been known to produce the opposite effect. He concluded that the stimulation caused constriction of the smooth muscle in the walls of the arteries.[58] This established the existence of vascular vasomotor

---

[49] Jackson's emphasis on regional vascular anatomy was an important element in his later thinking about stroke, so part of our concept of stroke derives from this 'discarded' book.

[50] See C.U.M. Smith 1992, pp.69–70; for an extensive biography see Rupke 1994.

[51] See Jensen 1988; C.U.M. Smith 1997, 1999; and Owen et al. 2009.

[52] See Rupke 1993.

[53] See C.U.M. Smith 1997.

[54] See Greenblatt 1965, p.365, and footnotes 77 and 78 in that article.

[55] On p.45, he cited 'more than 200 cases of epilepsy and other convulsive diseases'.

[56] Jackson 1863a, p.24. Although the thalamus was thought to be related to visual function, Jackson and others found that in hemiplegia due to lesions in the basal ganglia the lesions usually involved the thalami, so they began to question the supposedly sensory nature of the thalami. See Jackson 1865f, p.301; on p.302, Jackson quoted Todd to the same effect.

[57] Jackson 1863a, pp.24–25; Jackson's parentheses, my square brackets.

[58] See Aminoff 1993, pp.132–134; Laporte 1996.

nerves, and he assumed (correctly) that the same system exists in the cerebral arteries. In his pathophysiological theory he conceived of the vasomotor nerve system as an extensive reflex network, intracranial and extracranial, which could respond to a large variety of afferent (incoming) stimuli.[59]

In the *Suggestions* section on 'Epilepsy' Jackson referred to Brown-Séquard's vasomotor theory. He said that there are many 'epilepsies', but their primary involvement is with the fourth, 'occipital vertebra', because that is the region that includes the medulla and the 'pneumogastric' (vagus) nerve and so controls the heart. Then he proposed that many seizures are caused by 'sudden and total stoppage of the heart'. In this regard, he said: 'Most physicians think that epilepsy is due to disease of the medulla oblongata. So that my calling it disease of the sensori-motor centre of the occipital vertebra … may be a difference of words only.'[60] Now obviously there is more than a semantic divergence in a proposal that some seizures are due to cardiac standstill. Jackson's theorizing had rather run amok. Nonetheless, it is important to recognize the motive for his overreach. He was trying to understand the pathophysiological events that lead to seizures, including 'certain links in the chain of the paroxysm'. In epilepsy, he said, 'the sensitive fibres going to a diseased part of the brain, act not according to their proper correlation, producing a simple reflex action, but, as it were, the stimulus runs on to another part of greater or more central vitality, and induces diseased action'.[61] Here, in embryonic form, we see one of the crucial elements in Jackson's later formulation of seizure pathogenesis. We still think about normal actions running out of control to produce an epileptic paroxysm whose clinical pattern is determined by the normal functions of the system in which it is occurring.

At the beginning of his pamphlet Jackson used the example of hemiplegia to explain what he was trying to do: 'I wish then to be able to think of it [hemiplegia] as a disease of a certain centre which commands a certain tract of the body'.[62] And later he said that 'disease occurs in physiological tracts as well as in geographical ones'.[63] By 'physiological tracts' he meant integrated systems of gray matter and fibers that subserve distinct functions, such as the motor system. In contradistinction, 'geographical' refers to anatomical proximity without regard to function. For example, if two separate nerves run through the same hole in the base of the skull, and a disease process (e.g., a tumor) invades that foramen, the different functions of the two nerves will both be disrupted, because they happen to suffer the consequences of being in geographical proximity. But there is not necessarily any physiological connection between them. This 'geographical' anatomy was known in some detail by the early 1860s, but knowledge of neurophysiology was far less advanced. Jackson felt the constraining effect of that ignorance when he tried to organize his clinical notes in a physiologically meaningful way.[64]

The *Suggestions* as a Reflection of Jackson's Innate Conservatism, 1863

Beyond pathophysiology, there is a broader observation to be made about the *Suggestions*. Jackson's choice of Owen's theory as the basis for his scheme was made primarily because he

[59] See Greenblatt 2003, pp.798–800.
[60] Jackson 1863a, pp.43–45; see also Chapter 8.
[61] Jackson 1863a, p.44.
[62] Jackson 1863a, p.1; my square brackets.
[63] Jackson 1863a, p.20.
[64] Jackson 1863a, p.1.

found the theory to be useful for his immediate needs. But his choice of Owen's theory was also consistent with his innate conservatism. Owen was, after all, on the opposing side in the debates about Darwinian evolution. Hutchinson tells us that Jackson was innately conservative, politically and socially, somewhat in the mold of Samuel Johnson (1709–1784).[65] Unlike Johnson, however, Jackson had an intense dislike of open conflict or even the semblance thereof.[66] While it is true that there was little in Darwin's *Origin* that was relevant to Jackson's immediate needs, I think he would have hesitated to use Darwin's ideas when they were so controversial. His close friend, Thomas Buzzard (1831–1919), attributed some of Jackson's personality to his Yorkshire roots, which made him, paradoxically, 'cautious in drawing conclusions, but when convinced, sturdily indisposed to change them, except under the influence of more or less overwhelming evidence; at the same time eminently reasonable, and far from displaying undue obstinacy.'[67] Throughout his life Jackson exhibited this tendency to keep to the old idea until he was thoroughly convinced that a new conclusion was necessary. At the same time he was constantly probing the old ideas with new data.

A Lecture on Method, June 1864

In 1864 Jackson began to publish original contributions that brought him notice in the medical community. Before we look at those early papers, however, we need to address the unfinished business of Jackson's revised approach to neurological disease, which he promised in the Preface of the *Suggestions*. Throughout the remainder of his career he made only a few references to the *Suggestions*,[68] but with regard to method there was an obvious successor. In June 1864 he delivered a lecture 'On the study of diseases of the nervous system' at the London Hospital.[69] Its tone indicates that he was talking to medical students. Despite his relative youth (age 29), he was a decade older than the students, and he addressed them with the solicitous air of an experienced clinician-teacher. He began with a Baconian paraphrase whose first part could have been the motto on his coat-of-arms, if he had one.

> "It is easier," Lord Bacon says, "to evolve truth from error than from confusion" … in the study of Disease it is better to have even a mechanical arrangement, than to work without a plan. But I hope, that the method I am about to submit to you, is in some sense a natural system, rather than an artificial scheme."[70]

---

[65] Hutchinson 1911, p.1553.

[66] This is seen in the tone of Hutchinson's 'Recollections' (1911). Jackson's younger colleagues, James Taylor (1859–1946) and Charles Mercier (1852–1919), both recalled that Jackson did not like to disparage anyone; see Taylor in Jackson 1925, pp.16–17; and Mercier in Jackson 1925, p.43.

[67] [Jackson, J.H.] 1911, p.952.

[68] See, e.g., Jackson 1864i, p.358, which contains a long quotation from the *Suggestions*; also Jackson 1866p, p.273. In Jackson 1866f, p.660, footnote (a), Jackson used the term 'limb' from the *Suggestions* but without citing that title. In 1870g, p.191, there is a phrase about the 'physiological regions of the limbs of one side'.

[69] Jackson 1864h; see also York and Steinberg 2006, pp.10–11.

[70] Jackson 1864h, p.146. I could not find the Baconian source of Jackson's paraphrase when I quoted it in 1977 (Greenblatt 1977, p.414), and I still can't find it. In 1888 Jackson (Jackson 1888c, p.61) presented a more nuanced view of Bacon's supposed inductivism. When Harvey Cushing (1869–1939) visited Sir William Broadbent in July 1900, there was a portrait of Jackson in the waiting room. Cushing reported to his father that Broadbent and Jackson were 'lifelong friends. H.J.'s [Hughlings Jackson's] motto was "Error is preferable to Confusion," [and Broadbent's motto was] "Chaos is preferable to Error," and hence they had many discussions …' (Fulton 1946, p.164). With attribution to Bacon, but not to Jackson, Cushing repeated Jackson's paraphrasing of Bacon almost *verbatim* in one of his early papers (Cushing 1905, pp.83–84).

What Jackson meant by 'artificial scheme' is not clear, but he was probably complaining about the contemporary emphasis on empirical nosology, because he challenged that approach directly in the later 1860s. With regard to epilepsy and most diseases, classification was a primary concern from the eighteenth century and beyond.[71] Thus abjuring nosology, Jackson went on to 'insist on one thing as an essential preliminary in the study of disease, and markedly essential in the study of diseases of the Nervous System, viz: – a knowledge of Anatomy'. And later in the same paragraph he said, 'diseases of the Nervous System are not more obscure, than those of the chest or abdomen. It is the anatomy that is difficult.'[72] His use of the word 'anatomy' here means functional anatomy. I have underlined the last sentence in the quotation because it denotes his recognition of the limitations of that knowledge at the time. Hence,

> … Just as we study, as physiologists and anatomists, the vegetative life of general tissues, the structure of organs for special functions, and the universal harmony of most diverse functions in individuals, so we ought, as workers in the field of Practical Medicine, to study every case that comes before us; as presenting
>   1. Disease of Tissue. (Changes in Tissue.)
>   2. Damage of Organs.
>   3. Disorder of Function.[73]

These three categories can be rearranged into a succinct statement of how physicians have been taught to think about the etiology of disease since the early nineteenth century: disease of tissue causes damage of organs, which in turn causes disorders of function. So Jackson's method was not original. It was, however, a clear statement of the clinico-pathological method, and he used it to good effect. As York and Steinberg put it, Jackson 'showed that it was possible to diagnose focal pathology in the central nervous system'.[74]

Most of the rest of Jackson's lecture consisted of examples of how his method would lead to clear thinking. For example, syphilitic tissue damage is the same regardless of which organ it attacks, but its clinical appearances may be quite dissimilar in different organs. Toward the end of the lecture he used the example of hemiplegia to show how many different kinds of tissue damage can all produce the same clinical phenomenon if the same organ is damaged. That is, the same clinical presentation of left hemiplegia may result from (1) syphilitic disease of the right hemisphere, causing dysfunction of the striatum, (2) embolism of the right middle cerebral artery, (3) hemorrhage into the right striatum, or (4) tumor in the right striatum. He had started to think about method as early as October 1861.[75] In the Preface to his *Suggestions* he promised that he would try again, with 'aid from Pathology', as well as from Physiology'.[76] During 1863 the main themes in his writings were seizures and various forms of paralysis, including unilateral seizures and hemiplegia. In his first paper of 1864—before publication of the lecture on method—he started to present some original observations.

---

[71] See Temkin 1971, pp.247–252, 285–291.
[72] Jackson 1864h, p.147; my underlining.
[73] Jackson 1864h, pp.146–147; Jackson's parentheses.
[74] York and Steinberg 2006, p.10.
[75] Jackson 1861f, p.290.
[76] Jackson 1864h, p.iv.

The Beginnings of Originality: Hemiplegia, Unilateral
Seizures, and Language Disorders, 1864

In January 1864, Jackson began to address 'loss of speech' as a neurological phenomenon.[77] It was this addition of language disorders to his intellectual stew that eventually led to his mature conceptualizations. However, there are still many controversies about language and its disorders, so my definitions cannot be as straightforward as my previous descriptions of neuroanatomy.

Definition Section 4—Language and Its Disorders[78]

Language—an arbitrary system of communication between individuals, which typically links sound to meaning. Languages can be conducted in other *modalities*, e.g., reading in the visual modality.

Speech—language in the aural modality. Jackson often used 'speech' to mean roughly what we mean by 'language'. The concern, in his time and ours, is to understand the biological basis of all forms of human language.

Speech production—there are three different groups of biological structures for production of aural language:

  (1) the vocal apparatus, including lungs, vocal cords, pharynx, tongue, lips, etc.;
  (2) the neural structures that directly control the vocal apparatus, including the relevant cranial nerves, their brainstem nuclei, the motor system (cortical and subcortical); and
  (3) the brain structures that process outgoing (efferent) speech above the level of the purely motor. Part of the problem here is to distinguish between brain structures that subserve general intelligence and those that process premotor information which is specific to auditory language. The latter is primarily *Broca's area*. An old-fashioned but still useful distinction is to say that components (1) and (2) are the mechanisms for production of spoken utterances (whose disorder is called *dysarthria*), whereas (3) is the basis of *internal* speech, i.e., in the brain.

Almost everything in this section is still subject to vigorous investigation and debate. For example, some people say that all language production is motor processing, until one reaches the level of cognition, whatever that is. In any case, the above discussion has concerned only speech production—the motor side of auditory language. On the sensory side, we also receive language in the aural modality.

Speech reception—has three groups of anatomical components:

  (1) the *end organ* structures that receive sound, including the external ear, the tympanic membrane ('ear drum'), the middle ear ossicles (sound- conducting bones), and the cochlea deep in the inner (bony) ear;
  (2) the neural structures that transmit signals from the cochlea into the brain, including the cochlear part of the eighth cranial nerve, the cochlear nuclei and other nuclei in the brainstem, Heschl's gyrus on the dorsum of each temporal lobe, and the white matter tracts that make these connections; and

---

[77] Jackson 1864a.
[78] With many thanks to Marjorie Perlman Lorch for extended discussions.

(3) the brain area(s) that receive and somehow interpret the sounds as communication. This process may start in *Heschl's gyrus*, but *Wernicke's area*, just posterior to Heschl's gyrus, is thought to be the major site for this function.[79] Beyond Wernicke's area, the connections are myriad, but at least one connecting pathway is commonly accepted, i.e., the *arcuate fasciculus*, which connects Wernicke's area to Broca's.

Disorders of speech: the aphasias—a large variety of aphasic syndromes has been described since the later nineteenth century, but there is now general agreement that the main distinction is between disorders of speech production and its reception.

Broca's aphasia (also called *motor, expressive,* or *anterior* aphasia)—the main clinical feature is, to use Jackson's words, 'loss of speech', albeit seldom total. There is marked reduction in *fluency* (roughly, words per minute) and many mistakes in words (*paraphasias*). The brain lesions that cause this syndrome are usually centered in or include Broca's area, but they generally extend well beyond the lateral third frontal gyrus that carries Broca's name. Since those lesions are also in or near the primary motor cortices and their tracts, there is a high correlation with contralateral hemiplegia, as Jackson observed.

Wernicke's aphasia (also called *sensory, receptive,* or *posterior* aphasia)—initially these patients may be nonfluent, but they evolve to a syndrome of normal or high fluency and their speech is difficult to interpret. Often it is just *jargon.* They have little *comprehension* of what is said to them, nor do they realize that they are making no sense to others. The lesion is usually centered in or close to Wernicke's area, but the same controversies arise about the extent of the lesions, which can be very large.

Mixed/global aphasias—clinical syndromes involving a mixture of Broca's and Wernicke's elements are very common. *Global aphasia* refers to severe impairment of both comprehension and production of aural language, although complete mutism is uncommon.

Cerebral dominance for language—*dominance* is the term for the clinico-pathological correlation of language disorders with damage to only one side of the brain, usually the left. Pure right brain dominance is quite unusual. Most left-handed people have some degree of *mixed* dominance. *Cerebral specialization* for language refers to anatomical asymmetries that can be correlated with language dominance. The brains of about 2/3 people will show these side-to-side differences if they are carefully sought, but data about this phenomenon began to become available only in the very late nineteenth century, and some of it is still controversial.

I never said this would be easy! And at the bedside these things are messy. It is much more difficult than the above outline would imply, because patients' individual presentations are seldom so clear-cut. Even so, we are now sufficiently equipped with the basics so we can begin to investigate Jackson's role in the development of these distinctions. His early encounter with aphasia had a profound impact on his theorizing, because it led him to think about some fundamental issues.

---

[79] However, Carl Wernicke's (1848–1905) classic description of the aphasia that comes from damage to 'Wernicke's area' was published in 1874, a decade after the events that we will be discussing in this chapter.

Jackson's Early Observations on Aphasia: Before His Knowledge of Broca, January 1864

In the *Medical Times and Gazette* (*MTG*) of January 30, 1864, Jackson devoted one-and-a-half columns to his own 'Clinical remarks on hemiplegia, with loss of speech – its association with valvular disease of the heart'.[80] His interest in aphasia arose from his prior interest in hemiplegia. At the outset he 'remarked that in nearly all the cases of loss of speech that he had seen ... there had been hemiplegia'. Seeking a neurological explanation for the loss of speech, he said:

> ... [it] was frequently pointed out at this [National] Hospital by Dr. Brown-Séquard, [that] the defect is not one of talking, but rather of language ... in some extreme cases Dr. Brown-Séquard used to point out that the patient had lost altogether the power of expression, not by oral language only, but even by making signs. One patient who was admitted into the Hospital ... could only say "no" and "yes," and these words at the wrong time.[81]

Jackson went on to state that there is always 'some defect of talking' with hemiplegia, because of facial weakness, but 'Loss of speech cannot be too carefully distinguished from loss of power of articulation'.[82] Thus, because of his early exposure to Brown-Séquard, Jackson had a prior understanding of the critical linguistic and neurological categories for the motor side of internal speech. At this point he said nothing about the sensory/receptive side, and there is no evidence that Brown-Séquard had anything to say in this respect.

We might ask where Brown-Séquard had learned what he taught. The most likely suspect is Jean Baptiste Bouillaud (1791–1881). He was a colorful, politically liberal, and highly respected professor of medicine in Paris, starting in 1831. Bouillaud remained steadfastly adherent to some parts of Gall's organology, especially with regard to localization of language in the 'anterior' (frontal) lobes bilaterally. For this he had independent, clinico-pathological evidence.[83] There is no record of any direct contact between Bouillaud and Brown-Séquard. However, Brown-Séquard was a medical student in Paris from 1838 to 1846, and he remained there until his first sojourn to America in 1852.[84] So there was ample opportunity for a bright young student to become acquainted with the ideas of a popular professor.[85]

Bouillaud is generally given credit for making the crucial distinction between the neurology of internal versus external speech,[86] because he located some motor aspects of speech production in the white matter of the frontal lobes, while ascribing word memory to the cortex.[87] Since no one else is a candidate for such credit, I conclude that Brown-Séquard's knowledge of language disorders was derived from Bouillaud, which means that in some

---

[80] Jackson 1864a.

[81] Jackson 1864a; my square brackets.

[82] Jackson 1864a.

[83] See Brown and Chobor 1992.

[84] Aminoff 1993, pp.14–21.

[85] For a more complete argument about the likely connection between Bouillaud and Brown-Séquard see Greenblatt 1970, pp.557–558. The Critchleys (1998, p.151) contend that my proposed connection is 'too tenuous to be plausible', and they are correct that I cannot prove my case. However, I think the historical circumstances make it quite plausible; one does not have to be tutored directly by a prominent professor in order to absorb his ideas.

[86] See Riese 1947, p.324; Marx 1966, pp.337–338; and Harrington 1987, p.37. Harrington (1987, pp.216–217) states that Jackson's view of this distinction was not the same as Bouillaud's, but she cites a Jacksonian paper of 1874, which was written after Jackson's ideas had a decade to develop. When Jackson first learned the distinction from Brown-Séquard, presumably he received Bouillaud's version.

[87] See Clarke and O'Malley 1996, pp.488–491; and Finger 2000, pp.137–139.

sense it came from Bouillaud's furtherance of organology. Even in the academic community of Paris the old bogeyman was only partially suppressed, and the same applies to London.

Theorizing the Connection Between Aphasia and Hemiplegia: The Syndrome of the Middle Cerebral Artery, January–April 1864

Getting back to Jackson's first paper of 1864, his method compelled him to look for some way to explain the connection between 'loss of speech' and hemiplegia. To account for the apparent link he had another observation:

> Recently it occurred to him, that in all the cases of this kind that he had seen (seven), there was valvular disease of the heart ... Of course, there is no physiological connection betwixt disease of the aortic or mitral valves and paralysis on *one* side of the body ... But the coincidence is, probably ... that, as is well known, vegetations may be detached from the diseased valves and plug up the middle (and anterior?) cerebral arteries ... the connexion is a mechanical one ... This middle cerebral artery supplies the corpus striatum (the upper part of the motor tract, disease of which so often produces hemiplegia), and also part of the hemisphere. We have, then, paralysis of motion, as evidenced by the hemiplegia, and defect of mind, as shown by loss of speech. Many physiologists and Physicians have considered the anterior [frontal] lobes to be the part of the brain in which resides the faculty of speech ...[88]

This passage requires consideration of two kinds of localization, vascular and neurological. First the vascular. The runaway 'vegetations' (emboli) are still reckoned as a common cause of stroke. Immediately after the above passage, Jackson said, 'Dr. Kirkes long ago pointed out that in heart disease hemiplegia from plugging of the middle cerebral artery was not uncommon.'[89] So the idea of embolic stroke already existed, though Jackson and his generation did not use that term for it. Their term was *apoplexy*, which commonly referred to bleeding into an organ, especially the brain.[90] As we now use the word 'stroke', it means a neurologic deficit due to focal death of brain tissue. But the details of the deficit—the signs and symptoms—can have no significance if there is no knowledge of brain localization to correlate with them. In this sense, Jackson was advancing knowledge of the *syndrome of the middle cerebral artery* by pointing out that it can have at least two components: (1) contralateral weakness or paralysis, and (2) loss of speech. In light of Jackson's *Suggestions*, it would appear that his thoughts about regional vascular supply to the brain had some of their origin in his 'discarded' vertebral theory.

With regard to neurological localization, the last sentence in the above (indented) quotation is key. The 'Many physiologists and Physicians' who accepted frontal lobe localization for speech were using a phrenological idea. Moreover, 'faculty of speech' is also phrenological,

---

[88] Jackson 1864a, p.123; Jackson's parentheses, my square brackets.

[89] The German pathologist Rudolf Virchow (1821–1902) usually gets credit for being the first to describe cerebral emboli, in 1846–1856 (Garrison 1929, p.571), but William S. Kirkes (1823–1864) is sometimes recognized for publishing the observation independently in 1852; see Greenblatt 1970, pp.558–559. There is no comprehensive book on the history of stroke. Fields and Lemak's (1989) small volume does not mention Jackson, Kirkes, or the middle cerebral artery. Schiller (1970) provides some coverage of the nineteenth century. The more recent chapter by Storey and Pols (2010) is useful but limited in scope.

[90] See Dunglison 1860, p.873.

because phrenology was based on the 'faculty psychology'.[91] Its use in phrenology resulted in a 'mosaic' view of how the faculties are located in the different regions of the brain. Since each faculty was assigned to a tightly defined area of cortex, the resulting montage had the appearance of mosaic tiling, as seen on phrenological busts. However, this is not to say that Jackson accepted phrenological theory beyond the 'faculty of speech'.

Further along in his remarks of January 1864, Jackson said, 'Talking may be divided into three things – articulation ... for sounds, speech for words, language for the expression of ideas. The mind ... forms the ideas, the memory furnishes the words, and the tongue, lips, etc., turn them out as certain recognized sounds.' After giving some clinical examples, he continued:

> When the defect begins in language, it would imply ... general loss of power of mind, so that a person cannot express himself either by talking, writing or by signs. When in speech he forms ideas, but his memory cannot find the words for them and he re-turns to the primeval language of signs; when his tongue, larynx, etc., are paralysed, he cannot talk well ... in short, defect of ideas, defect of words, defect of sounds. In thus entering minutely into these differences, Dr. Jackson said he did not attempt to claim any great amount of precision. The subject was to him far too obscure to induce him to dogmatise.[92]

The operative statement here is the cautionary note in the last sentence. The subject was indeed 'obscure'. Simply talking about ideas and about memory for words does not define the relationship between them. Jackson was suggesting that only memory for words is located in the frontal lobes,[93] while intelligence was generally assumed to be located diffusely in the hemispheres. As always, when he took up the challenge of this conundrum his primary investigational tools were clinical observation and clinico-pathological reasoning.

In another clinical report, dated April 30, 1864, we find statements that bear on two of Jackson's major themes, seizures and aphasia. He described a patient who had onset of focal seizures beginning in the left face, associated with visual dimming, scintillations, and sometimes loss of consciousness.[94] To explain the conjunction of these symptoms, he invoked the idea of disturbance in the territory of the left middle cerebral artery. Later in the article he defined the disturbance as arterial 'spasm', and he postulated spasm in the anterior cerebral artery as the cause of the olfactory aura in some seizures.[95] Hence, he was generalizing the idea of focal disturbances of arterial flow as the cause of specific neurological dysfunctions, dependent on the normal functions of the disturbed tissue. This was an incremental but crucial step in our concept of cerebrovascular pathophysiology. Whether anyone else had preceded Jackson in this way of thinking is not clear to me, but certainly he was among the first to figure it out.[96]

---

[91] See Young 1970, pp.17–23, and further.

[92] Jackson 1864a.

[93] Similar ideas had circulated earlier, e.g., by Robert Dunn (1799–1877); see Lorch 2016, pp.195–198.

[94] Jackson 1864b, p.481, col.2.

[95] Jackson 1864b, p.482. The olfactory nerves, bulbs, and tracts are supplied by ethmoidal branches of the external carotid artery; some olfactory cortex is supplied by the anterior cerebral.

[96] See Storey and Pols 2010, pp.408–410.

An Original Observation on Right Hemiplegia and Aphasia, April 1864

The same report of April 30, 1864 also contains another original observation.

> Dr. Hughlings Jackson has already observed that whenever loss of speech occurs with hemiplegia the hemiplegia is on the <u>right</u> side. A note on this subject will be found in this journal for January 30, but Dr. Jackson has now had under observation about twenty-eight cases, and he still thinks it plausible, if not highly probable, that the cause is embolism of the left middle cerebral artery. He intends, then, to investigate the sequence of symptoms in the paroxysm, and the subsequent mental condition of a patient who has epileptiform convulsions in the left and right side[s] respectively.[97]

Again, two of Jackson's early interests are interwoven here: seizures and aphasia. With regard to seizures, he intended to 'investigate the sequence of symptoms in the paroxysm', which soon became the key to his understanding of epilepsy's pathophysiology. This was his first explicit statement about this approach. In the *Suggestions* there are some prescient statements about seizure patterns, and Jackson had previously described the sequence of motor involvement in focal seizures in his reporter's columns,[98] but here he was laying out a deliberate strategy. When he wrote about investigating the 'subsequent mental condition' of a postictal patient, he was referring to the patient's linguistic status in relation to the side of the seizure.

The issue of laterality in relation to 'loss of speech' was about to become pivotal, so we need to be clear about the sequence of events to April 30, 1864. In that publication Jackson was drawing a connection between loss of speech and *right* hemiplegia, implying *left* brain abnormality.[99] As of April 30, he did not have any autopsy evidence—just the clinical observation of the side of the hemiplegia. Nonetheless, he seemed to know that he was on to something important. In fact, he was about to become involved in one of the most iconic events of modern neurology. To understand what happened we need to go back to where it started, in Paris.

First Encounters with Broca and the Edge of the Mind-Brain Problem

The central figure was a Parisian surgeon, Paul Broca (1824–1880) (Fig. 3.2),[100] who had founded the Société de Anthropologie in 1859.[101] In the spring of 1861 there was a debate in the Société about brain size and intelligence—a common topic of discussion at the time. Bouillaud's son-in-law, Ernst Aubertin (1825–1893), brought up the related issue of language localization, promoting Bouillaud's claim for the frontal lobes. It was then that Broca encountered a severely aphasic patient (Leborgne), whom the Bicêtre hospital staff called 'Tan', because that was the only word he could utter. Before he died on April 17, 1861, Tan

---

[97] Jackson 1864b, p.482; my square brackets and underlining.
[98] The earliest are in Jackson 1861b, p.650 (June 22, 1861).
[99] Jackson 1864a. He referred back to this paper, but there is nothing in it about laterality.
[100] For biography see Schiller 1979; also Greenblatt 1984, 2006.
[101] Jackson was a founding member of the Anthropological Society of London in 1863; see Lorch 2016, p.194, footnote 7.

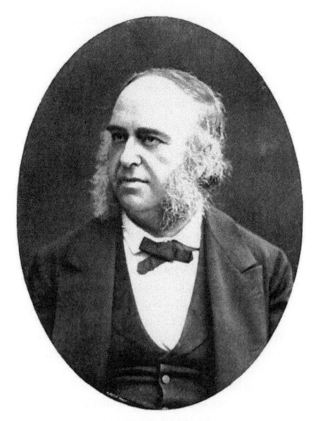

Fig. 3.2 Paul Broca.
(Reproduced under a Creative Commons Attribution 4.0 International (CC BY 4.0) from Wellcome Collection.)

was examined by Broca and by Aubertin. At autopsy he was found to have a large left brain lesion (softening) centered in the area that now carries Broca's name.[102] Six months later another similar patient (Lelong) was found to have a smaller lesion in the same area. Broca's original term for the language deficit was 'aphémie' (aphemia), but 'aphasia', proposed by Armand Trousseau in 1864, soon supplanted it.[103]

By 1863 Broca had collected a total of eight autopsied cases of *aphémie*. In reporting them to the Société de Anthropologie, he said it was 'Remarkable how in all these patients the lesion was on the left side. I do not dare to draw any conclusion from this and am waiting for new data.'[104] Given the legacy of Bichat's laws of symmetry,[105] bilateral symmetry was an article of French biological faith, so Broca's hesitation is understandable. By 1865 he had dozens of cases, and he said definitively, 'we speak with the left hemisphere' ('*nous parlons*

---

[102] Broca 1861. There are many versions of this story, including Schiller's biography of Broca (Schiller 1979, pp.165–211). Finger's very readable version (Finger 2000, pp.137–154) follows Schiller's. A detailed contextual analysis of these events is given by Lorch 2011.

[103] Trousseau 1864. The *BMJ* of February 27, 1864 ([Broca] 1864) contained a report of a letter that Broca sent to Trousseau concerning the correct word to express 'loss of voice', but 'aphasia' is not mentioned, nor is this letter cited by Jackson. See also Greenblatt 1970, p.563. While validating this sequence of events, Lorch 2011 has shown that aphasia was a minor issue in the Parisian debates for many months after Broca's reports.

[104] Schiller 1979, p.194.

[105] Harrington 1987, p.53; and Leblanc 2017, pp.30–33.

avec l'hémisphère gauche').[106] There were many controversies besetting all of this, including competing priority claims about the discovery of cerebral dominance for language.[107] Here it will suffice to return to Jackson in the relative calm of unmindful London. Later in 1864 he wrote that 'no one in England' had been interested in the issue of language laterality in the brain.[108] That is, until Jackson's prepared mind chanced upon it.[109]

Jackson's First Notice of Broca, May 1864

Recall now that Jackson published his preliminary observation about loss of speech and right hemiplegia in the *MTG* of April 30, 1864. On May 21, 1864, the *BMJ* published a letter from Jackson, dated May 2.[110] It started with his comments on another physician's case of right hemiplegia and aphasia, which had been reported in the *BMJ* on April 30, 1864.[111] Jackson repeated his observation about the laterality of his own cases and his embolism theory, and then he said, 'M. Broca believes that disease of the brain *on the left side only* produces loss of speech; and, if I were to judge from the cases under my own care, I should think so too.'[112] From there he went on to discuss his developing theory of epilepsy, as it bore on the laterality issue. The following passage shows how his ideas about different clinical problems developed in close relation to each other.

> I think I can shew [sic] by records of numerous cases that when, in severe epileptiform seizures, convulsions affect the right side of the body, there is, after the paroxysm, greater mental defect, and a greater loss of speech, than when the left side is convulsed. In the former – temporary spasm of the branches of the left middle cerebral artery – there are the symptoms faintly marked, which are, as it were, more permanently written down in the defect of speech and hemiplegia which follow complete blocking up of the artery … there are good reasons for believing that epileptiform seizures are due not to general spasm of the blood-vessels of the brain, but to spasm in certain definite arterial regions, or possibly in regions mapped out by vasomotor nerves.[113]

After he made his point about the etiology and laterality of postictal loss of speech, Jackson returned to his main subject.

> M. Broca points out a particular part of the brain, where, he believes, the faculty of speech resides; but I can only surmise that it is in some part of the brain supplied by the left middle

---

[106] Broca 1865. An English translation of this entire paper is in Berker et al. 1986, where the quoted passage is on p.1068, col.1. See also Greenblatt 1984; Henderson 1986; Harris 1991, 1993; and Eling 1994, pp.41–58.

[107] See Schiller 1979, pp.192–202; Finger and Roe 1996; Roe and Finger 1996; Leblanc 2017; and Chapter 5.

[108] Jackson 1864j, p.464; this paper was published sometime between August 1864 (see his Case V, p.418) and October 1864, because it was reviewed in the *BMJ* of November 5, 1864 (see Jackson 1864k). On pp.464–465, Jackson contrasted Trousseau's and Broca's views on 'M. Broca's hypothesis' as respectively 'conservative' and 'radical'.

[109] Two British physicians who took early interest in language disorders were Ramskill (see Lorch 2004a) and Frederic Bateman (1824–1904) of Norwich (see Radick 2000), but neither published before Jackson in Jackson 1864c. For further on Ramskill see Chapter 5.

[110] Jackson 1864c.

[111] The case was Fletcher 1864.

[112] Jackson 1864c, p.572; Jackson's italics.

[113] Jackson 1864c, p.572.

cerebral artery. Of course, a clot or a tumour in this region would produce the same results as plugging of the artery ...

I may briefly say, that by defect of speech I mean, not difficulty of articulation, but want of brain-power either to form ideas or to find words ... This mental symptom has been described by Trousseau under the name of *aphasia*. I have heard Dr. Brown-Séquard describe it many times ...[114]

This shows that by late April 1864—a year before Broca's definitive statement about left cerebral dominance for language—Jackson had found his way into the French debate, although we don't know exactly when or how he found it. Brown-Séquard could be a suspect, but he had left London for America in July 1863.[115] Jackson's reference to Trousseau in the above points to the possibility that he was reacting to a small news item in the *BMJ* of February 6, 1864. This was a single paragraph that summarized the 'learned letter' which Broca had addressed to Trousseau regarding the best word 'to express *loss of voice*'.[116] It was part of the episode that led to Trousseau's selection of *aphasia* in preference to Broca's *aphemia*.[117] Since Jackson could read French, he might have traced the subject to its source. Harrington has followed this line of argument to suggest that a different French author, Jules Parrot, was Jackson's *entrée*,[118] but this idea suffers the same paucity of evidence as the others.

Early Differences with Broca: Establishing Boundaries and Independence, Mid-1864

In the middle of 1864—probably as late as August—Jackson published a long review paper on 'Loss of speech: Its association with valvular disease of the heart, and with hemiplegia on the right side ... arterial regions in epilepsy'.[119] The bulk of the paper's 84 pages consist of case reports and repetitions of his speculations about embolism and/or spasm in the middle cerebral artery. But there are some new elements: (1) thoughts about the relationship of his findings to Broca's, (2) evidence that his search for a better understanding of aphasia was starting to draw him into the literature of psychology and linguistics, and (3) his self-proclaimed stance of conservatism on these controversial matters. At the beginning of the paper he was careful to establish boundaries between Broca's data and his own.

The chief physiological results of the following observations I arrived at independently, but on every point of importance I have been anticipated by M. Broca. Therefore, what

---

114 Jackson 1864c, p.572; Jackson's italics.

115 Gooddy 1964, p.192.

116 [Broca] 1864; italics in original. For the period 1861 through mid-1864, my search of some leading British medical journals turned up only this mention of Broca on February 6, 1864 (Greenblatt 1970, p.563, footnote 22), before Jackson's first published reference to Broca on May 21, 1864 (Jackson 1864c). Lorch (2004a, p.129) subsequently conducted a similar review of a larger number of journals and came to the same conclusion. See also Chapter 5.

117 Trousseau 1864. This episode is discussed in Schiller 1979, pp.199–200; Henderson 1990; Pearce 2002; and Leblanc 2017, pp.130–136.

118 Harrington 1987, pp.207–208. I have not found any mention of Parrot by Jackson.

119 Jackson 1864j. It appears that Jackson began to write this paper before July 1864, because he said on the first page that he had seen 34 patients, but in a brief paper of July 23, 1864 (J64-04) he claimed to have seen 41. On the other hand, in it (J64-10, pp.417–418) he stated that he saw two of the patients in August 1864. This volume of the 'London Hospital Reports' was reviewed in the *BMJ* of November 5, 1864. The reviewer would have needed at least a few weeks to write his review and get it into print, so (in agreement with York and Steinberg 2006, p.45) I conclude that the entire volume 1 of 'Reports' was published in September or October 1864.

I have to do is simply to bring forward my work as evidence bearing on his views. Besides, M. Broca has studied the subject from another point of view, and has arrived at more precise results than I can possibly deduce from observations which are clinical only. M. Broca believes that disease of the left side of the brain only, produces loss of Language; and more-over [sic], he locates the faculty of Articulate Language in a very limited part of that hemisphere. My observations tend to support the first hypothesis, and, in a general way, the second. The Convolution of Articulate Language of Broca is but one of many convolutions supplied by the left middle cerebral artery ... Therefore, my observations must necessarily be indefinite evidence as to the exact seat of the faculty of language, or of articulate language, but fairly definite as to the side of the brain in which these faculties reside.[120]

On the next page Jackson made peremptory riddance of priority claims:

I have premised the above as to priority, simply to have done with it, and in order that I may give with more freedom, and in my own way, the steps by which I arrived at the results announced in this paper ... although I have in a great part of my subject worked quite independently, I lay no claim to priority on any point of importance.[121]

In other words, he prized his independence, but he viewed priority claims as bothersome intrusions in the pursuit of the truth. The truth that he wanted to pursue was a deeper understanding of phenomena on both sides of the mind-brain equation. Later in the paper Jackson gives us some insight into his thoughts about the neurological basis of the association of hemiplegia with loss of speech.

Now, the strangeness of this association – the loss of a purely mental faculty with paralysis of the limbs on one side – made me think frequently on the subject, and seek for some explanation of the concurrence of the two symptoms. For here are ... two incoherent symptoms ... coming on suddenly together. Then, apart from this, I often wondered how it was that there were no well-defined mental symptoms in cases of embolism of the middle cerebral artery. This vessel supplies the corpus striatum, the highest part of the motor tract, and hence the hemiplegia was easily accounted for; but it also supplies a vast tract of convolutions, and, therefore, one would à priori expect to find decided symptoms of mental failure. (This difficulty still remains in respect to cases of plugging of the right middle cerebral artery.)[122]

It was this line of speculation that led Jackson to the psychological literature. In his paper on 'Loss of speech' we find the first clear instances of his use of psychological terminology, and he gives us some of his sources.[123]

---

120 Jackson 1864j, p.388.
121 Jackson 1864j, p.389.
122 Jackson 1864j, p.402; Jackson's italics and parentheses.
123 The sources were listed on pp.390, 395, 396, 398, etc. An intriguing example occurs in a footnote to his discussion of paraphasias (mistakes in words) and recurrent utterances (repeated stock words or phrases): 'Just as we analyse various defects in Expression, so we ought to be careful not to confound the varieties of disorders of its corresponding opposite, Perception' (p.398). In fact, Jackson's case reports included a few who probably had Wernicke's aphasia (Cases XII and XIII, pp.430–431).

The Psychology of Language and Jackson's First Encounter with the Writings of Herbert Spencer

One of Jackson's most important sources was Broca himself, because Broca was also struggling with psycholinguistic issues. According to Jackson, 'M. Broca speaks of two kinds of loss of language: first, a loss of the General Faculty of Language; and second, a loss of the faculty of Articulate Language'.[124] Jackson seemed to state this distinction of faculties without quite accepting it. He was focused on an effort to understand the underlying neurological mechanisms of the psychological phenomena. In a long footnote,[125] he quoted a source with an intriguing title, *An Essay on Physiological Psychology*, by Robert Dunn.[126] Dunn's Chapter IV is largely devoted to speech and language.[127] He accepted Gall's localization of speech in the frontal lobes, and he gave many references to the French literature on the subject. All in all, it appears that Dunn's little book may have been a significant contributor to Jackson's thinking on the subject, but it was published in 1858, 3 years before Broca's first paper on language localization. In any case, there was another source.

Hughlings Jackson's first references to the writings of Herbert Spencer are found in his discussions of two cases in his paper on 'Loss of speech' of 1864. In those reports he was trying to understand the recurrent utterances of chronically nonfluent aphasics. The patient in Case XX could say only ' "yes", and "oh! yes", in different tones'. About this patient Jackson remarked, ' "All speech", says Herbert Spencer, "is compounded of two elements – the words and the tones in which they are uttered – the signs of ideas and the signs of emotion".'[128] Describing the second patient (Case XXVI), Jackson said:

> ... She could say "yes" and "no," but then she said these words with no bearing on the question asked. When spoken to she replied in one continuously repeated jargon, "Committymy – pittymy." She used these words as if they had some real meaning, and kept continually trying to make herself understood ...
>
> Here was voice, and also articulation; but not language, or at least, it was a language which could express emotion only ... "Cadence," says Herbert Spencer, "is the involuntary commentary of the emotions on the intellect." ... It was indeed, a commentary with the text almost suppressed.[129]

For Jackson an intellectual journey of many decades began here, almost *en passant*, with a few small steps of commentary. At the time, he apparently did not feel any necessity to cite the exact source of his Spencerian quotations. They were originally published in an essay on 'The origin and function of music', which first appeared in 1857.[130] It was reprinted in Spencer's collected *Essays: Scientific, Political and Speculative* in 1858, and that is where Jackson found it.[131] We don't know how he came upon Spencer's essay, but

---

[124] Jackson 1864j, p.391.

[125] Jackson 1864j, p.404

[126] Dunn 1858; Jackson quoted from p.72. For further on Dunn see Richards in Matthew and Harrison 2004, vol.17, pp.322–323; Lorch 2009; and Lorch 2016.

[127] See pp.66–75.

[128] Jackson 1864j, p.440.

[129] Jackson 1864j, p.448.

[130] *Fraser's Magazine* 56:406,1857.

[131] Spencer 1858, pp.359–384. In 1965 I could only cite both places of publication of Spencer's essay, without knowing where Jackson had found it (Greenblatt 1965b, p.374, footnote 105). In researching the present book (in

I suspect the book title may have piqued his interest when he was burrowing around in a bookstore.[132]

A Declaration of Neutrality

Jackson's apparently accidental discovery of Spencer exemplifies his lifelong intellectual eclecticism. At the same time, he maintained an innate conservatism, which he stated toward the end of his essay on 'Loss of speech'.

> There is ... in every one, a radical and a conservative element. Here the radical tendency, representing numbers of cases, urges me to conclude that the Faculty of Language resides on the left side of the brain. But a conservative respect for long-held principles prevents my coming to this conclusion. The one points to facts I have independently observed, and to their confirmation by the previous observations of M. Broca. The other urges that the observations are not yet numerous enough, and that the evidence of mine (wanting autopsies) is not sufficiently exact ... whilst I am anxious on the one hand to insist ... that when hemiplegia attends loss of speech it is almost invariably on the right side, I am ... equally anxious to investigate still further ... whether this peculiarity may not be due to some slighter physical difference ... it is difficult to understand how disease of *one* hemisphere ... can produce speechlessness. If one hemisphere be the duplicate of the other ... there ought to be disease on both sides in complete speechlessness.
>
> I therefore neither accept the old view that the brain is a double organ, nor the new one that the faculty of language resides in the left hemisphere only ... My object is to be a mere witness, especially as there are very great advantages in being neutral.[133]

Of course, an active participant cannot be 'a mere witness'. The fly-on-the-wall is not supposed to join the conversation. The above is a clear expression of one of Jackson's most fundamental traits. Thoughtful conservatism remained a hallmark of his approach throughout his career. In fact, a conservative outlook was a good fit with his political and social environment.

2008), I found his later citation (in 1866) of Spencer's essay on music in Spencer's *Essays* of 1858; see Jackson 1866a, p.175. Strictly speaking, we can know only when Jackson first *published* something about Spencer.

[132] Spencer 1858, p.379, italics in original; also footnote 105 in Greenblatt 1965b, p.374. Jackson made an interesting error of omission because Spencer actually said: '*cadence is the commentary of the emotions upon the propositions of the intellect*'. Jackson began to use 'propositionizing' in 1866 (Jackson 1866a, p.175), but there is no evidence that he took it from Spencer.

[133] Jackson 1864j, pp.463–464. A more complete quotation of this passage is provided in Greenblatt 1970, p.565.

4

Enlarging Prospects and Evolving Ideas

Seizures, Language Disorders, and Associationism, 1865–1867

Marriage and Professional Life, 1860–1865

In 1861 the major event in flourishing Britain was the death of Queen Victoria's consort, Prince Albert, after 21 years of marriage and nine children. His loss sent the Queen into mourning for the rest of her long life. Jackson's immediate lot was a happier one. On July 25, 1865, he married his first cousin, Elizabeth Dade Jackson (1838–1876) (Fig. 4.1). They had known each other from childhood, and their courtship was rumored to have lasted for 11 years. The marriage was childless but otherwise very happy. The newlyweds set up housekeeping at 28 Bedford Place, Russell Square, near Queen Square. In 1868 they moved to No. 3 Manchester Square, in London's West End, close to medically fashionable Harley Street.[1] Since Jackson took on the responsibilities of marriage within the upper middle class mores of his time and place, we can surmise that he was feeling comfortable about his situation and optimistic about his prospects. In 1865–1866 he moved deeper into London's medical life.[2]

In the mid-century the city harbored a multitude of medical societies. They were relatively informal groups by comparison to the long-established colleges.[3] One of the first societies that Jackson joined was the Pathological Society of London, where he became a member in the session of 1865–1866.[4] The Pathological Society was devoted to furthering medical science by pursuing the clinico-pathological method. From the beginning of his career as a medical reporter Jackson had often quoted cases from the Society's *Transactions*.[5] His participation in the group was probably due to the influence of Hutchinson, who had joined the Society in 1852–1853.[6] Also *circa* 1865, Jackson

---

[1] The Critchleys (1998, pp.171–173) say that the Jacksons moved to Manchester Square after the death of Mrs. Jackson's mother, which occurred on December 27, 1867. A letter from Jackson to the editor of *The Lancet* (Jackson 1868e) is addressed and dated 'Bedford-place, Russell-square, March, 1868'. The Jacksons' next-door neighbor at 2 Manchester Square was Julius Benedict (1804–1885), an immigrant German-Jewish composer and conductor who was knighted in 1871 (online *Wikipedia*, accessed October 20, 2011).

[2] During the cholera epidemic of 1866, Jackson told Hutchinson that he had been 'engaged by Government to report on Cholera' (see Hutchinson 1947, p.80), but we have no other information about his work on the problem (see Critchley and Critchley 1998, p.42).

[3] See Bailey 1895; Peterson 1978, pp.18–21, 134–135, 266–268.

[4] In the *Transactions of the Pathological Society of London 17*:xi, 1866, for the 'Session 1865–66', Jackson is listed as a member, whereas he is not listed in the *Transactions 16*, 1865, for the session 1864–1865.

[5] See Jackson 1861a, pp.197, 199; Jackson 1861c, p.59; Jackson 1863f, pp.213–215.

[6] The Society's *Transactions* 6:xii, 1855, notes Hutchinson's election in the session of 1852–1853. In the *Transactions 10*:ii, 1859, he is listed on the Society's Council for 1858–1859.

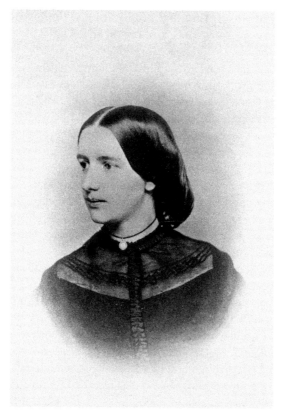

Fig. 4.1 Mrs. Hughlings Jackson (Elizabeth Dade).

joined the Hunterian Society of London, again following in Hutchinson's wake.[7] On the other hand, presumably it was Laycock who recruited him to the Medico-Psychological Association *circa* 1866.[8]

Jackson's published output for 1865 was diminished as compared to 1864 and 1866, likely due to two factors. The first, of course, was his marriage. The second is more germane to the development of his thought. He seems to have used 1865 and part of 1866 as a kind of reading period, when he immersed himself in the authors of the 'association psychology',[9] and others, in an attempt to understand language disorders. However, this is not to say that he was entirely unproductive in 1865. His pace of writing slowed, but his restless mind continued to churn.

---

[7] Jackson presented a paper (Jackson 1866i), which was 'Read before the Hunterian Society April 19, 1865'. Hutchinson had joined the Hunterian Society in 1853; he became its President in 1869 (see Hutchinson 1947, p.36).

[8] See the earliest list of 'Members of the Association' in the *Journal of Mental Science 12*, for 1866–1867, where Jackson is listed as a member. He was listed as an Auditor for 1869–1870, when Laycock was President and the annual meeting was in York (*Journal of Mental Science 15*:326). The Association is now the Royal College of Psychiatrists (Bewley 2008, p.49).

[9] For an explanation of the 'association psychology' (associationism), see further in this chapter, and Definition Section 7 in Chapter 5.

Prelude to a Unified Pathophysiology: Epilepsy and the Brain, *circa* 1865

To us, one of Jackson's most fundamental contributions is not immediately obvious. It is easily lost in plain sight because it is how we think, i.e., how we organize our thoughts when we approach a clinical problem. We assume that neuroclinicians have always tried to analyze problems within the structure of a single, coherent pathophysiological framework. Not so. One of the great strengths of Galenic medicine was its unified pathophysiology, which was based on Galenic physiology. In the Renaissance, the work of Vesalius and Harvey started to undermine the validity of Galenic theory, but it was not fully replaced by modern scientific medicine until approximately 1870.[10] From the seventeenth century until that time, there was something of a free-for-all in the realm of physiological theory. This was certainly true for the functions and dysfunctions of the nervous system, because Galenic humoral neurophysiology was ultimately incompatible with the newer, solidist system of neurology that had been proposed by Willis in the seventeenth century.

Modern neurophysiology began to emerge in the early nineteenth century, with the demonstration of the separate sensory and motor roots by Charles Bell (1774–1842) and François Magendie (1783–1855). Brown-Séquard was a significant contributor to this process in the mid-century. The thrust of Jackson's *Suggestions* was to find a way to think about neurological disease within a unitary framework. The *Suggestions* didn't work because its vertebral framework was flawed. By 1865 Jackson had some of his own theories about normal neurological function, but they can best be described as premodern. The cerebral cortices remained largely *terra incognita*. Since knowledge of brainstem function was improving in the 1860s, this put the basal ganglia in the middle—on the edge of the known world, so to speak—and Jackson's ideas reflected this state of incomplete knowledge. In a lecture on hemiplegia, he showed that hemiplegia can be due to a lesion anywhere along the motor tract in the brainstem,[11] but localizing the lesion in the basal ganglia was more difficult.

Jackson's Cerebral Physiology in 1865: Uncertainties and Inconsistencies

Despite the statements of Carpenter and others about the separate functions of the striatum and the thalamus, Jackson lumped them together as the highest part of the motor tract. The lesions that are found in autopsies of hemiplegic patients are usually too large to allow reliable conclusions about how much damage has occurred in each of the two adjoining structures.[12] In his lecture on hemiplegia in 1865, he said that the thalamus opticus would be 'better called *non*-opticus, as it is not the centre for sight'. He 'put together the corpus striatum and the thalamus opticus ... because I have not been able to make out what the difference is betwixt the hemiplegia from disease of the corpus striatum and disease of the thalamus opticus'.[13]

---

[10] See Temkin 1973, p.191; Greenblatt 1991.
[11] Jackson 1865f, pp.318–331.
[12] See Jackson 1863a, pp.24–25.
[13] Jackson 1865f, p.301; on p.302 Jackson quoted Todd to the same effect.

When he discussed the relationship between the basal ganglia and the cortices in 1865 Jackson was not always consistent. In a short case report he described a woman who died 2 years after a large stroke that had caused right hemiplegia and aphasia. At autopsy he found 'healthy' frontal lobes. Even so, the disease 'was far too extensive to help us to determine anything precisely as to the seat of speech'. Nonetheless, 'The probability is, that the convolutions near the corpus striatum have to do with guiding muscles in articulation'.[14] This sounds like he was willing to consider the existence of some kind of motor function in the cerebral cortices. Contrariwise, in an ophthalmological paper of 1865, he described a man whose autopsy showed extensive syphilitic disease over the *right* hemisphere but not on the left. He had left hemiplegia, left-sided seizures, and other problems, but intact language.[15] The disease on the right involved,

> ... among others, a particular convolution, the fellow of which in the left hemisphere is, according to M. Broca, the seat of the faculty of articulate language... I have greater (and increasing) doubts than I had as to the propriety of using the term "faculty" at all, and greater doubts still as to the possibility of locating any faculty, if there be one, in a particular convolution ...[16]

Well, there you have it. The convolutions near the striatum probably 'have to do with guiding muscles in articulation',[17] but there is little possibility of locating any faculty in any 'particular convolution', because faculties don't exist. Now all of this is not quite as self-contradictory as it may seem, but neither is it terribly clear. In fact, it wasn't entirely clear to Jackson. His thoughts were evolving rapidly and not always with full coherence among them.

The Historiographic Challenge of Jackson's Developing Ideas

In following the development of Jackson's theories, a persistent challenge is the fact that his ideas about several different clinical phenomena developed in close apposition to each other. In the lecture on hemiplegia in 1865, he said: 'It is simply impossible to study defects of speech, defects of sight, and ... a certain class of cases of epilepsy, unless you know this form of paralysis well.'[18] What he meant was that hemiplegia, aphasia, hemianopsia, and unilateral seizures all involve dysfunctions in the same arterial territory. Accordingly, in analyzing Jackson's development at this early stage it would seem artificial to segregate discussions of those separate entities. In his mind, they should all be explicable within the same pathophysiological framework. On the other hand, it is impossible to discuss everything at once. The subjects have to be parsed for analysis, starting here with epilepsy.

---

[14] Jackson 1865e, p.284.

[15] Jackson 1865g, pp.442–446; since Jackson's paper includes a citation of the *Medical Times and Gazette* (*MTG*) of 'June 17, 1865', this number of Vol.4 of the *Royal London Ophthalmic Hospital Reports* (*RLOHR*) was probably published in the late summer or fall of 1865.

[16] Jackson 1865h, p.54. This article was a continuation of Jackson 1865g. It contains Jackson's description of an autopsy that was performed on another patient on 'Nov. 8, 1865' (p.77), so this first issue of Vol.5 of the *Royal London Ophthalmic Hospital Reports* (*RLOHR*) was probably published in late December 1865 or early 1866; it is dated 1865.

[17] Jackson 1865e, p.284.

[18] Jackson 1865f, pp.302–303.

Modern Definitions of Epilepsy and Epileptic Seizures

In any discussion of epilepsy and epileptic seizures it is important to distinguish between *nomenclature*, the names of clinical phenomena, and *classification* of disease phenomena as entities (nosology). Historically nomenclature came first, but more recently classification has driven nomenclature. From long before Jackson's time in the mid-nineteenth century, until the mid-twentieth, there was no broad agreement about nomenclature or classification. The first successful effort toward international consistency was achieved by Henri Gastaut (1915–1995) in 1964–1970, under the auspices of the International League Against Epilepsy (ILAE) and other international groups.[19] However, these 'official' classifications have changed almost every decade, and they will continue to do so.

To avoid this book becoming rapidly out-of-date, I will define and use some 'modern' terms as they were used loosely in the middle of the twentieth century. That was after the advent of electroencephalography (EEG),[20] but before the work of Gastaut and the ILAE, and before computerized imaging. In fact, many old-fashioned terms have been incorporated into the ILAE definitions, and many people have continued to use the old, unofficial terms with which they were familiar.

Definition Section 5—Seizures and Epilepsy

Epilepsy—a succinct definition says simply that it is 'the tendency to recurrent [epileptic] seizures'.[21]

Epileptic seizure—the clinical phenomena can be myriad, from very brief and minor alterations of consciousness (absence), or minor sensory symptoms, to full-blown grand mal convulsions. As recently as 2005, Jackson's *pathophysiological definition* of 1870 was quoted in the ILAE's classification: 'A convulsion is but a symptom, and implies only that there is an occasional, an excessive, and a disorderly discharge of nerve tissue on muscles.'[22] Three years later he gave an improved definition, which was more accurate for him and for us: '*Epilepsy is the name for occasional, sudden, excessive, rapid, and local discharges of grey matter*.'[23]

Jacksonian seizure—a seizure characterized by a *Jacksonian march*. Classically, these seizures start with repetitive movements in one body part (e.g., the thumb) and spread through adjacent parts (e.g., to other fingers, then wrist, arm, etc.). The term usually applies to motor seizures, but patients can experience Jacksonian sensory marches without motor activity. If the seizure spreads to the other side, and especially if it is followed by unconsciousness, it is said to have become *generalized* (see below).

Temporal lobe seizure—another old term for this type is *psychomotor* seizure. Both terms are descriptive: *temporal lobe* for the usual (not exclusive) localization of the myriad *psychomotor* manifestations. In Gastaut's classification, they were *complex partial* seizures,[24] and that term has retained some popularity. Late in his career, Jackson called

---

[19] Gastaut et al. 1964; Gastaut 1970. On the history of classifications see Wolf 2009, and Engel 2013, pp.14–32.
[20] See Zifkin and Avanzini 2000, and Millett 2001.
[21] Aminoff 1993, p.148; my square brackets.
[22] Jackson 1870g, p.162. Jackson's definition is quoted in Fisher et al. 2005, p.471. See Chapter 6.
[23] Jackson 1873y, p.331; Jackson's italics. See Chapter 7.
[24] Gastaut et al. 1964, pp.298–300; Gastaut 1970, p.106.

them *uncinate fits*.[25] Another old (and much-loved) Jacksonian term for the complex behaviors with altered consciousness in these seizures is 'dreamy state'.[26]

Generalized seizure—*generalized* refers broadly to clinical phenomena that indicate bilateral brain involvement, either at the onset of the seizure or later in its course. At the onset there may be bilateral *grand mal* convulsions or, at the other end of the spectrum, brief *absence* spells (*petit mal*). Seizures with focal onsets may spread to become generalized.

An operational assumption in the clinical analysis of seizures—when the onset of a seizure is focal, we conclude that the responsible brain lesion is in some location in one cerebral hemisphere. This can be established if there is a clear motor onset, as in a Jacksonian seizure. However, the onset can be sensory or behavioral, and that localization can be harder to determine. Even in the case of a seizure that appears to begin with bilateral phenomena (including alteration of consciousness), the current (Jacksonian) assumption is that the abnormal brain activity has started in one place and generalized so quickly that the initial spread was not observed.

These attempts at definitions of seizure types show that it is perhaps too easy to combine and confuse semiology, etiology, and pathophysiology. In its literal sense, *semiology* is the science of the observable manifestations of disease, but the word is now commonly used to mean simply the signs and symptoms of some condition; e.g., the 'semiology' of a Jacksonian seizure is the observable motor march. Likewise, strictly speaking, *etiology* should mean the science of the causes of disease. However, the word is now widely used to mean the actual cause(s) of the tissue change. So we say that the 'etiology' of a Jacksonian seizure is the type of pathological lesion (infection, stroke, tumor, etc.) that has affected some neurons and thus altered their normal physiology. *Pathophysiology* is the functional connection between etiology and semiology. So the abnormal synchronous discharge of a restricted group of neurons in the motor cortex will produce an abnormal expression of the normal functions of that piece of brain tissue. The discharge is the pathophysiological event. As it 'spreads' to adjacent motor cortex, it is said to 'recruit' normal neurons in the abnormal firing. The Jacksonian march appears because adjacent parts of motor cortex exhibit exaggerations of their normal functions progressively.

Jackson didn't use the terms *semiology*, *etiology*, and *pathophysiology*, but in his lecture on method in June 1864 it is clear that he understood the concepts and their importance.[27] At this point in his story we are watching his early application of these ideas to epilepsy. It will be needful to keep them in mind as we look at Jackson's place in the history of epilepsy *circa* 1865, just when he was starting to create his own independent theories.

The Nosology of Epilepsy in the Mid-Nineteenth Century

In the earlier part of the nineteenth century one of the widely used classifications was 'idiopathic' versus 'sympathetic' types.[28] During the mid-century, a third class, 'symptomatic',

---

[25] Jackson 1898c, pp.586–587, and Jackson 1899a, p.79; see Chapter 12. More recently, *uncinate* has referred specifically to psychomotor seizures that begin with an olfactory aura.

[26] See Jackson 1876u, p.702.

[27] Jackson 1864h.

[28] Temkin 1971, p.272; and see 'Nosology' in Temkin's Index, p.463.

was commonly added. 'Thus, there seemed to be three kinds of epilepsy: (1) idiopathic, originating from the brain itself; (2) sympathetic, having its seat somewhere else in the body; and (3) symptomatic, occurring in dentition, smallpox, and other conditions.' In the 1830s and 1840s Marshall Hall (1790–1857) and others made the concept of reflex action in the brain the subject of serious study. It was applied to epilepsy, but without much satisfaction. Overall, 'the nosological concept of epilepsy had disintegrated, and it became necessary again to define its meaning'. Most of the attempts at redefinition were exactly that—efforts 'to modify the meaning of the older terms'.[29] In London, J. Russell Reynolds (1828–1896) published an important book on epilepsy in 1861.[30] He considered only idiopathic epilepsy to be 'genuine'. For Reynolds, it was 'a disease entity per se' and never involved unilateral manifestations or retention of consciousness.[31]

In the 1860s and 1870s, 'the majority [of medical authors] paid little attention to partial convulsions caused by gross anatomical lesions of the brain'.[32] However, we have seen that Jackson began to take an interest in these phenomena as early as 1861.[33] By 1864 they were a major focus of his attention. He thus joined a small group of like-minded clinical investigators, whose first member in the nineteenth century was Louis-François Bravais (1801–1842). He had described the Jacksonian march in 1827, but he was primarily interested in 'establishing a new type of disease . . .', so 'he did not venture upon an explanation of what he had observed'.[34] Another of Jackson's forerunners was Richard Bright (1789–1858).

> Bright studied cases of "Jacksonian epilepsy," observed their connection with impaired sight, paresthesia and weakness of the convulsed parts, noticed the presence of consciousness, and associated these symptoms with local lesions affecting the surface of the brain . . . on the side opposite to the one convulsed. Moreover, Bright did not separate these cases from "epilepsy," even if he tried to point out their clinical and anatomical peculiarities.[35]

All in all, 'Bravais' thesis was little read, and even Bright's observations did not receive the attention they deserved'.[36] In Jackson's time, the short-list of others who did take notice of unilateral seizures includes Carpenter, Todd, and Wilks. Carpenter was important because he had formulated 'Dr. Carpenter's theory of the function of the sensori-motor ganglia',[37] which we saw in Chapter 3. It postulated a relay function of the striatum in the descending motor tract, which was a minority opinion. Since Jackson accepted it, he could claim that the location of the lesion in unilateral motor seizures was in the basal ganglia, rather than on the surface of the hemispheres. However, according to Wilks, 'Morbid changes in the cortex of the brain . . . accounted for practically all cases of epilepsy whether partial or general'. This claim constituted 'an almost complete break with the accepted theory of irritation of the medulla oblongata and pons Varolii',[38] a break that Jackson also made by 1865, albeit with less finality.

---

[29] Temkin 1971, pp.278–289.
[30] Reynolds 1861.
[31] Temkin 1971, pp.289–291. On Reynolds' neurology see Eadie 2007a.
[32] Temkin 1971, p.316; my square brackets.
[33] Jackson 1861b.
[34] Temkin 1971, pp.306–307.
[35] Temkin 1971, p.311. Bright's work antedated the term 'Jacksonian epilepsy'.
[36] Temkin 1971, p.311.
[37] Temkin 1971, p.314.
[38] Temkin 1971, p.315. For more on Wilks see Pearce 2009a and 2009b.

Todd's Pathophysiology of Epilepsy

Among Jackson's immediate predecessors, Todd was the most significant, because he offered an explanation for the common clinical phenomenon of postictal motor weakness, which is still known as 'Todd's paralysis'.[39] After suffering generalized motor seizures most patients appear exhausted. They often sleep. This condition is intuitively understandable as exhaustion. 'Todd's paralysis', on the other hand, is the postictal phenomenon of focal motor weakness or paralysis in the muscles that were affected by a seizure. It is a common feature of the semiology of Jacksonian seizures—called 'epileptic hemiplegia' by both Todd and Jackson.[40] Todd explained his 'humoral theory of epilepsy' by stating: 'that the peculiar features of an epileptic seizure are due to the gradual accumulation of a morbid material in the blood, until it reaches such an amount that it operates upon the brain in ... an explosive manner ...'.[41]

In Todd's theory, when the explosive activity occurs in the hemispheres there is disturbance of consciousness, whereas motor convulsions are due to involvement of the quadrigeminal bodies (in the dorsal midbrain). Regarding postictal paralysis, Todd postulated that the relevant parts of the brain are left in a weakened state after a seizure, due mainly to a condition of 'weakened nutrition'.[42] In the first of Jackson's bylined reporter's columns in the *Medical Times and Gazette*, dated June 22, 1861, he mentioned Todd at least four times, and he cited Todd's 'Clinical Lecture "On Diseases of the Nervous System"'.[43]

The combination of Todd's discharge theory and Wilks' correlation of brain surface lesions with epilepsy could have led to locating the discharge in the cortices. Nonetheless, in 1865 Jackson could not quite make this leap, although he did reject the older theory of the medulla as the site of origin of epilepsy. And he suggested an alternative: 'I feel confident that in many cases, the cause of epileptic seizures is disease of the cerebrum.'[44] Recall, however, that the basal ganglia are part of the 'cerebrum'. During the years 1866–1870 Jackson struggled with the implications of assigning any motor function to the cortices. In fact, there was a part of his background that had the potential to lead in that direction. Laycock had postulated that the entire neuraxis, including the cortex, functions on a reflex basis. He had presented this view in the 1840s, a decade before Jackson's contact with him at the York Medical School.

Laycock's Universal Reflex Theory and the Uniformity of Nature

Laycock and the History of Reflex Theory

When modern neurophysiology began with the work of Bell (in 1811) and especially Magendie (in 1822), on the separate functions of the dorsal and ventral spinal nerve roots,[45] neither Magendie nor the great German physiologist Johannes Müller (1801–1858) had a clear notion of how sensory input is processed to motor output in the central

[39] See Lyons 1998, pp.20–22; and Lyons 2000.

[40] Temkin 1971, p.313; Jackson 1870g, p.169.

[41] Quoted in Temkin 1971, p.312. Todd also discussed 'epileptic hemiplegia' extensively in Todd 1855, pp.196–213.

[42] Temkin 1971, p.313. Todd's idea of focal postictal tissue exhaustion should not be confused with Charles Radcliffe's theory that seizures in general are caused by (or related to) 'enfeebled power of the nervous centres' (Temkin 1971, p.332). Jackson also accepted Radcliffe's theory; see Jackson 1866k, p.329, and Jackson 1868y, p.21.

[43] Jackson 1861b, p.649.

[44] Jackson 1865f, p.328,

[45] See Cranefield 1974, pp.xiii–xvi. and above in this chapter.

nervous system.[46] With experimental work between 1832 and 1850, Marshall Hall (1790–1857) showed that segmentally mediated spinal reflexes are modified by the influence of more rostral structures. Hall postulated the existence of an 'excito-motory' system in the spinal cord and medulla.[47] It was separate from the 'cerebral' system and had no connection with the 'will'.[48]

With apologies to Hall, in 1845 Laycock restated more forcefully a position that he had first asserted in 1841. He said: 'that the brain, although the organ of consciousness, was subject to the laws of reflex action, and that in this respect it did not differ from the other ganglia of the nervous system'.[49] In other words, Laycock proposed that the entire neuraxis functions on the same reflex principle, including the cerebral hemispheres. This idea got some limited attention in the scientific world.[50] It had its conceptual basis in a mode of thought that was well known in the first half of the nineteenth century.

Laycock and the Uniformity of Nature (Uniformitarianism)

The metaphysical foundation for Laycock's reflex proposal was the idea of the 'unity' or 'uniformity' of nature. It was also known by the mouthful's expression 'uniformitarianism'.[51] This premise holds that everything in the natural world is subject to the same laws of nature, including man. By contrast, Christian cosmology placed man—or at least his immortal soul—in a special relationship to God and therefore subject to special canons. On the continent uniformitarianism was a feature of German 'romantic biology' in the early nineteenth century, and it had adherents in France as well.[52] In both countries it was generally opposed to Christian theology. In England, on the other hand, the relationship of uniformitarianism to theology was different, because the uniformity of nature argument was used to support the existence of God through the tradition of natural theology. Some difficulties for natural theology were raised by Charles Lyell's work in geology and by the uniformitarian leanings of Chamber's *Vestiges*.[53]

Laycock was potentially exposed to uniformitarianism in many different venues, because he took his medical education and training in York, London, Paris, and Germany, from 1827 through 1839. Given his adherence to uniformitarianism, its application to the universality of the reflex was straightforward: 'I was led to this opinion by the general principle, that the ganglia within the cranium being a continuation of the spinal cord, must necessarily be regulated as to their reaction on external agencies by laws identical with those governing the functions of the spinal ganglia and their analogues in the lower animals'.[54]

---

[46] See McHenry 1969, pp.183–190.

[47] See Clarke and Jacyna, p.128.

[48] See Clarke and O'Malley, p.347.

[49] Laycock 1845, p.298. See also Amacher 1964, pp.171–173; and Greenblatt 1965, pp.376–368.

[50] Laycock's work had a significant impact on Carpenter; see Clarke and Jacyna 1987, pp.127–128, 140–147. Two of his papers (Laycock 1845 and Laycock 1855) were discussed extensively in the *Edinburgh Review 103*:423–452 (no.209, January–April).

[51] See Mayr 1982, pp.375–379; Mayr says that the British philosopher William Whewell (1794–1866) invented the word 'uniformitarianism' in 1832.

[52] Clarke and Jacyna 1987, pp.2–3, 38–46; and see 'Unity of nature' in their Index.

[53] See Mayr 1982, pp.375–379, 381–385. For an interpretation of the 'uniformity of nature' in the later Victorian period see Stanley 2014.

[54] Laycock 1845, p.298; see also Clarke and Jacyna 1987, p.141; and Leff 1991.

Jackson's Limited Use of Laycock's Theory

So now the question is, how much was Jackson affected by uniformitarianism and/or by Laycock's universal reflex theory? It is easy to dispose of uniformitarianism, because we can see by implication that Jackson did not practice that creed. If he had, he would have been much less hesitant to locate motor processes in the cortices. In reading Jackson's papers I have not encountered any kind of uniformitarian assumption or argument.[55] One could posit that uniformitarianism might have crept into his thought as part of the baggage with Laycock's reflex theory, but the validity of that proposition would depend on the degree of Jackson's acceptance of Laycock's theory, and the evidence for the latter is quite modest.

In Jackson's writings from 1861 through 1865, I have found only two brief citations where Jackson referred explicitly to 'the doctrines of Professor Laycock on the reflex function of the brain'. In his paper on 'Loss of speech' in 1864, Jackson speculated that the recurrent utterances ('interjectional expressions') of aphasics might be explained by Laycock's theory.[56] In 1865, he offered a similar speculation about the 'Involuntary [verbal] ejaculations following fright – subsequently chorea' in a case that was likely Tourette's syndrome.[57] In the *Suggestions* there is an assumption that the mechanism of function within segments is reflex, but there is no citation of Laycock. Rather, when the *Suggestions* was published in early 1863 Jackson was under the influence of Brown-Séquard's theories about vasomotor reflexes.

Thus, as of 1865 Jackson did not accept uniformitarianism. He mentioned Laycock's reflex theory, but infrequently and always for limited purposes. On the other hand, he was clearly searching for some way to bring order out of chaos in neurological pathophysiology. When he encountered language disorders and Spencer in 1864 his intellectual eclecticism led him home, so to speak, to a native English mode of analysis.

The Conundrums of Language Lead to the Associationists

At the end of Chapter 3 we saw that in 1864 Jackson was puzzled by the many controversial aspects of aphasia, so he explicitly declared his neutrality about the uncertainties. Neutrality, however, need not imply passivity. It appears that in 1865 he focused his reading to help with the problem. Through this effort he began to find his way to the 'association psychology'. It gave him a perspective on the reason for his discomfort with some of Broca's positions.[58]

---

[55] In 1876, referring to the hemispheric 'centres which are the substrata of mental states in man ...', Jackson said (Jackson 1876e, p.130, footnote (*c*)): 'There is reflex action here, too, but it is imperfect ... reflex action "breaks down" in the very highest centres.'

[56] Jackson 1864j, p.454.

[57] Jackson 1865a. Dewhurst 1982, pp.21–25, gives the case this diagnosis. The chorea-like syndrome described by Georges Gilles de la Tourette in 1885 became widely known only in the twentieth century; see Kushner 1999.

[58] The following three sections are derived largely from Young 1970. There is some confusion about 'associationist'. The history to be outlined here is about the English 'association of ideas', which is generally called 'associationism'. Its continental cousin is also called 'associationism' (e.g., Guenther 2015, p.10), but that is better described as 'connectionism'. The latter was fathered by Theodor Meynert (1833–1892) and Carl Wernicke in the 1870s and beyond. However, it is not clear that by 'Drawing on the language of the association psychology' (Guenther 2015, pp.9, 34) they were consciously engaging the English tradition. I believe it is this kind of confusion that led the late Arthur Benton (1909–2006), a preeminent neuropsychologist, to say (Benton 2000, p.186), 'Jackson opposed the prevailing associationist theory at every major point', which is wrong or at the least confusing. Benton was using 'associationist' as synonymous with 'connectionist'. See also Goldenberg 2013, p.1, footnote 1, and p.50, footnote 5.

Brief History of the Association Psychology (Associationism) in Philosophy, 1749–1865

'Associationism' refers to the theory of the 'association of ideas' (the 'association psychology'). Some of its elements can be found in Aristotle.[59] In the late seventeenth century, John Locke's analysis of the human mind was 'explicitly formulated by Locke in opposition to *a priori* reasoning and the Cartesian doctrine of innate ideas ...'. He 'sought to demonstrate that all knowledge and all experience could be accounted for by combinations of sensations and perceptions ...'.[60] As a coherent system to explain how the human mind works, associationism is usually traced back to the Yorkshireman David Hartley (1705–1757), in his *Observations on Man* of 1749.[61] He connected 'his psychological theory with postulates about how the nervous system functions. His sensations were paralleled by vibrations (derived by analogy to Newtonian mechanics) of "elemental" particles in the nerves and brain ...'[62]

According to Hartley, as summarized by Young: 'The relations among sensations, ideas, and muscular motions as well as the faculties of memory, imagination, fancy, understanding, affection, and will are accounted for ... in terms of <u>repetitive</u> associations ...'[63] I have underlined '<u>repetitive</u>' because a basic principle of association psychology was the requirement for repetition of a sensation in order to solidify memory of the sensation and its associated ideas. After an idea has been implanted in the mind—and by implication in the brain—it could be revived by an incoming sensation that is similar to an existing one. In historical perspective, 'associationism was to be the ... opponent of faculty psychology ... its elementary task was to reduce faculties to aggregates of elementary sensory units'.[64]

In the early nineteenth century the leading advocate of associationism was James Mill (1773–1836). In his *Analysis of the Phenomena of the Human Mind* (1829) Mill applied himself 'to extending and completing Hartley's doctrine. Hartley had been concerned to prove the validity of the associationist view. Mill assumed it, and later writers in the school could extend a doctrine which was taken as a settled starting point.'[65] James Mill's son, John Stuart Mill (1806–1873), asked the question 'Not ... how far the law extends ... but how much of the apparent variety of the mental phenomena it is capable of explaining ...'[66] With the Mills, associationism reached the limit of its development as an introspective, philosophical endeavor.[67] From there it was advanced by Alexander Bain (1818–1903) and Spencer, who amalgamated associationism to the biological science of the mid-nineteenth century, albeit still from their armchairs.

---

[59] See Buckingham and Finger 1997.

[60] Young 1970, p.95; Young's italics, my square brackets.

[61] Hartley 1749. See also Ribot 1874, pp.35–43; Herrnstein and Boring 1965, pp.326–406; Young 1970, pp.94–100; and Rylance 2000, pp.84–86. For more recent studies of Hartley see Smith 1987; Allen 1999; and Glassman and Buckingham 2007.

[62] Young 1970, pp.95–96.

[63] Young 1970, pp.96–97; my underlining.

[64] Young 1970, p.95.

[65] Young 1970, p.97.

[66] J.S. Mill, quoted in Young 1970, p.98.

[67] Not everyone agreed that associationism was so fundamental; see Henry L. Mansel's *Metaphysics* (Mansel 1866, pp.244–248). Jackson read Mansel in the later 1860s (Jackson 1868u, p.527). He was still pondering Mansel's metaphysical problem in 1874; see Jackson 1874e, p.64, footnote (d).

Alexander Bain: Associationism and the Neuroscience of the Mid-Century

Bain spent most of his life in Aberdeen, Scotland, where he was professor of logic at the University in 1860–1880.[68] He 'has been credited with writing the first "comprehensive treatise having psychology as its sole purpose". His two-volume systematic work, *The Senses and the Intellect* (1855) and *The Emotions and the Will* (1859), was the standard British text for almost half a century ... His work ... is the meeting-point of experimental sensory-motor physiology and the association psychology.'[69] Bain recognized the importance of integrating contemporary knowledge of the nervous system into analyses of mind. However, his most important work was done before the advent of modern neuroscience in the 1870s. Initially he followed Flourens and denied cortical excitability. After he published *On the Study of Character, Including an Estimate of Phrenology* in 1861, he accepted the general idea of cortical localization for psychological faculties, but he tried to transform 'the psychology of phrenology in order to bring it into conformity with his own associationist view'.[70] Although he came close to accepting the idea of motor representation in the cortices, Bain never quite got there.[71] Nonetheless, he:

> ... provided a discussion of motor phenomena which gave the association psychology a balanced sensory-motor view. The bias of the Lockian tradition had been toward the sensory side, ... [which resulted in neglect of] motor phenomena, and overt behavior ... Bain's analysis of motor phenomena was the first union of the new physiology with a detailed association psychology in the English ... tradition and he thereby laid the psychological foundations of a thoroughgoing sensory-motor psychophysiology.[72]

One way to understand Bain's contribution is to go back to Locke's theory of the development of the human mind. If we start with a *tabula rasa*, then somehow the mind has to be populated by sensory data from the environment. When a person encounters any new object, the ultimate reality of that object is not necessarily 'proven' by its secondary qualities, which are perceived by the special senses of vision, sound, etc. Our knowledge of three-dimensional reality, said Bain, depends on the sense of touch, which meets *resistance*. Until his analysis, all afferent information about the external world was considered to be sensory. By the 1850s, when Bain was writing, the distinction of *motor* versus *sensory* had a physiological basis, *à la* Bell and Magendie. Bain argued that exploring resistance necessarily involves muscular movement, which is a *motor* activity. Jackson's conception of language as a motor phenomenon is derived from Bain's position.[73] In 1874 Jackson said:

> To Professor Bain I owe much. From him I derived the notion that the anatomical substrata of Words are motor (articulatory) processes... This hypothesis ... gives the best anatomico-physiological explanation of the phenomena of Aphasia *when all varieties of this affection*

---

[68] Herrnstein and Boring 1965, pp.592–593, mention that a chair in logic was as close as anyone could come to a chair in (nonexistent) psychology in 1860.

[69] Young 1970, p.101; the quotation inside this quotation is from Murphy 1949, p.107.

[70] Young 1970, p.104.

[71] Young 1970, pp.106–107.

[72] Young 1970, p.114; my square brackets.

[73] This paragraph is based on Young 1970, pp.93–95 and 114–121; see also Jones 1972. There is no evidence that Jackson read Locke directly, but he did read *about* Locke; see J78-07, p.310, footnote 1.

are taken into consideration ... because it helped me very much in endeavouring to show that the "organ of mind" contains processes representing movements, and that ... there was nothing unreasonable in supposing that excessive discharge of convolutions should produce that clotted mass of movements which we call spasm [seizure].[74]

Here Jackson explained how his analyses of aphasia and epilepsy were dependent on each other. In the phrase 'From him I derived' Jackson didn't say that he *took* the 'notion' from Bain, but rather that he extended from it independently. Bain's book that most influenced Jackson was *The Senses and the Intellect* of 1855. In it Bain said only a little about language and its acquisition. There was no statement that preceded Jackson's view of individual words as fundamental units of analysis.[75] Jackson's derivation from Bain was more by analogy than deduction. If afferent signals can be motor in some way—as signals from muscle—then incoming words can likewise be motor. Jackson used Bain's view of muscular resistance sparingly, but the motor aspect of words was a constant theme.

George Henry Lewes and Herbert Spencer: Associationism and the Evolutionary Biology of Adaptation

Among Bain's friends were two other exponents of associationism, J.S. Mill and George Henry Lewes (1817–1878) (Fig. 4.2). Lewes was the *de facto* husband of the novelist George Eliot (*née* Marian Evans, 1819–1880), which has not always redounded to his advantage—he was sometimes known as 'Mr. George Eliot'.[76] Nonetheless, Lewes was a significant figure in his day.[77] We might describe him as a science writer, although, like Spencer, he considered himself to be a scientist.[78] Lewes' book that would have attracted Jackson's attention was *The Physiology of Common Life*, two volumes that were published in 1859–1860. The second volume was largely a review of the state of neuroscientific knowledge as of 1860, but there was little reference to associationist ideas and certainly no new contributions.[79] Lewes

... strove to integrate contemporary trends in philosophy, psychology, and physiology ... Lewes' particular contribution lay in showing how contemporary German physiological data could be integrated with British evolutionism and associationism... Lewes was a prolific and effective popularizer. His texts on physiology were read all over Europe. Ivan Sechenov and Ivan Pavlov in Russia credited their reading of Lewes's *Physiology of Common Life* in part with their decision to become scientific psychologists.[80]

[74] Jackson 1874aa, pp.347–348; Jackson's italics and parentheses, my square brackets.

[75] Bain (1855, pp.428–435) discussed 'VOCAL OR LINGUAL ACQUISITIONS' entirely at the psychological level. My cursory survey of Bain 1859 revealed nothing about words as fundamental units.

[76] See Williams 1983.

[77] Reed 1997, pp.145–156, gives a sympathetic *précis* of Lewes' contributions, saying (pp.145–146): 'Lewes is nowadays almost invisible ...' See also Bell 1981, and Rylance 1987.

[78] In the mid-nineteenth century, 'scientist' was not entirely evolved from 'natural philosopher'; see Heyck 1982, pp.62–63; and Cahan 2003, p.4. Lewes acquired a partial medical education; see Ashton 1991, p.14. He was apparently a competent microscopist (see Lewes 1860, pp.270–272), and he did some simple biological experiments in the process of writing *The Physiology of Common Life* (e.g., see Lewes 1860, pp.177–181). Huxley felt that Lewes was a competent popularizer but an incompetent scientist; see Lightman 2007, pp.359–361. Price 2014 is a helpful guide to Lewes' ideas and publications.

[79] Association as a reflex was discussed in Lewes 1860, p.204. In his Preface to this second volume (p.vi), Lewes said, 'It is in the chapters on the Nervous System that the greatest amount of dissent from current opinions will be found ...'.

[80] Reed 1997, p.145.

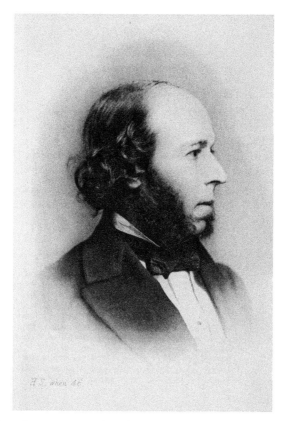

Fig. 4.2 George Henry Lewes at age 50 (1867). (© iStock/ilbusca.)

Lewes and Spencer (Fig. 4.3) began a long friendship in 1850, when they talked about *Vestiges*. At the time, Spencer rejected the 'development hypothesis', which Lewes accepted.[81] Spencer met Eliot in 1851. A life-long bachelor, he was nevertheless the matchmaker for Lewes and Eliot.[82] In turn, it was Lewes who introduced Spencer to psychology and philosophy.[83] All three of these writers—Eliot, Lewes, and Spencer—were initially interested in phrenology. Spencer's first book, *Social Statics*, was published in 1851. His 'argument is based on a distinctly phrenological view of man … Each faculty grows by exercise and dwindles from disuse. Happiness results from "the fulfilment of their functions by the respective faculties".[84]

In the early 1850s Spencer experienced two intellectual conversions: (1) from the faculty psychology of phrenology to associationism,[85] and (2) from uncertainty to full acceptance of 'the development hypothesis'.[86] The central dynamic of evolutionary biology is its use of adaptation to the environment as an explanation for why and how species evolve. According to Spencer, the two biological mechanisms that mediate adaptation are (1) 'the physiological division of labour' by different structures within the individual organism, which drives

---

[81] Spencer 1904, vol.1, p.348.
[82] Spencer 1904, vol.1, pp.63–64; for further on 'Spencer and His Circle' see Jones and Peel 2004, pp.1–16.
[83] Young 1970, p.162.
[84] Young 1970, pp.153–154.
[85] Young 1970, pp.165–166.
[86] Spencer 1852; see also Perrin 1993, p.171.

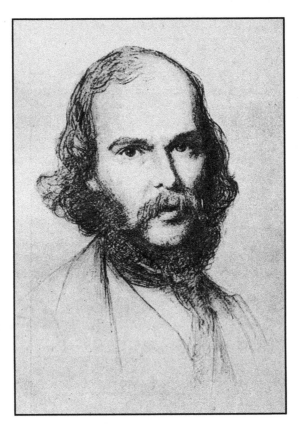

Fig. 4.3 Herbert Spencer at age 46.
(PAUL D STEWART / SCIENCE PHOTO LIBRARY.)

(2) the tendency of each organism to increase its complexity, i.e., to change its internal organization 'from homogeneity to heterogeneity'.[87] So species evolve by increasing the complexity of the division of physiological labor among their internal structures. These two principles were incorporated into associationism in the first edition of Spencer's *Principles of Psychology*, published in 1855.[88] The basis of this book was Spencer's 'conception of psychology as a biological science of adaptation'.[89] What made it 'biological' was his assumption that all of the principles of adaptation apply to operations of the brain *and* the mind. This is a straightforward uniformitarian position, which Spencer took from the same continental sources as Laycock, although less directly.[90]

Looking back from 1899, Spencer said that in 1853 he realized that one of *The Principles of Psychology*'s 'leading views' was 'the idea that the growth of a correspondence between inner and outer actions had to be traced up from the beginning; so as to show the way in which Mind gradually evolves out of life'.[91] This illustrates two important aspects of Spencer's

---

[87] Young 1970, pp.167–168.
[88] In historical perspective (Peel 1975, p.571), '*The Principles of Psychology* (1855) was a real milestone in the history of the subject, marking its transition from a heavily epistemological phase to one in which it was closely dependent on physiology. In it Spencer paved the way for Wundt, William James, and Pavlov.'
[89] Young 1970, p.169.
[90] Young 1970, pp.168. Laycock read French and German, whereas Spencer used translations and English language commentators.
[91] Duncan 1911, p.546; my underlining.

thought. First, he used the term 'correspondence' to describe the relationship between the internal states of the organism and its external environment. States of mind thus become 'correspondences', and adaptations are changes in correspondences.[92] Second, the underlined phrase encapsulates a theory of mind as *emergent* from the activities of the brain. This position on the mind-brain problem is reductionistic and was always considered to be materialistic. Jackson eventually developed a different view of the mind-brain relationship, but he had to consider Spencer's view in the process. Since we are trying to understand Jackson's thought as of 1865, I will briefly follow the further development of Spencer's principal publications to that year and a little beyond.

Bain and Spencer were each writing their respective treatises in the early 1850s, but their styles were entirely different. Whereas Bain laid out what was known about neuroscience and then applied what he could to associationism *a posteriori*, Spencer tried to derive his conclusions *a priori*. Needless to say, many readers did not find this to be convincing, but Spencer soon conceived a grand scheme. In late 1857, he decided to create a multivolume 'System of Philosophy',[93] based on his theory of evolution. It would encompass all of the biological and social sciences. To support this effort, in 1860 he proposed to publish a series of ten volumes: 'Quarterly installments were to be issued to subscribers; and volumes . . . were to be issued for the general public as they were completed.'[94] This project became a consuming passion. He turned down prestigious professorships because 'He could not spare the time'.[95]

The first fascicle of Spencer's *A System of Philosophy* was issued in October 1860.[96] The whole first volume was titled, logically enough, *First Principles*. It was issued in 1862, but Jackson seldom mentioned it. The first volume of the next in the sequence, *The Principles of Biology*, came out in 1864 and the second in 1867.[97] Jackson apparently became a subscriber to the series in time to receive the first fascicles of the second edition of *The Principles of Psychology* in December 1867.[98] The two volumes of the second edition of *Psychology* were published in 1870 and 1872.

Jackson and Associationism to 1865

Given this background on Spencer and associationism, the question arises whether Jackson was influenced by any of it early on, and the tentative answer is: not really. Direct proof could be either citations of associationist authors and/or finding associationist modes of thought in his analyses. There was none of the latter before 1866. Regarding citations, Jackson cited Lewes by name five times in his *Suggestions*. Four of those instances were concerned with Lewes' concept of 'sensibility', especially in the spinal cord, and the fifth was also about the cord.[99]

---

[92] See Collins 1889, pp.216–226, for a *précis* of Spencer's extensive expositions of 'correspondence' in his later writings. For further on 'adaptation' see Collins, pp.89–91.

[93] By 1870 he was calling it *A System of Synthetic Philosophy*.

[94] Perrin 1993, pp.37–38.

[95] Perrin 1993, p.39.

[96] Perrin 1993, p.41.

[97] Perrin 1993, pp.969–970; Spencer coined 'survival of the fittest' in the first volume.

[98] See Jackson 1868l, p.178; see also Perrin 1993, p.119. Before he received these fascicles, Jackson frequently referred to the first edition of the *Psychology*; e.g., in J66-06, p.661.

[99] Jackson 1863a, pp.9, 10, 26. Lewes 1860, vol.2, discussed 'sensibility' extensively.

At the end of Chapter 3 we saw that Jackson first cited Spencer in 1864, but he was referring to some specific points about recurrent utterances in aphasics. It does appear that this was how Jackson first made intellectual acquaintance with Spencer, but Jackson's reading of Spencer in depth is not evidenced before 1866. The same holds for Jackson's citations of Bain, so there is no indication that Jackson had any in-depth knowledge of associationism before 1865–1866. The possibility remains that he could have imbibed associationism from his environment in London, where anything was possible but nothing is discernable. We have descriptions of the medical and scientific interests of the leading thinkers in York, but they tended toward the practicalities of patient care and industrialization.[100] A potential exception to this statement is Laycock.

Most historians of associationism do not consider Thomas Laycock to be a significant contributor to that tradition,[101] although he is sometimes recognized as an early advocate of physiological psychology.[102] Laycock was an adherent of associationism in the same way as the Mills—he simply assumed its validity. In a paper of 1845, there is a paragraph labeled 'The association of ideas', where Laycock declared: '... the true explanation of the association of ideas is to be found in the doctrine of the reflex functions of the brain'.[103] In Laycock's *Mind and Brain* (1860), there is no discussion of associationism. Nonetheless, 'The psychological concepts expressed [in the book] were in complete accord with the tendencies of association psychology. All mental operations were described as involving nothing more than ... the combining of sense-perceptions with each other. The nature of mental processes was determined entirely by the nervous processes concomitant to them.' In sum, 'Laycock did not take his psychology from one or two men, but as a doctrine which pervaded his cultural *milieu*'.[104]

Since we know that Jackson had been exposed to Laycock's reflex theory, we can presume his exposure to uniformitarianism, but he did not find either of those doctrines helpful in his quest to understand neurological function and dysfunction; likewise with regard to Brown-Séquard's vasomotor theories. Thus, to the end of 1864 Jackson maintained his intellectual independence in the form of indeterminacy about the functions of the cortices and the localization of language. His mind was open to new ideas, so the next question is:

What Did Jackson Read in 1865?

More specifically, who was Jackson reading that he hadn't read before? Of course, we can know only who he cited. As usual, it's hard to prove a negative, but we do have Hutchinson's recollections of Jackson's early reading habits, and Hutchinson does not mention any author directly in the associationist tradition.[105] Fortunately, Jackson himself has come to our assistance. In a paper about 'temporary loss of speech', dated April 28, 1866, he said: 'The books to read to make us feel the importance of single cases of loss of speech as flaws of mind were those of Max Müller, Herbert Spencer, J.S. Mill, etc.', and the 'etc.' included Bain.[106]

---

[100] See Matthew 1981, 'Science and Technology in York 1831–1981', in Feinstein, pp.30–52; and Parsons 2002, pp.39–62.

[101] Laycock is not mentioned as a major contributor by Warren 1921, Young 1970, or Ribot 1974.

[102] See Hearnshaw 1964, p.20; and James 1998, p.491.

[103] Laycock 1845, p.311.

[104] Amacher, p.177; my square brackets.

[105] Hutchinson 1911.

[106] Jackson 1866d, p.442; see also [Jackson] 1866, p.261, where Jackson listed Spencer, J.S. Mill, Bain, Lockhart Clarke (see Chapter 6), 'Whately', William Thomson, Max Müller, and others.

Table 4.1 Jackson's citations of three associationist authors, 1864–1868.

	1864	1865	1866	1867	1868
Bain	0	0	4	1	3
Lewes	0	0	1	0	0
Spencer	3	0	11	3	11

Friedrich Max Müller (1823–1900) was an Oxford philologist who delivered two series of *Lectures on the Science of Language* at the Royal Institution of Great Britain, London, in the early 1860s.[107] We don't know if Jackson attended Müller's lectures, but it is easy to see how their title might have attracted his attention. Müller was interested in the phylogenetic development of language in humans, but he disputed Darwin's claim that it could have developed out of animal 'language', whose existence he denied.[108] So Max Müller came down on the conservative side in the debates about Darwinian evolution—another potential reason why Jackson might have found him attractive. However, Jackson cited him only infrequently, and the same is true for J.S. Mill.

Starting in 1866, the extent of Jackson's assimilation of Bain, Lewes, and Spencer can be seen in Table 4.1. To create it I simply counted the number of times the name of each author appeared in print in Jackson's writings of each year. It supports my conclusion that in 1865–1866 Jackson began to read and absorb the two most important associationist authors of the time, Bain and Spencer. The results are seen in his writings of 1866 and beyond.[109]

Following a New Analytic Approach, 1866–1867

At the beginning of Chapter 3, I said that Charcot and Jackson both used the clinico-pathological method in a 'reverse' manner to try to figure out the normal functions of the damaged neural structures they were studying. In his 1865 lecture on hemiplegia Jackson said, 'It is of very great importance to define the border-land of our ignorance and knowledge as sharply as we can, and not to conceal it by the use of names which have a loose meaning'.[110] In other words, he wanted to understand pathophysiology, rather than promulgating empirical classifications and naming of diseases. It would be impossible to create a unified pathophysiology without knowledge of normal functions. In late 1866 he said this clearly: 'To establish the laws of healthy muscular movements, and of those variations in them which occur in certain altered states of nerve tissue and nervous organs, is a thing of fundamental importance for the progress of the Medical Physiology of the Nervous System.'[111]

Regardless of the type of disease Jackson was studying, it turned out that the basic physiological issue was cerebral localization. He was not inclined to accept strict localization of

---

[107] Müller 1861, and Müller 1864.

[108] See Richards 1987, pp.203–205.

[109] In Jackson 1875o, p.578, he said that 'in every paper written during and since 1866 ... ' he had '*always* written on the assumption that the cerebral hemisphere is made up of processes representing impressions and movements', and he attributed this 'implication' to Spencer.

[110] Jackson 1865f, p.298.

[111] Jackson 1866p, p.254. See also p.266, and Jackson 1869a, pp.307–308. He had a 'written scheme' to follow in examining the 'physiology of [the] nervous system' in his patients (see Jackson 1865c, p.626), but I don't know what was in it.

language, as evidenced by his view that: 'It is probable that the so-called faculty of language "'resides" wherever mind resides, and that language is but an outward form of thought'.[112] On the other hand, he also said: 'Although I have grave doubts as to the localisation, or even as to the existence of any such faculty as that of language or of articulate language, it is not contradictory to say that … disease in only one region of the brain causes defect of speech. Facts force me to this conclusion.'[113]

This was the essence of the challenge—the force of the clinical facts in the face of physiological uncertainty. Part of the difficulty was Jackson's reluctance to localize anything in the cortices—perhaps due to a residual distaste for phrenology—versus the undeniable fact that something about speech is disturbed by damage in one part of the cortex and not in another. What associationism brought to Jackson's struggle was a coherent way to think about this conundrum. Hence my analysis will be concerned primarily with how Spencer and the other associationists affected Jackson's investigation of the relationships between disorders of language and movement, on the one hand, and the nature of localization, on the other. Part of the issue comes down to the question of exactly what it is that might be localized.

Language and Localization in Early 1866

The effects of Jackson's reading in 1865 began to show only modestly in his first publication of 1866.[114] It seems to be a continuation of the 'Loss of speech' paper of 1864,[115] where he had quoted Spencer on the distinction between intellectual and emotional language.[116] In 1866 he came up with the fundamental idea of a 'proposition', which remained central to his thinking about language for the rest of his life. In discussing the case of a man who had right hemiplegia and severe Broca's aphasia, Jackson said:

> … It is not safe … to conclude that a patient who has lost speech is regaining power of language because he begins to swear … By such words no part of a proposition can be conveyed; that is, they add nothing to precision of expression in delivering an idea … Where no proposition is conveyed, there is no intellectual language.[117]

So a proposition delivers an idea. It is not clear whether Jackson took 'proposition' directly from another source or simply used it as he found it in the English language. In any case, the use of 'proposition' in this way was common at the time. J.S. Mill discussed it extensively.[118] To support his argument Jackson quoted Max Müller and another lesser known philologist, Robert G. Latham (1812–1888).[119] In addition, Jackson again quoted Spencer's article on 'The Origin and Function of Music', which he had cited in 1864.[120] This time, however, he had been

---

[112] Jackson 1866d, p.442.
[113] Jackson 1865h, p.55.
[114] Jackson 1866a.
[115] Jackson 1864j.
[116] For a brief discussion of the previous history of this distinction see Harrington 1987, pp.215–216. As she says, issues of priority are probably moot.
[117] Jackson 1866a, p.175.
[118] See Mill 1851, vol.1, pp.18–22, and beyond.
[119] Jackson did not give references for his quotations from Max Müller or Latham. The latter was probably Latham 1856, where the entire first half is concerned with 'Propositions'.
[120] Jackson 1866a. Here Jackson began to express the special deference to Spencer that continued throughout his lifetime.

thinking about the physiological meaning of the linguistic distinction between emotional and intellectual language. Discussing a patient who had severe nonfluent aphasia, Jackson said:

> … having reference to Spencer's views, … we may conclude that our muscles may be used in two kinds of language, one intellectual [voluntary] and the other emotional [involuntary]. But the muscles may, in some cases of disease of the hemisphere, be readily put in action for most purposes, when they cannot be used to make signs by words or by pantomime.[121]

Substituting 'voluntary' for 'intellectual' and 'involuntary' for 'emotional' shows how Jackson was relating the problem of localization in language disturbances to similar problems in motor disorders. Thus, a tentative answer to the problem of what might be localized is: something related to the guidance or use of muscles for particular actions. Doubtless Jackson would have recoiled at the idea that a proposition might be localizable, since it exists in the mind. On the other hand, a few months later, in 1866, he did refer to 'the anterior lobe of the cerebrum … [as] … the chief organ of intellectual life'.[122]

Motor Disorders, Broadbent, and Brain Organization, Mid-1866

I have already noted that Jackson brought together evidence from many different kinds of neurological disease in his effort to sort out these vexing issues. This makes for a wonderful intellectual stew, but it is difficult to isolate the individual ingredients, so now we need definitions of some terms related to motor disorders.

Definition Section 6—Movement Disorders and Motor Disorders

Movement disorder—currently this term refers to almost any clinical entity whose primary manifestation is some kind of abnormal movement, with the important exception of seizures/epilepsy. Included in this group are Parkinson's disease, the choreas,[123] dystonias, and a host of others. One general feature of most of these conditions is an established or suspected etiology involving the basal ganglia. Seizures and seizure disorders are not generally included in this rubric because their pathophysiology is thought to be different (primarily cortical) and because they are the professional province of a separate neurological subspeciality, epileptology, which is distinct from the subspecialty of 'movement disorders'. Very roughly, Jackson and his contemporaries used *chorea* (singular) to mean approximately what we mean by 'movement disorders' (plural).

Motor disorders—in contradistinction to 'movement disorders', this term has only a generic meaning in current usage. I will arbitrarily use this term—'motor disorders'—to refer to the group of clinical motor phenomena that interested Jackson, including hemiplegia, chorea, and seizures.[124] Remember that in the 1860s, the definition of epilepsy did not include nonmotor phenomena, although various auras were known to precede motor seizures.

---

[121] Jackson 1866a, p.175; my square brackets.
[122] Jackson 1866e, p.660; my square brackets.
[123] See **hemichorea** in Definition Section 3 (Some Unilateral Clinical Phenomena) in Chapter 3.
[124] See Jackson 1866p, p.255, footnote (*), where he used 'disorders of motion' and 'motor disorders' interchangeably.

At this point in Jackson's story we have reached early 1866. However, he had been thinking about brain organization and motor disorders since 1862, or maybe earlier, so now it is necessary to go back and look at some of those developing ideas. In his *Suggestions* of early 1863, Jackson pointed out that 'ordinary hemiplegia' in most cases is incomplete, since the forehead and trunk muscles are not usually affected, and 'All the sensitive nerves escape. I think we find only paralysis of the muscles of the limbs ... Is this another way of saying that those muscles less under the control of the will escape, and hence that the corpus striatum and thalamus opticus are able to direct (voluntarily) the limbs only?'[125] In his 'Loss of speech' paper of 1864, Jackson added the observation that the leg is usually involved less than the arm in hemiplegia, so 'I think it is pretty certain that the corpus striatum is *chiefly* the motor centre for the arm, and that it sends comparatively few motor fibres to the muscles of the leg'.[126] The same observations were analyzed extensively in his '*Lectures on hemiplegia*' of 1865.[127]

For Jackson the explanation for these observations came from William Broadbent, whose paper was titled 'An attempt to remove the difficulties attending the application of Dr. Carpenter's theory of the function of the sensori-motor ganglia to the common form of hemiplegia'. It was read at the Medical Society of London in December 1865 and published in April 1866.[128] Carpenter's proposal was the idea that the striatum and the thalamus are the subcortical, hemispheric ganglia for the motor and sensory tracts. This theory was not widely accepted, so Broadbent was trying to bolster an otherwise unpopular idea that Jackson had initially adopted. In his paper Broadbent said that he was responding to Jackson's clinical observations on hemiplegia, as presented in Jackson's '*Lectures on hemiplegia*' of 1865.[129]

To explain the clinical observation that axial muscles are relatively spared in the 'common form of hemiplegia', Broadbent postulated that muscles which regularly act together with their homologues on the other side of the body will be controlled by nuclei in the striatum that are strongly connected by 'commissural fibres' from side to side, whereas those that act 'independently' (voluntarily/unilaterally) have no such connections. Thus, for the less voluntary muscles there will be, in effect,

> ... *a single nucleus. This combined nucleus will have a set of fibres from each corpus striatum, and will usually be called into action by both, but it will be capable of being excited by either singly, more or less completely according as the commissural connection between the two halves is more or less perfect.*[130]

Thus, according to Broadbent the nuclei of the two sides of the corpora striata can function as a single nucleus because there are strong interhemispheric connections between them.

---

[125] Jackson 1863a, pp.24–25; he made the same observation on p.1. See also Greenblatt 1977, pp.417–418.

[126] Jackson 1864j, p.419, footnote.

[127] Jackson 1865f, pp.303–312. In cortical strokes, this difference between arm and leg involvement happens because the arm is represented in cortex that is supplied by the middle cerebral artery, whereas the smaller leg area is in the territory of the anterior cerebral artery. Jackson knew the location of the anterior cerebral artery, but he did not know about the function of the tissue it supplies.

[128] Broadbent 1866. In a letter of December 9, 1865, Broadbent said, 'I read the paper at the Medical Society [of London], but there was not a soul present who could understand it' (Broadbent 1909, p.92). Apparently Jackson was not in the audience. On Broadbent 'as a neurologist' see Eadie 2015.

[129] Jackson 1865f; see also Greenblatt 1977, pp.418–420.

[130] Broadbent 1866, p.477; italics in original.

Damage on one side would still leave the other side able to drive the same muscles on both sides. He did not identify the commissural connection, and now we know that such a connection does not exist.[131] Nonetheless, Broadbent had offered a plausible explanation of how the system works to preserve axial and other involuntary movements when a lesion in one striatum has abolished unilateral voluntary motion. This theory explained Jackson's earlier observation that in ordinary hemiplegia 'those muscles less under the control of the will escape, and hence that the striatum and thalamus are able to direct (voluntarily) the limbs only?'[132] Broadbent's idea even accounted for the varying extent of paralysis, by postulating different densities of commissural connections for different movements, depending on their degrees of independence.

Jackson first referred to Broadbent's 'hypothesis' in print on April 28, 1866,[133] and he again took notice of Broadbent in a paper dated June 23, 1866. In the latter he explained its basics in a short footnote.[134] Broadbent's quasi-quantitative way of thinking about differing degrees of weakness in hemiplegia accorded well with Jackson's speculation that greater defects of language are associated with more extensive tissue damage in the region of the striatum:

> … the difference in the execution of voluntary and involuntary movements is very striking in some cases of loss of speech … [it] probably depends on the difference in quantity of brain damaged near to … the highest part of the motor tract, the point of emission of the orders of the "will" to muscles and to centres for muscular groups.[135]

Bain's Place in Jackson's Study of Localization in Language Disorders, June 1866

The above quotation is taken from Jackson's seminal paper of 1866, 'Notes on the physiology and pathology of language'. It contains the first solid evidence of how far he had worked his way into the associationist literature and the extent to which it had started to affect his thinking. Even the title carries interesting implications. His use of 'physiology' in this context implies that there is a normal physiology of language, as distinct from a psychology. The question was, how is the nervous system arranged so that some patients who cannot use certain muscles to voluntarily articulate words can still use those same muscles to perform involuntary actions or even to perform different voluntary movements?

Jackson's 'Notes' seem to be exactly that: case reports, citations, quotations, analytic ideas, etc. They pop up in no discernable order, as if by free association. This incoherence reflects the unsettled state of his thoughts. Nonetheless, he was following an underlying theme. It is exemplified by his enthusiasm for Broadbent's hypothesis. He was trying to focus on the *motor* aspect of loss of speech—i.e., on articulate language—as distinct from the intellectual (propositional) part, which entails mind. Because loss of articulate speech and motor

---

[131] Carpenter 1855, pp.525–526, said (incorrectly) that the corpus callosum connects the corpora striata and the thalami, and the anterior commissure also connects the corpora striata. Jackson seemed to talk about bilateral cerebral representation in Jackson 1866f, p.660, footnote (a).

[132] Jackson 1863a, pp.24–25; Jackson's parentheses.

[133] Jackson 1866d, p.443.

[134] Jackson 1866f, p.660.

[135] Jackson 1866f, p.660.

disorders both involve motor functions, they could potentially share a common physiology and pathophysiology. It was that potential connection that Jackson was trying to explore. In this regard, Bain had more to offer than Spencer.

In applying sensory-motor physiology to associationism, Bain brought an emphasis on the motor side. In *The Senses and the Intellect*,[136] he raised a basic question about how the brain is organized to direct the entire spectrum of motor activities, from the involuntary to the fully volitional. And then Bain said:

> There is a power in certain feelings or emotions to originate movements of the various active organs. A connexion is formed either by instinct or by acquisition, or by both together, between our emotional states and our active states, sufficient to constitute a link of cause and effect between the one and the other. And the question is whether this link is original or acquired. [137]

Bain answered his own rhetorical question by claiming to show that all motor activity originates from inborn patterns or instincts—truly volitional movements must be acquired by further education of the preexisting patterns. Hence the spectrum of types of motor actions, from the completely automatic to the completely voluntary, depends on their degrees of education. Jackson found this idea useful for understanding clinical phenomena.[138] In describing a patient with severe aphasia, he said:

> These patients can do things which require scarcely ... any education to do, or for which ... the centres exist ready to co-ordinate muscles. It would seem that the centres for the emotional and the semi-voluntary and involuntary actions are in the pons, medulla oblongata, and spinal cord; but where the power is that sets them a-going is not clear.[139]

So Jackson was localizing the center(s) for involuntary movements below the midbrain—a position that would have been agreed by his colleagues. Then he went on to a less-settled problem:

> There are plenty of facts to show that in disease of the corpus striatum those muscles less under the control of the "will" escape, and that through this, the highest part of the motor tract, we are able to direct our *limbs* voluntarily... there is no more difficulty in supposing that there are convolutions near the corpus striatum for superintending those delicate movements of the hands which are under the ... control of the mind, than there is one, as Broca suggests, for movements of the tongue in purely mental operations.[140]

Looking back from 1884, Jackson said: 'Twenty years ago ... it occurred to me that convolutions represent movements – a view I have taken ever since.'[141] This point about cerebral representation of *movements*, rather than muscles, was a fundamental contribution.

---

[136] The first edition of 1855 was cited in Jackson 1866o, p.605, although the second edition of 1864 was available.
[137] Bain 1855, p.292.
[138] In Jackson 1866f, p.660, Jackson said: 'On the education of voluntary movements Bain has some most valuable remarks ..', but he gave no specific citation to Bain.
[139] Jackson 1866f, p.660.
[140] Jackson 1866f, p.660; Jackson's italics.
[141] Jackson 1884b, p.592.

Adjudicating '*my disagreement with M. Broca*', June 1866

In the above, Jackson again seemed to be allowing some intrusion of motor control into the cerebral cortices, which had been the biological province of the 'will'.[142] This time, however, with Bain's help he had a physiological conception that could lead to more precise analysis. What he was really trying to define was his thinking on the pathophysiology of loss of speech, *vis-à-vis* Broca. His statements about Broca were always deferential, but he stood his ground intellectually.

> … I believe less in some of the views propounded by Broca than I did … Yet I cannot but think that my disagreement … [is] to a great extent due to different ways of putting the same thing… I think, then, that the so-called "faculty" of language has no existence, and that disease near the corpus striatum produces defect of expression (by words, writing signs, etc.) … because this is the way out from the hemisphere to organs which the will can set in motion … disease of the convolutions near the corpus striatum is the cause of chorea, which, as regards the limbs, is not so much a disorder of mere motion as disorder of those movements which are voluntary and educated, or at least co-ordinated.
>
> On the education of voluntary movements … chorea is a rare disease either before these movements have been learned or after they have been fully acquired. Unilateral epilepsy seems to replace and sometimes … to displace chorea, and both run into actual hemiplegia occasionally.[143]

Although Jackson didn't say it, one might infer from this that he was willing to allow the existence of 'educated' motor functions in the cortices close to the striatum.[144] Chorea, in his view, occurs when there is a lesion in neural structures that have been partially educated. Unilateral seizures and ordinary hemiplegia involve more educated functions, and the same is true for aphasia.

Getting back to the problem of language, later in the paper Jackson returned to the theme of the 'great difference betwixt ataxy of articulation [dysarthria] and uttering wrong names for things [paraphasia]'.[145] In a footnote to this section he recommended four chapters in Spencer's *Principles of Psychology*, because 'The facts related in this paper seem to me to be in harmony with certain views Mr. Spencer has put forward … '.[146] Then he quoted from one of his papers of early 1865, where he had discussed 'Involuntary [verbal] ejaculations following fright – subsequently chorea' in a patient who may have had Tourette's syndrome.

> "It is in some classes of cases of disease of the nervous system hard to say where obviously motor symptoms end and where the purely mental ones begin. Thus there is (in cases of hemiplegia on the right side) every gradation betwixt, on the one hand, a total loss of power to express ideas, or a loss of knowledge of the relation of words to things, and on the other, apparently scarcely more than an ataxy of articulation …" [147]

---

[142] He repeated this statement about articulatory (motor) functions in the cortices at the end of these 'Notes' (Jackson 1866h, pp.661–662).

[143] Jackson 1866f, p.660; my square brackets.

[144] Here Jackson (1866f, p.660) again used Laycock's reflex ideas to explain lower order (emotional) expressions in aphasics. Since they are not fully voluntary/educated, their origin would not be in the cortical gyri close to the striatum.

[145] Jackson 1866f, p.661; my square brackets. Our term for 'ataxy' is 'ataxia', meaning poorly coordinated.

[146] Jackson 1866f, p.661, footnote (b). Jackson referred to the chapters on 'The Growth of Intelligence', 'Reflex Action', 'Instinct', and 'Memory' in Spencer 1855, pp.522–563.

[147] Jackson 1866f, p.661; Jackson's parentheses. His self-quotation is from J65-01, p.89.

This passage may seem inconsistent with a distinction between articulatory and aphasic disorders, and it is. It shows Jackson's predilection to view semiology on a spectrum. In this case, the basis of the spectrum was Bain's motor interpretation of associationism. Jackson said:

> It is not difficult to show that ataxy of articulation and so-called loss of memory for words are really defects of the same kind, and that the loss of the sign the speechless patient had for a thing is the loss of power to reproduce in his organs ... the *movements* he has learned for that sign ... and that damage near the corpus striatum affects language and thought, not because any so-called faculty resides there ... but because ... parts which help in making symbols are broken up. The fact that people do not put their tongues in motion when they think may seem to be a great difficulty; but ... it is not so great... This will be but a particular expansion of the views which Bain has long taught ... "When we recall," he says, "the impression of a word or a sentence, if we do not speak it out, we feel the twitter of the organs just about to come to that point. The articulatory parts – the larynx, the tongue, the lips – are all sensibly excited; *a suppressed articulation* is, in fact, the material of our recollection, the intellectual manifestation, the *idea* of speech."[148]

In the first part of this passage, Jackson was deliberately conflating two separate aspects of speech, i.e., memory for words and motor ability to produce words. Since he had not made this distinction previously, and he quoted Bain in the same paragraph, it is reasonable to conclude that he had absorbed Bain's view of motor function in relation to language. In this view, we think of a word by a process of stimulating the motor arrangements for pronouncing the word without actually saying it. Jackson accepted Bain's conception, and he applied it immediately to an analysis of Broca's statements.

> M. Broca makes the following remarks ... in a pamphlet he was good enough to send to me a year or two ago. (Extrait des *Bulletins de la Société Anatomique*, juillet, 1863.) "To explain how an aphemic understands spoken language, without meanwhile being able to repeat the words which he comes to understand, one would be able to say that he has lost, not the memory of words, *but the memory of the means of coordination which one employs to articulate words*."[149] The use of the word memory in the sense of its being a distinct faculty, is, I think, likely to lead to some confusion. Spencer says, "... such a succession of states [*motor impulses*, the results of conflicting impressions] constitutes *remembrance* of the various motor changes which thus become incipient – constitutes a *memory*." ... "Thus then the nascent nervous excitements that arise during this conflict of tendencies, are really so many *ideas* of the motor changes which, if stronger, they would cause ... and thus memory necessarily comes into existence whenever automatic action is imperfect." According to this definition, memory is the obtruding of some of the motor impulses on the consciousness, but I suppose M. Broca means by memory of words the connexion the seats of motor impulses ... for words have with what other part of the nervous system ... sets them a-going.[150]

---

[148] Jackson 1866f, p.661; Jackson's italics. In Jackson 1866o, p.605, footnote (*), Jackson gave this quotation again, with a citation to Bain 1855, p.334; it is found there with only *idea* italicized.

[149] The English quotation from Broca (within Jackson's quotation marks) is my translation from the original French in Jackson's paper.

[150] Jackson 1866f, p.661. The italics and square brackets are Jackson's; my underlining. Jackson gives no citation for his quotation from Spencer. Presumably he was quoting from *Principles of Psychology*, 1 ed., 1855, because he referred to it on the same page in another context. After this passage Jackson said, 'Dr. Fournié has also written admirably on this subject ...', but he turned away from further details. Presumably this is a

Despite the conciliatory tone at the end of this difficult passage, there was a basic difference between Jackson's views and Broca's, although they did share some assumptions. As Jackson pointed out, Broca regarded the normal cerebral arrangements for articulation as a form of memory, consistent with the faculty psychology. Jackson agreed with Broca that memory is a part of mind, and they were agreed that mind is widely distributed in the entire brain, especially in the hemispheres. On the other hand, Broca could not see aphasia as a motor disturbance, but Jackson did.[151] At this stage, Jackson was beginning to see the motor aspect as a neural mechanism *sui generis*, i.e., as a primary form of brain organization. Toward the end of the paper Jackson said: 'I think it will be found that the nearer the disease is to the corpus striatum the more likely is the defect of articulation to be the striking thing, and the further off, the more likely is it to be one of mistakes of words.'[152] What he seemed to be asserting is that real mistakes in words, where the propositional value of words is degraded, are *mental* mistakes and therefore assumed to be due to disease of the whole cortex—at a remove from the striatum. The undertone of inconsistency is due to his difficulty with the concept of 'mind'.

At this early stage in Jackson's development, he had not yet partitioned 'mind' away from 'brain' as utterly immiscible but parallel entities (psychophysical parallelism), so he still thought about the mind-brain relation in the ordinary dualistic way. The above passages show his inconsistency about the relation at this time. That is, he didn't always draw the line between mind and brain clearly or at the same metaphysical boundary. However, he did have a sense of discomfort about the problem. With regard to 'defects of expression', he said: '... we must think of them as defects of mind, as well as of that part or phase of mind which enables us to think aloud in words ... for the brain is not only the "organ of mind", but it is the nervous system of the nervous system ... words, especially such as "mind", sensory, motor, &c., fetter our thoughts as well as define them.'[153]

Jackson expressed his discomfort with Cartesian dualism at a meeting of the Harveian Society of London in October 1866, when he commented on a paper by psychiatrist Henry Maudsley (1835–1918). Jackson observed that many symptoms of 'coarse disease' (e.g., hemorrhage and tumors) of the brain 'stand betwixt the two artificial extremes which are conveniently, though arbitrarily, distinguished as physical and psychical symptoms'.[154] His pragmatic resolution of the problem (parallelism) came many years later, impelled by his absorption of Spencer's theories.

Spencer's Growing Influence on Jackson: Evolution and 'Physiological Units', Late 1866

Toward the end of 1866 Jackson's writings began to exhibit Spencer's pervasive influence. On December 1 of that year, a reporter for *The Lancet* gave an account of Jackson's 'Case of disease of the left side of the brain, involving the corpus striatum, etc.; the aphasia

reference to Édouard Fournié (1833–1886), *Physiologie de la voix et de la parole*. Paris: Adrien Delahaye, 1866. Jackson again referred to Fournié in similar contexts in 1869 (Jackson 1869m, p.481) and in 1877 (Jackson 1877n, p.606).

[151] See Young 1970, p.144.
[152] Jackson 1866f-06, p.662.
[153] Jackson 1866f, p.660.
[154] Jackson 1866m, p.587; see Maudsley 1866.

of Trousseau; clinical remarks on psychico-physical symptoms'.[155] The reporter said of Jackson:

> He thinks that a study of Mr. Herbert Spencer's works will show the extreme importance of working at the whole of the physico-psychical symptoms we meet with ... from those grossly motor, as defects of articulation, to those purely "mental," as incoherence. He believes that observations on this plan will help to demonstrate the truth of many of the views Mr. Herbert Spencer has put forward in his 'Principles of Psychology'.[156]

Jackson gave no page citation in Spencer's *Psychology*, but it likely would have included the section on 'The Nature of Intelligence', where Spencer said: 'Out of a great number of psychical actions going on in the organism, only a part are woven into the thread of consciousness ...' And on the following page, Spencer started his consideration of 'The gradual rise of this distinction between the psychical and the physical life'.[157] His analysis invoked the factors of: (1) evolution from homogeneous to heterogeneous, (2) physiological division of labor, (3) gradual emergence of consciousness, and (4) the serial nature of conscious thought.

At the bottom of all this was Spencer's conception of evolution. He 'reintroduced' the word 'evolution' in 1857,[158] 2 years before the publication of Darwin's *Origin* in 1859.[159] Spencer initially used 'evolution' in the general sense of progress,[160] so the word was not exactly synonymous with the *Vestige*'s and others' use of 'development hypothesis'. This may explain an interesting absence in Jackson's writings—he never used 'development hypothesis'. His first published use of 'evolution' was in the case report of December 1, 1866, where the reporter said that Jackson 'urges strongly that we should from cases of chorea, epilepsy, paralysis, and defects of speech try to learn something towards establishing the Laws of the Evolution of Movement and Sensation'.[161] As Jackson was then using 'evolution', it did not necessarily have the same broad meaning that it would have had in Darwinian evolution. He used it in a more technical sense, i.e., as roughly equivalent to 'functional anatomy of phylogenetic and/or ontogenetic development'. For his clinical purposes, he wanted to know only the pattern ('Laws') of how the phenomena present themselves. He was not interested in evolutionary adaptation *per se*. This is seen in a passage where he began to exhibit his early thoughts about the hierarchical organization of the nervous system, in connection with his data about hemiplegia and aphasia *and* his reading in Spencer:

> The difficulty of articulation with hemiplegia ... is not to be analysed onto difficulty in pronouncing palatals ... nor dentals, nor labials, for there is no paralysis of any corresponding divisions of the articulatory organs. It is a defect in a higher series of anatomical possibilities.*
>
> * On the evolution of movements I have spoken several times, especially as regards the arm-nervous-system, *i.e.*, from nerve-trunks supplying muscles directly, to the corpus striatum. From this centre we shall, I hope, be able to trace another series of evolutions of movements, those of speech and thought.[162]

---

[155] Jackson 1866o.

[156] Jackson 1866o, p.605; my underlining.

[157] Spencer 1855, pp.495–496.

[158] See Perrin 1993, p.186; also Taylor 2007, pp.58–59.

[159] Darwin did not use the word 'evolution' in the *Origin*, but widespread use of the term began soon after the *Origin* appeared; see 'evolved' (used once) in Barrett et al. 1981, p.239.

[160] See Perrin 1993, pp.34–35, 186.

[161] Jackson 1866o, p.605. The same desideratum is found in another review paper that was published in late 1866; in Jackson 1866p, p.257, Jackson referred to his paper of November 24, 1866 (Jackson 1866m), so Jackson 1866p must have been published no earlier than December 1866 and probably later.

[162] Jackson 1866p, pp.289–290.

Let me try to interpret these two passages. Before Jackson had fully absorbed Spencer's evolutionary view of the nervous system, he had concluded that the striatum is primarily a center for arm function, more than leg, because the *voluntary* movements of the arm are more affected by damage to the striatum. Now comes the Spencerian element. Since *voluntary* implies *consciousness*, and consciousness itself evolves, the striatum must be the product of a higher level of evolution than the rest of the nervous system below the cortices. Jackson thus hoped that further analysis of this progression would clarify the location and function of the neural structures involved in speech and language. The reporter said of Jackson, 'From the corpus striatum, inwards and outwards, he would begin his anatomical studies of Medical Psychology'.[163] This kind of thinking is not found in Jackson's writings before he made intellectual acquaintance with Spencer. Its origin is linked closely to another Spencerian idea.

Spencer's 'Physiological Units' and Jackson's 'First Symptom', 1866

Spencer had a highly abstract conception of 'physiological units', which was ultimately crucial to Jackson's quest for understanding all neurological disorders, including aphasia.[164] By 'unit' Spencer meant generic 'units of analysis', that is, the categories into which we divide natural phenomena so we can study them. Prime examples given by Spencer are the molecule as a unit in chemistry and the cell as the morphological unit in biology. He then defined the physiological unit as intermediate in scale between the chemical and the morphological. Physiological units are composed of 'immensely more complex' aggregates of molecules, such that:

> … in each organism, the physiological units produced by this further compounding of highly compound atoms, have a more or less distinctive character… In each case, some slight difference of composition in these units, leading to some slight difference in their mutual play of forces, produces a difference in the form which the aggregate assumes.[165]

So physiological units are aggregates of whatever structures at whatever size are necessary to carry out some function for the organism. It was characteristic of Jackson's genius that he was able to convert such amorphous generalities into useful constructs. Indeed, he insisted that such conceptualization is methodologically required.

> Unless a man can put the particular phenomena he himself sees under more general Laws, or unless he tries to do this, he can scarcely be said to know or to be studying a thing in any very valuable sense… the knowledge the physician has of defects of articulation, of chorea, and of epilepsy, and that the psychologist has of incoherence and delusion should aim to be Physiological* Units, each different but each related to a wide common knowledge of such Laws … as those of the Evolution of Sensation and Movement in organisms.[166]

---

[163] Jackson 1866o, p.605.

[164] Jackson's first published reference to Spencer's 'Physiological Units' is found in his comments on Maudsley (1866) at the Harveian Society (Jackson 1866m), concerning 'the causes of insanity', where the topic of discussion was genetic inheritance (Jackson 1866m, p.587). Other Jacksonian references to 'Physiological Units' are found in Jackson 1866n, p.585, and Jackson 1866p, p.256–257, 265. See also 'Units' in Collins' Index (Collins 1889, p.570) and 'units of analysis' in Young's Index (1970, p.278).

[165] Spencer 1864 (vol.1), pp.182–183; see summary in Collins 1889, p.88.

[166] Jackson 1866p, p.256. The asterisk on 'Physiological*' referred the reader to 'Mr. Spencer's work on Biology', without further citation, so presumably he meant Spencer 1864.

Later in the same paper Jackson made one of his most important and original contributions to epileptology. Discussing 'aura' in 'Unilateral epileptiform fits', he said: ' "First symptom" is a better term, as it involves no theory, and yet gives us hints as to the desirability of studying what functional region or part of the brain is first disordered, in order that we may seek … where the epileptic process begins in the brain …'[167] Of course, 'First Symptom' does involve a theory, as seen in a long footnote on 'aura*':

> * … When [in] the spasm [seizure], of the hand, "partial fits" are witnessed, it will be found that they are not of one anatomical set of muscles, as of extensors or flexors, but there is one contending spasm of all the muscles which go to the hand. It is a defect in the highest range of Evolution. The study of hemiplegia leads me to the belief that the whole of the arm is represented in each part of the corpus striatum … and I think the phenomena of unilateral chorea and of some unilateral epileptiform seizures also illustrate this. I imagine that however much the hand may appear to suffer alone, it suffers in the most highly developed and the part most represented of the *whole* limb. In general every act is a physiological unit in Spencer's sense of the term.[168]

Even before he met Spencer's 'physiological unit', Jackson was well along on the road to this understanding of the aura, but Spencer's unit helped give 'aura' the status of an analyzable entity. More to the point, Jackson's statement about motor representation of 'the whole of the arm' being 'in each part of the corpus striatum' makes sense in the context of Spencer's units. Jackson's insight about the localizing value of the 'first symptom' was also a direct product of (1) his focus on the importance of unilateral symptoms, and (2) his tripartite method, which emphasized tissue changes. Just before the above two quotations, he said: 'It is most important to give a place in our thoughts to the slightest one-sided symptom … in order that we may seek … where the epileptic process begins in the brain, and thus get a clear idea of where to look, after death, for those minute abnormal changes which are the permanent part of that unknown process.'[169] At least as early as 1866 he suspected that the holy grail of epileptology is 'those minute abnormal changes'. In some ways, we're still looking for them.

Jackson's Ideas about Motor Disorders and Normal Brain Function in 1867

Jackson's furious pace of publication in 1866 slowed somewhat in 1867. To the extent that he had a theme for 1867, it was seizures and epilepsy, sometimes interpreted through his recently acquired Spencerian lens. In February and March of 1867 he published a two-part 'Note on the comparison and contrast of regional palsy and spasm',[170] where 'spasm' meant any kind of abnormal movement, but the emphasis was on seizures. Notably, he delivered his message in a style that was more direct than earlier, indicative of growing confidence in the value of his own opinions. He proposed to disregard nosology and to work at pathophysiology, because that would be the only profitable approach.

---

[167] Jackson 1866p, pp.282–283.
[168] Jackson 1866p, p.283; my square brackets and underlining.
[169] Jackson 1866p, pp.282–283.
[170] Jackson 1867a, J67-02.

I fear we too frequently arrange our thoughts on cases according as the symptoms *approach* supposed types – such as genuine epilepsy, real chorea, &c. Thus we hear it discussed whether genuine epilepsy is always attended by loss of consciousness, or necessarily involves spasm of muscle … and … of a particular case, whether it be a case of genuine epilepsy or not… I fear that students – it was so in my own early medical career – imagine there is some entity of which epilepsy is the proper name.[171]

Instead, Jackson suggested

… a more positive method of inquiry than we usually adopt – namely, an examination, in many differing cases, of the whole of the states of muscles in the various parts – face, arm, and leg – of the region the corpus striatum governs, and of their conditions in Time, *from health*, through nearly continuous irregular movements and occasional spasm, to permanent palsy.[172]

This comparative approach, he said, would allow the study of 'cases of palsy, spasms, irregular movements and tremors as *departures* from what we can learn about the healthy condition of a region of the nervous system and the outward parts this region governs'.173 He was primarily interested in applying his tripartite method to the problems of pathophysiology.

… cases of disease should be classified triply according to (1) changes of Tissues, (2) damages of Organs, and (3) disorders of Functions. But in most cases of convulsions … we do not know either (1) the tissue changes, or (2) the organ where the tissues are changed. We have these gaps … to fill before we can fully classify cases of "genuine" epilepsy. And I fear we shall not be able to make minute investigations of nervous matter in such cases … until we work more elaborately at (3) signs of disorder of function, and thus find where it is hopeful to search for slight changes which, whilst they elude common examination *post mortem*, the disorder of function during life declared to exist. But I fear genuine epilepsy is at present an insoluble problem. I would begin … with a simpler kind of convulsion.[174]

In fact, Jackson had been following his own counsel. Over the preceding few years he had been working toward understanding the pathophysiology of seizures, and now—in early 1867—he had started to carry the analysis in a promising direction.

… I think … that in chronic fits, in which the physiological symptoms are related to gross disease of one hemisphere, the diffused changes are *permanent*, and that the *occasional* <u>disorderly expenditure of force</u> (acquired by *continuous* nutrition) occurs in some periodical wave over the whole system – an attempted equilibration of a degraded part … in which the part degraded is like a note out of tune.[175]

In this passage we should note that Jackson used the term 'disorderly expenditure of force' without saying anything explicit about the nature of that force. There is no evidence that he

---

171 Jackson 1867b, p.295; Jackson's italics
172 Jackson 1867b, p.295; Jackson's italics.
173 Jackson 1867b, p.295; Jackson's italics.
174 Jackson 1867b, p.296.
175 Jackson 1867b, p.296; Jackson's italics and parentheses, my underlining. His 'nutrition' is roughly our 'metabolism'.

thought of the phenomenon as strictly electrical. At the time, 'force' was still used to mean 'energy' in our terms, though 'force' was gradually going out of style.[176] Jackson's conception invoked the gradual and *normal* accumulation of force from *normal* nutrition. Thus normal force produces a motor *disorder* only when it is released in a 'disorderly' manner. Todd's humoral pathophysiology of epilepsy involved accumulation of 'a morbid material in the blood'.[177] He thought that seizures are set off when abnormal material is released within the brain in an explosive manner. By contrast, in Jackson's view, as of 1867, unilateral seizures are the result of *aberrantly released but otherwise normal metabolic processes*. This conception fulfilled the requirement of his tripartite method for an explanation of its third element, disorder of function, and he continued to think along the same lines through the year.

In December 1867, Jackson published another paper in two parts: 'Remarks on the disorderly movements of chorea and convulsion'.[178] There he began to show the increasing depth of Spencer's influence on his conception of normal physiological function.

> ... the word function has a threefold meaning when used in speaking of the healthy nervous system. (1) It is the function of nervous matter to store up force for *future* expenditure. (2) It is the function of nerve units, in expending their stored up-force; to develope *certain orderly* and more or less complex movements. (3) It is the function of nervous matter forming the nerve units of particular organs to expend the stored-up force in developing certain ... complex movements *in correspondence* with special ... excitations, which bring the local movements into harmony with the entire organism.[179]

In a footnote Jackson continued his analysis, using Spencer's distinctively theoretical and 'artificial separation' of processes in '(1) time, (2) movement, and (3) relations of local movement and local time to the succession of bodily movements and mean time ...'.[180] Spencer's theories thus helped Jackson to extend his ideas as they evolved, but he was not basing them entirely on Spencer. He had a large mass of clinical data on which to ground his thoughts.

> In complete hemiplegia there is no disorder of function, as there is no function at all: all nerve tissue is *destroyed*. But in hemichorea and hemispasm [unilateral seizures] there must be some kind of [living] nerve-tissue [remaining], or there would not result even the *disorder* of function. It is equally clear that nerve-tissue must be faulty, or this disorder could not result. 1. The ill-nourished nerve-tissue is more unstable, over-ready, "excitable;" there is discharge too soon; its Time is shortened. 2. The movement resulting from the ill-timed discharge is a disorderly movement – an unintelligent action. 3. The ill-timed disorderly movement is not the result of a proper "motive," (d)[181] but will follow an excitation of a less special or of a more general kind.[182]

---

[176] See C. Smith 1998, pp.1, 176; Sourkes 2006, p.32.
[177] Quoted in Temkin 1971, p.312.
[178] Jackson 1867h and Jackson 1867i.
[179] Jackson 1867h, p.642; Jackson's italics and parenthesis.
[180] Jackson 1867h, p.642, footnote (a). There he cited the first edition of Spencer's *Psychology* (Spencer 1855, pp.412, 414–415).
[181] In footnote (d) Jackson explained: 'Each movement is conceived to have its proper motive. This is seen in its least complex form—the lowest types of reflex action. A simple sensation provokes a simple movement. The motive is in its highest manifestations when a movement ... follows on the excitation of that varying and complex state which is called the "will". (See Spencer on "The Will", op. cit.)' Since there is nothing about 'motive' in Spencer's chapter on 'Will' (Spencer 1855, pp.612–620), nor is 'motive' listed in Collins' Index (1889, p.561), I conclude that 'motive' was Jackson's invention. It sounds teleological, and it did not appear again in his writings.
[182] Jackson 1867h, p.643; Jackson's italics, my square brackets.

In this passage Jackson's use of '*destroyed*' and '*disorder*' can be correlated directly to his later ideas of 'negative' and 'positive' lesions, although he first applied the latter pair to neurological phenomena in print only in 1875.[183] Here in 1867 he had the conceptions of negative and positive phenomena without those particular words. Negative symptoms for Jackson are those which result from the absence of the function(s) of dead or non-functional tissue, and positive symptoms are caused by abnormal activity of tissue that is still living but dysfunctional. These conceptions are integral parts of his pathophysio-logical framework—and ours—but his use of the concepts and the words was not original with Jackson. They were in the air that he was breathing, because Brown-Séquard and Russell Reynolds had both used the concepts around 1860.[184] I will sometimes use 'nega-tive' and 'positive' for convenience, remembering that for Jackson the words themselves are anachronistic until 1875. Utilizing these conceptions, and his comparative method, he tried to work out the physiological implications of the different semiologies of hemichorea and unilateral seizures:

> ... the irregular movements of the arm in cases of hemichorea are not mere jerks and spasms – not incoherence of muscles, but incoherence of more complex and more specialized muscular movements... one difference betwixt unilateral irregular movements and unilateral spasm [seizure] is, that the former results from an instability of nervous matter, composing units of a higher degree of complexity ... In convulsion, the *whole* of the muscles are contending *at once* ... In chorea, movements of muscles follow in rapid succession. But how the two come to differ in time – the "explosions" in one being in con-tinuous succession, and in the other abrupt and occasional – is not accounted for except by supposing that the correspondence with external coexistences increases with the increased correspondence with external sequences.[185]

Here Jackson was trying to explain some of the different semiologies of unilateral movement disorders, versus unilateral seizures, by invoking his early version of Spencerian hierarchies. He was postulating that the abnormally continuous movements of chorea are more com-plex and therefore of a higher evolutionary order than those of unilateral seizures. But still he could not account for the differing instabilities of nervous tissue, which are paroxysmal in seizures and continuous in chorea. This kind of analysis was leading him to think more deeply about the organization of the nervous system—about localization in the striatum and in the cortices.

---

[183] Jackson 1875ll, p.111; see Berrios 1985, p.95. Of course, we don't know exactly when Jackson began to use these terms in his thoughts or in his teaching.

[184] See Berrios 1985. The terms 'negative' and 'positive' were first published obscurely by Russell Reynolds in 1858 and again more visibly in 1861 (Reynolds 1861, pp.9–10). Berrios points out that Reynolds' conception of negative and positive symptoms was based partly on waning nineteenth-century vitalism, which Jackson ignored. Reynolds was Jackson's colleague on the staff of the National Hospital from 1864 to 1869 (see Holmes 1954, pp.36, 96). Also in 1861, Brown-Séquard (1861, p.29; see also Aminoff 1993, pp.43–45) approximated the concepts of negative and positive symptoms, though he referred to them as: '1. Symptoms of cessation of function ... [and] 2. Symptoms of irritation'. In Jackson 1867h Jackson did not cite either Brown-Séquard or Reynolds, nor did he use their terms. In Jackson 1867h (pp.111–112, footnote 1) Jackson identified older sources. Pearce (2004) claims that Jackson derived his ideas about negative and positive symptoms from Spencer, but he quotes only Jackson's papers from 1881 and later.

[185] Jackson 1867h, p.643; Jackson's italics, my square brackets. Note the Spencerian wording.

Spencer and Associationism in Jackson's Developing Ideas about Cerebral Localization, December 1867

The second part of Jackson's 'Remarks' of 1867 had an addition in its title: 'Remarks on the disorderly movements of chorea and convulsion, and on localisation'.[186] This was the first publication in which he addressed the issue of localization *per se*. Since the section on localization comes after his ideas about pathophysiology, it would appear that he was reasoning from the abnormal to the normal, starting with the assertion that 'no one denies that the hemisphere is the chief seat of the mind, and that through the corpus striatum the rest of the nervous system acts on the limbs'.[187] Thus assuming the motor function of the striatum, he went on to observe: 'In incomplete hemiplegia … there is not palsy of part of the arm, but partial paralysis of the arm … So it seems that each movement of the arm is represented in each part of the corpus striatum, or conversely that each part of the corpus striatum represents the movements of the limb as a whole.' So according to Jackson in 1867, in partial hemiplegia all movements are weak to the same degree (which is wrong), rather than some movements being weaker than others. Applying this principle to the whole brain, he said, 'we see how it happens that disease of the forepart of the anterior [frontal] lobe, of the posterior [occipital] lobe, and of the hemisphere above the lateral ventricle [parietal lobe], need not produce any defect of the psychico-physical processes which constitute the phenomena of language'.[188]

Jackson was reasoning that if damage to any limited part of the striatum produces the same pattern of equal, partial weakness, regardless of which part is involved, then there must be representation of all affected body parts equally throughout the striatum. However, he had generalized a bit too much about clinical phenomena. It is common to see limited retention of many movements in partial paralyses, but usually some movements are more affected than others. Some years later he recognized this neurological truth and used it to further his explication of localization. However, in December 1867, he was still working with his view of hemipareses as being uniform in their degrees of weakness of all movements. Thus we are now encountering the beginning of the process by which he eventually arrived at his mature ideas about cortical localization. His next step was to follow the implications of his analysis of striatal motor localization into the adjacent cortices immediately 'above' the striatum.

> Just as in the arm-nervous-system there is a gradually increasing complexity from the delivery of nerves to muscles through interweaving of nerves in nerve trunks to an interrelation so great in the corpus striatum, that damage to a small part of this organ weakens the whole of the limb, and yet destroys no single movement – so we may infer that, continued from the corpus striatum, deeper [higher] in brain – further in mind – are still more complex arrangements of motor processes, reaching a minute degree of interrelation and a vast width of association … and becoming at length so complete that a quantity of brain may be destroyed without any special mental defect resulting.[189]

---

[186] Jackson 1867i; my underlining.

[187] Jackson 1867i, p.669.

[188] Jackson 1867i, p.669; my underlining. In 1869 (J69-13, p.481) Jackson stated explicitly that it is movements, not muscles, that are represented in the hemispheres. See Chapter 5.

[189] Jackson 1867i, p.669; my square brackets and underlining.

In association theory the operations of any part of the mind-brain can involve only sensory and motor signals. Hence it follows that there must be 'complex arrangements of motor processes' that are 'deeper in brain', i.e., in the hemispheric cortices. Now if Jackson had actually reached this conclusion at the time, it would be quite remarkable. In fact, he had not yet gotten that far, probably because he did not see this implication as clearly as I am stating it. Nonetheless, his thoughts were developing in that direction, as evidenced in another footnote.

> (b) The principle of localisation I have adopted seems to be the one which Herbert Spencer has put forward. He has given an illustration which is ... essentially the same as the one I have given ... Spencer says ("Principles of Psychology," p.607):- "No physiologist who calmly considers the question in connexion with the general truths of his science can long resist the conviction that different parts of the cerebrum subserve different kinds of mental action. Localisation of function is the law of all organisation whatever: separateness of duty is universally accompanied with separateness of structure, and it would be marvellous were an exception to exist in the cerebral hemispheres."[190]

Immediately before the Spencerian text that Jackson quoted in the above, Spencer had said: 'in their antagonism to the unscientific reasonings of the phrenologists, the physiologists ... have gone to the extent of denying or ignoring any localization of function in the cerebrum ...'[191] All in all, Spencer was leading Jackson to localization in the hemispheric cortices, in part through Spencer's incomplete rejection of phrenology. In the sentence to which the above footnote (b) is attached Jackson said: 'The foregoing [about the arm-nervous-system] does not imply that there is no localisation in any sense of the word, although it does imply that there is no localisation in the sense phrenologists suppose. (b)'[192]

Jackson's footnote (b) warrants further discussion on two points. First is the wording of his remark about the similarity of his example and Spencer's. Jackson seems to imply that he first worked out his illustration of the 'arm-nervous-system' and then he discovered its similarity to Spencer's example. This is entirely possible but hard to prove. Comparing Jackson's example with Spencer's text near the place that Jackson cited does confirm Jackson's statement about their similarities.[193] In sum, I submit that the tone of Jackson's wording in the first sentence in footnote (b) is another illustration of his vehement insistence on his intellectual independence, despite his acknowledgment of Spencer's lead in many important matters.[194]

The second and larger point about footnote (b) is related to the contents of the penultimate chapter of Spencer's *Principles of Psychology*, from which Jackson took his Spencerian quotation. There Spencer offered an extensive discussion of the claims of phrenology.[195]

---

[190] Jackson 1867i, p.669, footnote (b). Jackson's quotation of Spencer is accurate in its wording, but there are minor changes in spelling in Jackson's version.

[191] Spencer 1855, p.607.

[192] Jackson 1867i, p.669.

[193] Jackson cited Spencer 1855, p.607, for the Spencerian quotation in footnote (b), but the example is actually on p.608. The main difference is that Spencer did not include the striatum in his example. Knowledge of that structure's function was poor in 1855, when Spencer's *Principles of Psychology* was first published; see Carpenter 1855, pp.498–499, 524–525.

[194] In 1881 (Jackson 1881h, p.332), after mentioning several authors on epileptic insanity, including Spencer, Jackson said: 'The foregoing must not be taken as an admission that I have not worked quite independently at most parts of the subject.'

[195] Spencer 1855, pp.606–611.

Considering that he had earlier been an acolyte to that creed,[196] Spencer's critique is both thoughtful and damning. More important for Jackson, however, is Spencer's accompanying elucidation of his views on localization. Since Jackson referred the reader back to 'Mr. Spencer's views on localisation', we can presume that he agreed with Spencer's formulations. Following his associationist/evolutionary premises, Spencer began with a seeming truism about brain organization for behavior.

> That an organized tendency toward certain complex aggregations of psychical states, sup-poses a structural modification of the nervous system ... no one ... can doubt... the com-bination of any set of impressions, or motions, implies a ganglion in which the various nerve-fibres concerned are put in connection. To combine the actions of any set of ganglia, implies some ganglion in connection with them all. And so on in ever-ascending stages of complication: the nervous masses concerned, becoming larger in proportion to the com-plexity of the co-ordinations they have to effect.[197]

The point that Spencer had grasped is the necessity for coordination of centers with related functions in any scheme of brain organization. Following Sir Charles Scott Sherrington (1857–1952), we moderns would call it 'integration'.[198] From an evolutionary standpoint, any center ('ganglion') that integrates the functions of two others is hierarchically 'higher' than the ones that it integrates. The main phrenological proposition that Spencer accepted was an insistence on some kind of 'separateness of duty' of different parts of the hemispheric cortices.[199] This concept follows logically from the idea of the division of labor in physio-logical systems. Spencer exhibited his uniformitarian faith when he asked rhetorically 'Can it be ... that in the great hemispherical ganglia alone, this specialization of duty does not hold?'[200] In his view the phrenologists had the right idea, but very much in the wrong form, and they were irritatingly rigid about it.[201] From his theoretical reasoning he surmised that localization must have some kind of graded quality between cortical areas with different functions. He argued against the phrenologist's '*precise* demarcation of the faculties', saying that: 'The only localization which we may presume to exist ... is one of a comparatively vague kind ... which does not suppose specific limits, but an insensible shading-off'.[202]

> As every more complex aggregation of psychical states, is evolved by the union of minor aggregations previously established ... it follows that that which becomes more especially the seat of this more complex aggregation ... is simply the *centre of co-ordination* by which all the minor aggregations are brought into relation. Hence, that particular portion of the cerebrum in which a particular faculty is said to be located, must be regarded as an agency by which the various actions going on in other parts of the cerebrum are combined in a particular way.[203]

---

196 See above in this chapter, and Young 1970, pp.151–167.
197 Spencer 1855, pp.606–607; 'ganglion' here simply refers to masses of gray matter.
198 Sherrington 1906.
199 Spencer 1855, p.607.
200 Spencer 1855, p.608.
201 Spencer 1855, pp.608–609.
202 Spencer 1855, p.609; Spencer's italics, my underlining.
203 Spencer 1855, pp.610–611. This is an associationist precursor of Sherringtonian integration, which the faculty psychology lacked. Spencer never quite said that the phrenologists ignored the problem of integration ('co-ordination'), but I think he understood it.

Spencer wrote this loquacious passage in 1855—13 years after Flourens' supposedly fatal attack on phrenology.[204] In France at that time, ideas of cortical localization had been so tainted that respectable scientists and physicians feared for their respectability if they espoused anything that smacked too much of it—and the same applied to a lesser extent in Britain. Even in 1867—6 years after Broca's first publication on aphasia—Jackson was still subject to this feeling, especially given his general conservatism. On the other hand, he was subscribing to Spencer's view when he wrote the sentence that ends with 'there is no localisation in the sense phrenologists suppose'.[205] So it appears that reading Spencer's analysis of phrenology gave Jackson an opportunity to rethink his own attitude toward cortical localization, and he was gradually accumulating clinical evidence.

Going back now to the remainder of Jackson's 'Remarks' of December 1867, he was still presuming that motor 'representation' existed only up to the striatum and not in the cortices. But some of his clinical observations were beginning to contradict the idea that all movements represented in the striatum are represented equally.

> We find now and then in hemiplegia that when there is a trifling degree of power in moving the upper arm and flexing the elbow, the power to move any one of the fingers may be absolutely lost. The movements of the hand – the most intelligent part of the limb – must be at once more represented, and more specially represented, than the coarser movements of the limb. For the same reason ... the arm suffers more and longer than the leg in hemiplegia ... in unilateral convulsions the "aura" nearly always begins in the hand; sometimes, however, in the side of the face, and rarely in the leg. So the speculation is that, although each movement is everywhere represented, <u>there are points where particular movements are specially represented</u>.[206]

In our contemporary neuroscience, the above conception about special representation of 'particular movements' is not valid for the gray matter of the striatum,[207] but it is valid for the motor cortex. What are in the cortical tissue are aggregations of neurons whose activities in different places elicit different movements. Thus there will be many more aggregations for the hand, and especially for the fingers, than there are for the relatively crude movements of the arm and shoulder. If focal seizures arise by equal chance from any piece of tissue that might be damaged and unstable, there is a much greater chance that a part of the limb with more abundant representation will be involved. That is why focal seizures occur with the relative frequency that Jackson observed, i.e., hand more than face, more than leg, etc. However, it is important to realize that Jackson's statement above in 1867 did not draw this quantitative conclusion about *amounts* of tissue devoted to representation of the movements of different parts of each limb. Rather, Jackson made only the qualitative statement that is underlined above. Still, the idea that different movements may have points of special representation is here getting a foot in the door to Jackson's thought, because he had stated previously that all movements are represented equally in all parts of the striatum. Indeed he did make some quantitative speculations about the representation of language in the cortices.

> But it is not supposed ... that the faculty of language, ... in any sense of the term, resides solely close upon the cerebral side of the corpus striatum. The speculation I hold ... is that

[204] Flourens 1842. See also Ackerknecht and Vallois 1956.
[205] Jackson 1867i, p.669.
[206] Jackson 1867i, p.669; my underlining.
[207] See Kandel et al. 2000, p.854–857; and Nolte 2002, pp.464–473.

the different degree of the symptoms produced depends on the different *quantity* of the brain damaged "round about the *highest part of the motor tract*, the corpus striatum – the point of emission of the orders of the 'will' to the muscles" (*Lancet*, November 26, 1864). I would now put it that <u>the quantity of defect produced is proportionate to the quantity of nervous tissue injured</u>, but that the defect varies inversely in quantity – to speak metaphorically – as the square of the distance of the disease from the corpus striatum.[208]

It follows from the above that language is more intensely represented in the cortical tissue close to the striatum than it is in cortex that is further away. Hence, the above statement is entirely consistent with Spencer's conclusion that cortical areas are demarcated only by 'an insensible shading off'.[209] In Spencer's mind, all of this follows from the principle of the uniformity of nature, but Jackson was still reluctant to take that logic to the point of allowing motor representation in the cortices. One source of his reluctance is still a valid point.

> <u>Whilst we may localise the damage which makes a man speechless, we do not localise language</u>. It will reside in the whole brain (or whole body), and, although the nervous arrangements for its most exterior manifestations lie close to the corpus striatum – possibly ... largely in "Broca's convolution" – they will be continuous with the most complex and most widely related sensation and movements in every part of the brain.[210]

The logic of Jackson's first sentence still stands. Localizing the damage that disrupts the system is not necessarily the same as localizing or otherwise defining the entire system. On the other hand, only humans exhibit language in its full complexity. In 1867 the clinico-pathological method was the only way to investigate the neural basis of language. In his quest for a better understanding of normal and abnormal language, Jackson stepped onto a larger stage in 1868.

---

[208] Jackson 1867i, p.669; Jackson's italics, my underlining. Jackson's self-quotation is from Jackson 1864l, where there are no italics.
[209] Spencer 1855, p.609.
[210] Jackson 1867j, pp.669–670; my underlining.

5

Aphasia, Localization, and a National Reputation, 1868–1869

In retrospect Jackson arrived on the national scene in British medicine in 1868. His early reputation came largely from his work on language disorders, which began in 1864. In August 1868 his rising reputation was established when he participated in a 'debate' with Paul Broca at a meeting of the British Association for the Advancement of Science (British Association or BA) at Norwich. Before I get into the substance of the debate I will first describe the expansion of Jackson's activities during the 3 years leading up to 1868.

Professional Life, 1865–1868

For the rapidly growing middle class, Victorian society in the late 1860s was increasingly open—though surely not really egalitarian—so access to higher standing was increasingly possible. Of course, achieving upward mobility was never easy. Probably because of his grandfather's generous endowment,[1] Jackson seems to have enjoyed a niche in the upper ranks of the middle class from the earliest days of his residency in London. In the British medical community, 'The formation of a professional elite' was an ongoing process throughout the nineteenth century.[2] However, having a position in the upper middle class was no guarantee of membership in the medical elite, because such membership was quite restricted. 'If senior status in a London teaching hospital is used as an index of success, then for most of the nineteenth century, the inner circles of elites numbered no more than 180 – five percent of all London practitioners …'[3] Senior status meant appointment as 'full' Physician or Surgeon to one of the major London hospitals, which numbered approximately eleven at mid-century, including the London.[4] These staff positions were usually not salaried. The incumbents were expected to earn their livings in private practice. The Assistant Physicians treated outpatients, and the full Physicians supervised the inpatient treatment that was actually carried out by the house officers.[5]

In some ways Jackson's career followed the general pattern for advancement into the medical elite,[6] and in some ways it did not. As a graduate of the provincial York Medical School, he was denied the automatic access afforded to medical graduates of Oxford and Cambridge ('Oxbridge'). Beyond that, the common practice in the awarding of consultantships at leading hospitals was the appointment of 'old boys', men who had

---

[1] See Chapter 2.
[2] Peterson 1978, pp.136–193.
[3] Peterson 1978, p.137.
[4] Peterson 1978, p.142.
[5] Holmes 1954, pp.25–26.
[6] As described by Peterson 1978, pp.136–193.

been house officers at the same hospitals where they were appointed. On the other hand, Jackson had Hutchinson to lead the way at the London. Hutchinson achieved the position of Surgeon to the London in 1863, the year when Jackson was appointed Assistant Physician at age 28. Otherwise Jackson's sequence of appointments was mostly in keeping with the usual pattern.

> Qualifying at age twenty-one, the aspirant to consulting status stayed in London, serving in minor hospital posts, seeking the beginnings of practice, and making what connections and income he could. At age twenty-six, he became a fellow of his [Royal] College and, with luck, by age thirty he might be appointed assistant physician or surgeon at one of the London hospitals. For most young men this decade was primarily a time of surviving and waiting for posts that would secure their future as consultants. Promotion to full physician or surgeon came typically at age forty, and election to Royal College office by age fifty.[7]

Jackson had indeed qualified at age 21, in 1856. He had returned to York for 3 years (1856–1859), but otherwise his path was largely true to the above form. He became a Fellow of the Royal College of Physicians in 1868, a little late at age 33, probably because he was not an Oxbridge graduate.[8] Promotion to Physician at the London came in 1874, at age 39. In 1885 he was exactly 50 when he became a Member of the Council of the Royal College of Physicians.[9] Since Jackson was appointed Physician to the National Hospital in 1867, at age 32, the question arises whether he was actually ahead of the curve. By and large, the answer is no. Despite the National Hospital's noteworthy beginnings, it remained very small in the 1860s.[10] It began to blossom into its position of prominence in the world of neurology only in the 1870s, and neurology did not begin to be recognized as a specialty until the 1880s or later.[11]

Language Disorders and Brain Organization on the National Scene, 1864–1868

Jackson's ascent to the British medical elite was atypical in one significant respect—scientific achievement was not usually considered in decisions about hospital appointments in the 1860s. Scholarly contributions gradually gained more weight as the decades went by, so Jackson was in the vanguard of that trend.[12]

---

[7] Peterson 1978, p.137; my square brackets.

[8] Restriction of fellowship to Oxbridge graduates had been abolished in 1835, but that old boy network was too large and too strong to simply collapse; see Cooke 1972, p.804.

[9] Jackson served on the Council 1885–1887. He was a Censor of the College in 1888 and 1889; see Critchley and Critchley 1998, p.184. The Council is a central part of the governing structure of the College; the Censors' Board is a disciplinary body, which also has some responsibility for admission of candidates to examination (see Cooke 1972, pp.1153, 1156, 1164, 1174). The Censors are members of the Council.

[10] Holmes 1954, pp.17–18.

[11] See Lorch 2004a, pp.125–126, and Casper 2014, pp.13–23. By 'recognized' I mean in practical terms within the medical profession. Casper shows that 'official' recognition by the relevant medical and governmental bodies was delayed well into the twentieth century.

[12] See Peterson 1878, pp.172–173, 187; and Weisz 2006, pp.27–28.

Recognition of Jackson's Work on Disorders of Language, 1864–1867

It is difficult to reconstruct something so ephemeral as the historical reputation of a single person at a given time, except in the case of highly celebrated individuals, and Jackson was never that famous. However, a useful approximation of his standing is available in the form of published comments about his work. In Chapter 3 we saw that he began to take an interest in language disorders in January 1864,[13] at least 4 months before he became aware of Broca and the French debates about language.[14] Later in 1864 he remarked that 'no one in England' had previously paid attention to the deliberations in Paris or to the issue of cerebral domin-ance.[15] The remainder of this section and the next will examine the verity of that statement. To investigate the issue, there are two separate series of published records to follow. One is the news reportage about the Parisian debates in the British medical press,[16] and the second is the record of relevant British cases in their own journals.

To follow the British reports about the French discussions it is necessary to be familiar with two distinct parts of the continental controversies: (1) the Dax priority claims about dominance, and (2) Trousseau's introduction of the term 'aphasia'. With regard to Dax, recall that Broca's correlation of language disorders with lesions in the frontal lobes occurred in 1861. At that time he did not make any observations about left cerebral dominance. Broca first broached the issue of dominance in 1863, and he enunciated the principle of left hemisphere dominance in 1865.[17]

On March 24, 1863, the *Bulletin* of the Academy of Medicine of Paris contained a notice that the Academy had received a sealed package from a rural physician in Sommières, near Montpellier. In it, Gustave Dax (1815–1893) claimed that his late father, Marc Dax (1770–1837), had stated the principle of left cerebral dominance for language in a paper presented to a medical conference in Montpellier in 1836.[18] Some contents of the 'sealed' claim were leaked in 1864, and a final (not unanimous) report was issued by a committee of the Academy in December 1864.[19] Since Broca's first recorded public remarks about the possibility of left dominance were made on April 2, 1863,[20] it is possible but not likely that Broca would have known about the elder Dax until after he made his own speculations on dominance. At the

---

[13] Jackson 1864a.

[14] Jackson 1864c.

[15] Jackson 1864j, p.464.

[16] In searching the popular British medical periodicals of that time, I found only two small, unconnected news items that might contradict Jackson's statement about 'no one in England'. They are in the *British Medical Journal* (*BMJ*) 1:161 and 534, dated February 6 and May 14 1864. This statement is based on searches of the indices of the *British and Foreign Medical Review*, the *BMJ*, *The Lancet*, and the *Medical Times and Gazette* (*MTG*) from 1861 through June 1864; see Greenblatt 1970, p.563, footnote 22. For this book, I repeated these searches in the *BMJ*, *Lancet*, and *MTG* from 1864 through 1868. Lorch (2004a, p.129) conducted a more thorough review of six journals and came to the same conclusion, with the one problematic exception of a paper by Jabez Ramskill, Jackson's colleague at Queen Square (Ramskill 1864; Lorch 2004a). Ramskill's paper was published in the London Hospital's *Clinical Lectures and Reports* for 1864, after Jackson's paper on 'Loss of speech'. Ramskill gave no citations to any of his contemporaries. He used Broca's term 'aphemia' (Ramskill 1864, p.484), but without attribution and mainly to state that his three patients were dysarthric, not aphemic. It is impossible to know where he got the term. Presumably Jackson started to talk about the French debate shortly after he learned about it in May 1864. This first volume of the London Hospital *Reports* was apparently published in September or October 1864; see Chapter 3.

[17] See Chapter 3, section on 'First Encounters'.

[18] See Schiller 1979, p.194, and footnotes 46 and 47 on his p.301. Schiller points out that the same issue of the *Bulletin* contained Broca's application for membership in the Academy of Medicine, including 'The annotated bibliography of Broca's work . . . which contains his tentative views on the left versus the right hemisphere . . . It must have been given to the printers some time ahead'. So Broca's independence from Dax seems to be well substantiated.

[19] See Finger and Roe 1996, pp.808–809.

[20] See Schiller 1979, p.194 and footnote 44.

time, Broca was awarded priority in most people's minds. Recent scholarship has concluded that Marc Dax probably did deliver the paper as his son claimed. However, it was never published, nor were its contents otherwise publicized, until his son sent it to Paris in 1863.[21] In 1866 a reporter covering a case of Jackson's said, 'The almost constant association of loss of speech with hemiplegia of the *right* side has been discovered three times independently ... by M. Dax, M. Broca, and by Dr. Hughlings Jackson'.[22] Presumably the reporter was repeating what Jackson had said.[23]

In the long run, the historical role of Armand Trousseau (1801–1867) was more important, because it was he who introduced the term 'aphasia'. Trousseau was a participant in the debates from 1862, largely in opposition to Broca's localization of 'aphemia' to the lateral third frontal gyrus. In January 1864, Trousseau introduced 'aphasia' to substitute for 'aphemia', because he asserted that the latter actually means 'infamy' in ancient Greek. Since Trousseau was Professor of Clinical Medicine at the Paris medical school, he had a bully pulpit. 'Aphasia' prevailed.[24] All of this occasioned some highly wrought philological exchanges in the French Academy of Medicine, which the British medical press chronicled irregularly and with puckish delight.

In Chapter 3 we saw that the *BMJ* published the first British notice about the French debates on February 6, 1864. It described Broca's addressing 'a learned letter to M. Trousseau', wherein Broca is reported to have asked Trousseau's opinion about the best word 'to explain *loss of voice*'.[25] Another brief report in the *BMJ* of May 14, 1864, again referred to Trousseau's role in the nomenclature debates, without reference to the earlier notice or to Broca or Jackson.[26] The *MTG* carried stories about the French arguments on December 24, 1864, and May 6, 1865.[27] At the end of 1864 Jackson's contributions were discussed in a leading French journal's piece about the debates at their Academy of Medicine.[28]

On July 1, 1865, the *BMJ* devoted nearly a full page to a juicy debate at the Academy of Medicine between Bouillaud and another academician, Alfred Velpeau, mainly about a prize that Bouillaud had offered earlier.[29] And on July 15, 1865, another report in the *BMJ* began with the piquant observation that: 'The love which our French medical academician friends have for learned and eloquent and deep discussion of what we may call impossible questions, has been well exemplified in the long debates on Aphasia in the Academy of Medicine'.[30] There were no further reports about the French debates in the major British medical periodicals, with one intriguing exception. On September 1, 1866, the *BMJ* carried a long 'Leading Article'—really an extended editorial—titled simply 'Aphasia'.[31] Although it was unsigned, it could have been written only by Jackson. No one else in Britain would have written about

---

[21] See Schiller 1979, pp.192–197; Cubelli and Montagna 1994; Roe and Finger 1996; Finger 2000, pp.145–147; Leblanc 2017, pp.87–108.

[22] Jackson 1866o, p.606; italics in original.

[23] In 1872 Jackson referred to 'the hypothesis of Dax and Broca' (Jackson 1872q, p.598, footnote (c)), and in 1874 he referred to 'the researches of Dax and Broca' (Jackson 1874b, p.19).

[24] See Schiller 1979, pp.199–200; Henderson 1990. Jackson first used Trousseau's name and '*aphasia*' in print in 1864 (Jackson 1864c, p.572), when he first acknowledged Broca; see also further references to Trousseau in J64-10, pp.461, 462, 465.

[25] *BMJ* 1:161, 1864.

[26] *BMJ* 1:534, 1864.

[27] *MTG* 2:679, 1864; and 1:473–474, 1865.

[28] Fritz 1864; see also Joynt 1982, p.100. Fritz was apparently discussing Jackson's paper of November 26, 1864 (Jackson 1864l), because he mentioned that Jackson had 70 cases, and Jackson had not previously reported that many.

[29] *BMJ* 1:670, 1865. For details about the prize see Finger 2000, pp.137–139.

[30] *BMJ* 2:40, 1865.

[31] [Jackson] 1866.

the subject so extensively without mentioning Jackson's name. He used the editorial 'we', and in one place he quoted 'a writer in a commentary (*Lancet*, Nov. 26th, 1864)', alluding to his own earlier paper.[32] The main thrust of the editorial was an exhortation against the tyranny of nosology, which Jackson feared would be encouraged by the debate over 'aphemia' versus 'aphasia'. In the last paragraph he declared resoundingly:

> We need constantly to be going back to [real] things, or the names we use will become our masters rather than our servants ... We must use some technical words; but whilst willing to sacrifice part of our freedom for the sake of order, we ought surely not to give up altogether the government of our thoughts, on thought itself, to a tyrant of yesterday.[33]

Strong words for an ordinarily restrained Victorian. Probably Jackson felt emboldened by the anonymity of an editorial, but I doubt that his colleagues had any difficulty identifying its author.

Reports about Language Disorders in British Journals, 1864–1867

Looking back at the British medical scene in 1864, we cannot give Jackson all of the credit for instigating the journalistic reports on aphasia. They started before he knew about the Parisian debates. However, he does get the lion's share of credit for initiating the series of British case reports, because he started the series with his own cases, *and* he asked his readers to publish theirs.[34] The first response that I have found was published by James Russell (1818–1885), a prominent physician in Birmingham. Apparently Russell and Jackson had met in April or May, and Russell was favorably impressed. Starting in the *BMJ* of July 23, 1864, Russell described 38 relevant cases and concluded that his data supported the idea of left dominance for speech.[35] He prefaced his series with the observation that

> Any statement by so laborious and accurate a student of cerebral pathology as Dr. Jackson must be received with much respect; and he had interested me in the subject by a conversation a short time before his letter appeared. I am therefore led to present the result of an examination of my case books, as a contribution towards the inquiry which Dr. Jackson invites.[36]

Another publication related to Jackson's growing reputation was an item in the 'Reviews and Notices' column of the *BMJ* on November 5, 1864, where the entire first volume of the London Hospital's *Clinical Lectures and Reports* was extensively reviewed.[37] Nearly a quarter of the review was devoted to Jackson's paper on 'Loss of speech'. About it, the reviewer said:

> ... the main points ... have already been brought before the profession [by Jackson]. In his most important speculations, he has been anticipated by M. Broca, as he mentions; but

---

[32] Jackson 1864m.

[33] [Jackson] 1866j, p.261; my square brackets.

[34] Jackson 1864c, p.572.

[35] Russell 1864a, 1864b, 1864c. The series of reports was published from July 23 to October 8, 1864. In the final paper (p.410), Russell said that he supported 'Dr. Jackson's hypothesis – definite functional regions, associated with the particular arterial divisions ...'.

[36] Russell 1864a, p.81.

[37] Jackson 1864k.

<u>much merit remains with him</u>. He was the first in this country to remark the association of loss of speech with right hemiplegia; and from this and other observations in epilepsy, etc., he arrived independently at the conclusion, or hypothesis rather, that the faculty of language was seated in the *left* cerebral hemisphere.[38]

After these mildly chauvinistic remarks, the reviewer went on to gently criticize both Jackson and Broca for inconsistencies in their terminologies. This must have been rather heady stuff for a young man only 5 years arrived from the provinces. And there was more to come. From late 1864 through 1867 there were many papers on aphasia in British medical journals. After 1866, Jackson's name often was not mentioned. Nonetheless, the message continued to circulate, with or without the name of the original messenger. Practicality allows discussion of only three articles that have particular historical significance.[39]

One of the important early British papers on aphasia was published in *The Lancet* on May 20, 1865, by Frederic Bateman (1824–1904) of Norwich.[40] He gave an account of a 51-year-old man who had sudden and severe nonfluent aphasia, but little else. After 6 months the patient was partially recovered. Bateman cited Jackson in his brief historical review of British commentators, but the main value of this paper was its review of the continental literature. A more original contribution was published in 1866 by Jackson's friend, Walter Moxon (1836–1886), in the *British and Foreign Medico-Chirurgical Review*.[41] He tried to explain unilateral left hemisphere dominance by postulating that earlier use of the right side in development leads to earlier 'education' of the left hemisphere, including the brain areas that control the organs of articulation. Moxon's paper did not mention any name in the associationist pantheon, but a recent study of Moxon connects his use of 'education' directly to that tradition.[42] At the beginning of Moxon's paper he said: 'no observations have for many years excited in the medical world more intense and general interest than those of M. Broca, upon the coincidence of loss of speech with paralysis of the right side, which have been brought before the profession in England by Dr. H. Jackson, in a comprehensive and able record of cases'.[43] Jackson responded quickly to Moxon's idea about 'education' of the left hemisphere. He accepted Moxon's position, while conjecturing that '... both sides are probably educated, but ... the left is the one that begins to act'.[44]

One of the most interesting commentaries on Jackson's developing ideas was published on December 14, 1867, by H. (Henry) Charlton Bastian (1837–1915), who became a staff colleague of Jackson at Queen Square in that same year. Bastian presented the autopsy results of a 62-year-old woman with renal disease. She had sudden onset of right hemiplegia and nonfluent aphasia, with a few recurrent utterances. She died 8 days later. Autopsy showed diffuse vascular disease, with multiple emboli to the right lung and left brain. The right hemisphere was normal. On the left the cerebral infarcts were entirely limited to the cortical gray

---

[38] Jackson 1864k, p.524; Jackson's italics, my square brackets and underlining.

[39] I surveyed the *BMJ*, *Lancet*, and *MTG* and found: *Lancet* 2:605, 1864 (Barlow); *Lancet* 2:605–606, 1864 (Davies); *BMJ* 1:268, 1865 (news item); *BMJ* 1:209–210, 1866 (Sanders); *BMJ* 1:567–568, 1866 (Russell); *BMJ* 2:276–277, 1866 (Russell); *BMJ* 2:180–181, 1867 (Bramwell), *BMJ* 2:419–421, 1867 (Bateman); Bateman 1865; Bateman 1867; *Lancet* 1:656–657, 1866 (Sanders); *Lancet* 2:145–146, 1866 (Fox); *MTG* 1:377, 1866 (Sanders); *MTG* 1:155–156, 1867 (Ogle); *MTG* 1:537, 1867 (Peacock); *MTG* 2:459–460, 1867 (Peacock); *MTG* 2:670, 1867 (Simpson); *MTG* 2:706–707, 1867 (Ogle); *MTG* 1:57–59, 1868 (Wilks); *MTG* 1:75, 1868 (Simpson); *MTG* 1:87–88, 1868 (Bruce). Jackson acknowledged some of these writers, and others, in his 'anonymous' editorial on aphasia in 1866 ([Jackson] 1866j, pp.260–261).

[40] Bateman 1865; on his role in the later 1860s and 1870s see Radick 2000, and Lorch 2008.

[41] Moxon 1866. Hutchinson 1911, p.1552, certifies Jackson's friendship with Moxon.

[42] Buckingham 2003, p.297.

[43] Moxon 1866, p.481.

[44] Jackson 1866f, p.661.

matter, leaving the subcortical structures intact, including the striatum. There were many hemorrhagic infarcts in the left frontal and parietal lobes, including a large lesion in Broca's area, and another, even larger one in the medial frontal lobe.[45]

Bastian saw two separable problems in this case: localization of the lesions causing (1) the aphasia, and (2) the hemiplegia. Regarding the 'loss of speech',[46] Bastian noted that one of the large lesions was in 'the place indicated by M. Broca as the seat of articulate language'. However, there were even more extensive lesions elsewhere on the left, so a definite conclusion was not possible. Like Jackson, he seemed to view the degrees of deficits as representing a spectrum between 'loss of the power of articulation' and 'an abolition of verbal memory'. Also like Jackson, he had a problem with the 'hypothetical faculty of language'. To account for his patient's findings, Bastian discussed three possible theories, including (1) Brown-Séquard's vasomotor reflex theory, (2) Jackson's vasomotor theory, derived from Brown-Séquard's, and (3) his preferred theory, i.e.,

> ... the suggestion of Dr. Wilks, that hemiplegia may be produced by an extensive lesion of the grey matter of the convolutions of the opposite hemisphere, the mechanism of its production being direct, and immediately dependent upon a destruction or morbid change in the *volitional centre*, which formerly presided over the movements of the opposite half of the body.[47]

In this passage Bastian had put words in Wilks' mouth—or at least in his pen. Wilks did not use the term *'volitional centre'*. Indeed, he had only 'hinted at the possibility that fibers of the motor tract might run downward directly from the cerebral cortex, and that damage to the hemispheres might cause epileptic fits without intervention at the corpus striatum'.[48] Wilks' 'suggestion' was actually correct, but in the late 1860s the cortices were still the territory of the 'will' in the minds of most physicians. Insofar as 'volitional' connoted 'motor', they could not conceive of materialistic motor functions in the cortices. The same presumption was part of the underlying difficulty in the next phase of the debate about language localization.

Jackson and Broca at the British Association, Norwich, August 1868

On August 15, 1868, an item in the news columns of *The Lancet* proclaimed:[49]

M. BROCA AT NORWICH
A very interesting discussion on Aphasia is likely to take place at the British Association meeting [scheduled to open on August 19] at Norwich. M. Broca, whose anatomical

---

[45] Bastian 1867. The patient was admitted to St. Mary's Hospital and examined by 'Dr. Alderson', presumably James Alderson (1794–1882), who became President of the Royal College of Physicians in 1867 (see Brown 1955, pp.2–3). Bastian did not examine the patient himself, although it appears that he performed or observed the autopsy.

[46] Bastian did not use 'aphasia' or 'aphemia' in this paper. In an address in 1868, Jackson also claimed that he 'never uses the terms aphasia, aphemia, etc.' (Jackson 1868n, p.275), but that promise was impossible to keep (see Jackson 1868q, p.358). All of the brief quotations in this paragraph are taken from Bastian 1867, p.545.

[47] Bastian 1867, p.545; italics in original. On p.546, Bastian stressed that he had only recently made acquaintance with Jackson's theory. Bastian gave no citation to Wilks; it is found in Wilks 1866, pp.168–169.

[48] Temkin 1971, p.333.

[49] My analyses in this section and the next are concordant with and partially derived from Lorch 2004b (abstract) and Lorch 2008. See also Leblanc 2017, pp.168–178.

researches in connexion with aphasia have done so much to clear up that difficult subject, will be present, and will doubtless speak in the discussions on Dr. Hughlings Jackson's paper on the same topic. It will be no small attraction to the meeting that visitors will thus have the opportunity of immediately comparing the best English and the best French views on the pathology of this remarkable disease.[50]

Thus was heralded the 'Great Confrontation' that probably never happened—at least no one has ever produced evidence to show that it did.[51] To avoid confusing context and content, I will devote the remainder of this section to the historical events as best we can reconstruct them. The next section will deal with the actual content of what Broca and Jackson each said. About the order of the presentations, which turned out to be important, the reports in three different journals agreed.

> Three papers were read upon the Seat of the Faculty of Articulate Language; viz:
> *The Physiology of Language*. By J. Hughlings Jackson, M.D.
> *Seat of the Faculty of Articulate Language*. By M. Paul Broca.
> *The Power of Utterance in Respect of its Cerebral Bearings and Causes*. By R. Dunn, Esq.[52]

According to the brief summaries in the *BMJ*, Jackson largely restated his previous positions, i.e., (1) the distinction between 'intellectual and emotional' language, (2) the 'leading' role of the left hemisphere, and (3) the differences in the clinical syndromes of language disturbance in relation to the size of the lesion and its distance from the striatum. He postulated that the recurrent utterances of many aphasics are remnants of the 'leading sensori-motor process when the brain was suddenly damaged'.[53] Broca then

> ... demonstrated, by means of a diagram and plaster of Paris casts, his view of localisation of articulate language in the third frontal convolution of the left side, and argued for the corpus striatum as merely the medium of connexion ... He argued for an original organic force which determined the left side of the brain rather than the right ... [and he proposed a four-part] ... terminology for expressing the various forms of defective speech.[54]

---

[50] *Lancet* 2:226, 1868; my square brackets. An earlier, general notice appeared in the *Lancet* on July 25, 1868 (2:121). It listed Broca among the expected foreign guests and said, 'The meeting promises to be one of very great interest'. In *The Times* of London, on Monday, August 17, 1868 (p.40), there was an announcement about the BA meeting. It included Broca's name in the long list of 'foreign visitors'. The invitation to Broca was issued by Bateman, who practised in Norwich (see Lorch 2008, p.1660; also Schiller 1979, p.203).

[51] Robert Joynt (1982) was apparently the first to express scepticism about this iconic event. The mythical part may have originated with Head (Lorch 2008, p.1665). In Schiller's discussion of the events at the BA (1979, pp.203–205) he says nothing about any debate. The Critchleys (1998, p.93) agree with Joynt. Lorch (2008, pp.1660–1663) has laid out convincing evidence against an actual debate between Broca and Jackson, to which conclusion my analysis concurs.

[52] *BMJ* 2:259 (September 5, 1868); this is the same as Jackson 1868o, p.259. In addition, the *Lancet* (August 29, 1868) (British Association 1868) and the *MTG* (2:275–276, September 5, 1868; same as Jackson 1868n, pp.275–276) give the same order of the presentations. The official *Report* of the meeting (British Association 1869, p.120) lists Broca's and Jackson's contributions only by title and in that order, but it includes an abstract of Dunn's paper (pp.114–115). The *Lancet* introduced the authors and titles with the remark that, 'The interest of the medical philosophers culminated in the three following papers ...' (British Association 1868, p.293).

[53] *BMJ* 2:259 (September 5, 1868); this is the same as Jackson 1868p, p.259.

[54] *BMJ* 2:259, 1868; my square brackets. Presumably Broca's 'original organic force' meant that dominance is inborn, not that Broca invoked crude vitalism.

Finally, 'Mr. Dunn argued for the dependence of utterance upon the corpus striatum ...' His lengthy paper argued against exclusively left-sided dominance.[55] By all accounts, after the formal papers, 'A very animated discussion took place'.[56] Combining the names of the discussants from the reports in the three weekly journals, there was a total of nine individuals who got into the act, plus Broca, *but not Jackson*.[57] So the question arises whether Jackson was actually present for the discussion, and the evidence for his absence is more compelling than for his presence.

At the end of its report, *The Lancet* said: 'It must be stated that Professor Broca, in reply, combated with great ability the objections to his theory ...'[58] If Jackson had said anything in the discussion, surely the reporter would have noted it, especially since there was an undertone of national pride in *The Lancet* reports. Indeed, nationalistic sensitivities might explain why the reporters were careful not to lament Jackson's apparent absence. Either he said nothing in the discussions or he wasn't there. His absence seems more likely, because he would have been called upon if he were in the room.

All of this makes sense in light of the contrasting positions and personalities of the two supposed antagonists. In 1868 Broca had reached the pinnacle of French academic medicine. He had been elected to the Academy of Medicine *and* Professor in the faculty of medicine in 1867. He got there because he thrived in the vicious rough and tumble of that environment,[59] so defending himself at the BA would have presented only a linguistic challenge. In the same year, 'Broca's views [on aphasia] took their final shape. After that he practically ceased to study this thorny and slippery subject'.[60] By 1868, Broca's primary interests in anthropology and surgery were reclaiming his attention.[61] During the BA meeting Broca attended various sessions, and he offered comments on some of the papers.[62]

At age 33, on the other hand, Jackson was 11 years younger than Broca and still very much on the make in London, albeit quietly. At smaller medical gatherings Jackson had shown a ready willingness to comment on others' papers,[63] and in print he guarded his intellectual independence with fierce precision. However, he was congenitally nonconfrontational. Moreover, his 'dread of being bored was extreme', and 'It was almost impossible to induce him to incur the risk of having to sit through a lecture or long speech'.[64] He disliked ceremonial occasions and large meetings, and there was a surfeit of both in Norwich.[65] Another factor, I suspect, was the pre-meeting publicity and its attendant expectations.

From the available evidence I conclude—tentatively—that Jackson delivered his paper, perhaps listened to Broca's paper, maybe to Dunn's, and then he fled. Indeed, the possibility

---

[55] *BMJ* 2:259, 1868; for longer summaries of Dunn's paper see Jackson 1868n, pp.276–277, and British Association 1869, pp.114–115.

[56] British Association 1868, p.293.

[57] *The Lancet* listed the discussants as Bateman, Hughes Bennett, 'Dr. Humphrey, of Cambridge', 'Mr. Gilson and Professor Voit' [probably a misspelling of Vogt] (British Association 1868, p.293). In addition, the *BMJ* (Jackson 1868o) listed 'Dr. J. Thompson Dickson' and 'Dr. Crisp', and the *MTG* (Jackson 1868n) included 'Professor Carl Vogt', 'Dr. Crisp', and 'Sir Duncan Gibb'. On Dickson see Eadie 2007d, and Chapter 7.

[58] British Association 1868, p.294.

[59] See Schiller 1979, pp.84–89, and Greenblatt 2006.

[60] Schiller 1979, pp.201–202; my square brackets.

[61] See Schiller 1979, pp.201–202; also Joynt 1982, pp.100–101; Henderson 1986; and Leblanc 2017, pp.177–193.

[62] British Association 1868, p.293.

[63] See e.g. Jackson 1866m.

[64] Hutchinson 1911, p.1553.

[65] Lorch 2004b states that there were 2,000 people at Norwich. Howarth 1931 gives average figures that accord approximately with Lorch, especially given that there was also an International Congress of Prehistoric Archaeology at Norwich, which probably diverted the attention of Broca and others from the main event at the BA; see British Association 1868, p.291.

arises that Jackson may not have been in the audience for Broca's presentation.[66] Based on the reports of the meeting in *The Times* of London, Jackson's was the last paper on Monday, August 25, in the session of the 'Department of Anatomy and Physiology'. Broca's was the first on the next day, Tuesday, August 26, so the 'animated discussion' would have happened on the day after Jackson's presentation. Since the Monday session ended after Jackson's paper, he could have easily slipped away then or the following morning, thus avoiding the possibility of an uncomfortable confrontation with anyone.[67] We get no hint of any of this from the reports of the BA meeting in *The Lancet*. Shortly after the meeting ended, that journal said: 'The discussion of the physiology of language by Dr. Jackson and Professor Broca, is too large and important a matter to be dealt with here; but on a future occasion we shall give an analysis of Dr. Jackson's paper, and of the debate which followed.'[68] True to its promise, on September 19 *The Lancet* devoted nearly a full page to an editorial on the subject. It began by declaring:

> The Norwich discussion raises once again the question of the intimate physiological nature of that curious cerebral change which produces the disease known under the various names of aphasia ... There has seldom been, in the history of medical polemics, a more <u>singularly tangled controversy</u> than this ...
>
> If we endeavour now ... to get at the solid facts and principles which still remain ... it is not impossible to see how the idea of aphasia first fashioned itself, and the form which the doctrine is likely ultimately to assume.[69]

The editorial went on to review the discoveries of Dax and Broca (in that order) and the 'semi-phrenological view' of Bouillaud. Rejecting any '"simple" explanation of the whole affair', *The Lancet* asserted:

> ... there was at first a general disposition to settle this matter of aphasia by a rude application of a bastard phrenology. <u>If there be one writer more than another to whom medicine is indebted for having first drawn attention to the insufficiency of this kind of view, it is Dr. J. Hughlings Jackson.</u> He it was who ... insisted first, that language was a very much more complicated faculty than had been assumed; and, secondly, that if a large number of fatal cases of aphasia showed lesions about the neighborhood of the third frontal convolution, that was as much as to say that a large proportion of those cases had lesions in the immediate surroundings of the corpora striata, i.e., in the most important centre and meeting place of the various fibres of the brain.[70]

The implication here is not very subtle. According to *The Lancet*, the French made the original observations about aphasia, but they tried to understand it by 'rude application of a

---

[66] See Lorch 2008, pp.1664–1665.

[67] See *The Times*, Tuesday, August 25, 1868, p.9, which reported that for Monday, August 24, the papers to be read in the 'Department of Anatomy and Physiology' were by Rolleston, Richardson, Crum Brown, Jackson, Broca, Dunn, and Dickson, in that order. For the following day, Tuesday, August 25, *The Times* (Wednesday, August 26, p.4) began the same kind of list with Broca. Furthermore, *The Times* of August 27, 1868, p.8, said that the Department of Anatomy and Physiology would begin its session of Wednesday, August 26 with Dickson's paper, since that is the one previously listed to follow Dunn. This confirms that much time was consumed by the discussion after Dunn's paper on August 25.

[68] *Lancet* 2:286 (August 29, 1868).

[69] *Lancet* editorial 1868; my underlining.

[70] *Lancet* editorial 1868; my underlining.

bastard phrenology'. Now Jackson (i.e. England) was leading the way to its clarification. Since the English were inclined toward associationism, rather than the faculty psychology, such a claim could be valid, at least with regard to their respective systems of psychological theory. In truth, of course, the entire subject has always been a 'singularly tangled controversy'.

Before I go on to my analysis of Jackson's developing thoughts, let me insert a reality check. *The Times* (London) gave no coverage to the papers on aphasia or to the debates about it. Following each day's sessions, *The Times* devoted extensive space to the ceremonies at the BA and to many of the papers. The subjects it reported in detail were mainly in fields that we would call technology and public health, i.e., practical stuff. In line with the longstanding interests of the British intelligentsia, there was significant attention paid to geology and archaeology, and 'Darwinism' got some notice.[71] Presumably *The Times*' editors felt that aphasia held little interest for most of its readers. Since the BA was not primarily a medical organization, none of this should be surprising. Still, the conclusion remains that problems in the science of physiology, including the brain, did not command much attention from the reading public.

Aphasia and Brain Organization at the BA, Norwich, August 1868

In their respective addresses at Norwich, Broca and Jackson described similar clinical presentations of their aphasic patients. They were both seeing the same range of clinical phenomena. This is to be expected—they were both astute observers. What was different was their conceptualizations of how to understand what they were seeing. Broca's primary objective was to suggest a new classification and nomenclature for the different types of clinical appearances. His first and fourth groups were, in our terms, (1) language disturbances associated with dementias and (4) dysarthrias. He wanted to call them 'alogia' and 'alalia' respectively. In his second group he described patients with impaired intellect and 'loss of speech', which he wanted to name 'verbal amnesia'. Broca's third group of patients would now be said to have Broca's aphasia. Ignoring Trousseau's offer of 'aphasia', Broca still wanted to call their condition 'aphemia'.[72] So, at bottom, he was interested in clinical classification, though he emphasized that 'Loss of speech is not a particular disease...'.[73]

With regard to localization, Broca insisted only that the posterior left third frontal convolution (now 'Broca's area') is important. He did mention that the lesions in his second and third groups (now Wernicke's and Broca's aphasias) are probably close to each other; and he explained cases of aphasia with lesions in the 'Island of Reil' (insula), but not in the third frontal convolution, by postulating that the insular lesion cut off Broca's area from the striatum. In other words, he did not make any direct connection between the insular lesion and the patient's clinical presentation. Interestingly, Broca said little about dominance.[74]

Jackson's more physiological orientation is clear from the beginning of his paper. He started with a discussion of the hemiplegia that is frequently seen in association with aphasia. It involves mainly voluntary movements: 'This kind of paralysis depends on damage to the

[71] See *The Times* of August 20, p.6; August 21, p.4; August 22, p.4; August 24, p.7; August 25, p.9; August 26, p.4; August 27, p.8; August 28, p.9. Bellon 2011 (pp.416–417) states that after Darwin's earlier struggles with his critics, 'Darwinism received its triumphant settlement as the theory of the scientific establishment' at the BA's meeting in Norwich in 1868.

[72] Schiller 1979, pp.201–203; see also J68 15, p.259.

[73] Schiller 1979, p.202. In 1869 Broca again offered the same classification; see Henderson 1986, p.611.

[74] Schiller 1979, p.203.

very highest parts of the motor tract – viz., the corpus striatum ... In other words it shows loss of function of a motor centre, which is *embedded in the cerebral hemisphere*; or, to speak metaphorically, which *lies close upon mind*...'[75] When 'intellectual' and 'emotional' language 'are separated by disease', he said, for intellectual language, 'It is the power of intellectual expression by "movements" of any kind which is impaired – those most special, as of speech, suffering most; those of simple sign-making least...'[76] With that background he defined two classes of patients with defects of intellectual language:

> *Class* I. – Severe cases in which the patient is speechless or nearly so, or in which speech is very much damaged. In the worst of these cases the patient can only utter some one unvarying word or two words, or some jargon ... In these cases power to read write and make simple signs is impaired ...[77]

In our terms, the patients in Jackson's Class I are *nonfluent*, probably a mixture of severe Broca's aphasics and some mixed and global cases. They are contrasted to Jackson's

> *Class* II. – Cases in which there are plentiful movements but wrong movements, or *plenty of words but mistakes in words*.
>   Under Class II. He points out that taking the phenomena of many cases, we find evidence of damage to sensori-motor processes, higher or lower in evolution according to (*a*) Complexity of movements. (*b*) Width of interrelation. (*c*) Number of associations from ataxy of the grosser movements of articulation to an 'ataxy' of movements embodying ideas.[78]

Then Jackson gave a fascinating description of the spectrum of '*mistakes in words*', from 'Ataxy of articulation – often an unintelligible gabble' to paraphasias in 'processes so high in complexity, (interrelation and association) there is usually a traceable similarity ... betwixt the phrase used and the one intended'.[79] Again, in our terms the patients in Class I are *nonfluent*, and those in Class II are *fluent*. Fluency is now our first criterion in the classification of aphasias. Broca also made essentially the same distinction. The idea that Jackson's Class II (fluent) patients were largely sensory (receptive) aphasics was amply confirmed a little later in his paper, when he posited a series of rhetorical questions about the clinical findings in the two classes. The questions show how he examined his aphasic patients *and* how he analyzed the results.

> (*c*) Do the patients know what is said to them?
>   It is usually held that "aphasic persons" do. The author thinks they usually do when they are speechless except for some unvarying jargon [in Class I, nonfluent] ... but that when ... they have free but disorderly utterance so high as mistakes in words [Class II, fluent] they often do not understand, *i.e.*, quickly understand words said to them?
>   (*d*) Can the patients repeat words said to them?

---

[75] Jackson 1868p, p.237; Jackson's italics. My summary of Jackson's paper is based largely on the abstract in *The Medical Press and Circular* (Jackson 1868p; also reprinted in Lorch 2008, pp.1666–1670), because it is more detailed than the abstract in the *MTG* (Jackson 1868n).

[76] Jackson 1868p, p.237; Jackson's italics.

[77] Jackson 1868p, p.237.

[78] Jackson 1868p, p.237; Jackson's italics.

[79] Jackson 1868p, p.237.

They cannot in Class I.; in Class II. they can, with or without blunders.

The author supposes the reason in (c) and (d) to be:

That in Class I. [nonfluent], the sensori-motor arrangements for speech are destroyed in their lowest processes by limited disease near to, and involving the corpus-striatum. The sensory aspect of the sensori-motor processes of mind is not reached. It is the "way out" which is broken up.

That in Class II. [fluent], the sensori-motor processes are impaired but not destroyed, and that the change is not limited to the region of the corpus-striatum, but reaches deeper [higher] in brain.[80]

In his answer to (c) Jackson was clearly describing the poor auditory comprehension of patients with fluent aphasia, but that is our way of thinking about the clinical phenomena, not his. At this stage in his development he simply had the idea that sensory processes somehow penetrate 'deeper in brain' than their motor counterparts. Getting back to the motor side, although Jackson did not accept Moxon's explanation of dominance, he did apply Moxon's associationist view of 'educated movements' to the physiology of speech.

The movements of speech are educated movements and thus differ widely from those movements which may be said to be nearly perfect at birth, such as those for respiration, smiling, swallowing, &c. All the muscles represented in the corpus striatum unilaterally require a long education, and the most special of these are those engaged in the movements of speech, and next those of the arm ... the term "Intellectual language" merges in the larger term "Special movements acquired by the individual," and the term "Emotional" language in the term "Inherited movements," (common to the race) ...[81]

Using this distinction, Jackson applied Spencerian hierarchical analysis to aphasics' recurrent utterances and other verbal 'ejaculations'. There is, he said, 'an ascent in 'compound degree' from the 'common explosive oath' to 'actual propositions', until the 'difference betwixt voluntary and involuntary utterance is effaced'.[82] From there he continued his discussion of recurrent utterances.

The above-mentioned series of phenomena show ... that there are sensori-motor processes for words somewhere, though usually the "will" cannot get at them.

This somewhere can scarcely be on the *left* side of the brain, for damage of this side has made the man speechless. These involuntary utterances are, [Jackson] supposes the result of action of the *right* side. In other words, he thinks that the left is the leading side, and the right the automatic.[83]

In this passage, and again later, Jackson proposed that the right (nondominant) hemisphere has a function in speech processing that is 'automatic', i.e., involuntary. He continued to

---

[80] Jackson 1868p, p.238; my square brackets and underlining. When he introduced his dual classification of the aphasias, Jackson said, 'In the first class [nonfluent] the author supposes that the sensori-motor processes for speech are more or less *destroyed*; in the second [fluent] that they are *unstable*' (Jackson 1868p, p.237; Jackson's italics).

[81] Jackson 1868p, p.238.

[82] Jackson 1868p, p.238. For an explanation of 'compound' in association theory see Definition Section 7 in this chapter.

[83] Jackson 1868p, p.238.

operate on this assumption, but it was only an assumption. He had no clinical or clinico-pathological evidence for it. He simply went on to the related issue of:

THE WILL

[Jackson] then tries to shew [sic] the relation of the so-called "will" to the rest of the sensori-motor processes, and this time takes his illustrations from the stock words or phrazes [sic] which the patients always use ... it is probable that the stock phraze [sic] was the leading sensori-motor process, when the brain was suddenly damaged ...

He then speaks of Spencer's views on the "will," and ... in accordance with those views, calls the "will" the *leading* sensori-motor process of the moment – there being no such separation as Will *and* Mind.[84]

Here the toe of materialistic physiology is getting into the door of the last bastion of the immaterial 'will' in the cerebral cortices. But this materialistic claim is valid only when one accepts the following proposition: If the will is a sensori-motor process, and will and mind are equivalent, then mind is a sensori-motor process. This was the position of the associationists, and it was Spencer who was leading Jackson to venture in this direction, although Jackson was still quite tentative about it. Rather than following out the consequences of his remarks about the will, he turned back to an earlier issue:

THE LEFT SIDE OF THE BRAIN THE LEADING SIDE, THE RIGHT THE AUTOMATIC

... [Jackson] does not think as Dr. Moxon does, that the left side of the brain only is educated, but that both are educated ...

Although the cerebral hemisphere[s] are twins, the left may, if we accept Gratiolet's[1] statement, be said to be the first born. It is born with the lead ...[85]

The French neuroanatomist, Pierre Gratiolet (1815–1865), was a participant in the original discussions about language localization in Paris in 1861.[86] A few years earlier he had published a major treatise on comparative neuroanatomy. According to Jackson's description,

Gratiolet's observations show not only that the *frontal* convolutions ... of the left side are developed in advance of those on the right, but that the [right] sphenoidal [temporal] and *occipital* convolutions ... are in advance of those of the left. May we not suppose that the right is the leading side, and the left the automatic side for "educated sensation?"[87]

Gratiolet's claim of earlier development of the left frontal lobe, as compared to the right, was later shown to be wrong. At the time, however, Jackson thought he had found a

---

[84] Jackson 1868p, p.238; Jackson's italics.

[85] Jackson 1868p, pp.238–239. On Gratiolet see Leblanc 2017, pp.49–61, etc.

[86] See Schiller 1979, pp.166–177. For a brief biography see Haymaker and Schiller 1970, pp.39–43. For more on Gratiolet's role in the debates of 1861 see Lorch 2011 and Leblanc 2017.

[87] Jackson 1868p, p.239, footnote 1; Jackson's italics, my square brackets and underlining. Jackson's first published notice of Gratiolet was in June 1866, when he said, 'M. Baillarger quotes from Gratiolet a statement to the effect that the frontal convolutions on the left side are in advance of those on the right in their development. Hence ... the left side of the brain is sooner ready for learning. It is the elder brother' (Jackson 1866f, p.661). On August 15, 1868, Jackson repeated the same wording, adding the phrase 'and takes the lead through life' at the end (Jackson 1868l, p.179). So it appears that by the time of his presentation at the BA, Jackson had looked into Gratiolet's writings for himself. Harrington 1987, p.57, footnote 6, provides a translation of the crucial passage from Gratiolet.

morphological asymmetry to correlate with his clinical and pathological evidence of left cerebral dominance for speech. I get the sense that one possible motivation for his plea ('May we not suppose') was an effort to 'save the appearances' of biological symmetry by assigning a function to the seemingly neglected right side. It appears to be a case of biological egalitarianism—if the left frontal lobe has such an important role in speech output, surely the right must also be important for something else. Jackson's assignment of automatic function(s) to the right hemisphere is entirely speculative. He offered no clinical data to support it—only the assumption that automatic speech must come from the right hemisphere, because sufficient damage to the left can make a man 'speechless', i.e., without voluntary, propositional speech.[88]

At this point in his paper at the BA, Jackson turned rather abruptly to the basic problem underlying all of these issues—the nature of cerebral 'LOCALIZATION'—and he started with a delightful Victorian analogy.

> The author [Jackson] does not attempt to localize language in any limited spot. The object is to find in <u>mind</u> the latitude and longitude of the defect, and in <u>brain</u> the corresponding latitude and longitude of the *damage* – the corpus striatum being the Greenwich.
>
> Destruction of parts of the hemisphere at a distance from the motor tract *need* produce no *obvious* mental symptoms of any kind. An equivalent quantity of destruction of parts near the (left) corpus striatum will, however, cause defects of intellectual expression. He thinks that the quantity of defect depends generally on the (1) quantity of destruction of tissue, and (2) on its nearness to … the corpus striatum … (The author here quotes Mr. Dunn, who has long held essentially similar opinions).
>
> … He believes … [his] principle of localization is essentially the same as that given by Spencer.
>
> Taking the corpus striatum and optic thalamus as the illustration, the author speaks of the "localization of the limbs." He thinks the facts supplied by an observation of many cases of damage to these [striatal] bodies show –
>
> 1. That both the arm and leg are represented throughout these bodies.
> 2. That there is an order of representation according to the "intelligence" of parts.
> The arm is *more* represented than the leg, the hand than the arm, and the thumb and first [index] finger than the rest of the hand.
> 3. That there is also a representation of speciality, there being localities where even the less intelligent parts have the leading representation.[89]

This long passage is a prime example of Jackson's 'comparative' method at work in the combined study of epilepsy and aphasia, where he had plenty of clinical evidence. That evidence supported his application of Spencer's 'units' in the localization of motor function, which included speech.

> … putting the above another way. He thinks that pathology shows the corpus striatum to be made up of physiological units – this term he takes from Spencer – each representing potentially the whole of the limb. Yet that there are not repetitions of exactly similar units, but that each unit superintends a *different* movement of the *whole* limb.

---

[88] Jackson 1868p, p.238.
[89] Jackson 1868p, p.239; Jackson's italics and parentheses, my square brackets and underlining.

So admitting that speech resides in each part of the brain, he supposes that there are points – probably in Broca's convolution – where the most immediate processes for talking are *specially* represented, and that there will be others near the corpus striatum where other acquired "faculties" – for instance, the movements of the arm for playing the violin, &c., &c., are *specially* represented, but that there is no localization in the sense that one part superintends one thing and no other.[90]

The last clause is a rejection of oversimplified, phrenological thinking. The first part of the quotation shows that Spencer's idea of 'physiological units' was central to Jackson's increasingly sophisticated view of graded and overlapping localization.[91] This is a place where a piece of speculative Spencerian philosophy is woven into the fabric of modern neuroscience, because Jackson's conception of localization is immanent in Spencer's physiological unit. His mature theories of localization were developed directly from this starting point.

The Status of a Unified Cerebral Pathophysiology, August–September 1868

Overview of Jackson's Unified Cerebral Physiology and Pathophysiology as of August 1868

By late August 1868, Jackson had a conception of the combined pathophysiologies of unilateral phenomena that was sufficiently comprehensive to be called 'unified', and it was beginning to attract the attention of his contemporaries. In historical context, it represents an intermediate stage in his development. Unfortunately, to the extent that there was unification it was in Jackson's head, not in his writings. He never presented a complete synthesis of his views in any single publication. For 1868—and for the remainder of his career—one has to piece together the whole from its scattered parts. I will now do this as of 1868, but I wonder whether Jackson himself ever took a similar overview of his entire conceptual scheme. By forcing his ideas into a single outline, I may be giving them a coherency that they really didn't have. This is a particular concern with regard to his views of normal brain function. On the other hand, the cohesion of Jackson's ideas—or lack thereof—is one of the main themes of this book.

The Cortex and the Motor System

In 1868 Jackson and his contemporaries still perceived the hemispheric cortices to be the province of the mind. Parts of the mind included memory, intellect, and especially the 'will'. Following the tenets of association theory, Jackson held that all mental processes are sensorimotor. There was little problem in conceiving of sensory perceptions penetrating into the cortices ('deeper in brain'), because that idea carried no implication of materialism. On the other hand, the motor side of 'sensori-motor' was problematic. Allowing the presence of motor activity into the hemispheric cortices would violate a centuries-old principle, because motor activity was thought to be corporeal and therefore mechanistic. For Jackson the problem was especially acute, because his view of physiology, normal and abnormal, was increasingly focused on the motor system. In fact, the will had a quasi-motor aspect, because

---

[90] Jackson 1868p, p.239; Jackson's italics.
[91] York and Steinberg 2007, pp.17–18, describe Jackson's localization theory formally as 'weighted ordinal representation'. Walshe 1961, p.22, used 'graded, overlapping'.

it could direct the actions of the motor system through the striatum. By implication, this meant that there had to be connections from the cortices to the striatum, but Jackson did not address that issue in the period up to 1868. The will simply had a requisite relay in the striatum, and then the motor system extended down to the brainstem, spinal cord, and muscles. In sum, the physiological relationship between the motor functions of the striatum and the motor aspects of the nearby cortex remained undefined.

Localization in the Striatum

In accordance with his Spencerian approach, Jackson postulated a specific form of localization for motor functions in the striatum. By 1867 he understood that what is represented in grey matter are movements, not individual muscles, although this conception was not stated explicitly until 1869.[92] Moreover, in his view it was mainly voluntary, unilateral movements that are represented. Movements that occur bilaterally and simultaneously are less voluntary and so are less represented. Following Broadbent, Jackson accepted the (inaccurate) idea that there are strong interhemispheric connections of the parts of the corpora striata that represent the less voluntary movements. This meant that the combined representations in the two corpora striata were thought to function as a single nucleus for automatic movements.

Jackson's earlier view of the localization of voluntary movements in the striatum held that all such movements were represented everywhere to an equal degree. By August 1868 he was beginning to think that maybe the striatum is not so egalitarian—some movements probably have more representation in one part than in another. Using Spencer's physiological units, he conceived of a multitude of networks, each for a different movement. Whether he grasped the modern notion that the same neural cells might participate in many different networks is uncertain; it seems to be implied but it is not explicitly stated. In any case, highly voluntary movements would have more and stronger networks than less voluntary, automatic movements, but all voluntary body movements would be represented to some degree throughout the contralateral striatum. Although Jackson lacked the neuron theory, his conception of graded and overlapping localization has been amply confirmed by modern neuroscience—in the cortex but not in the striatum. It first appeared in recognizable form at the BA in August 1868.

Hierarchical Organization and Dominance

Jackson thought about movements in a spectrum, from purely automatic (involuntary) to highly voluntary. Following Moxon, he explained this spectrum in terms of the degrees of postnatal education of the neural substrate that are required to bring the voluntary movements to functional maturity. All of this fitted nicely with the increasingly hierarchical view of cerebral organization that he was imbibing from Spencer.

Concerning *left hemispheric dominance for language*, Jackson adopted Gratiolet's embryological claim that the left frontal brain areas develop before those on the right, so the left (including Broca's area) is educated ahead of the right. Here again there is the potential for a slippery slope toward allowing motor processes to extend above the striatum, because Jackson was suggesting the possibility that the cortices closest to the striatum might be involved in directing the voluntary movements of articulation. This meant that cortex at

---

[92] See Jackson 1867i, p.662: '... each movement of the arm is represented ...'; and Jackson 1869m, p.481: '... the units of the corpus striatum do not represent groups of muscles of the arm, but movements of the whole limb'. In 1873 (Jackson 1873k, p.531), he used a pithy analogy: 'The nervous centres represent movements, not muscles; chords, not notes.'

a greater distance from the striatum was more involved with purely intellectual activity. In that way, localized functions were creeping into the supposedly equipotential, hemispheric cortices. It is possible that Jackson was not aware of this tendency, but I think it's more likely that he chose to follow it wherever it might lead. Indeed, he seemed to be abandoning equipotentiality when he raised the possibility that the right hemisphere is more highly educated for sensation and perception.

Neural Tissue: Its Metabolism, Vascular Territories, and Vasomotor Innervation

There was no widely accepted neuron theory until approximately 1891, so Jackson's ideas were formulated in the pre-neuron era. The microscopic techniques of the mid-century showed only that neural tissue was composed of two kinds of structures: 'fibers' or 'filaments' *and* 'cells' or 'globules'.[93] Jackson and his contemporaries thought about cells and fibers as separate entities. In 1868, the nature of the connections between the cells and the fibers was just beginning to arouse the serious attention of microscopists.[94] When Jackson discussed neural events at the histological ('minute') level, he usually referred to 'nerve tissue' or 'neural tissue', without specifying its constituents. This is seen in his definition of the biological purpose of such tissue: 'It is the function of <u>nervous</u> <u>matter</u> to store up force for *future* expenditure.'[95] This force was derived from nutrition supplied by the blood. At the time he could not have had any deeper understanding of neuronal metabolism, and he could not have known about synapses, membranes, or the blood–brain barrier.

On the other hand, Jackson had a conception of vascular territories in the brain, as he showed in his *Suggestions* of 1863. In February 1869, he expressed his thoughts 'on the importance of considering the relations parts have by their arterial supply. Arteries give to parts which have no relationship by continuity of duties, a relationship by community of nutrition.'[96] As long as the cortices were thought to be equipotential, knowing which artery supplied which cortical part had little practical value. But knowing that the left middle cerebral artery supplies Broca's area is important if we think that that area has some function that might be disturbed when it is damaged. Since Jackson attributed a central role to the striatum, the fact that the left middle cerebral artery supplies the left striatum was significant.

'Community of nutrition' was important for another reason. Because of his friendship with Brown-Séquard, Jackson gave extra attention to the existence and reflex nature of the vasomotor nerves in the cerebral arteries. Thus he developed an idea about '*arterial integration*. My speculation is, that the cerebral arteries in health have to do with the *orderly development* of the functions of nerve centres, and that their contraction is one factor in the *disorderly development* of the phenomena of chorea, convulsion, etc.'[97] In our terms, Jackson thought (correctly) that constriction of the cerebral arteries could affect the metabolic rate of tissue and thereby control the tissue's rate of function. Extending Brown-Séquard's ideas about vasomotor reflexes, Jackson went on to a more specific formulation. According to his theory, any lesion that irritates its vascular bed could cause reflex vasospasm in the entire territory of the middle cerebral artery, including the ipsilateral striatum.[98] In theory the same phenomenon could occur in any vascular territory, but little was known about the functions

---

[93] See Definition Section 1 in Chapter 3.
[94] See Shepherd 1991, pp.27–55; and Schmahmann and Pandya 2007, pp.250–256.
[95] Jackson 1867h, p.642; Jackson's italics, my underlining.
[96] Jackson 1869a, p.307.
[97] Jackson 1868r, pp.302–303; see also Jackson 1868l, pp.177–178.
[98] Vasospasm is constriction of arteries by contraction of the muscle in their walls. For Jackson's more extended explanation of his theory see his section on 'Arterial regions of the brain' in Jackson 1868l, pp.177–178.

of cortical or subcortical tissue in the distributions of the anterior and posterior cerebral arteries.[99]

Principles of Neurological Pathophysiology

Jackson may have learned the distinction between completely destructive versus disruptive (incomplete) lesions from Brown-Séquard, or he may have derived it on his own.[100] Dead tissue can produce only negative symptoms—its clinical manifestation can be only the absence of its function(s). In Jackson's experience, destruction of tissue was often due to either 'coarse disease' (e.g., tumors or inflammatory lesions) or interrupted blood supply (stroke).[101] On the other hand, tissue that is alive but dysfunctional may produce positive symptoms. These are clinically observable phenomena that are alterations or exaggerations of the normal functions of that tissue, e.g., focal seizures or recurrent utterances in aphasics. This understanding of living but dysfunctional neural tissue was a unifying concept, because it explains the pathogenesis of many different clinical phenomena by relating each one to an abnormality in a specific area of the brain. This goal of reductive explanation is part of the background for the prescription to:

'First Localize the Lesion'

As explained in Chapter 1, a basic rule of neurology is our instruction to students: 'First localize the lesion, then decide the pathology.' Experienced clinicians can often identify the anatomical location *and* the pathology of a patient's complaint quite quickly, based on their knowledge of common clinical patterns. But all of us fall back on this fundamental rule when the origin of a patient's problem is not obvious.[102] In his lecture on method of June 1864, Jackson showed that he understood the importance of locating lesions in the central nervous system by physiological reasoning. He gravitated toward the study of unilateral phenomena because their clinical focality implied the possibility of anatomic specificity.

Interpreting Unilateral Phenomena in a Coherent Framework

From the beginning of his work in the early 1860s Jackson viewed hemiplegia, unilateral seizures, hemichorea, and aphasia as different manifestations of similar localizations in the striatum. By August 1868 he could use his evolving principles to advance his interpretations. Hemiplegia is a negative phenomenon, because, according to Jackson's localization at the time, it is due to complete loss of function of the contralateral striatum. Unilateral seizures and hemichorea, on the other hand, are positive phenomena; they result from instability of dysfunctional but living neural tissue. However, they are clinically and physiologically different, he said, because motor seizures commonly manifest as gross, often antagonistic movements, whereas choreic movements show some apparent coordination and therefore they are more highly educated. He explained the greater frequency of seizures involving the face or thumb/hand by reference to his recently reformulated theory of graded and overlapping localization, where there are more assemblies of neural tissue ('units') devoted to those parts of the body that perform more complex, voluntary movements.

---

[99]   In March 1869 Jackson summarized the state of knowledge about vascular territories and stroke: 'The middle cerebral artery is said to be more often plugged than any other cerebral artery. But symptoms of plugging of the other cerebral vessels – excepting the arteria centralis retinae – are not yet known' (Jackson 1869g, p.236).

[100]   See Chapter 4.

[101]   See Jackson 1866m, p.587; and below in this chapter.

[102]   A statement similar to the instruction to 'first localize' is given by Felix von Niemeyer (1820–1871) in Niemeyer 1870, p.29 (*Clinical Remarks*).

Jackson also saw the clinical aspects of aphasia as a spectrum. Since propositionizing is a function of the mind, patients who produce large amounts of mistaken or meaningless speech have mental defects, he said. This may be due to cortical damage at a distance from the striatum, but it cannot be localized any further. On the other hand, patients who produce little or no language generally seem to have intact minds, although they have lost the ability to remember words or to articulate them. Empirically, the latter type of patient is often found to have damage in or near Broca's area in the left inferior third frontal gyrus. Since this area is close to the left striatum, Jackson reasoned that Broca's cortical area may contain some representation of articulation, which in his scheme was a highly educated function.

As of August 1868 Jackson thought that relatively localized cortical damage in or near Broca's area produces a deficit of 'articulatory' (expressive) language, whereas more widespread damage at a distance from Broca's area may produce relatively little expressive deficit, because there is such a wide field of undifferentiated cortex still devoted to the mind. He explained the recurrent utterances of nonfluent aphasics as the products of instability in the partially educated tissue of the nondominant hemisphere, rather than invoking a role for residual tissue on the dominant left side. At this point in his development, he had not given any sustained attention to the phenomena of clinical recovery. In any case, language output is a highly educated, voluntary activity, so its neural representation is highly unilateral.

The Physiology and Pathology of Chorea

In all previous studies of Jackson's ideas, including my own, chorea has been the neglected stepchild, probably because his contribution was ultimately unfruitful. However, Jackson didn't know that the pathophysiology of chorea would remain a conundrum into the twenty-first century. His ideas about it were part of his developing conceptual framework. As early as 1864 he postulated that chorea is due to embolization of small branches of the middle cerebral arteries, 'which supply convolutions near the corpus striatum. There is no more difficulty in supposing that there are certain convolutions superintending those delicate movements of the hands, which are under the immediate control of the mind, than ... there is ... as Broca suggests, for movements of the tongue in purely mental operations.'[103]

Although Jackson's view of Broca and the mental–physical divide changed markedly over the years 1864–1868, his position on the pathophysiology of chorea did not change. In October 1868 he published a review of his previous 'Observations on the Physiology and Pathology of Hemi-Chorea'. With regard to his 'hypothesis' about hemichorea, he held that 'in chorea, nerve-tissue forming the convolutions near to the corpus striatum, is in parts diseased ... [It] is *not* destroyed, but is unstable.'[104] So, as early as 1868, he was willing to allow the existence of motor representation in the peri-sylvian cortex to explain the highly complex *motor* manifestations of chorea, because he analogized them to the motor phenomena of aphasia.

'Hemispherical co-ordination', August–September 1868

With the above perspective we can now go on to the continuing evolution of Jackson's main ideas. In the *MTG* of August 15, 1868—just before the BA at Norwich—he began to

---

[103] Jackson 1864j, p.459.
[104] Jackson 1868r, p.295; Jackson's italics, my square brackets. In 1885 (Jackson 1885b) Jackson was still struggling to sort out the many theories about the pathophysiology of chorea.

publish a series of 'Notes on the physiology and pathology of the nervous system'. They continued to appear over the next 14 months.[105] Cerebral dominance and interhemispheric relationships claimed most of his attention in his 'Notes' of August–November 1868. From December 1868 through October 1869, his focus was mainly on unilateral seizures and localization.

When Jackson used the term 'Hemispherical co-ordination'[106] he was not referring to our idea of integrative signals going back and forth between the hemispheres through the corpus callosum. Rather, he meant only that each hemisphere has functions that *complement* the other, thus to create a whole functional entity, but without specifying the anatomical connection.[107] When he first encountered the puzzling phenomenon of left cerebral dominance for language output in 1864, he said that if 'it should be proved by wider evidence that the faculty of expression resides in one hemisphere, there is no absurdity in raising the question as to whether perception – its corresponding opposite – may not be seated in the other'.[108] Four years later, in his paper at the BA and in his 'Notes' of August 1868, he again speculated that if the left frontal lobe is dominant for the motor aspect of language, then the right hemisphere may be dominant for processing incoming sensations and 'perception – educated sensations'.[109]

At the BA Jackson again cited Gratiolet to support his view of the hemispheres' complementarity.[110] However, in September 1868 he had to report that 'the observations of Vogt do not confirm Gratiolet's statement as to advanced development of the *left* frontal convolutions of the brain'.[111] Jackson then cited some French authors, including Broca, who seemed to offer other anatomical evidence for the idea of hemispheric complementarity in the form of left frontal dominance for language output and right posterior dominance for perception.[112] In the end, he had to abandon this line of argument, but he kept the idea of hemispheric complementarity on other grounds, which were largely associationist.

A Digression on Association Theory

As long as 'mind' was allowed to remain in neurophysiology, integration of the two hemispheres' activities could be accomplished by that metaphysical entity. In the absence of the mind, however, the mechanism of hemispheric integration had to be either ignored or specified. For Jackson and his Victorian colleagues, mind and brain were both understood in the terms of association theory. Definition Section 7 presents some aspects of associationism as Jackson received them from Bain, Carpenter, and Spencer.

---

[105] Jackson 1868l, Jackson 1868m, Jackson 1868q, Jackson 1868u, Jackson 1868v, Jackson 1869e, Jackson 1869i, Jackson 1869m.

[106] Jackson 1868m, p.208.

[107] Harrington 1987, p.223, also uses the word 'complementary' to describe Jackson's view of the relationship between the functions of the two hemispheres.

[108] Jackson 1864l, p.604.

[109] Jackson 1868m, p.208.

[110] Jackson 1868p, p.239.

[111] Jackson 1868q, p.358, footnote (a). 'Vogt' is Carl Christoph Vogt (1817–1895), not the later and more famous husband-and-wife team of Oscar (1870–1950) and Cécile (1875–1962) Vogt. Jackson did not give his source for Carl Vogt's statement. On Carl Vogt see Finger 1994, pp.162, 301–302. Despite Carl Vogt's apparent negation of Gratiolet's claim, Jackson continued to cite Gratiolet's conclusion; see Jackson 1873d, p.233; and Jackson 1874e, pp.64–65.

[112] Jackson 1868q, p.358, footnote (a).

Definition Section 7—Some Fundamentals of Association Theory

Association of ideas—as originally formulated by Hartley, based on Locke, the mind at birth is gradually populated by sensations and ideas from the environment. When ideas occur consistently together, or in regular succession, they become associated through what Bain, Carpenter, and others called the

'**Law of contiguity**'—which states that 'Two or more states of consciousness [ideas], habitually existing together or in immediate succession, tend to cohere, so that the future occurrence of any of them is sufficient to <u>restore or revive</u> the other'.[113] In regard to 'all the higher exercises of our Reasoning faculties', Carpenter further described the '*law of similarity*'. It says that 'any existing state of consciousness tends to <u>revive</u> previous states that are similar to it'.[114] So arises the concept of the

Revival of ideas—which is central to associationism's explanation of how the mind functions. After the work on the reflex by Bell, Magendie, Müller, and Hall in the 1820s and 1830s, the notion of the reflex as a physiological, brain-based **sensori-motor process** entered associationism, especially through the writings of Bain. Words are ideas, and they are also 'motor processes' because they are brought into consciousness by 'faint' activation (revival) of the cerebral representations for their production in speech, even if they are not pronounced aloud. This faint revival is sometimes called **nascent excitation**. It applies to our recollections of all ideas, a process that Bain regarded as motor.

The motor aspect of the 'muscle sense'—the vague idea that there are sensory signals from the muscles to the brain was extant in the first part of the nineteenth century,[115] although the relevant histology and physiology were not worked out until much later. In the mid-nineteenth century, as outlined in Chapter 4, Bain emphasized the motor aspect of our knowledge of the primary qualities of the physical world. He argued that we learn about it when we meet resistant objects, which require muscular (i.e. motor) effort to explore, including eye movements.

Compound association—Bain devoted an entire chapter of *The Senses and the Intellect* to this subject.[116] It involves 'the case where several threads, or a plurality of links or bonds of connexion, concur in reviving some previous thought or mental state ... Associations that are individually too weak to operate the revival of a past idea may succeed by acting together ... [In] a very large number of our mental transitions a multiple bond of association is at work ...'[117]

In the same 'Notes' of September 1868, where he had to discount Gratiolet, Jackson repeated his associationist assertion that, 'We think by help of words – i.e., – by acquired arbitrary signs – and these are motor processes'.[118] Regarding this 'need of *motor* signs for thought', he referred back to quotations from Bain, Spencer, and Thomson, which he had

---

[113] Carpenter 1855, p.575; my underlining and square brackets. See also Bain 1855, pp.318–410.

[114] Carpenter 1855, p.576; my underlining. J.S. Mill wrote about 'resemblence' [*sic*], employing the basic distinction of 'Likeness and Unlikeness' (Mill 1851, vol.1, pp.74–77).

[115] See Young 1970, pp.97, 114; and Clarke and Jacyna 1987, pp.116, 121, 298.

[116] Bain 1855, pp.544–570; Bain 1864, pp.558–584. Spencer apparently did not use 'compound' in any extensive way, because the term is not found in Collins' (1889) Index. Jackson did not comment on the meaning of 'compound'. However, he used 'compound degree' in Jackson 1868p, p.238, and in Jackson 1868q, p.358.

[117] Bain 1855, p.544; my square brackets.

[118] Jackson 1868q, p.358.

given in a paper of 1866.[119] And in another footnote Jackson explained his reason for extending motor functions further into the realm of thought.

> This distinction betwixt articulation and speech is, I think, an unreal one ... The "organ of language," if there be such a thing, will extend ... from the articulatory muscles to its merging in general mind ... the only differences in ataxy of articulation, mistakes of words, and disorder of ideas, are differences of "compound degree." "The mental recollection of language is a suppressed articulation ready to burst into speech." (Bain)[120]

All of this was worked out further in Jackson's next 'Notes', published on November 7, 1868. They continued his effort to understand normal brain processing of language.

Toward a More Unified Cerebral Physiology and Pathophysiology, November 1868–October 1869

'Language and Thought—The Duality of Mental Processes', November 1868

The article 'Language and thought – the duality of mental processes'[121] was Jackson's first detailed effort to create a theoretical model of neurolinguistic processing. It was short, dense, sometimes inconsistent, and ultimately incomplete. Moreover, it was *neuro*lingusitic only insofar as he tried to relate involuntary processes to the right hemisphere and voluntary ones to the left. What he really wanted to apprehend was the linguistic basis of propositionizing. This was a new element that he brought to association theory. To understand how he was thinking, we have to start by suppressing our own knowledge of neurocognitive processing, because we know about human 'split brains'.[122] From those patients we have learned that there is a parallel stream of cognitive activity in the nondominant hemisphere, but it can't express itself under normal conditions, i.e., when the corpus callosum is intact. Jackson probably would have welcomed this finding, but it's not what he meant.

About dominance, Jackson first explained his idea of sensory processing ('Sensation and Perception') in the nondominant hemisphere and its relationship to the dominance of the left hemisphere for the motor aspect of language output ('Expression'). A long footnote at the beginning of his paper is actually his (misplaced) introduction, because it defined his terms in accordance with association theory:

> ... It is needful to say how the term "perception" is to be understood ... *The psychical, like the physical, processes of the nervous system, can only be functions of complex combinations of motor and sensory nerves.* I have ... guarded myself against being understood to imply

---

[119] Jackson 1868q, p.358, footnote (b); Jackson's italics. Jackson referred to Jackson 1866f, where he had quoted Spencer's statement of the associationist position on the motor aspect of memory (Jackson 1866f, p.661). For Jackson's reference to 'Dr. William Thomson, the present Archbishop of York' see Jackson 1866f, p.662; it concerns the mechanism of memory in the deaf and blind.

[120] Jackson 1868q, p.358, footnote (d); Jackson's parentheses. In Jackson 1866f, p.661, he gave a different quotation to the same effect from Bain, but he gave no citation and I have not been able to find the wording of either in Bain 1855, nor has Lorch found it (personal communication).

[121] Jackson 1868u, p.526.

[122] Gazzaniga et al. 1962; these are patients whose cerebral hemispheres have been disconnected by surgically cutting ('splitting') the corpus callosum ('callosotomy').

that sensation and movement exist separately, although ... I speak of them as separate ...
it is not implied that Sensation and Perception are altogether different. A Perception is a
complex and yet an orderly development of impressions ... from *many different* sense surfaces, and when I speak of a sensation arousing a perception involuntarily I simply mean
that, for instance, a noise or a touch may at any time make *actual* in the higher parts of the
nervous system ... a *unit*, which is at all times potential, formed out of *many* impressions ...
In perception ... several sensations ... have yielded, so to speak, their own personality into
the formation of a <u>higher unit</u> which we can then distinguish as a perception.[123]

In the first part of this passage Jackson deliberately conflated the physical and the psychical,
because they have the same neurological basis in sensori-motor processes. A perception is
a compound 'higher unit' that is composed of multiple sensations, but all such higher compounds ultimately consist only of sensori-motor elements.[124] Association theory would predict that a perception can be called into cognitive existence by the arrival of its constituent
sensations. Immediately after the above, Jackson continued, with reference to aphasia:

Similarly in Expression, the corresponding opposite of Perception, we find in a certain disorder of articulation (from disease of the higher parts of the nervous system ...) that the defect
is not of the muscles of the palate alone, nor of those of the tongue alone, etc., not of all of these
grouped together. It is a disorder of a <u>complex unit</u> for the whole process of articulation.[125]

The physiological basis for Jackson's conception of a 'complex unit' for expression was his idea
that a unit contains representations for movements, not for individual muscles. Continuing
in the same lengthy footnote, he explained the neural basis of consciousness in associationist
terms, but he defined 'will' only by reference to verbal synonyms.

I adopt the expression "thread of consciousness" for those of our always possible sensori-
motor processes, which are for the time *actual*, and into which sensations or perceptions
are continually bringing modifications.
      I may here say something on the use of the words "will," "voluntary," etc. Although we
"will," in the sense that we do what we like, provided there are no external hindrances, we
do not desire as we like ... [*] ... I must use some such word, and I use the words "will," etc.,
pretty much as "effort," "reflection," etc., are used.[126]

Here, in 1868, Jackson secularized the will to the extent that it had no transcendental
meaning. Nonetheless, he retained it in his neurologically based version of associationism
even when he could not define it. To put it another way, associationism had difficulty ac-
counting for spontaneous thought, because the theory is grounded in the idea of a sensori-
motor *reflex*, which in turn implies the necessity of an incoming stimulus for anything to
happen. As long as the idea of 'will'—noun or verb—remains in any system of brain science,
there is no requirement for the existence of any other integrating mechanism.[127]

---

    123 Jackson 1868u, p.526; Jackson's italics, my underlining.
    124 In the older associationist usage, a perception is one form of 'idea'.
    125 Jackson 1868u, p.526, footnote (a); Jackson's parentheses and italics, my underlining.
    126 Jackson 1868u, p.526, footnote (a). Within this passage, where I placed the bracketed asterisk [*] Jackson
referred to 'Spencer on the "Will". "Principles of Psychology", Lockhart Clarke on "Volition", *Psychological Journal*,
Nos. 8, 9, and 10'. Presumably he was referring to Spencer 1855, pp.612–620, and to Clarke 1862.
    127 Jackson's next mention of 'will' is in Jackson 1874c, p.43, where he called 'the 'stimulus of the "Will"' a 'hackneyed
expression'. It appears that between 1868 (Jackson 1868u) and 1874 he avoided the word altogether, at least in print.

With Jackson's definitions as background, we can now go on to his effort to explain the '*doubleness* of mental processes', which proposed that both hemispheres are involved in linguistic processing. At the beginning of 'the duality of mental processes' he said that he was actually talking about 'two pairs' of parallel processes.

> ... the pair Expression and Perception are really two pairs – (1) Involuntary and (2) Voluntary Expression, and (1) Involuntary and (2) Voluntary Perception ... I was led to this supposition by a consideration of the phenomena of some cases of speechlessness the result of damage to one [usually the left] side of the brain ... of the cases of persons who cannot revive words *voluntarily.* What follows is mostly ... an attempt ... to make clearer what I have ... spoken of crudely as a double revival of "images," "concepts," etc.[128]

These ideas have their origins in Jackson's clinical observations on the recurrent utterances of aphasic patients. Some aphasics with severe left hemisphere damage can produce a few words, but not full propositions. Those observations were his hard data. Since he was about to stray from the path of the factual, he confessed 'that most of what follows is speculative ... much of ... [it] ... is accepted doctrine, and the only point I wish ... to urge is the <u>*doubleness of mental processes*</u>'.[129] Having thus made prior atonement for his sin of speculating, Jackson turned to the part of the subject that really interested him—an analysis of propositionizing.

> Words serve not only in speech, but in thought ... But I think it is not sufficiently exact to speak of Thought as "internal Speech."
>
> It is [also] not enough to say that Speech consists of Words. It consists of words *referring to one another in a particular manner* ... A proposition – *e.g.,* Gold is yellow – consists of two names, each of which, by conventional contrivances of position ... modifies the meaning of the other.(b)[130] All the names in a random succession of words may ... excite perceptions in us, but not perceptions in any relation to one another deserving the name of thought. The several perceptions so revived do not make a unit ...
>
> When we apprehend a proposition, a *relation between two things* is *given* to us ... We receive in a *twofold* manner, not the words only, but the order of the words also.[131]

This passage makes no reference to neural structure or function. It is a purely linguistic exercise, with the individual word as the unit of analysis. In the next paragraph Jackson introduced a neural element, by reference to the right and left hemispheres.

> ... in the process which leads to outward speech ... [as] propositions – there is a double revival of words – automatic revival prior to voluntary revival ... the *automatic* revival occurs first, and on the *right*, and the voluntary revival afterwards on the *left*, side of the brain. Concepts, images, perceptions, or whatever they may be called ... develope [*sic*] words automatically in no order, or rather in their own order, on the right side of the brain. Words are, or may be, objectively considered on the left – put into new relations – made into propositions. I wish to speak of the links *between* these two revivals. The links are ... the perceptions of which the words are the arbitrary signs.[132]

---

[128] Jackson 1868u, p.526; the parentheses, square brackets, and italics are Jackson's.
[129] Jackson 1868u, p.526; Jackson's italics, my square brackets and underlining.
[130] Footnote (b) was a reference to Waitz 1863, p.241, which was an ethnological discussion of language structure.
[131] Jackson 1868u, pp.526–527; Jackson's italics, my square brackets.
[132] Jackson 1868u, p.527; Jackson's italics, my square brackets.

Jackson was proposing that when incoming perceptions arrive in the form of words, they revive words automatically (involuntarily). This process begins in the right hemisphere, but conscious (voluntary) revival in the left hemisphere is necessary to form a proposition from the random array of words in the right hemisphere. In the second half of the above he was essentially asking how the random words in the right hemisphere get into meaningful order in the left. Here he had encountered the basic conundrum of the sensori-motor model in associationism. It can explain a simple proposition but not anything more subtle, like poetic complexity. Be that as it may, he gave a further explanation in another footnote.

> Although I must speak, for convenience, of the two sides [of the brain] being respectively voluntary and involuntary, I do not think there is any abrupt difference ... there are all degrees betwixt automatic action and that kind of imperfect action which is the dawn of "will." (See Spencer's "Psychology," chapter "Will").[133]

Now if there is no 'abrupt' distinction between involuntary and voluntary, then presumably both kinds of activity occur in both hemispheres, albeit in different degrees. Since the medium of thought (propositionizing) is dual (i.e., movements and sensations), and occurring in both hemispheres, the 'will' emerges as mind. This conclusion goes back to the sensori-motor basis of associationism, which Spencer extended to explain 'will' as emergent.[134] Perhaps sensing that his readers would have difficulty following his argument, Jackson tried to restate it.

> To repeat, there is first involuntary revival of perception, afterwards there is or may be voluntary revival. And of the voluntary revival it must be added that the perception, besides being modified, is or may be put in a new order with others. Indeed, it is necessarily modified by being put in a new order, as words are in a proposition. But what is the intermediation betwixt these two different perceptions? ... It is movement – *i.e.*, the movement of words.[135]

The phrase 'movement of words' is ambiguous. Is he referring to the motor aspect of words stored in the brain and available for revivification (our 'lexicon'), or does he mean the process by which words are supposedly moved between the hemispheres? He gave an example which shows that he was referring to both the motor *and* the sensory aspects of word storage.

> Let us see how the hypothesis applies to what follows [after] hearing the word "horse" in a proposition ... There have long been permanent modifications of my brain which make it possible to another person at any time to *compel me* to have in my consciousness, at least momentarily, unless I am strongly preoccupied, some kind of notion of horse. He excites certain changes in the "grooves" of those permanent modifications of my brain which are always with me ... What is the nature of this ever-present modification ... [at] any time to be awakened by the noise "horse," to give me a notion of horse? Is it a sensory or is it a motor process? ... I think there must be both a motor and sensory process.[136]

---

[133] Jackson 1868u, p.527, footnote (c); my square brackets. The citation is to Spencer 1855, pp.612–620.

[134] Collins 1889, pp.205, summarizes Spencer 1870, pp.190–192, on the subject of mind as emergent: 'the development of Mind is fundamentally an increased integration of feelings on successively higher stages, along with which there go increasing heterogeneity and definiteness; and these traits answer to traits in the evolution of the nervous system ...'.

[135] Jackson 1868u, p.527; my underlining.

[136] Jackson 1868u, p.527; Jackson's italics, my square brackets.

On the last page of Jackson's paper on 'the duality of mental processes' he summarized his views about the neurology of thinking: 'My notion is that we not only think by help of arbitrary *motor* signs (words), but by help of arbitrary perceptive signs, and that we have permanently in our brain organised forms of the latter, just as we have organised forms for the former – movements of words.'[137] Now even if we accept Jackson's model of hemispheric complementarity, we are left with no explanation of how perceptions and/or words actually get from the right to the left, since the 'will' is no longer admissible. A similar problem continues to bedevil modern neuroscience—we still have no comprehensive theory of how the brain integrates all of its incoming data to make propositional sense out of it. We presume that the ultimate explanation will be some form of connected localization, involving functions carried out by connected networks of neural structures. The earliest *theoretical* conception of localization as we now know it was derived by Jackson from his detailed study of unilateral seizures.

The Sequence of the 'March' in Unilateral (Jacksonian) Seizures, December 1868

In Jackson's 'Notes' of December 19, 1868, the precision of his clinical observations on unilateral seizures offers a sharp contrast to the highly theoretical nature of his speculations about language and cognition. Even so, he began with a caveat.

> I wish now to remark on the sequence under which parts [of the body] are most frequently affected in a single paroxysm of unilateral convulsion ... It is most important to observe convulsive paroxysms minutely; but it is obviously difficult to observe them precisely. It must be understood that the following only purports to give what is ... the *usual* sequence in *one* variety of those convulsions which begin unilaterally. I never forego an opportunity of watching patients in fits, but the opportunities are rare, and the observations are painfully difficult to make.[138]

In his next paragraph, Jackson used the term 'march'[139] to describe the sequence of movements in focal seizures. To the best of my knowledge this is the first place where he used that word in the context of motor seizures—although he had used the same term to describe a 'march of the sensation' in mid-1868.[140] Then he went on to describe the motor march.

> The muscles acting unilaterally are first seized, then those acting bilaterally, and lastly the unilateral muscles of the opposite side. *But the sequence is not a simple sequence. I have*

---

[137] Jackson 1868u, p.528. A year later (in Jackson 1869m, p.481, footnote (b); Jackson's italics), Jackson said, '... I have perhaps too much taken it as settled that motor processes constitute the verbal signs by which we think, and that there is necessarily a nascent reproduction of movements for words when sounds of words fall on the ear ... Dr. Charlton Bastian has ... [*] ... advanced the hypothesis that we think by aid of *sounds* of words ... it will be necessary to give a careful consideration to the recently expressed views of Dr. Bastian, which I hope shortly to do.' In the place where I have put the asterisk ([*]), Jackson referred to Bastian 1869a and Bastian 1869b. In 1874 (Jackson 1874a, p.348, footnote (a)), while discussing the 'phenomena of Aphasia', Jackson said in a footnote: ' ... Dr. Bastian, a physician whose opinion on any such subject deserves the greatest respect, has vigorously and very ably combated Bain's opinion, and ... my explanation of the phenomena of Aphasia founded on it ...'.

[138] Jackson 1868v, p.696; Jackson's italics, my square brackets.

[139] See Definition Section 5 in Chapter 4. See also York and Koehler 2000. Bravais used 'march' in 1827. Jefferson 1935, p.150, quotes Bravais' thesis in (translated) English, but there is no evidence that Jackson took the word from Bravais.

[140] Jackson 1867l, p.330. This long paper was actually published in 1868; at its end Jackson cited Prevost 1868 (p.394). Prevost (p.393) described a patient who died on January 24, 1868.

tried by use of figures to show at what stage in the <u>march</u> of the convulsion of the unilateral muscles of the side first convulsed the bilateral muscles begin to be involved.

Then there is an order of involvement of the unilateral muscles of the side first affected. But this again is not a simple sequence ... Let us say ... that the spasm begins on the right side, and let us limit the illustration to those cases in which the thumb and index finger are the parts first affected. It is important to bear this in mind, as I think the mode of beginning makes a great difference as to the <u>march</u> of the fit. When the fit begins in the face, the convulsion in involving the arm may *go down* the limb.[141]

When Jackson said that the sequence of the march is not '*simple*', he meant that one body part may start to move *before* the seizure in an adjacent part has ended. Table 5.1 shows his sequence data in graphic form. It is rearranged from his original, semi-narrative presentation. By looking vertically down the columns of the progressive stages, arbitrarily labeled 1–5 by Jackson, one can see which body parts are typically involved at each stage, but the

Table 5.1 Jackson's summary of the order of involvement of muscles in a convulsive march beginning in the right thumb and index finger. Rearranged in graphic form from his outline (Jackson 1868v). Items in quotation marks are from Jackson's text.

Anatomical parts involved	Stages				
	1	2	3	4	5
'*Unilateral Muscles of Right Side*'					
'Arm – Thumb and index finger	X				
whole of fingers and forearm		X			
upper arm'			X		
'Face – Cheek drawn up		X			
eye closed			X		
both eyes to right				X	
head to right'					X
'Leg – Thigh			X		
leg'				X	
'Sometimes the leg is affected before the face'					
'*Bilateral Muscles*'					
'The occipito-frontalis'				X	
'The two buccinators, the orbicularis oris, the right zygomatici, and depressor anguli oris'					X
'The thoracic and abdominal muscles'					X
'*Unilateral Muscles of the Left Side*'					

'The unilateral muscles of the opposite side commence to move when the chest begins to be decidedly involved.' ... 'I am unable to say anything as to the order of the march in the second side – i.e., whether it begins in the hand or foot and then goes up, or vice versa.'

---

141 Jackson 1868v; Jackson's italics, my underlining.

chart shows only the patterns of onset, not the seizures' durations. However, in this paper he did not attempt to analyze their physiological implications.

And he added further clinical comments:

> ... it is not asserted that the several parts which are seen to move one after another are not really affected simultaneously, but simply that whilst some are visibly affected, others are not apparently affected ...
>
> It is to be observed that the spasm may cease at any stage, there being often only a little twitching of the hand. <u>Slight seizures are sometimes called "partial fits" or aurae</u>.[142]

The last, underlined sentence carries an important implication: for Jackson, 'Slight seizures' and 'aurae' are epileptic seizures. That is, they are manifestations of the same basic pathophysiology as more 'complete' unilateral seizures. In his era when concern with nosology implied that such phenomena were not 'genuine', this was new. At the end of the next quotation we will see that Jackson was also leaning toward an explanation of generalized ('genuine') epilepsy by the same basic process. His pathophysiology was gradually becoming more unified.

> It does not follow of necessity that both hemispheres are affected one after the other when the spasm affects one side of the body after the other ... the unilateral muscles of the two sides are represented in each side of the brain, although unequally and perhaps differently represented ... convulsions beginning unilaterally resemble and differ from those more general convulsions which set in without warning or are preceded by an obscure sensation in the head or by a strange feeling at the epigastrium. The latter kind of convulsions are sometimes called "genuine" epilepsy, or idiopathic epilepsy.[143]

Jackson's last 'Note' of 1868 ended here, leaving us hanging on the possibility of a breakthrough in his thinking about *three* kinds of seizures: unilateral (Jacksonian), generalized, and (in mid-twentieth-century terms) 'temporal lobe' or 'psychomotor' seizures. Change was coming, but in his usually cautious way. A true Yorkshireman will not be unduly hurried.

Method, Physiology, and Pathophysiology in the Gulstonian Lectures, February–March 1869

In early 1869, Jackson gave the three prestigious Gulstonian Lectures on 'Certain Points in the Study and Classification of Diseases of the Nervous System'. They were 'Delivered at the Royal College of Physicians' and published as abstracts in the *BMJ* and *The Lancet*.[144] The first two lectures are of a piece, concerned with method, physiology,

---

142 Jackson 1868v; my underlining.
143 Jackson 1868v.
144 Jackson 1869a, Jackson 1869b, Jackson 1869c, Jackson 1869d, Jackson 1869f, Jackson 1869g. The listed dates of these publications are February 27, March 6, and March 13. The dates of the actual lectures would have been no more than a few weeks before their publication. The current spelling of the still-continuing lectures is 'Goulstonian', but 'Gulstonian' was common until the end of the nineteenth century.

and pathophysiology. In the third lecture he discussed some specific pathologies, and he began to relate their clinical manifestations to his developing principles. His first lecture started with an updated version of his tripartite method, which he had initially presented in 1864.[145]

> ... we should study each case of nervous disease in a threefold manner: as it shows (1) damage at a certain point in a sensori-motor tract (Organ); (2) as it is an instance of local change of some wide-spread Tissue; and (3) as it is one of disorder of Function. He takes the word organ to imply, not only nervous centers, but – illustrating by motor organs – the nerves to the muscles they are known to govern.[146]

Jackson's advancing definition of a neurological 'organ' is worth noting. It is not just a collection of cell bodies in grey matter, but rather an entire functional system, which constituted a '"unit of action" of the nervous system'.[147] In his *Suggestions* of 1863, and especially in his lecture on method in 1864, he had emphasized the importance of thinking about disordered physiological states in relation to their underlying normal physiology. However, he had not said anything specific about using pathophysiology to get at the normal, which, in Chapter 3, I called a 'reverse' use of the clinico-pathological method. Now, in his first Gulstonian lecture of 1869, he recognized what he was doing.

> ... the general scientific world will more and more look to us for facts as to the physiology of the nervous system, and especially for more precise facts on the relation of mind to brain, such as cases of defect of speech supply ... whilst as medical men we endeavour in particular cases to find the organ damaged, we should as physiologists endeavour to trace the differences of speciality in the ascending line of function from the spinal cord to the cerebral hemisphere. By a careful study and comparison of the effects of damage by disease to each of the geographical regions of the nervous system we shall ... reach a knowledge of the fundamental plan of structure of the nervous system, and thus find out what is the general principle of localisation throughout the nervous system.[148]

The final clause about the 'general principle of localisation' evokes uniformitarianism, because it seems to assume that there *is* localization throughout the system, and yet Jackson had not fully accepted that idea. He still did not apply it above the striatum. In discussing the striatum, he continued to say that that structure 'lies close upon the organ of mind', so its disorders will

> ... give us a clue to the true interpretation of cases which it is the custom to call aphasic ... and to a knowledge of the principle of localisation and of the action of the two hemispheres in mental processes ... the lecturer endeavoured to account for the paradox that – assuming the so-called faculty of language to "reside" in every part of the brain – damage

---

[145] Jackson 1864h, pp.146–147.
[146] Jackson 1869a, p.307.
[147] Jackson 1869c, p.345.
[148] Jackson 1869a, p.307. The same point was repeated in Lecture II (Jackson 1869c, p.345), where Jackson said that by arriving 'at a better knowledge of the plan of composition of one nervous organ, we may fairly use this knowledge as a means of further investigation'.

near to the [left] corpus striatum did, and that damage distant from that body did not, destroy speech. <u>This part of the lecture does not admit of brief abstract</u>.[149]

The underlined sentence is the lament of a very frustrated reporter—and so he might well have been, because Jackson was inconsistent about the supposed uniformity of the 'principle of localisation' in the nervous system. Are the hemispheric cortices part of the system or aren't they? He devoted much of Lecture II to answering this question with a resounding yes and no. He did not accept—or even mention—any phrenological idea of parcellation of functions of the hemispheric surfaces. Rather, he said that the two hemispheres are different in their functional organizations. His observations on unilateral seizures and his concept of localization in the striatum had 'led him to a modification of Broadbent's hypothesis'.

> ... taking one side of the brain, the right, ... the muscles acting unilaterally, both of the left and of the right side of the body, are represented in the right side of the brain, but the muscles of the left side of the body are especially represented there – 1st, more in quantity, for they are more affected when the hemisphere discharges: 2ndly, first in time (instability), for they are affected before those of the right side.[150]

Jackson did not say exactly how he had modified Broadbent's hypothesis, nor can I be sure about what he meant, but I think he was trying to save Broadbent, while attempting to account for dominance. Again, however, there is ambiguity. In the above passage he used the word 'brain', not 'corpus striatum', whereas Broadbent's original hypothesis referred specifically to the latter.[151] My accusation of ambiguity is based on the fact that, without resolving the issue, his text moved rather quickly from Broadbent to aphasia.

> There is ... a difference betwixt damage to the corpus striatum and damage to the hemisphere just above it – viz., that whilst damage to *either* of the corpora striata produces ... the same effect – viz., loss of the most voluntary movements of the limbs on but *one* side of the body, damage to *but one side* of the brain – usually the left – will destroy voluntary speech altogether ... in the highest sensori-motor processes we cannot expect that there will be two sides for the "cessation of automatic action and the dawn of volition," which is, Spencer says, one and the same thing. The two brains cannot be *mere* duplicates if damage to one only will make a man speechless. For those processes, than which there are none higher, there must surely be one side which is leading.[152]

The root cause of Jackson's difficulty was his continuing reluctance to assign motor functions of mind to the cortices. Indeed, his third Gulstonian lecture did not start where the second left off. Rather, he went back to pick up the neglected second part of his tripartite method, i.e., damage to tissue. In his ophthalmological work over the preceding years, Jackson had recognized a clinico-pathological correlation between '<u>optic neuritis</u>' and 'coarse disease' of the brain.[153] Within the latter category he included the gross changes of syphilis, large hemorrhages, tumors, and other mass lesions. These he contrasted to

---

[149] Jackson 1869a, p.308 (*Lancet*); square brackets '[left]' in original; my underlining. The *BMJ* (Jackson 1869b) said, 'This part of the Lecture scarcely admits of brief abstract'.

[150] Jackson 1869c, p.345.

[151] Broadbent 1866.

[152] Jackson 1869c, p.345; Jackson's italics.

[153] Explained in Chapter 6.

'minute' changes in tissue. The latter were observable, if at all, only at the histological level. Nonetheless, Jackson's empirical correlation of optic neuritis with coarse disease was correct. Moreover, as he stated in Lecture III, knowing whether a patient has coarse or minute disease is important, because the outlook for patients with seizures is worse when they were caused by mass lesions.[154]

At the end of his discussion Jackson summarized the usual complaints of patients who have coarse disease, but he was careful to point out that 'none of them are "localizing" symptoms'.[155] This refers to the clinical phenomena that allow us to 'first localize the lesion'. Here, in 1869, is the place where I have found Jackson's first use of the term 'localising', although it is clear that he understood the concept when he discussed the meaning of the epileptic aura in 1866.[156] Of course, a sign or symptom can have localizing value only if the normal function(s) of the abnormal tissue is known. By 1869 he was expressing this desideratum quite clearly.[157]

'Localisation' and 'The Unit of Constitution of the Nervous System', June and October 1869

Jackson's 'Notes' of June 5, 1869, were titled simply 'On localisation'. The piece was actually his response to a published query from Frederic Bateman about Jackson's intellectual relationship to Broca.[158] Jackson's answer contained nothing new in that respect—he rejected the faculty psychology and its mosaic form of localizing. But he issued a challenge to himself and his contemporaries. He recommended careful study of 'the seemingly strange cases where extensive destruction of parts of the cerebral hemispheres occurs without obvious symptoms', because such cases would 'supply us with materials towards determining *the plan of structure of nervous organs*'.[159] He gave no instructions about how to accomplish this difficult task, but he did explain himself further in the last of this series of 'Notes'.

A 'Note' on 'The Unit of Constitution of the Nervous System' appeared on October 23, 1869.[160] At the outset Jackson said, 'The following is intended as a continuation of the article on "Localisation."' At first it is difficult to see the connection between the two articles, but the key is Jackson's concern with understanding '*the plan of structure of nervous organs*'. In Chapter 4 we saw that he took the idea of a 'physiological unit' directly from Spencer, starting in 1866. At that time he applied it in his studies of language disorders and seizures. In 1868 he used the idea in explaining his view of localization in the striatum and his notion of perceptions as compound sensations.[161] Now, in October 1869, he implied

---

[154] Jackson 1869f, p.380.

[155] Jackson 1869f, p.380.

[156] See Chapter 4; Jackson used 'localising' extensively in Jackson 1871h, p.342.

[157] Charcot also understood it in a nosological context; see Goetz et al. 1995, pp.76–77.

[158] Jackson 1869i. Bateman's paper (Bateman 1869, published May 8) was 'Read before the Medical Society of London, February 1, 1869'. On p.488, footnote (*c*), Bateman reviewed some of Jackson's statements in Jackson 1864j, and then said, '... it would be extremely interesting to know whether this painstaking observer is still to be ranked among the supporters of M. Broca's views'. Lorch (personal communication) points out that Bateman's query might have arisen because Jackson did not debate Broca directly at the BA in 1868.

[159] Jackson 1869i; Jackson's italics. In his final paragraph he again referred to Spencer's concept of localization, citing Spencer 1855, p.607, which he had quoted in Jackson 1867i, p.669, footnote (b).

[160] Jackson 1869m. Jackson's use of Spencer's 'unit' has never caught the attention of his commentators, including me until now. The idea was central to the development of his thought.

[161] Jackson 1868u, p.526; which is quoted above in this chapter.

quite directly that he was offering a new extension of the original idea, because he gave it a new name.

> The term Constitution I borrow from chemistry.
>
> By this term I do not mean a unit of Composition (a) – consisting of an arrangement of afferent fibres, ganglion cells, efferent fibres, *etc.* – but a unit containing those in such balance of relations that they serve harmoniously in complete actions.[162]

The point of the first sentence in the above is that it was *he* who borrowed the 'term Constitution'. Jackson's footnote (a) gives a reference to Spencer's *Principles of Psychology*, second edition, which is largely a summary of Spencer's reading in the neuroscience of the time.[163] When Spencer dealt with the histology and physiology of the neural cells and fibers in mediating reflexes, he had written:

> These coupled nerves, with the ganglion-cell acting as a direct or indirect link between them ... appear to form a compound structure out of which the nervous system is built – its <u>unit of composition</u>. But this is not so. By multiplication of such arcs we may get a multitude of separate nervous agencies, but not a nervous system. To produce a nervous system there needs an element connecting each such nervous arc with the rest ...[164]

In our Sherringtonian terms, Spencer was saying that reflexes must be *integrated* in order to create the coordinated actions that the organism requires to react successfully to its environment, which was essentially what Jackson was saying. Spencer's text goes on to describe the role of neural elements that we would ascribe to connecting neurons. In Jackson's text it is clear that he was not referring to this kind of simple neural arrangement when he used the term 'constitution'. Rather, he had in mind a more extensive kind of integrated neural apparatus.

> ... the units of the corpus striatum do not represent groups of muscles of the arm, but movements of the whole limb. Entering into the composition of the unit of constitution of the nervous system, there will be the skin impression, the sensory nerve, the centre, the motor nerve, the sensory nerves from moving muscles, and from tracts of the skin stretched or relaxed by the movement ... in the lower processes these several things are concerned in each action, and ... it is inferable that a *corresponding* process takes place in speech and thought.[165]

Jackson's insight about the cerebral representation of movements, rather than individual muscles, goes back to 1867,[166] but here in 1869 he was able to give it better definition by thinking about it in terms of Spencer's physiological units. He went on to apply his idea of a 'unit of constitution' to hearing a word—how it is processed through the ears, and thence through the auditory nerve to 'some unknown centre ("the brain") [via] nerve fibres to the

---

    [162] Jackson 1869m, p.481. In his text immediately after this passage Jackson gave a chemical example of 'composition' versus 'constitution'.

    [163] Spencer 1870, vol.1, pp.2–142. The apparent chronological discrepancy—Jackson in 1869 cited Spencer 1870—is explained by Jackson's receipt of a prepublication installment of Spencer's book.

    [164] Spencer 1870, vol.1, p.28; my underlining.

    [165] Jackson 1869m, p.481; Jackson's italics.

    [166] See Jackson 1867i, p.662.

nervous arrangements superintending the movement of the word'.[167] And within association theory there is even more complexity.

> ... the speculation of units of constitution supposes us to have particular auditory sensations (of the sounds of words) in fixed, although acquired, association with particular movements for words ...
> But the whole of the elements of the unit have not been considered in the above illustration. It frequently happens that these sensori-motor processes occur in succession. For instance, after the particular auditory and articulatory sensori-motor process serving for the *word* "ball," there follows another sensori-motor process, a subjective image of the thing ball ... By what means is it that these two sensori-motor processes occur in sequence? There must be an organic connexion of some kind.[168]

We have seen that Spencer was also looking for an organic mechanism to explain the coordination of simple reflexes into adaptive reactions to the organism's environment. Likewise, in the above passage Jackson was looking for a universal form of 'organic connexion' to explain the temporal succession of movements at all levels. As an instance of processes that involve 'succession', Jackson offered the example of walking.

> When a large movement ... occurs as one of a series ... its range and degree have definite relations to the range and degree of those before it and after it ... The unit of the sensori-motor arrangement, by the excitation of which one movement results, must then have *organic* connexions with the units of the sensori-motor arrangements, by excitation of which the movements before and after result. Similarly there must be an organic connexion betwixt the units of the two sensori-motor arrangements for the word "ball" and the image "ball," as the two are in indissoluble association. If the nervous system is built on one plan – mental and physical being but convenient names for large degrees of difference – the organic connexion will be of the same kind in all cases.[169]

Again using the example of walking, Jackson defined the components of a physiological unit that would account for temporal succession in that activity.

> My speculation is that in gross movement the "return" nerves from the muscles moving and from the skin stretched or relaxed by the movement serve in the excitation of the next movement, and that correspondingly return nerves from the nervous arrangements for the movement-word "ball" serve to revive the visual image and ocular movement, which constitutes the mental representatives of the object "ball" ...
> So far, then, I believe that in every action, whether it be a gross movement, as in walking, or a process above actual movement, as thinking, the whole elements of units are concerned.[170]

Unfortunately, the term 'whole elements of units' is not clear. Is he saying that there are units which superintend other, more elementary units, or would it be the case that such 'lower'

---

167 Jackson 1869m, p.481; Jackson's parentheses, my square brackets.
168 Jackson 1869m, p.481; Jackson's italics, my underlining.
169 Jackson 1869m, p.481; Jackson's italics.
170 Jackson 1869m, p.481; my underlining. This is Sherringtonian thinking before Sherrington.

units can also be part and parcel of the more complex units that integrate the overall activities of the combined units? Some hint of how he might have answered this question is given in the next part of his text, which also shows his associationist stripes.

> But it is, I conceive, plain that single units would not suffice for giving <u>relations of likeness and unlikeness</u>; and this is what is fundamental in all mental operations ... It is by an alternation of two sensations and two movements that we obtain an idea of the coexistence of two external objects; and I suppose, we speak and think by the "same method of parallax" – by an alternation of words and perceptions.[171]

According to both J.S. Mill and Spencer, an organism's ability to make the binary distinction of likeness versus unlikeness is fundamental to how it investigates and reacts to its environment. Mill made the distinction an integral part of association theory in the first edition of his *System of Logic* (1843),[172] and Spencer discussed it in the first edition of *The Principles of Psychology* (1855).[173] Presumably Jackson took it from Spencer. Jackson's use of the term 'single units' in the above quotation is clarified a little in the final paragraph of that paper, where he introduced another dimension of the subject by pointing out, 'It is evident that the whole nervous system is double ...'. But the two halves are not simply duplicates of each other, as shown by the hemispheric lesions that produce hemiplegia and loss of speech.

> ... A careful study of cases of disease of the nervous system has led me to conclude that *each* side of the brain contains processes for all classes of movements of *both* sides – (1) those which must act bilaterally; (2) those which may act alternately; and (3) those which can act independently – are all represented in (d) *each* side of the brain ... those muscles of both sides which are in their action bilateral only, are equally represented in each of the two sides of the brain ... the muscles of both sides which are alternate in their action have a less equal representation in each side, and ... those muscles of both sides which act independently as well as alternately and bilaterally have a very unequal representation in each of the two sides.[174]

This is hemispheric localization in the sense of anatomical specialization—the two hemispheres are not exact duplicates of each other. On the other hand, Jackson was saying that both hemispheres are involved when any movement occurs, including highly voluntary, unilateral movements. His text immediately following the above ends this 'Note' with a summary statement of his physiological conclusion.

> The facts supplied by diseases of, and experimentation on, animals seem to show that the representation of the two sides of the body in each side of the brain is more equal the lower we go. These facts, read with the phenomena of hemiplegia, point ... to the conclusion that

---

[171] Jackson 1869m, p.481; see also Jackson 1873a, p.84. I have not identified Jackson's source for 'method of parallax'.

[172] I have used Mill 1851 (the 3 ed.); see pp.74–77.

[173] Spencer 1855, pp.312–316. Both Mill and Spencer used 'similarity/dissimilarity' or 'resemblance' with slightly different meanings than likeness and unlikeness; see Definition Section 7 in this chapter.

[174] Jackson 1869m, pp.481–482; Jackson's italics. Footnote (d) is a uniformitarian statement: '... the whole of the nervous system and its parts are developed on the same fundamental plan'.

the units of the nervous system are, like the nervous system itself, double ... <u>The unit of action is double the unit of constitution</u>.[175]

As of 1869 Jackson conceived of the 'unit of constitution' as the complete neural apparatus for any given movement in one hemisphere, so the 'unit of action' that controls the movement is the 'double' combination of the units in each hemisphere. The 'unit of action' is integrative, even if he did not specify its neural mechanism.

---

[175] Jackson 1869m, p.482; my underlining. Jackson gave no hint about the source of his statement regarding 'experimentation on, animals', and this was before the work of Fritsch and Hitzig in 1870 and Ferrier in 1873 (see Chapter 7).

6

'A Study of Convulsions', 1870:
Background and Analysis

For Hughlings Jackson's entire career, 1870 was a high-water mark. In that year, at age 35, he published 'A study of convulsions',[1] which launched the conceptual foundations of modern epileptology. He had already earned a substantial reputation in the British medical community for his work on aphasia, and the positive notices of his 'Study' further enhanced his standing. The second part of this chapter will explore the paper and some of its antecedents. First, I will offer an overview of British society and culture, and Jackson's place in it, at the turn of the decade.

Jackson's Cultural and Professional Settings, *circa* 1870

British Society and Culture, *circa* 1870

In 1870 Britain was the world's only super power. It ruled an enormous empire that was largely at peace. From their secure island the British watched events on the continent with horror. After the Franco-Prussian war of 1870–1871, chancellor Otto von Bismarck consolidated the German Empire. The war was a disaster for France, which lost Alsace, Lorraine, and more than a modicum of pride. The French army surrendered after 6 weeks, in September 1870, but Paris held out under siege into the winter of 1870–1871. 'Broca was put in charge of an *ambulance*: a dozen sheds set up for war casualties'.[2] At l'Hôpital Salpêtrière 'teaching halted and acute care of the wounded and smallpox victims superceded normal routines…Charcot…remained at his Paris home and workplace throughout…'[3]

In Chapter 2 we saw that the period 1850–1870 has been called the British 'age of equipoise'—a time when its world seemed to be in peaceful and prosperous equilibrium. The age of the not-so-equipoised was coming. Its harbingers can be seen in the late 1860s.[4] But the Victorians in 1870 didn't know that they were nearing the end of an era, so for most people at the time the most important change was increasing prosperity. Certainly Hughlings Jackson would have had no reason for existential angst—his career and its prospects were thriving. In a letter of 1869, to his brother Thomas in New Zealand, he wrote:

I am getting on well as far as the spreading of my views on disease of the nervous system is concerned, but it takes a long time for a physician in London to get into practice, and for

---

[1] Jackson 1870g.

[2] Schiller 1979, p.237.

[3] Goetz et al. 1995, p.48. After the war, the patriotic Charcot 'refused to attend medical congresses held in Germany' (Guillain 1959, p.26).

[4] See Newsome 1997, pp.113–117; and Young 1953, pp.100–102, 107–108.

the present my pecuniary position is nothing very remarkable. However I suppose hard work and patience will tell in time and I feel very well satisfied on the whole.[5]

To Jackson's good fortune, his neurological 'views' were developing in harmony with some of the cultural trends that surrounded him. Another theme in Chapter 2 was the societal movement toward *secularization* in the nineteenth century, which accelerated in the later decades. The declining centrality of religion was crucial to the work of Jackson and his colleagues, because it liberated them from the lingering necessity to avoid charges of materialism.[6] While they could pursue ideas that seemed to lead in that direction, they were not required to be materialists. In fact, many of the culture's leaders in philosophy and science were not strict reductionists, nor were they atheists. They were agnostics. The word 'agnosticism' was coined by Huxley in 1869.[7] Lightman has defined it as 'a species of scepticism', whose adherents were skeptical about the limits of human knowledge, so 'The essence of the agnostic argument was epistemological'.[8]

Spencer had started to work out his version of agnosticism—with a different label—in the 1850s. 'The Unknowable' was an epistemological axiom in his *First Principles of* 1862.[9] It had a quasi-sacred quality, because Spencer and the 'other Victorian scientists who serenely shed their belief in the Christian God, passionately struggled to retain the moral interpretation of nature that the ancient creed had supported'.[10] This characterization certainly applies to the core group of agnostics who took some of their inspiration and arguments from Spencer, including Huxley, Leslie Stephen (1832–1904), John Tyndall (1820–1893), and William Clifford (1845–1879). These men thought through their issues in the 1860s and published their vows to agnosticism in the 1870s.[11]

The 1860s were preparatory to changes that became manifest in the 1870s,[12] so 1870 is a convenient historical marker. When the physiologist Michael Foster left London to establish the Cambridge School of Physiology in 1870,[13] his move was part of a larger trend toward the professionalization of science.[14] That process had a profound impact on the larger culture, because 'scientific developments were at the center of Victorian intellectual life …'[15] Among the educated classes, there was a parallel development: '… in the early and mid-Victorian periods (1830–1870), the English did not think of their society as having a separate, distinct class of people known as "intellectuals", but … in the late Victorian years (1870–1900), they generally adopted this concept …'[16]

The two groups—scientists and intellectuals—overlapped. Spencer would have claimed membership in both. Because of Jackson's increasing affinity for some of Spencer's ideas, it is important to understand Spencer's position in British society *circa* 1870. I say *some* of Spencer's ideas, because I have seen little evidence that Jackson was interested in Spencerian concepts that were not immediately germane to his analyses of neurological problems. This

---

[5] Critchley and Critchley 1998, p.49.

[6] An explication of secularization in relation to Huxley is given by Smith 1999.

[7] Huxley initially formulated his thoughts about agnosticism in 1860; see Huxley 1900, vol.1, pp.216–222. See also Lightman 1987, pp.10–13. For Huxley's recollection of how he invented the word see Huxley 1896, pp.237–240.

[8] Lightman 1987, p.15.

[9] Spencer 1862/1864, pp.3–123. On Spencer's 'universal postulate', see Francis 2007, p.179.

[10] Richards 1987, p.246.

[11] See Lightman 1987, pp.93–95 and further.

[12] See Poynter 1968, and Greenblatt 1991.

[13] See Geison 1972, and Geison 1978, pp.13–47.

[14] See Young 1985, p.128.

[15] Young 1985, p.133.

[16] Heyck 1982, Preface.

caveat notwithstanding, Jackson's frequent and deferential references to Spencer had the potential effect of tying some of his intellectual standing to Spencer's. In 1870, such a connection would have been all to the good, because Spencer's star was rising rapidly.

Spencer's Place in British Culture

Spencer's writings began to attract attention in the 1850s.[17] His *Social Statics* (1851) and the first edition of *The Principles of Psychology* (1855), along with numerous essays, all contained elements of his early evolutionary thinking. Since the development hypothesis and Chamber's *Vestiges* were the subjects of widespread discussion, Spencer's ideas found a large audience. Following the publication of *First Principles* in 1862, his reputation 'began to soar'.[18] He became a member of the inner circles of London's scientific intelligentsia. In 1864 he was among the founders of the highly influential X Club, 'which consisted of a set of mutual [scientist] friends who were to become prominent in their respective fields of research …'. The group eventually 'wielded tremendous power in the scientific world'.[19]

By the late 1860s, Spencer had become 'a celebrity known to the middle class reading public at large'.[20] His reputation peaked in the 1870s and 1880s. He was considered to be a genius, because he pursued the idea of evolution into nonbiological realms where the more cautious Darwin did not venture. Spencer's consuming project, the Synthetic Philosophy, was unique. 'No other contemporary monument to the belief in the continuity of matter, life and thought, and laws governing them, could remotely equal it in volume and laboriousness of construction'.[21] Most important for our purposes, he 'made it possible to enlist the philosophy of mind under the banner of science'.[22] So the question arises, how much personal contact did Jackson actually have with the scientists and intellectuals who lived in the same areas of central London?

Jackson's Contacts with Spencer and Lewes

About Jackson's contacts with Spencer, valuable information is provided by the Critchleys. They found two letters in private hands *from* Spencer *to* Jackson. The first was dated November 26, 1866',[23] almost 2 years *before* the 'debate' at the BA in Norwich. It was written in response to a letter that Jackson had sent to Spencer, apparently regarding some of Jackson's observations and ideas about language and heredity. Spencer thanked Jackson for enclosing 'a copy of the Medical Journal containing the remarks to which you draw my attention'.[24] With regard to Jackson's views on heredity, Spencer finished politely by saying,

[17] My summary of Spencer's standing over time is based on Kennedy 1978, Richards 1987, Perrin 1993, Jones and Peel 2004, Francis 2007, and Smith 2007.

[18] Peel 2004, p.128.

[19] Lightman 1987, p.94. Spencer was also a member of the elite Athenaeum club, where Huxley, another X clubber, was also a member. At the X Club, it is said that, 'When Spencer claimed to have once written a tragedy, Huxley replied that he knew the denouement: "a beautiful theory killed by a nasty, ugly, little fact"' (Taylor 2007, p.22). See also Barton 1998.

[20] Jones 2004, p.6. Spencer's celebrity status in the United States, and his hypochondriacal tendencies, are described exhaustively in Werth 2009.

[21] Burrow 2000, p.44; see also Chapter 4 section on 'What did Jackson read in 1865?'

[22] Francis, p.185.

[23] Critchley and Critchley 1998, pp.54–55.

[24] Critchley and Critchley 1998, pp.54–55. They think the paper Jackson sent was Jackson 1866f. I am inclined to nominate Jackson 1866g, because Jackson 1866f was in the *Medical Times and Gazette*, whereas Jackson 1866g was

'I propose to reserve them in the hope of hereafter turning them to use'.[25] What happened to Spencer's hopeful promise is not clear, but the existence of Spencer's letter shows that (1) early in Jackson's career he was quite willing to point out his own contributions, even to a very prominent person, and (2) Spencer took Jackson's ideas seriously enough to comment on them in detail.

The second letter found by the Critchleys was from 1903,[26] near the time of Spencer's death, but there is other evidence of substantial contact with Jackson. In the second edition of Spencer's *Principles of Psychology* (1870), Spencer wrote that, in contrast to the cerebellum, '... the *cerebrum* predominates in creatures showing, like ourselves, the power of adapting throughout long periods ...*' And the footnote said: '* Let me here draw attention to papers in the *Medical Times and Gazette*, for December 14 and December 21, 1867, in which Dr. Hughlings Jackson has published some facts and inferences that quite harmonize with these interpretations, in so far as the common function of the great nervous centers is concerned'.[27]

Because Spencer was famously stingy about crediting his sources, his detailed citation of Jackson's papers is remarkable. It may be due to the fact that Jackson cited Spencer generously. Other snippets of evidence about contact between Jackson and Spencer are found in 1873,[28] 1883,[29] and, as mentioned, 1903.[30] Part of the difficulty in trying to investigate Spencer *vis-à-vis* Jackson arises from the fact that when Spencer was old, 'he recalled the vast bulk of his correspondence and had it destroyed, preserving only that material by which he wanted to be remembered'.[31] However, there was an intermediary who probably did bring Spencer and Jackson together in person in the later 1860s or early 1870s. It was George Henry Lewes, whom we met in Chapter 4.[32]

---

in the *British Medical Journal*, and Spencer said 'Medical Journal'. Moreover, Jackson 1866f says little about how 'associated ideas become organised', which was part of Spencer's reply of November 26, 1866.

[25] Critchley and Critchley 1998, p.55.

[26] Critchley and Critchley 1998, p.55.

[27] Spencer 1870, vol.1, footnote on p.62. Spencer's citation of Jackson (Jackson 1867h and Jackson 1867i) has the correct dates; in York and Steinberg 2006, p.51, Jackson 1867h should be dated December 14, not December 24.

[28] Discussing an analogy between 'mistakes in words' and 'choreal movements', Jackson said: 'But I now think, as was several years ago suggested to me by Mr Herbert Spencer, that there is in some of the cases of mistakes in words, the mistake of making a more general for a more special symbol' (Jackson 1873x, p.189). 'Several years ago' could have been 1866 or later.

[29] On January 9, 1883, Spencer wrote to an American supporter: 'I enclose some pages from the *Medical Times and Gazette* [6 Jan.] sent to me the other day by Dr. Hughlings Jackson' (Duncan 1911, p.227; Spencer's italics and square brackets). There is no article by Jackson in the *MTG* of January 6, 1883. The Critchleys (1998, pp.55–56) think the paper that Jackson sent was J82-08 (November 15) and J82-09 (November 22), and that would make sense. The subject of Jackson's two papers was his concept of dissolution in the nervous system, which Jackson derived from Spencer in the 1870s and 1880s. In his letter Spencer expressed some surprise—but not disapproval—about Jackson's conclusions.

[30] Shortly before Spencer's death on December 8, 1903, he and Jackson exchanged letters about 'Weismann's experiments' (Critchley and Critchley 1998, p.55; their footnote 6 on p.200 gives the date of Spencer's letter as '8th December 1903', but Spencer died early that morning; see Duncan 1911, p.477). August Weismann (1834–1914) was a physician-biologist who rejected the Lamarckian theory of inheritance of acquired characteristics (see Mayr 1982, pp.698–707). Jackson used Spencer's Lamarckian views from the 1860s; see Jackson 1866m, p.587; and Jackson 1868y, p.233, footnote concerning the mechanism of genetic inheritance.

[31] Francis 2007, p.vii; I have no reason to doubt this statement, but Francis gives no reference for it, and I have not found its source.

[32] Using the Eliot papers at Yale (which I have also reviewed through 1872), Raitiere (2012, chapters 8 and 11) claims that Spencer and Jackson did meet, and often, because Raitiere thinks that Spencer was Jackson's patient. The evidence for that is highly circumstantial (see Greenblatt 2017), but I agree with Raitiere's claim that the two men were probably in contact through Lewes. See also Chapter 9.

In the 1860s and 1870s, Eliot and Lewes lived together without formal marriage in a house called, paradoxically, 'The Priory'.[33] It was in the Regents Park section of central London, about a mile from Jackson's home in Manchester Square. They often entertained groups of friends and visitors at meals, especially Sunday lunch. By the later 1860s, those gatherings had become famous. Invitations were highly prized, especially by 'a varied group of "worshippers" of George Eliot's genius'.[34] In Lewes' diary of Sunday, June 20, 1869, 'Dr Jackson' is listed among the guests.[35] Since Lewes usually noted 'Mr and Mrs' when couples attended, the apparent absence of Mrs. Jackson raises some interesting questions.

Lewes and Eliot began their *de facto* marriage in 1854, when Lewes was long estranged—but not divorced—from his first wife. Those well-known facts disturbed the moral equipoise of the mid-Victorians. In the early 1860s, many women refused invitations to socialize at the Priory, so their husbands sometimes went alone. By the late 1860s, this reaction was less common but still in evidence.[36] I can only speculate that Mrs. Jackson's absence was an indication of that lingering disapproval, or perhaps she was just too modest about her own intellectual abilities in the setting of such a high-powered crowd. In any case, Jackson (alone) was a guest at lunch at The Priory at least twice in the early 1870s.[37] Given the mutual interests of Jackson and Lewes, it would seem likely that they would have met more often. Perhaps they did, but apparently not on any recorded occasions. Since Jackson had no patience for the frivolous, he might have found that Eliot's salons were not to his taste. It is also worth noting that Spencer's name is seldom found on the guest lists in Lewes' diaries.[38]

Lewes' consuming project for the last decade of his life was his five-volume treatise on *Problems of Life and Mind*, which was published from 1874 to 1879. Before publishing, he 'spent years amassing information ... [and] stuffing notebooks full of psychological case histories'.[39] In fact, many of those case histories were actually neurological, including one notation about Jackson's experience,[40] so it makes sense that his guest lists frequently included physicians who had neurological interests. Bastian seems to have been a favorite,[41] and Broadbent came for Sunday lunch on July 11, 1869.[42] Some days later, on July 23, Lewes recorded that he 'Called on Broadbent and spent the afternoon with him over the Brain. Showed me his discoveries of optic nucleus and convolutions having no direct central connections. Third convolution the most complex in its connections.'[43] Lewes' remark about the

---

[33] 21 North Bank; photo in Williams 1983, opposite p.154.

[34] Ashton 1991, p.252; and see further in pp.217–219, 251–253.

[35] Lewes' diary 1869, in Lewes, Beinecke/Yale, MS Vault Eliot Box 40. Other evidence (Lewes' reading lists) makes it clear that 'Dr Jackson' is *our* Dr. Jackson, not another one.

[36] Ashton 1991, pp.217, 252.

[37] On June 1, 1873 (Haight 1978, vol.9, p.97) and February 8, 1874 (Haight 1955, vol.6, pp.13–14). Since we don't have Jackson's personal papers, we can know about his appearances at The Priory only when he is mentioned in Eliot's and (usually) Lewes' correspondence, and the latter was not comprehensive about lunch guests.

[38] Lewes' diary 1871 in Lewes, Beinecke/Yale, MS Vault Eliot Box 42, says, 'Spencer and [Dr. T. Clifford] Allbutt to dinner' on February 8, but there is no other listing of Spencer through 1872.

[39] Ashton 1991, p.265. Lewes' collection included an abstract of Jackson's BA address (J68-16; see Lorch 2008, p.1661).

[40] Lewes, Beinecke/Yale, MS Vault Eliot Box 53, folder 17, 'Psychological cases' notebook, p.5: 'Dr Hughlings Jackson has had several patients who could swear but were unable to repeat the words of their emotional utterances when requested to do so.'

[41] Bastian came to dinner on May 23, 1868 (Lewes' diary June 1866 to May 1870 in Lewes, Beinecke/Yale, MS Vault Eliot Box 39). 'Dr & Mrs Bastian' were on the guest list for Sunday, June 27, 1869, and on other occasions in 1869 (Lewes' diary 1869 in Lewes, Beinecke/Yale, MS Vault Eliot Box 40).

[42] Lewes' diary 1869 in Lewes, Beinecke/Yale, MS Vault Eliot Box 40.

[43] Lewes' diary 1869 in Lewes, Beinecke/Yale, MS Vault Eliot Box 40.

'Third convolution'—presumably frontal—is indicative of his keen interest in the neurology of language. In his diaries he also kept lists of his readings. In 1871–1872 those lists contain at least four references to Jackson on 'Naming' or 'Aphasia'.[44]

Given Lewes' neurological interests, we would like to know how he became acquainted with Jackson, intellectually and personally. Several possibilities come to mind. First suspicion falls on Spencer, who knew about Jackson's interest in language and aphasia. Another possibility is the publicity about the Broca–Jackson episode at the BA in 1868. We have no indication that Lewes was there, but it is likely either that he was or that he followed reports of the sessions in the press. Since Jackson was gaining recognition at the time, Lewes might have taken notice of him in some other way. For Jackson's growing reputation, on the other hand, we have good evidence.

Jackson's Professional Situation, *circa* 1870

In 1868–1869 Jackson acquired important honors from the Royal College of Physicians of London. He had earned the College's membership by examination in 1861.[45] In 1868 he was elevated to its Fellowship, thus gaining the coveted 'F.R.C.P.'.[46] This title was prized because the powers-that-be in the English medical profession resided in that ancient body. In Jackson's case the honor was even greater, because, as we saw in Chapter 5, he was appointed Gulstonian lecturer for 1869. The candidates for this annual position are the 'four youngest Fellows',[47] so selection is in effect a designation of the most promising among them.

Now honors are nice, but it's usually life's day-to-day work that earns them, and Jackson did not lack for daily activities. His efforts to make a living were helped by his appointments at the London and Queen Square. He was also active in many of the local medical societies that sprang up in London in the nineteenth century. In addition to the three societies that he had joined in 1865–1866,[48] he became a Fellow of the Medical Society of London in 1868,[49] and it appears that he joined other groups at around the same time.[50] All the while he was publishing prolifically. Among his writings in 1868 were two book chapters which are indicative of his standing among his colleagues, because the chapters were requested by one of them.

---

[44] On April 23 and 25, 1871, Lewes noted 'Hughlings: Logic of Naming' (Lewes' diary 1871 in Lewes, Beinecke/Yale, MS Vault Eliot Box 42). In 1872 he noted reading 'Hughlings on "Naming"' (March 15); 'Hughlings' (March 16); and 'Trousseau & Jackson on Aphasia' (August 10) (Lewes' diary 1872 in Lewes, Beinecke/Yale, MS Vault Eliot Box 43).

[45] See Chapter 2.

[46] Brown 1955, p.161. In Critchley and Critchley 1998, p.39, the dates of Jackson's M.R.C.P. and F.R.C.P. are given incorrectly as 1860 and 1866.

[47] Email to me from Pamela Forde, archivist, RCP London, January 23, 2006.

[48] The Pathological Society of London, the Hunterian Society of London, and the Medico-Psychological Association; see Chapter 4.

[49] Minutes of the 'Tenth Ordinary Meeting, March 30th 1868', in the Medical Society of London Collection at the Wellcome Library, London.

[50] The Harveian Society (see J66-12); the Clinical Society of London (see J71-05); and the St. Andrews University Medical Graduates Association (see J68-23, and York and Steinberg 2006, p.56); for further on the St. Andrews Association see Blair 1987, pp.67–68).

Textbook Chapters 'On Apoplexy and Cerebral Hemorrhage' and on 'Convulsions', 1868

J. (John) Russell Reynolds (1828–1896) was Jackson's colleague on the staff of the National Hospital from 1864 to 1869.[51] In 1861 he had published *Epilepsy: Its Symptoms, Treatment, and Relation to Other Chronic Convulsive Diseases*.[52] With arguments that were reasonable at the time, Reynolds held that the word 'epilepsy' should be reserved for those cases that we would call generalized idiopathic, i.e., involving alteration or loss of consciousness, with or without observable movements, *and* without demonstrable lesion or cause. Everything else was labelled 'convulsions'. Of course, it was this 'everything else' that Jackson was studying. From 1866 to 1879 Reynolds edited a five-volume *System of Medicine*.[53] It was well received and widely used.

The combined neurological chapters constituted the first comprehensive textbook of neurology in English since the translation of Moritz Romberg's *Manual of the Nervous Diseases of Man* in 1853.[54] Reynolds' second volume was published in 1868. It included two chapters by Jackson: 'On Apoplexy and Cerebral Haemorrhage'[55] and on 'Convulsions'.[56] These two chapters are discussed here, in the context of *circa* 1870, rather than in their chronological place in Chapter 5, because neither contained anything new or different at the level of pathophysiology. Their focus was on clinico-pathological correlation, because Reynolds intended his *System* to be a practical guide to diagnosis, prevention, and treatment.[57]

The chapter 'On Apoplexy and Cerebral Haemorrhage' could more accurately be labeled 'Intracranial Hemorrhage'. It is more systematic than many of Jackson's writings. In our nomenclature, he discussed epidural, subarachnoid, and intracerebral hemorrhages in pathological terms that are close to ours. He also discussed subdural hematomas, but without knowing that they are anatomically *sub*dural, i.e., in the microscopic 'space' between the inner surface of the dura and the outer surface of the pia-arachnoid.[58] He thought that the blood in such lesions is in the 'arachnoid cavity',[59] but he understood the causal relationship between subdurals and trauma.

Jackson's chapter on 'Convulsions' in Reynolds' *System* immediately preceded Reynolds' chapter on 'Epilepsy'. Since Reynolds held views that might have been construed as opposed to Jackson's, the presence of Jackson's chapter in Reynolds' textbook tells us something about Reynolds. It confirms his reputation for fair-mindedness.[60] In fact, the two chapters are complementary, which presumably was Reynolds' intention. Within the spectrum of opinions on the subject, Jackson's ideas about seizures and epilepsy were still incompletely developed and not widely accepted, but Reynolds' chapter on epilepsy was arguably representative of the medical profession's views *circa* 1870. Hence I will review it for that perspective.

---

[51] Holmes 1954, pp.36, 96; see also [Reynolds] 1896, and Eadie 2007a.
[52] Reynolds 1861; see Temkin 1971, pp.289–291, and Buchwald and Devinsky 1988.
[53] Reynolds 1866–1879.
[54] See Eadie 2007a, p.312.
[55] Jackson 1868z; in Jackson 1868l, dated August 22, Jackson referred to this 'article *Apoplexy*' with a page number, so either the volume was published by then or he had the final page proofs. He was frustrated that he had to leave out 'nearly all illustrative cases' (see footnote on p.504).
[56] Jackson 1868y.
[57] See Reynolds' Preface to Vol.1.
[58] The true nature of subdurals was not worked out until the 1920s; see Sachs 1952, p.61.
[59] Jackson 1868z, p.509.
[60] See Eadie 2007, pp.310–311.

Reynolds' main thrust was the need for clarity, starting with nomenclature. He worried that the word 'epilepsy' had been abused to the point of uselessness:

> The older mistake was to apply the term to every case in which there were convulsions, appearing in a certain form, called "epileptic," "epileptoid," or "epileptiform;" the modern error is to use the word to denote a paroxysmal – *i.e.* occasional and sudden – loss or diminution not only of consciousness, but of any function of any organ ... [61]

Reynolds objected to terms like 'renal epilepsy' or 'epilepsy of the retina'. [62] He opined that, 'If good reason can be shown for getting rid of the word "epilepsy", I should rejoice to lose it from our nosology; but so long as the word is retained at all it should have a definite and intelligible meaning'.[63] He began his well-organized chapter with a

> Definition.– Epilepsy is a chronic disease of which the characteristic symptom is a sudden trouble or loss of consciousness, this change being occasional and temporary, sometimes unattended by any evident muscular contraction, sometimes accompanied by partial spasm [seizure], and sometimes by general convulsion.[64]

Within his definition Reynolds included mental and sensory auras.[65] He was particularly interested in interictal phenomena and the general health status of epileptic patients.[66] At the time it was widely believed that epilepsy is hereditary. Furthermore, another 'prevalent belief is that some form or degree of mental deterioration is necessarily associated with Epilepsy'.[67] To the contrary, Reynolds pointed out that 'statistics gathered from asylums' are likely to be skewed.[68] He had statistics from his own practice to show that inheritance and mental retardation are not so universal among epileptics.[69] In his discussion of 'Pathology' Reynolds adhered to the conventional wisdom: 'That the seat of the primary derangement is the medulla oblongata, and upper portion of the spinal cord ...' Physiologically, 'the derangement consists in ... [a] perverted readiness of action of these organs [medulla and cord]; the result of such action being the induction of spasm in the contractile fibres of the vessels supplying the brain, and ... [other regions]'.[70]

Jackson, on the other hand, was placing the abnormality in the striatum. He ignored the issue of the brainstem, saying simply, 'there is a Corpus Striatum Epilepsy, the analogue of Corpus Striatum Paralysis ...'[71] Although autopsy evidence for his localization

---

[61] Reynolds 1868, p.251. In this chapter on 'Epilepsy' there is no use of 'genuine', but Reynolds did use 'Epilepsy proper' on p.269 and 'epileptoid' on p.278.

[62] Jackson had used 'epilepsy of the retinae' (Jackson 1866d, p.443). He also used 'epilepsy' quite broadly (e.g. Jackson 1866g, p.328). In 1877 (Jackson 1877r, p.704) he said, 'I used to call ... these classes of cases [of 'sudden defect of sight'] epilepsy of the retina; but for many years I have abandoned this fallacious expression altogether, and now call them cases of epileptic amaurosis'.

[63] Reynolds 1868, p.252; Eadie and Bladin 2001, pp.58–59, provide a summary of Reynolds' nosology as of 1861.

[64] Reynolds 1868, p.251; my square brackets.

[65] Reynolds 1868, pp.262–263.

[66] Reynolds 1868, pp.268–269; see also Buchwald and Devinsky 1988. On p.278 Reynolds said: 'When conspicuous and persistent changes in the functions of the nervous system occur during the interparoxysmal period, we may infer the existence of structural disease.' He said this while maintaining that the site of the abnormality is in the brainstem.

[67] Reynolds 1868, p.269.

[68] Reynolds 1868, p.254.

[69] Reynolds 1868, pp.269–270.

[70] Reynolds 1868, pp.275–276; my square brackets.

[71] Jackson 1868l, p.178.

was lacking, he suggested a way to explain its absence. In 1867, he had described the case of a woman who suffered right-sided seizures a few days after a fall.[72] At autopsy, reported in 1868,

> There was blood in the arachnoid "cavity" on the left side. The bulk of it … lay in one spot over the frontal convolutions, and was so placed as, <u>I imagined</u>, to squeeze the corpus striatum, which body at the autopsy seemed to be otherwise undamaged. It is to the local anaemia which this mechanical pressure brought about that I attribute the local … *instability of nerve-tissue permitting the occasional disorderly* expenditure of force which constitutes the permanent factor in "epilepsy" … the addition of the words "corpus striatum" being to state where in this epilepsy the … disorderly expenditure occurred.[73]

So by 1868 Jackson's thinking about the localization of the lesion(s) in epilepsy had advanced part way up the neuraxis to the striatum, but not into the hemispheres. At the time, of course, none of this was as clear as I am stating it, and none of it was evident in his chapter on 'Convulsions', presumably because he wanted to be respectful of Reynolds' opinions. The result was a discussion of seizures that did not include his most advanced thoughts. In effect, he apologized for this acquiescence when he said, 'I beg the reader to bear in mind that this paper does not pretend to consider the whole subject of Convulsion, but only the relation Convulsion has to immediate professional action …'[74]

The complementarity of Jackson's chapter to Reynolds' is apparent in Jackson's opening paragraphs, where he distinguished between convulsions and epilepsy, albeit without mentioning the issue of consciousness. However, he was not enthusiastic about the nosological distinction.

> It cannot be kept too much in mind that a Convulsion is a symptom, not a disease …
>
> Convulsions occur in association with obvious organic changes in the nervous system of the most varied kinds, such as cerebral haemorrhage, intracranial tumours, and softening of the brain … Finally, there are a large number of convulsive seizures which, for want of knowledge … we are obliged to dismiss to the supposed definite groups of clinical symptoms, with the title of epilepsy or epileptiform.[75]

The last sentence separates Reynolds' 'Epilepsy' from Jackson's 'Convulsions', but the phrase 'obliged to dismiss' implies that the separation is arbitrary. Jackson did not think that alteration or loss of consciousness is a valid discriminator. In fact, he did not discuss the issue of consciousness in his chapter, nor had he given it any substantive attention in his publications throughout the 1860s. Presumably this is because he had no useful data about the physiological basis of consciousness, so he had no way to analyze its alterations. He and his contemporaries could only assume that consciousness is a function of the whole brain. In his

---

[72] Jackson 1867l, pp.352–355.

[73] Jackson 1868l, p.179; Jackson's italics, my underlining. The idea of local cortical tissue pressure squeezing the underlying striatum was tenuous. In 1876 (Jackson 1876v, p.290, footnote 1) Jackson acknowledged the criticism of 'Dr. Mickle', saying, 'I should not nowadays draw such an inference'. Presumably Mickle was William Julius Mickle (d.1917); see Brown 1955, pp.323–324. Jackson gave no citation for him.

[74] Jackson 1868y, p.241.

[75] Jackson 1868y, p.217.

preliminary remarks he invoked his tripartite method: 'But in many cases of Convulsions, as in so-called idiopathic epilepsy, whilst we know (3) the disorder of function, we know little as to (1) the organ affected, and nothing at all of (2) the minute changes on which the disorder of function depends.'[76]

So in 1868 Jackson was beginning to think that all seizures probably share the same underlying pathophysiology. However, in his chapter he quickly turned away from those thoughts to a long section on 'Convulsions in Children'.[77] About this he said: 'There is nothing pathologically different in the Convulsions of adults and the Convulsions of children. I say pathologically—for there are doubtless some physiological peculiarities in the abnormal states of muscles in children, due to disease attacking the nervous system whilst [it is] being quickly developed.'[78] Thus, he was sensitive to the importance of growth and development in children, and he lamented that 'our ignorance of the immediate causes of children's Convulsions is more profound than our ignorance of their causes in adults'.[79]

Throughout the 1860s Jackson made no direct references to Reynolds' publications, not even in his chapter on 'Convulsions' in Reynolds' *System*.[80] In his reporter's columns of 1861–1863 Jackson had used the word 'genuine' only twice that I've been able to find.[81] In 1866 he seems to have begun an occasional campaign against the term. He referred pejoratively to 'our idea of the almost metaphysical conception "genuine" Epilepsy',[82] and in 1867 he called 'genuine epilepsy' an 'insoluble problem'.[83] In December 1868 he was getting closer to the idea that all seizures share the same etiology.

> In subsequent notes ... I shall ... try to point out how convulsions beginning unilaterally resemble and differ from those more general convulsions which set in without warning or are preceded by an obscure sensation in the head or by a strange feeling at the epigastrium. The latter kind of convulsions are sometimes called "genuine" epilepsy, or idiopathic epilepsy.[84]

In 1869 Jackson published nothing more about the issues of 'genuine' epilepsy and consciousness, but in 1870 he delivered the 'notes' that were promised in the above quotation. This foundational paper was titled simply 'A study of convulsions'.[85] To construct his unified pathophysiological framework for all seizures, he brought together a *mélange* of ideas from many different sources. The following section will describe two related subjects in Jackson's thought that have so far been ignored—his concepts of (1) 'minute' and (2) 'coarse' disease of the brain.

---

[76] Jackson 1868y, p.218.
[77] Jackson 1868y, pp.219–241.
[78] Jackson 1868y, p.219; my square brackets.
[79] Jackson 1868y, p.220.
[80] The 'favor' was returned, since Reynolds gave no citations of Jackson in his chapter on 'Epilepsy'. Most of Reynolds' citations were to Continental authors.
[81] Jackson 1861a, p.198; and J62-02, p.223.
[82] Jackson 1866p, p.266.
[83] Jackson 1867b, p.296; full quotation in Chapter 4.
[84] Jackson 1868v.
[85] Jackson 1870g.

Some Additional Background to 'A Study of Convulsions'

'Changes in Tissue' in Jackson's Tripartite Method

In Chapter 4 I discussed the origins of Jackson's conception of instability in neural tissue, which he adapted from his predecessors, especially Todd. However, until now I have neglected Jackson's ideas about the nature of the microscopic changes that constitute the unstable focus.[86] Historically, we can trace the histological idea back to two elements: (1) his tripartite method, which led him to postulate the existence of (2) 'minute' histological changes in the focus. As applied to seizures, the latter was an original contribution.

As we saw in Chapter 3, Jackson first outlined his tripartite method in June 1864.[87] To advance the study of neurological disease, he had proposed to analyze each case in terms of (1) 'Disease of Tissue. (Changes in Tissue)', (2) 'Damage of organs', and (3) 'Disorder of Function'.[88] Over the years he repeated this mantra frequently. Concerning epilepsy, two related questions are: (1) how did he come to emphasize tissue changes, and (2) how did that emphasis lead to his idea of 'minute' changes as epileptic foci?

The theory of the primacy of tissue—rather than organs—came into biomedicine with the work of Xavier Bichat at the turn of the nineteenth century.[89] In the 1830s, the development of achromatic microscopes led to the establishment of cell theory by the botanist Matthias Schleiden in 1838 and the physiologist Theodor Schwann in 1839.[90] In 1858, when Jackson was still a house officer in York, Rudolf Virchow (1821–1902) brought cell theory into pathology and revolutionized the fundamentals of that entire field.[91] Jackson did not read German, but Virchow's *Cellular Pathology* appeared in English translation in 1860.[92] He certainly knew about Virchow no later than 1862, because his reporters' column with Hutchinson described a lecture on Virchow by Jackson's friend, Samuel Wilks, in the *Medical Times and Gazette* of July 12, 1862.[93] Wilks called histology a new and 'distinct branch of science'.[94] However, in the nervous system the power of Virchow's conception was constrained by the absence of the neuron theory, which did not come about until the 1890s.[95] Of course, this difficulty can be fully appreciated only in retrospect. At the time, the workers in the field simply kept working.

Lockhart Clarke and 'Minute' Tissue Changes in the Brain

One of those workers was a now-obscure figure with the auspicious name of Jacob Augustus Lockhart Clarke (1817–1880).[96] He is not entirely unknown, because neuroanatomists still

---

[86] The importance of Jackson's thoughts about 'minute' tissue changes became clear to me only when I read him chronologically. Those ideas were not previously analyzed by Walshe (1961), by me (Greenblatt 1977), by the Critchleys (1998), or by York and Steinberg (2006).

[87] Jackson 1864h.

[88] Jackson 1864h, p.147.

[89] Garrison 1929, pp.444–445.

[90] See Bradbury 1967, pp.191–199. On cell theory see Garrison 1929, pp.454–457.

[91] See Bynum et al. 2006, pp.121–122; and Garrison 1929, pp.570–571.

[92] Virchow 1860. At the London Hospital Medical College, Jackson was Lecturer on Pathology 1859–1869 and Demonstrator of Practical Physiology and Histology 1864–1870. These dates are approximations; see Greenblatt 1964, p.161.

[93] See Greenblatt 1977, p.414, footnote 9. The report of Wilks' lecture was not signed by either Hutchinson or Jackson, but presumably both would have known their column's contents.

[94] Wilks 1862, p.32; the subtitle of this lecture is 'On Virchow's theories'.

[95] See Definition Section 1 in Chapter 3; also Chapter 5.

[96] See Haymaker and Schiller 1970, pp.16–19; also [Clarke] 1880a, [Clarke] 1880b, and Clarke 1880c. He usually signed his publications as 'J. Lockhart Clarke'.

recognize 'Clarke's column' (or 'Clarke's nucleus')—a distinct group of neurons in the dorsal horn of the thoracic spinal cord.[97] Clarke described this structure in 1851, after he had developed a new method of hardening and clearing tissue for microscopy.[98] Those achievements led to his Fellowship of the Royal Society in 1854. He practiced in the Westminster (Pimlico) district of London, but never with great success. Apparently his focus was always on his science. His obituary described him as 'a man single of purpose, of noble independence and honesty, wholly free from ambition, and wanting in that knowledge of the world necessary for making way in it'.[99] Although Jackson proved to be wiser in the ways of the world, there would have been a deep sense of comradeship between these two men. So how, and when, did they meet?

The first evidence of a connection between Jackson and Clarke is from 1864, when Jackson stated that Clarke had sent him two cases of aphasia. Jackson saw the patients in June 1864 and included them in his paper on 'Loss of speech' of that year.[100] In December 1864 Jackson performed an autopsy 'On a case of disease of the posterior columns of the cord—locomotor ataxy (?)'. Clarke did an extensive histological workup of the spinal cord, and their joint paper was published in June 1865.[101] Later, in 1865, Jackson used 'some magnificent preparations lent me by Lockhart Clarke ...' in his 'Lectures on hemiplegia'.[102] I suspect that around this time Jackson may have been tutored by Clarke in histological technique, because Jackson described his own efforts at microscopic examination of three cases in 1865.[103]

Clarke's histological work had a crucial impact on Jackson's early thinking just when Jackson's originality was in the flux of its beginnings. Musing about his case of 'Involuntary ejaculations following fright—subsequently chorea' in 1865, Jackson said: 'Perhaps a minute examination of nervous tissue on Lockhart Clarke's plan might show some change in the motor tract or convolutions near it ... we may hope to discover what the disease of apparently healthy tissue in such diseases as chorea is.'[104]

So what was 'Lockhart Clarke's plan'? In 1863 he published another in his series of 'Notes of Researches on the Intimate Structure of the Brain'.[105] He usually investigated the spinal cord and brainstem, but this article was largely devoted to the '*Structure of the Cerebral Convolutions*' and their underlying white matter. According to Clarke the gray matter of the cortical convolutions is laminated into 'no less than *eight* distinct and concentric layers'.[106] There is no mention of any 'specific plan' in this paper, nor in the immediately preceding paper of the same series.[107] Jackson's next mention of minute tissue changes was in late 1866.

---

[97]   See Nolte 2002, p.233; also Pearce 2003, pp.48–50.

[98]   Clarke 1851; see also Bracegirdle 1978, pp.61, 83, 319. Clarke's use of Canada balsam resin to mount specimens gave much improved detail.

[99]   Clarke 1880b. Clarke was raised by his widowed mother in France. He quoted French and German authors liberally, and he published papers in those languages.

[100]   See Jackson 1864j, p.449.

[101]   Jackson 1865b; 'locomotor ataxy' is now known as (syphilitic) tabes dorsalis. Two years later Clarke and Jackson gave an early and accurate description of syringomyelia (Jackson 1867m), which is a degenerative cavitation of the center of the spinal cord; see Ramachandran and Aronson 2012, who state (p.60) that Clarke 'was attended during his last illness by John Hughlings Jackson ...'

[102]   Jackson 1865f, p.328.

[103]   See Jackson 1865c, p.627; and Jackson 1865h, pp.72, 78. The patients were autopsied in February, October, and November 1865.

[104]   Jackson 1865a. As discussed in Chapter 4, the patient possibly had Tourette's syndrome.

[105]   Clarke 1863.

[106]   Clarke 1863, p.716. He did most of this cortical research on the occipital ('posterior') pole, but he also stated (p.721) that the cellular structure is different in sections of cortex near the sylvian ('longitudinal') fissure. Since the late nineteenth century cytoarchitectonics has generally recognized six layers, but the neuroanatomist-psychiatrist Theodor Meynert (1833–1892) described large areas with eight layers; see Hakosalo 2006, p.177.

[107]   Clarke 1861.

It is most important to give a place in our thoughts to the slightest one-sided symptom ... in order that we may seek ... where the epileptic process begins in the brain, and thus get a clear idea of where to look, after death, for those <u>minute abnormal changes which are the permanent part of that unknown process.</u>[108]

Somewhere in the time between Jackson's reference to 'Lockhart Clarke's plan', on January 28, 1865, and the above quotation of later 1866, he developed his enduring hypothesis about 'minute changes'. My theory about the genesis of this innovation depends on a temporal coincidence. In Chapter 4 I discussed Jackson's use of Spencer's 'physiological units'.[109] Jackson's first published reference to them was contained in a report of his remarks on October 18, 1866,[110] so Jackson had encountered Spencer's 'units' by that date. We don't know the exact publication date of the above quotation, but internal evidence shows that it could not have been before December 1866.[111] It follows that Spencer's 'units' were part of Jackson's thinking by the fall of 1866, *before* his statement about minute tissue change in epileptic foci. In addition, he had been well versed in Clarke's histological studies of the cortex in 1865. Hence, Jackson's familiarity with Spencer's concept of a 'unit' could have been part of the inductive process that led Jackson to the idea of a microscopic focus in 1866. Further evidence for this proposition will come out when we see the larger importance of Spencer's 'units' for Jackson's thinking in 'A study'. And there is another factor in my theory.

In the time between the above quotation (1866) and his 'A study of convulsions' (1870), Jackson occasionally brought up the idea of 'minute' tissue changes, but without elaboration.[112] The idea seems to have lain largely fallow in those 4 years. Still, he continued to formulate a related idea about the gross pathology of unilateral seizures. I will deal with 'coarse disease' shortly, but it comes up now because Jackson sometimes contrasted it to 'minute' changes.[113] From numerous autopsies he knew that there is often focal disease of the brain when the patient has focal signs in life. Thus, in cases with focal seizures but no ostensible disease he reasoned that there must be a focal abnormality somewhere—if not grossly visible, then possibly microscopic.[114] I submit that this concoction of ideas in Jackson's fertile mind is the source of our current conception of epileptic foci—at the least it makes a credible story. In any case, he also stressed the importance of visible, 'coarse' disease, so we need to know more about the origins of his thoughts on that subject.

'Double Optic Neuritis' and 'Coarse' Disease of the Brain

When Jackson began to take an interest in ophthalmoscopy in the early 1860s, one of his main objectives was to observe the blood vessels in a living human organ that is directly connected to the brain.[115] Influenced by Brown-Séquard's vasomotor theories,[116] Jackson was also interested in the problem of 'amaurosis'. We still use this term to refer to blindness that

---

[108] Jackson 1866p, p.282–283; my underlining.

[109] See Chapter 4, section on 'Jackson's Ideas about Motor Disorders and Normal Brain Function in 1867'.

[110] Jackson 1866m, p.587.

[111] The dating of this paper (Jackson 1866p) is discussed in Chapter 4.

[112] See e.g. Jackson 1867b, p.296; Jackson 1868y, p.218; Jackson 1869f, p.380.

[113] See e.g. Jackson 1866p, pp.264–265. About the term 'coarse disease', in 1870 Jackson said (Jackson 1870g, p.178, footnote): 'it is used as the opposite of minute changes'.

[114] See quotation from Jackson 1867b, p.296, in Chapter 4.

[115] See Jackson 1862f, p.599; and Jackson 1863r, pp.10–11.

[116] Jackson 1863r, p.13.

is episodic or transient and not due to structural abnormality in the eye itself, i.e., amaurosis fugax. In the mid-nineteenth century, 'amaurosis' was used more broadly to mean loss of vision, but not necessarily with an episodic or transient element.[117] Given Jackson's detective-like instinct to solve neurological mysteries, the allure of this one is easy to understand. In his writings of 1863–1865, he struggled to comprehend the pathophysiology of amaurosis.[118] At the time, he was doing ophthalmoscopic examinations on large numbers of patients with all manner of neurological disease.[119] By late 1865 he began to see a pattern with regard to 'double optic neuritis'.[120] This is an instance when Jackson came to the correct conclusion for what we now recognize was the 'wrong' reason.

'Optic neuritis' now refers to inflammatory changes in the appearance of the optic nerve inside the back of the eye, where the nerve enters the globe (eyeball) and its entering 'head' can be seen through the ophthalmoscope. 'Inflammatory' means that the abnormality is due to a local irritative process within the tissue of the nerve. This abnormality is usually unilateral, but not always. However, changes induced by raised intracranial pressure (ICP) can look very much the same as optic neuritis. Swelling of the optic nerve head (papilla) is called papilledema. It can be more pronounced in one eye than the other, but usually the appearances are similar in each eye, because the cause is diffusely raised pressure inside the cranium. Hence, papilledema is usually bilateral—'double' in Jackson's terminology. Despite their similar appearances, the clinical implications of the two conditions can be quite different, because the presence of papilledema indicates raised ICP, which is often ominous. In Jackson's day, papilledema was not recognized as such. When it was seen it was thought to be optic neuritis.[121] Among the small group of clinical investigators who were interested in this problem in the 1860s,

> ... only Hughlings Jackson ... perceived that optic neuritis was not a uniform disease... [he] realized that in addition to optic neuritis concomitant with profound visual loss, a condition was present called neuritis, yet two of the cardinal signs of inflammation were lacking: there was no pain, and there was no loss of function ... Jackson had to insist many times, before his observation of swollen discs with intact vision was generally accepted ... The separation of patients with optic neuritis into those with good vision and those with bad vision countered the prevalent practice of classifying optic nerve disease by measuring diopters of disc swelling. Even Jackson's perspicacity did not prevent him from adopting an unwieldy theory of reflex vasomotor action to explain the swollen disc ...[122]

Our current understanding of papilledema is usually dated to 1911, when Paton and Holmes promulgated the idea that it is 'in its essential nature an *oedema*', due to back-pressure and obstruction in the venous drainage of the optic nerve, which in turn is due to raised

---

[117] Dunglison 1860, p.50, defined 'AMAUROSIS' as: 'Diminution, or complete loss of sight, without any perceptible alteration in the organization of the eye ...' The same definition was repeated in Dunglison 1874, p.39. Referring to a paper of 1866, Jackson later said (Jackson 1880o, p.969), 'The term "amaurosis" meant then atrophy which did not follow neuritis'.

[118] See Jackson 1863r, Jackson 1864b, Jackson 1864h, and Jackson 1865g.

[119] See Jackson 1865g, p.401 and footnote at asterisk.

[120] See Jackson 1868h.

[121] See Jackson 1868a, p.143; Jackson here used the word 'inflamed' and clearly described the appearance of 'optic neuritis', when it was actually papilledema. He also noted the frequent absence of visual loss in the milder stages of papilledema.

[122] Lepore 1981, p.178–179; my square brackets. In his reference 13, Lepore gives the date 1863 for the article that York and Steinberg (2006, p.47) list as '65–07'.

intracranial pressure.[123] This biophysical conception of ICP began to develop only at the turn of the twentieth century,[124] so no one earlier could have fully understood the pathophysiology of papilledema. Nonetheless, Jackson made an accurate correlation of 'double optic neuritis' with intracranial mass lesions on an empirical, clinico-pathological basis.

In late 1865 Jackson said, 'In all cases of [optic] neuritis in which I have made a *post-mortem* examination, there has always been found notable organic disease in the head'.[125] By 'organic disease' he meant grossly visible abnormalities, in comparison to 'minute' changes. In 1866 he began to use the term 'coarse disease', rather than 'organic disease', presumably to emphasize the contrast to findings at the histological level. He characterized a focal collection of coarse disease as a 'foreign body'.[126] We still use this latter term in the sense that Jackson meant it, as 'a mass out of its place'.[127] Throughout his career, Jackson took a special interest in neurosyphilis, partly because it was so common in his time, and especially because it was of particular interest to Hutchinson. Among its pathological phenomena are grossly visible lesions on the surfaces of the hemispheres, including inflammatory masses called gummas. However, Jackson understood that 'optic neuritis or epilepsy ... are [not] due to syphilis in any special manner. These two symptoms will occur in association with *any sort* of coarse disease of almost any part of the encephalon.'[128]

In essence, Jackson was correct in correlating bilateral papilledema with the existence of mass lesions or other gross pathology inside the cranium, although he knew that the correlation is not perfect. More to the present point, it was Jackson's early interest in ophthalmoscopy that led him to understand the role of 'coarse disease' in epileptogenesis.

'A Study of Convulsions', 1870: My Historiographic Approach

'A study of convulsions'[129] is the most important paper Jackson ever published—at age 35! His line of argument flowed mainly from his early clinical observations, to pathophysiology, and then to normal physiology. He was not entirely consistent about this, of course,

[123] Lepore 1981, p.179. In the year of Jackson's death (1911), his younger colleague, the ophthalmic surgeon Leslie Paton (1872–1943; see [Paton] 1943) provided the definitive explanation for the clinical entity (papilledema) that puzzled Jackson throughout his career.

[124] See Lepore 1982; Greenblatt 1997, pp.965–968; and Greenblatt 2003, pp.795–810.

[125] Jackson 1865h, pp.56–57, Jackson's italics, my square brackets. On p.64, referring to coarse intracranial disease, he mentioned 'the three symptoms of which I have spoken so much—headache, vomiting, and amaurosis ...' In Jackson 1866q, p.253, he described 'three symptoms, which very frequently come together, optic neuritis, vomiting, and severe headache. As a rule, these symptoms are produced by tumours ...' And in Jackson 1870g, p.178, he again said that when the three clinical phenomena are present 'I should then think it probable that ... [there is] ... a foreign body in the brain'. By the early twentieth century, and probably earlier, the combination of headache, vomiting, and papilledema was known as the clinical 'triad' of intracranial tumors (Cushing 1905, p.79). It appears that this maxim came from Jackson.

[126] Jackson 1866p, p.262. 'FOREIGN BODY' was defined in Dunglison 1860, p.401, as an 'Extraneous body', so the term was in use when Jackson applied it to neuropathology. In 1870 he said: 'I use the term "foreign body", as I use also the term "coarse disease", to include glioma, syphilitic nodules, hydatid cyst, blood-clot, abscess, &c...' (Jackson 1870g, p.178, footnote).

[127] Jackson 1866p, p.285.

[128] Jackson 1867k, p.50; Jackson's italics, my square brackets. He had made a similar statement in Jackson 1866p, pp.261–262. See also Jackson 1868h, p.392, which is the first instance I can find when he used the term 'double optic neuritis' (my underlining).

[129] In the *Selected Writings* there are at least four omissions in the text of 'A study': (1) on p.10 (pp.165–166 of the original) the original second paragraph of footnote 1 is missing. It contained a long discussion of Spencer; (2) on p.17 (p.176 in the original) a quotation from Reynolds (1861) is missing; (3) on p.23 (p.185 in the original) a long footnote about Trousseau is missing; and (4) after p.200 a figure (Plate I) is not reproduced.

and there is a problem with redundancy, both within the paper itself and in relation to his writings of the preceding years. I have tried to deal with this issue by creating an outline of the paper.

Outline of 'A Study of Convulsions'

As a piece of expository writing, 'A study' is better organized than most of Jackson's papers before 1870. This is readily seen in the outline (Table 6.1), which, as much as possible, is constructed with Jackson's original names for the sections within his article. In the column labeled 'New/old', items labeled 'New' in my opinion are original as they were presented in Jackson's 'Study', with the understanding that almost all of his ideas had predecessors. Hence, everything 'New' is a candidate for analysis here, though not all of the 'New' topics can be covered. The 'Old' items—already discussed in my *Overview* of August 1868[130] or in the Additional Background—will be brought up when needed to explain Jackson's synthesis.

'A Study of Convulsions', 1870: Analysis, Part 1:
Pages 162–185

Jackson began his paper with an iconic definition: 'A convulsion is but a symptom, and implies only that there is an occasional, an excessive, and a disorderly discharge of nerve tissue on muscles'.[131] Until early in the twenty-first century, the internationally accepted definition of epilepsy included a direct quotation from this sentence, along with the admonition that: 'This is the most difficult feature of the definition to apply in practice, because the electrical discharge is visible only under some circumstances of testing … Nevertheless, the definition assumes that such an abnormal electrical discharge could be ascertained under ideal circumstances'.[132] In other words, modern epileptologists are still struggling to fulfill the requirements of Jackson's definition. His idea of a localized focus[133] of instability in a limited piece of brain tissue has been simultaneously a unifying concept *and* an existential conundrum.

Disestablishing 'Genuine' Epilepsy

Immediately after his opening definition of 'convulsion', Jackson launched into his argument for ascribing all types of seizures to a unitary pathophysiology. He said that there are two 'classes' of 'chronic convulsions': (1) so-called 'genuine' or 'idiopathic', and (2) 'Those in which the fit begins by deliberate spasm on one side of the body, and in which parts of the body are affected one after another'.[134] He proposed to deal only with the second type: 'But

---

[130]   See 'Overview' in Chapter 5.
[131]   Jackson 1870g, p.162. Compare this sentence to the opening sentence of Jackson's chapter on 'Convulsions' of 1868: 'It cannot be kept too much in mind that a Convulsion is a symptom, not a disease' (Jackson 1868y, p.217; quoted above).
[132]   Fisher et al. 2005, p.471; my square brackets. See also Definition Section 5 in Chapter 4.
[133]   'Focus' was not Jackson's term, but the modern concept was clearly stated.
[134]   Jackson 1870g, p.162.

Table 6.1 Outline of Jackson's 'A study of convulsions' (1870g). Items in quotation marks are Jackson's original wording; phrases added by me are in square brackets.

	Pages	New/Old
[INTRODUCTION]	162–169	
[Definition of Convulsion]	162	New
[Disestablishing 'genuine' epilepsy—unitary pathophysiology]	162–163	New
[Instability versus destruction—comparing seizures to hemiplegia]	163–164	Old
[Motor functions in the cortices]	163–164	New
[Order of the march]	164–169	Old/New elements
[Larger grey matter representation of voluntary movements]	165–166	Old/New emphasis
[Molecular changes in discharge (Spencer)]	165	New
['*compound sequence*' of the march]	166	Old
REMARKS ON EPILEPTIC HEMIPLEGIA ['of Dr. Todd']	169–171	Old
REMARKS ON TONGUE-BITING—[no 'diagnostic value']	171–173	
DYSPEPSIA IN CHRONIC CONVULSIONS—[limit 'flesh food']	173	
ARREST OF FITS BY THE LIGATURE	173–177	
[Brown-Séquard on reflex 'external irritations']	175	Old/New emphasis
ABSENCE OF INSENSIBILITY IN CONVULSIONS	177–179	
[Due to 'minute changes'—rather than 'foreign body']	178	Old/?New
TEMPORARY DEFECTS OF SPEECH WITH CONVULSIVE SEIZURES	179–184	
[Aphasia is common with right face/tongue seizures]	179–180	Old
[Aphasia without agraphia is inconceivable, therefore hysterical]	180	New
['Mental' versus 'physical' is only 'degrees of difference' (same in J69-13, p.481, col.2)]	183	Old
CONVULSIONS BEGINNING IN THE FOOT	184–185	
THE CAUSE OF CONVULSIONS BEGINNING UNILATERALLY	185–204[a]	
1st. The seat of the internal lesion	186–193	
[Local symptoms denote a local lesion]	186–188	New emphasis
['The lump does not discharge']	188	New
[Diseased sylvian cortex produces the march]	188	New
[Cerebrum/mind/motor—uniformitarian associationism]	189	New
[Localization in levels—cortex and corpus striatum]	189–190	New
[Direct and indirect motor tracts from cortices]	190	New
[From 'unit' to graded, overlapping localization (*xyz*)]	190–191	New
[Co-ordination in Space and Time]	191	New
[Modification of Broadbent]	192–193	New
2nd. The nature of the changes in nerve tissue on which the spasm *directly* depends	193–195	
[Repeats: destruction versus instability]	193–194	Old
[All convulsions due to neural instability]	195	Old

(*continued*)

Table 6.1 Continued

	Pages	New/Old
3rd. The pathological process from which these local changes result	195–201	
'(*a*) Changes produced by embolism' [in the middle cerebral artery]	195–196	Old
'(*b*) changes diffused from coarse disease'	196–201	Old/New
4th. The circumstances which may determine a paroxysm	201–204	
['Paroxysm … determined by contraction of arteries']	203	Old/New emphasis
['Co-ordination' in space ('Simultaneous movements are brought about by combinations of fibres and cells')]	203	Old/New emphasis
['Co-ordination' in time is determined by vascular contraction]	203–204	Old/New emphasis
['Co-ordination is the function of the whole and of every part of the nervous system' (integration)]	203	New

[a] The subsection titles listed below are from Jackson's initial summary of this section, on pp.185–186. In the actual texts of these sections he changed the wordings of the subsections at the heads of the second, third, and fourth subsections.

although I thus limit myself to one class of cases, I contend that the title of my article is correct.* I trust I am studying the general subject of convulsion methodically when I work at the simplest varieties of occasional spasm …'[135] His emphasis on unilateral seizures was longstanding, but the collateral meaning of his text was new, i.e., all convulsions share a common etiology. Again the meat of his argument was in a footnote, which had a Spencerian flavor.

> * Those who say that the two classes differ "only in degree" make a remark the truth of which is admitted … But in what kind of degree do they differ? … in degree of evolution of the nervous processes which are unstable. A convulsion which is general, and in which the muscular regions are affected nearly contemporaneously, must depend on discharge of parts in which the nervous processes represent a more intricate co-ordination of muscles in Space and Time than those parts represent, which when discharged, produce a convulsion which begins in one limb and has a deliberate march. My speculation is that the first class differs from the second in that convolutions at a greater distance from the motor tract are discharged.[136]

Here Jackson was proposing that cortical discharges near the striatum are responsible for focal seizures, whereas discharges in hemispheric cortices away from the motor tract—later in evolution—are the cause of generalized seizures. In both classes the inciting event is a cortical discharge, so there is no fundamental difference between generalized and focal seizures. Now it would be ludicrous to claim that the nosological idea of 'genuine' epilepsy

[135] Jackson 1870g, pp.162–163.
[136] Jackson 1870g, p.162; my underlining.

disappeared immediately after 1870, simply because Hughlings Jackson said it should, but this is where its denouement began.[137]

The evolutionary element in the above quotation is the idea that cortical 'nervous processes'—whose discharge can affect the whole body simultaneously—must be evolved to control more of the body than those whose discharge affects more restricted parts. This was a premonition of his later conception of hierarchical levels in the brain. This idea of cerebral hierarchy was only embryonic in 'A study', but his statement that the discharges are in the convolutions was a change from his earlier thinking.

Extending Motor Functions into the Hemispheric Cortices, 1870: Part 1

Until 1870 and beyond, Jackson generally maintained his conviction that the striatum is the most rostral part of the motor tract. Nonetheless, as early as 1865, discussing a patient with hemiplegia and aphasia, he had said, 'The probability is, that the convolutions near the corpus striatum have to do with guiding muscles in articulation'.[138] In 1867 he added that 'deeper in brain ... are still more complex arrangements of motor processes',[139] where 'deeper in brain' meant further from—higher than—the striatum. In his second Gulstonian Lecture of 1869, speaking broadly about 'disease of the cerebral hemisphere', he said:

> On this higher level, however, there will, doubtless, be some kind of localisation ... Since – as Lockhart Clarke has pointed out – the structure of the anterior convolutions does differ from that of the posterior, they must serve differently in mind. Facts seem to show that the forepart of the brain serves in the motor aspect of mind, and we may fairly speculate that the posterior serves in the sensory.[140]

The last sentence in the above is the place where Jackson first began to work out his broad conceptions of anterior–posterior specializations of the hemispheres, paralleling the left–right specializations that had already appeared in his analyses of aphasia. Those speculations will be pursued in my later chapters. For now we might ask, what is the meaning of the 'motor aspect of mind' if it does not mean that there is motor representation in the hemispheric cortices, where mind is supposed to reside? To this question Jackson answered in terms of a unified pathophysiology.

> ... the most common variety of hemispasm [unilateral seizures] is a symptom of disease of the same region of the brain as is the symptom hemiplegia; *viz.* the "region of the corpus striatum." The loose term "region of the corpus striatum" is advisedly used. Hemiplegia shows

---

[137] See Temkin 1971, pp.349–351.

[138] Jackson 1865e, p.284; see also the same citation in Chapter 4.

[139] Jackson 1867i, p.669.

[140] Jackson 1869d; my underlining. This quotation is taken from the report of Jackson's second Gulstonian Lecture in the *British Medical Journal*; it is not included in *The Lancet*'s report of the same (Jackson 1869c). We would still agree broadly with the statement regarding the frontal lobes as compared to the parietal and occipital lobes. Jackson's reference to Clarke's findings apparently relates to Clarke 1863.

damage (equivalent to destruction) of the motor tract, hemispasm shows damage (equivalent to changes of instability) of the convolutions which discharge through it. Palsy depends on destruction* of *fibres*, and convulsion on instability of *grey matter*. <u>As the convolutions are rich in grey matter I suppose them to be to blame, in *severe* convulsions</u> ... But as the corpus striatum also contains much grey matter ... it may be sometimes the part to blame in slighter convulsions. Indeed if the discharge does begin in convolutions, no doubt the grey matter of lower centres ... will be discharged secondarily by the violent impulse received from the primary discharge.[141]

This was the place where Jackson first began to locate the discharging lesion for most types of seizures in the hemispheric cortices, although he did not entirely dismiss the corpora striata or other sites where gray matter is present. By allowing the possibility that there might be motor representation in the cortices close to the striatum, he was starting to give up the idea that the striatum is the most rostral part of the motor tract. At this point in his 'Study', however, he did not address that issue. He went on to a different problem.

Pathophysiology of the Discharge at the Molecular and Cellular Levels

It follows from the above quotation that the key to the pathophysiology of all seizures is understanding what is happening in gray matter. With his usual faith in the utility of clinical data, Jackson approached this issue by considering the implications of the motor march. He knew that the march is 'very significant in regard to what is under different aspects variously named "co-ordination", "grouping", "localisation", "plan of structure of nervous organs" ...,[142] i.e., motor integration. Referring to a principle that he had already enunciated, he said: 'Parts which have the most varied uses will be represented in the central nervous system by most ganglion* cells.'[143] In the footnote he offered his conception of the 'discharge', partly in terms that he took from Spencer's view of functional neurohistology.

* Although both the nerve fibre (axis cylinder) and the ganglion cell "store up force," it is the latter which stores it up in large quantity, and to instability of grey matter, therefore, will be chiefly owing the excessive discharges in convulsions.

Herbert Spencer ... supposes that "the masses [the grey matter] unstably constituted and conditioned, are seats of *destructive* molecular changes ... while the stably constituted and conditioned threads [axis cylinder] are the seats of molecular changes that are not destructive ..."[144]

---

[141] Jackson 1870g, pp.163–164; Jackson's italics, my square brackets and underlining. In the footnote at the asterisk Jackson said, '* The word "destruction" is scarcely the correct word to use ... it is not meant that the nerve fibres are necessarily broken up ... but simply that there is a change in them which *destroys their function*' (italics in original).

[142] Jackson 1870g, p.165.

[143] Jackson 1870g, p.165. Jackson hinted at this idea in Jackson 1866p, p.283. He stated it clearly in Jackson 1867i, p.669, and in Jackson 1868p, p.239.

[144] Jackson 1870g, p.165; the italics *and* the round and square brackets are all Jackson's. For this quotation from Spencer, Jackson cited ' "Principles of Psychology", 2nd edition, page 23'. This referred to Spencer's Vol.1, because Vol.2 was published in 1872.

Now we have to go back a few years, because there seems to be a contradiction about the functions of cells versus fibers. In my Overview of 1868, I stated that Jackson tended to conflate the two histological elements into terms like 'nerve tissue' or 'neural tissue'. Until the 1890s he could not have known how the cells connected to the fibers, so he thought about them separately. Since fibers are long, it seemed obvious that they convey signals, so fibers and cells could have different functions and dysfunctions. In a paper of October 1869 he wrote:

> Every nervous organ is made up of two elements – nerve fibres and cells. Palsy is owing to destruction of the former, and spasm to instability of the latter. The presumption is, that parts which have most varied, most widely associated, most independent actions have the greatest representation by ganglion cells, and that parts which have the least varied, &c. actions are most represented by fibres.[145]

This statement is different than his view of August 1868, because here in 1869 he was ascribing some 'representation' to 'fibres', and he seemed to imply that fibers can discharge on their own and thus cause seizures. Now we've already seen that in 'A study' Jackson was attributing some of this changed view to Spencer. Indeed, some of Spencer's morphological and physiological speculations had penetrated into Jackson's analyses. This is evidenced in the latter part of Jackson's footnote about Spencer.

> The following quotation is very important … the fact that parts which have most varied uses suffer most and first in convulsion is an illustration of the view expressed in the quotation [from Spencer]. "Each vesicle [cell], or each portion of grey matter … is *also a reservoir* of molecular motion which it gives out when disturbed … it follows that in *proportion to the number, extensiveness, and complexity of the relations* … that are formed among different parts of the organism, will be the *quantity* of molecular motion which the nerve-centres are capable of disengaging."[146]

Here Jackson went back to the functional primacy of cells. Despite the uncertainties about the respective functions of cells and fibers, both of Jackson's quotations from Spencer served to strengthen his conclusion that, 'Parts which have the most varied uses will be represented in the central nervous system by most ganglion cells'.[147] Spencer's conception of 'molecular motion' is essentially chemical, involving an interpretation of what was then known about proteins, colloids, and isomers.[148] By Spencer's logic, there will be more 'molecular motion' and thus more force associated with gray matter areas that represent more complex movements. Hence Jackson's designation of the cortex as the usual site of the discharges in both 'genuine' and focal seizures was based partly on his application of Spencerian evolution to the functions of the cellular elements in the cortices.

The modern definition of epilepsy assumes that the discharge is electrical.[149] However, there has been a small controversy about Jackson's conception of the events in the discharge.

---

[145] Jackson 1869l, p.140; my underlining.

[146] Jackson 1870g, pp.165–166; Jackson's italics, my square brackets. For the quotation from Spencer, Jackson cited 'Part 20 of his "System of Philosophy"'. Paragraph 20 in Spencer's *Psychology*, 2 ed. (Spencer 1870), pp.52–54, discusses this subject, but I cannot find the exact wording that Jackson quoted, either in Spencer's Paragraph 20 or in Spencer's other writings.

[147] Jackson 1870g, p.165.

[148] See Spencer 1870 (vol.1), pp.18–25.

[149] See Fisher et al. 2005, p.471: 'the definition assumes … an abnormal electrical discharge …'

Is it fundamentally an electrical phenomenon, is it chemical, or is it something else? Because 'discharge' sounds electrical, some authors have assumed that Jackson always had an electrical event in mind when he said 'discharge'. E.H. Reynolds makes this assumption.[150] He then goes on to show that Todd analogized the epileptic discharge to electricity in 1849, so Todd should get priority for this, rather than Jackson.[151] However, Reynolds is probably denying Jackson an honor that he would have rejected. York and Steinberg point out that Jackson 'never employed the terminology of electricity or polarity in describing epilepsy'.[152] Since chemistry was Jackson's 'first love', they propose that 'his conception of the epileptic discharge was chemical, not electrical'. Despite Jackson's apparent ratification of Spencer's chemical speculation, I submit that Jackson's notion was neither electrical nor chemical. It was more generic.[153]

To explain 'discharge' in 'A study' Jackson did not make any direct analogies to electricity or to chemical reactions. At one point he used the words 'discharge' and 'explosion' in sequential paragraphs—ostensibly as interchangeable.[154] A few pages later, with apparent approbation, he quoted Russell Reynolds' definition of the discharge as 'the peculiar organic condition upon which the paroxysm depends'.[155] Jackson's nonspecific view on this matter probably predated any influence by Spencer. To my reading, in 'A study' Jackson used 'discharge' only to indicate release of force (energy).[156]

'Eccentric' Stimuli and Focal (Jacksonian) Seizures

How the discharge is conceptualized is fundamental to understanding all epileptic phenomena, including the aura. Jackson recognized it as part of epilepsy in 1866,[157] and this interpretation of the aura was generally agreed by his contemporaries.[158] In his 'Study' Jackson addressed the pathophysiology of the aura in his discussion of 'Arrest of fits by the ligature'. Since ancient times it had been known that some Jacksonian seizures can be interrupted by tying a ligature around the limb proximal to where the march is starting.[159] Since Brown-Séquard explained all epileptic phenomena with his reflex theory, he thought about auras in that way.[160] Jackson accepted his mentor's idea, but with a critical change of emphasis.

---

[150] Reynolds 2001. Although I am rejecting Reynolds' view about Todd and Jackson, as based on a false presumption, Reynold's statement about the general neglect of Todd's experimental brain stimulation still stands. However, Todd's experiments were hardly definitive.

[151] Temkin 1971, pp.284–285, does not mention *electrical* discharge in his summary of discharge theories among Jackson's immediate predecessors 'around 1860'.

[152] York and Steinberg 2006, p.13.

[153] In 1866 Jackson speculated that a postictal, 'enfeebled hemisphere' could discharge 'tension' which it acquired from 'nutritive changes' (Jackson 1866p, p.263, second footnote). In 1876 he said (Jackson 1876v, p.280, footnote 1): 'I use such expressions as "store up energy" in the sense that the nerve cells are nourished by nutrient fluids containing potential energy; such expressions as "currents passing", &c., are used conventionally, and not as implying any particular hypothesis.'

[154] Jackson 1870g, p.174.

[155] Jackson 1870g, p.176, footnote.

[156] In Jackson 1873c, p.163, right column footnote, Jackson gave an explicitly chemical explanation of the seizure discharge—phosphorus is replaced by nitrogen. He explored this idea more extensively in J73-25, p.327. However, in Jackson 1875i, p.399, footnote (*a*), he said: '... such expressions as "store up force", "carry the current", &c., are used conventionally. I have no theory as to "nerve force", or force of any kind.'

[157] Jackson 1866p, pp.282–283; and Jackson 1868v, p.696.

[158] See Temkin, pp.306, 308.

[159] Temkin 1971, pp.39, 70.

[160] See Koehler 1994, especially p.192.

... it is unreasonable to suppose that a local irritation starting from the hand is the *sole* cause of the seizure – that it can provoke discharge in a *healthy* nervous system. It is to Brown-Séquard that we are indebted for our precise knowledge of the relation of <u>external irritations</u> to the production of convulsive paroxysms ... It may be supposed ... that in such cases of [Jacksonian] convulsion as I have described, there are ... two factors, (1) an irritation starting from the fingers which travels to (2) the part of the nervous system unstable, and then determines the discharge.[161]

The idea that abnormal stimuli in peripheral tissue ('eccentric' or 'external' irritations) can cause the onset of seizures is very old. It continued into the nineteenth century,[162] but it is not part of modern epileptology, and it was Jackson who started its elimination. He simply de-emphasized it by insisting on the necessity of a preexisting abnormality in central gray matter. Such a lesion could produce an aura, with or without an overt seizure. This line of thinking also led him to an explanation of interictal auras:

It indeed occasionally happens that an epileptic complains more to his doctor when his fits are diminished in number. It may be that when his serious troubles are lessened, he thinks of the smaller ones. But I suppose that before the abrupt explosion which constitutes the severe fits there are frequent minute discharges – too trivial to produce any visible effects, but enough to cause discomfort to the patient.[163]

'Absence of Insensibility in Convulsions'

Another longstanding problem that Jackson approached with similar logic was the clinical meaning of loss of consciousness in seizures.[164] The generally received opinion was 'that absence of insensibility in convulsions is some evidence that the internal lesion is organic, such for instance as tumor',[165] and Reynolds agreed.[166] We have seen that Reynolds excluded seizures without loss of consciousness from the category of 'genuine'.[167] As an empirical matter, Jackson agreed that he had never done an autopsy on a case of focal seizures without finding 'organic disease'. Nonetheless, he disagreed with the proposition that absence of unconsciousness *necessarily* indicates the presence of visible abnormality.

Such convulsions [without loss of consciousness] *point only to minute changes involving instability in the opposite hemisphere*. If the reader will not admit this, it suffices for the present argument to say that they only point to *local* changes of instability. They tell us nothing of the pathological processes by which that local instability results ...[168]

Jackson's position in the first sentence is still valid. That is, the clinical focality of a seizure indicates only where it is originating in the brain, not the type of pathology. He was able to

---

161 Jackson 1870g, pp.174–175; Jackson's italics and parentheses, my square brackets and underlining.
162 See Temkin 1971, p.290; and Eadie and Bladin 2001, p.132.
163 Jackson 1870g, p.174.
164 Jackson 1870g, pp.177–179.
165 Jackson 1870g, p.178; Jackson cited 'Dr. [Thomas] Addison' as the source of this statement.
166 Reynolds 1868, p.278.
167 Reynolds 1868, p.268; see also above in this Chapter.
168 Jackson 1870g, p.178; Jackson's italics, my square brackets.

make this crucial distinction because he had concluded that *all* seizures arise from '*minute changes involving instability*'. In this view, initial loss of consciousness in a seizure leads only to 'the inference that the discharge is of parts at a distance from the motor tract'.[169]

Aphasia and the Unity of the 'Mental' and the 'Physical'

With minute changes in epileptic foci in the background, Jackson went on to a long consideration of 'Temporary defects of speech with [focal] convulsive seizures'.[170]

> I have long observed of convulsions that when spasm begins on the right side there is defect of speech more marked than when it begins on the left ... when the spasm starts in the *face and tongue* of the right side, there usually is great defect of speech ... and there usually is not when it starts in the *right hand or right foot*.[171]

This was not new, but it gave him another opportunity to define his view of aphasia. He admitted that his own autopsy findings in cases of 'permanent *loss* of speech' due to 'destroying lesions' generally showed lesions in Broca's area. However, he felt 'that the absolute distinction made between cases of "genuine" aphasia and certain cases of difficulty of articulation* is at the least arbitrary, and I think misleading'.[172] And again in a footnote:

> * I cannot believe that there is any adequate reason for the popular separation of symptoms into "mental" and "physical." Everyone admits that there are degrees of evolution of sensori-motor processes, from those which are comparatively simple to those which are exceedingly compound, and the terms "physical" and "mental" may be convenient, but only as names for large degrees of difference.[173]

The most interesting part of this quotation is Jackson's use of 'Everyone'. In the midst of the ruckus about evolution in 1870, surely he was not referring to evolution's opponents or to the part of the literate population that was simply bewildered by the whole thing. I think 'Everyone' refers to Jackson's professional circle and to the writers that he was reading, especially Spencer. With his exaggerated use of 'Everyone' he was giving us his perception of his own milieu, in which Spencer's evolutionary associationism was coin of the realm. This was a major factor in his willingness to push motor processes into the hemispheres. In his writings before 1869, he had seldom made such statements about the identity of the mental and the physical.[174] His earliest, straightforward statement to this effect was published in late October 1869.[175] Jackson's apparent unification of the mental and the physical in 1870 shows the ascendency of the uniformitarian element in evolutionary associationism. We will see more of the same in the second part of Jackson's 'Study'.

---

[169] Jackson 1870g, p.182, footnote.
[170] Jackson 1870g, pp.179–184; my square brackets.
[171] Jackson 1870g, p.179; Jackson's italics.
[172] Jackson 1870g, p.183.
[173] Jackson 1870g, p.183; my underlining.
[174] See Jackson 1865a, p.89.
[175] Jackson 1869m, p.481; Jackson's statement was: 'mental and physical being but convenient names for large degrees of difference ...'

'A Study of Convulsions', 1870: Analysis, Part 2: Pages 185–204

The second half of Jackson's 'Study' was labeled 'The cause of convulsions beginning unilaterally'.[176] Using his conception of destructive versus destabilizing lesions, where the latter includes 'minute changes', he again denied the physiological reality of 'eccentric' causes of epilepsy.[177] Regarding such proffered causes for Jacksonian seizures, he said: 'The fact that the symptoms are local, implies ... that there *is* of necessity a *local* lesion'.[178] Therefore 'there must of necessity be some *place* where the nervous system is diseased, or the spasm determined by [eccentric] causes acting generally would not be local'.[179] On the other hand,

> I should not expect easily to discover the minute changes from which results only an *exaggeration of normal function*. It is the function of nerve tissue in health to 'store up' force and expend it in an orderly manner at the provocation of special excitations. The discharge of disease differs from the expenditure of nerve force in health, in quantity, and in that it is provoked by a more general excitation. And even in those cases where we do find a lump in the brain ... we do not discover the *very* changes on which the discharge depends. The lump does not discharge, but some ("softened") part of the brain near it—which part cannot be destroyed or it would not discharge at all ...[180]

Jackson's dictum 'The lump does not discharge' is fundamental to the modern clinical understanding of epilepsy, although I have never seen it quoted directly. In short, it says that seizures arise from brain tissue—period. This seems simple enough, but applying it in practice has not always been so straightforward. Jackson advanced its application by working out his pathophysiological framework to account for a wide variety of seizure phenomena. Part of this new framework was his evolving view of motor functions in the cortices.

Extending 'Sensori-Motor' Functions into the Hemispheric Cortices, 1870: Part 2

In the first part of his 'Study' Jackson entertained the idea that, 'As the convolutions are rich in grey matter I suppose them to be to blame, in *severe* convulsions ...'[181] In the second part he took the idea about the convolutions into the realm of the normal. For this he went back to an old theme, but with a new, comparative twist. Since the postictal hemiplegia after a Jacksonian seizure and the hemiplegia of stroke ('plugging of the middle cerebral artery') are clinically 'exactly' alike, they both imply 'local' disease 'in the region of the corpus striatum'.[182] From there, he said:

> ... when the fits begin in the hand ... if we do discover a gross lesion, it is found in the region of the corpus striatum – in the region of the brain supplied by the Sylvian artery ...

---

[176] See Table 6.1.
[177] Jackson 1870g, pp.186–187.
[178] Jackson 1870g, p.186; Jackson's italics.
[179] Jackson 1870g, p.187; Jackson's italics, my square brackets.
[180] Jackson 1870g, p.188; Jackson's italics and parentheses, my underlining.
[181] Jackson 1870g, pp.163–164; Jackson's italics.
[182] Jackson 1870g, p.188.

Some will reply that disease of *many* parts of the brain "will produce epilepsy." This is really irrelevant. I will not deny that disease in many parts of the encephalon "may produce epilepsy." I wish but to show that disease in the <u>Sylvian region</u> produces those convulsions which begin in one hand or in one side of the face, and which affect the side of the body they commence in . . .[183]

The transition from 'region of the corpus striatum' to 'Sylvian region' is critical, because the 'Sylvian region' includes the hemispheric cortex that is supplied by the middle cerebral artery. Jackson was not giving up on the striatum as a motor center. Rather, he was also allowing motor functions into the hemispheric, peri-sylvian cortex. Another long footnote contained essential background to those developing thoughts.

It is asserted by some that the cerebrum is the organ of mind, and that it is not a *motor* organ . . . It may then be asked, How can discharge of part of a *mental* organ produce *motor* symptoms only? . . . But of what "substance" can the organ of mind be composed, unless of processes representing movements and impressions; and how can the convolutions differ from the inferior centres, except as parts representing *more* intricate co-ordinations of impressions and movements in time and space . . .? Are we to believe that the hemisphere is built on a plan *fundamentally* different from that of the motor tract? . . . Surely the conclusion is irresistible, that "mental" symptoms from disease of the hemisphere are fundamentally like hemiplegia, chorea, and convulsions, however specially different. They must all be due to lack, or to disorderly development, of [normal] <u>sensori-motor processes</u>.[184]

Careful reading of this passage shows that 'the motor tract' implies purely motor functions below the hemispheres, whereas 'sensori-motor processes' in the hemispheres presumably refers to the combined 'sensori-motor' unit of associationism. So what Jackson was allowing into the hemispheres was a more complex entity than simple motor functions.

Although Spencer was cited only twice in 'A study',[185] the above shows his rising influence on Jackson's thought. Jackson could have asked the same questions and obtained the same answers at any time after 1865, but our cautious Yorkshireman needed more clinical data and more time for cogitation. He reached his conclusion that there are motor functions in the cortices only after he had fully absorbed Spencer's evolutionary associationism, including its uniformitarian basis. That is why he did not find the above arguments convincing until 1870. Thus it was Spencer who cleared Jackson's path to acknowledging the 'sensori-motor' functions of the cortices. And Spencer did more than that. His evolutionary outlook contributed directly to Jackson's analysis of how localization works at the physiological level.

Following Spencer's Evolutionary Physiology Deeper into Localization Theory

The basic elements of Jackson's mature theories about normal and disordered brain organization are found on pages 189–191 and 203 of his 'Study'. He started by asking a rhetorical question:

---

183 Jackson 1870g, p.188; Jackson's italics, my underlining.
184 Jackson 1870g, p.189; Jackson's italics, my square brackets and underlining.
185 In the same long footnote in Jackson 1870g, pp.165–166.

If … a square inch … of convolutions were cut away by the knife, there would be no loss of power, no paralysis. This is admitted. How then can discharge of this square inch produce violent convulsions? If lack of the part leads to no *loss* of function, how can discharge of that part lead to *excessive* function?[186]

To this paradox he replied:

As nervous processes ascend in complexity, the number of fibres of necessity increases, and at the same time the number of ganglion cells. Moreover, the ascent is not one of aggregation – different independent processes being tacked upon others. It is an evolution of the higher out of the lower … The facts supplied by cases of hemiplegia show that *each* part of the corpus striatum "contains" movements of the whole of the face, arm, and leg, although no doubt in each part the muscles of the face, arm, and leg are represented in <u>different degrees</u>, and are grouped in <u>different order</u>. In hemiplegia the loss is of a *certain* number of possible Simultaneous movements of the face, arm, and leg – the sum of a number of possible co-ordinations in Space. Similarly a convulsion on one side is the abrupt development of a certain number of possible Successions of movements of the face, arm, and leg – the sum of a number of possible co-ordinations in Time.[187]

In the first part of this paragraph, Jackson was expressing the embryonic idea that he later called 'levels'. That is, his conception of hierarchy in the nervous system was not simply a matter of 'different independent processes being tacked upon others'. At each higher level there is physiological reorganization of the representation of movements 'in different degrees' and 'in different order'. At the 'comparatively simple' level of the striatum, to which he still attributed hemiplegia, Jackson said:

Now palsy results from destruction of *fibres*, and of course the *fewer* fibres which go to a muscular region from a particular part of the nervous system,* the *more* that region is paralysed by a destroying lesion in that part. <u>In the ascent from the comparatively simple processes of the corpus striatum to the highly complex ones of the convolutions</u> there will necessarily be a great increase of fibres, and hence large destroying lesions in the hemisphere will result in no palsy, whereas palsy will follow lesions equally large in the corpus striatum. But the increase of complexity necessitates many ganglion cells, results in a large supply of explosive matter, and hence excessive discharge, producing severe convulsions … when this grey matter becomes unstable.[188]

The first sentence of this paragraph is a repetition of material in the first half of 'A study',[189] but the main point is Jackson's increasing commitment to 'complex' motor functions in the hemispheric cortices. This is seen in the body of the paragraph, where he talked about the 'highly complex [processes] of the convolutions', and in the asterisked footnote, where he speculated

---

[186] Jackson 1870g, p.189; Jackson's italics. Before the 1870s, ablative experiments on animals ('convolutions cut away by the knife') were uncommon, though Flourens' were well known; see Chapter 3; also Walker 1957. It is common to find cortical lesions with no clinical deficits in life.

[187] Jackson 1870g, pp.189–190; Jackson's italics, my underlining. A similar statement is found in Jackson 1869l, pp.139–140.

[188] Jackson 1870g, p.190. Jackson's empirical observation is true. Small lesions that involve the striatum and the motor tract at the internal capsule (see Definition Section 2 in Chapter 3) can cause much worse paralysis than larger ones in the cortices.

[189] Jackson 1870g, pp.163–164.

about motor fibers originating in the convolutions: '*It is not to be implied that all fibres run direct from the brain to the muscles. No doubt there are series of centres betwixt the convolutions and the muscles they move. Probably some fibres run direct.'[190] The footnote shows that he was beginning to think about the anatomical details of his proposal about sensori-motor functions in the peri-sylvian cortices. He was being led into the cortices by evolutionary theory, but his theoretical ideas had to be consistent with the clinical evidence. In the next paragraph he translated his observations on Jacksonian seizures into a conception of how movements of the body are represented both in the striatum and similarly at the next level up, in the cortex.

> Then it may be said that one convolution will represent only the movements of the arm, another only those of speech, another only those of the leg, and so on ... this is not the plan of structure of the nervous system. Thus, to take an illustration, the external parts [i.e., groups of muscles], x, y, z, are each represented by units of the corpus striatum. But the plan of representation is not that some units contain x largely only, as x_3, others y largely only, as y_3, but that *each* unit contains x, y, and z – some, let us say, as x_3, y_2, z, others as x_2, y_3, z, &c. When we come to the still higher evolution of the cerebrum, we can easily understand that, if the same plan be carried out, a square inch of convolution *may be wanting*, without palsy of the face, arm, and leg, as x, y, and z are represented in other convolutions; and we can also understand that *discharge* of a square inch of convolution must put in excessive movement the *whole* region, for it contains processes representing x, y, and z, with grey matter in exact proportion to the degree of complexity ...[191]

Now nothing about this difficult passage is easy to understand, so it requires elucidation:

(1) Jackson did not refer directly to phrenology, so it is hard to say that he was still slaying the old bogeyman. What is clear, however, is his *denial of simplistic localization*. In his theory, distinct functions are not represented in separately demarcated pieces of cortex, which would result in a phrenological, 'mosaic' pattern of localization.[192]

(2) In Chapter 4 we saw that Jackson first began to use Spencer's generic idea of functional 'units' in 1866, after his 'reading period' of 1865. By October 1869 the concept was integral to his thinking.[193] Earlier in this chapter I tried to show that it was an enabling component in his conceptualization of epileptic foci as 'minute changes'. The paragraph quoted above is transformative. It is the place where Jackson first gave Spencer's 'unit' a specified meaning in physiological terms. It follows that this contribution from Spencer is potentially contained within all subsequent theories of cerebral localization that may be derived from Jackson's.

(3) Jackson used the word 'unit' when he tried to explain his scheme of x's, y's, and z's. This is the starting place for his graded and overlapping (weighted and ordinal) theory of localization.[194] For the rest of his life he continued to use this theory with the same

---

[190] Jackson 1870g, p.190. Here Jackson was speculating about structural details of the corticospinal tract (see Definition Section 2 in Chapter 3). He still thought that there is primary motor localization in the striatum, i.e., that some fibers run from the corpus striatum to the muscles. In fact, there are no such connections. These uncertainties could be worked out only after the nature of the corticospinal tract was defined by Flechsig in 1876 (see Temkin 1971, pp.315–316) *and* with the advent of the neuron theory in 1891 (see Shepherd 1991, pp.177–193).

[191] Jackson 1870g, pp.190–191; Jackson's italics, my square brackets.

[192] See Chapter 3.

[193] See Jackson 1869l, pp.139–140; and J69-13.

[194] See York and Steinberg 1984; also Greenblatt 1988; York and Steinberg 1995; York and Steinberg 2006; Steinberg 2009.

meaning that it has in the above quotation. Therefore it is imperative to understand what he meant—and what he did not mean—when he tried to express his thoughts in this way, which I will label his '*xyz* theory'.

As Jackson worked out the implications of his theory over the years, its underlying conceptions did not change, but his way of writing it did vary—often to the reader's bewilderment. At times he used italicized capitals (X, Y, Z) to stand for the peripheral movements which were represented by corresponding units (x, y, z) in the brain. At other times the capital letters (A, B, C) stood for parts of the central nervous system, or the lower case x's, y's, and z's represented the peripheral (muscular) regions *and* their cerebral representations. Sometimes the attached numbers were subscript, as above, e.g., x_3, y_2, z; and sometimes the numbers were superscript, e.g., x^3, y^2, z. In general he called these combinations 'terms', rather than 'units', but none of these differences matters. They all meant the same thing. *The numbers were used to indicate only arithmetic multipliers*, not geometric. So x^3, y^2, z or x_3, y_2, z both meant three parts of x, two parts of y, and one part of z. They did not mean x to the third power, y to the second, etc.[195] If this is understood, the further development of Jackson's theory of localization can be followed without driving oneself to distraction.[196]

Viewed from 1870, the germinal idea of Jackson's localization theory can be seen in a long footnote in 1866.[197] His theory was consistent with Spencer's earlier, antiphrenological description of the soft boundaries in cortical localization as 'insensible shading off'.[198] And Jackson's theory of 1870 included additional Spencerian elements, the factors of Time and Space.

Integration of Movements: 'Co-ordination in Space' and 'Co-ordination in Time'

To begin his analysis of coordinations in Space and Time, Jackson posed another rhetorical question: 'Why, if the face, arm, and leg are represented together in the [same] square inch [of cortex], is the fit a sequence only? Why are not all these parts convulsed contemporaneously?[199] He answered with a discussion of how the brain mediates normal 'co-ordination' in space and time. I will first describe his theories about these normal functions (combining his pages 191 and 203), and then I will deal with his explanation of how normal brain organization determines the patterns of Jacksonian seizures.[200] He began with an admonition.

[195] In Jackson's use of Spencer's 'units', x alone, or x with any multiplier, could be a 'unit', as could xyz, with or without multipliers. In his *Principles of Psychology*, 1 ed., 1855, Spencer (1855) used a rather complex system of capitalized and lower case letters to try to explain 'Memory', but without multipliers.

[196] For other explications of Jackson's *xyz* theory see Greenblatt 1988; York and Steinberg 2006, pp.17–18; and Berkowitz 2018, p.450. When he used the *xyz* theory very briefly in 1888 Jackson (1888f, p.388, footnote 1) said: 'Nothing beyond rudest quantification is of course meant by these symbolisations, in spite of the employment of definite indices'.

[197] Jackson 1866q, pp.238–239.

[198] Spencer 1855, p.609; see also Chapter 4.

[199] Jackson 1870g, p.191; my square brackets.

[200] Jackson realized that he had to either salvage 'Broadbent's hypothesis' (see Chapter 4) or abandon it. In 1869 he had struggled with the inconsistency between his developing theory of cortical localization and Broadbent's assumption of the existence of subcortical commissural fibers. In his 'Study' he replaced Broadbent's assumption with the idea of *bilateral* hemispheric representation of automatic movements in the normal state, saying, 'Broadbent does not make an absolute distinction betwixt bilateral and unilateral movements ... I think there can be no doubt that the hypothesis is so far correct ... that the more muscles of the two sides act together, the more equally they are represented in the two sides of the brain, and the less they are paralysed on one side from disease of the opposite side of the brain' (Jackson 1870g, pp.192–193).

We are in the habit of considering degrees of range of paralysis – defects of co-ordination in Space – and too little degrees of disorderly succession of movements – disorders of co-ordination in Time … we may for analytical purposes consider each distinctly. <u>Co-ordination in Space</u> – the power of using several muscles together for one purpose – is brought about by groupings of fibres. <u>Co-ordination in Time</u> – the process by which one movement follows another – is brought about by relations betwixt ganglion cells … There must in health be fixed orders of simultaneous movements, and fixed orders of successions of movements.[201]

Some parts of this passage are likely to engender feelings of unease in us moderns—until we remember that Jackson did not have our neuron theory. He thought that fibers can generate their own signals, although the cells do it more intensely. Keeping this in mind helps to remove the confusion of saying, in the above quotation, 'Co-ordination in Space … is brought about by <u>groupings of fibres</u>', whereas 'Co-ordination in Time … is brought about by <u>relations betwixt ganglion cells</u>'. However, Jackson's units were not composed exclusively of cells or of fibers. Near the end of 'A study' he said,

Simultaneous movements are brought about by combinations of fibres and cells. <u>Successions of different movements [in time] are developed by contraction of arteries.</u> *Repetitions* of movements may be owing to repeated discharges of the *same* nervous process. But when one movement follows a different movement automatically, the discharge of the nervous process for the first movement develops the second movement by fibres to the vessels supplying the nervous process for that second movement.

I take it for granted that the arteries are arranged on some plan, or orderly nutrition would be impossible.[202]

So according to Jackson in 1870, coordination in Space is the result of the physical proximity of the components in each motor unit (in the *xyz* theory) to each other, but the physiology of time relations is mediated by arterial events. That is, when a motor unit discharges to generate a normal movement, part of its efferent signal is sent to 'fibres to the vessels supplying the nervous process for that second movement'. Thus, the discharge of the second unit is determined by changes in its metabolism ('nutrition'). This whole vascular idea seems foreign to us. Since the later nineteenth century we have presumed that the nervous system is capable of generating its own temporal relationships by a mechanism within itself.[203] On the other hand, Jackson's source for his vascular idea is not far to seek—it is part of the pathophysiology of Jacksonian seizures that he had worked out several years earlier.[204]

The usually accepted theory of the production of the paroxysm is that it is determined by contraction of arteries. (Brown-Séquard.) I have advanced the speculation that certain symptoms … follow the order of arterial regions, and that the *liability* to the convulsions which I have described in this paper – those at least beginning in the hand – is due to persistent changes in the region of the middle cerebral artery, and that the *paroxysm* itself is owing to a *local* vascular contraction.

---

[201] Jackson 1870g, p.191; my underlining.
[202] Jackson 1870g, p.203; my underlining and square brackets.
[203] See Debru 2006.
[204] See 'Overview' in Chapter 5.

It seems to me that the development of simultaneous movements and of movements in succession must depend on <u>different processes</u> both in health and in disease ...[205]

Indeed, he expected further study of unilateral seizures to clarify those 'different processes'.

In disease, the range of paralysis and the sequence of spasm will represent sums of fixed orders of co-ordinations ... When records of cases in which the spasm extends to the second side are obtained, the presumption is that sequences will be disclosed, which will show the time relations of physiological regions of the limbs of one side, to physiological regions of the limbs of the other side ...[206]

All of this amounts to a form of neural *integration*, which Jackson called 'co-ordination'.

It is ... of great importance to distinguish the two kinds of co-ordination [Space and Time]. It will not ... suffice to speak of co-ordination as a separate "faculty." <u>Co-ordination is the function of the whole and of every part of the nervous system</u>. And although each part co-ordinates different impressions in different time-relations ... the process ... is fundamentally the same – in breathing, walking, and thinking ...[207]

Here Jackson was describing coordination of the whole organism in a sensory-motor, reflex model, which he had derived from associationism. It evokes 'integration' in Sherrington's sense,[208] because Sherrington's conception of integration is in some measure derived from Spencer's and Jackson's concept of 'co-ordination'. This proposition will be examined again in Chapter 13. Here I will try to summarize Jackson's main ideas about brain function and dysfunction as of 1870.

Summary and Analysis of Ambiguities

Normal Brain Organization and Functions

At the histological level, Jackson and his contemporaries recognized 'cells' and 'fibres'. They understood that the fibers carry signals generated by the cells, but Jackson also stated that the fibers can generate signals on their own. Before 1870 he accepted the contested opinion that the most rostral part of the motor tract is the striatum, and he extended the 'sensori-*motor*' system into the peri-sylvian cortices, while retaining a central role for the striatum. In the motor system the more voluntary movements are represented by larger numbers of cells.

Jackson's cautious extension of the motor system into the hemispheric cortices was facilitated by his deepening commitment to the principles of Spencer's evolutionary associationism, including its uniformitarian assumption. It was this evolutionary outlook that led to his view of the motor system in the striatum as functioning at a lower level than the motor system in the cortices. Thanks to secularization, in 1870 Jackson could deal with the hemispheres in this materialistic way. The 'will' had been driven out of its last stronghold—there is

---

[205] Jackson 1870g, p.203; Jackson's italics, my underlining.
[206] Jackson 1870g, p.191.
[207] Jackson 1870g, p.203; my square brackets and underlining.
[208] Sherrington 1906.

no mention of it in 'A study'. However, it is important to note that Jackson did not point specifically to the *pre-rolandic* cortex as the primary location of voluntary motor control in the cortices. He said only that there are motor processes in *peri-sylvian* cortex, which is within the territory of the middle cerebral artery.

When Jackson inferred some details of normal brain organization from brain dysfunctions, especially motor seizures, Spencer's theoretical construct of 'physiological units' was integral to his thinking. As explained in Chapter 4, those 'units' were, in effect, any combination of histological and/or anatomical structures that work together to carry out a particular function. Thus, a group of fibers and cells that controls a limb movement (e.g., labeled *x*) could be a 'unit', and an aggregation of such groups to produce some combination of movements (e.g., *xyz*) could also be a 'unit'. Jackson proposed that spatial coordination of movements by the organism is the product of the activities of such units in connection with each other, but their temporal coordination is mediated by vasomotor effects on the tissue's metabolism. In our terms, the totality of these sensory-motor 'co-ordinations' by the nervous system would be integration, although he did not use that word.

Abnormal Function: The Pathophysiology of Motor Seizures

Jackson's pathophysiology of convulsions started with the distinction between positive and negative symptoms, which he had probably learned from Brown-Séquard in 1861.[209] The existence of positive symptoms has to mean that some tissue is alive, in contrast to negative phenomena, which must mean that neural tissue is destroyed or at least totally nonfunctional. In 1870 Jackson continued to maintain that the 'palsy' of hemiplegia is due to destruction of gray matter in the contralateral striatum. Although he was willing to locate some motor functions in the hemispheric cortices, in 1870 his *xyz* theory did not predict that destruction of large amounts of cortical tissue could also lead to hemiplegia. Indeed, he thought that damage to cortical tissue would often leave some representations of movements alive but potentially unstable. This instability could happen in the gray matter of the striatum, but it was more likely to occur in the cortices, because they contain much more gray matter, i.e., many more units representing movements. The timing of the pattern of the march, he thought, is determined by abnormal reactions in the vascular beds that control tissue metabolism ('nutrition').

All of this is background to Jackson's canonical definition: 'A convulsion … implies only that there is an occasional, an excessive, and a disorderly discharge of nerve tissue on muscles.'[210] In 'A study' he left the nature of the abnormal 'discharge' undefined, without saying whether it is electrical, chemical, or whatever. It is simply a normal unit discharging abnormally. He stated that convulsions can be associated with the presence of any kind of lesion, including 'softening' (stroke) and focal masses, but 'The lump does not discharge'.[211] Only neural tissue has the capacity to discharge, normally or abnormally. In the common situation where no lesion is found at post-mortem, Jackson postulated the existence of 'minute disease', i.e., changes at the histological level, although he could not see them. Thus was born the idea of a seizure 'focus'. Jackson did not use that term in 1870, but he applied the concept to all seizures. By making this generalization he hoped to disestablish the existence of the old nosological category of 'genuine' epilepsy. It died gradually, largely by judicious

---

[209] See Chapter 4.
[210] Jackson 1870g, p.162.
[211] Jackson 1870g, p.188.

application of benign neglect. The assumption of a central focus also laid to rest the antique idea of 'eccentric' foci.

Antiquities and Ambiguities
Although it is fair to say that 'A study of convulsions' is *the* foundational document of modern epileptology, it is still a historical text—written at a particular historical time—so it is equally fair to say that it is not thoroughly modern. Some parts of it are antiquated, in some places it is ambiguous, and some of its ambiguities are still with us. A prime example is Jackson's use of Spencer's 'physiological units' within his *xyz* theory. Since the *x*, the *y*, and the *z* are functional entities, separately or together, it is not clear whether individual cells and/or fibers can participate in more than one functional unit. Today we would make that assumption, but Jackson said nothing about it, which probably means that he had not considered the problem enough to make a statement. The question is important because the presence of the *xyz* theory in 'A study' makes the theory a part of our own thinking.

Another ambiguity is Jackson's antiquated theory of vasomotor reflexes as the controlling factors in the temporal sequencing of normal movements and focal seizures. The idea may not be totally antiquated, because at bottom it postulates metabolic factors in temporal sequencing. However, Jackson knew that the vasomotor nerves can activate only vasoconstriction, by stimulating contraction of the smooth muscle in the vessel walls. Vasodilation is a passive process, due to loss of vasoconstriction. So the question arises, how can the vasomotor system control temporal sequencing without active vasodilation? To put it another way, Jackson did not specify the vascular mechanism of temporal sequencing. With regard to the pathophysiology of seizures, since the early 1860s he had agreed with Radcliffe that seizures indicate an enfeebled state of the nervous system,[212] so apparently he assumed that vasoconstriction alone can cause seizures, but again the mechanism was not specified. This might also be relevant to another problem: i.e., how does focal discharge spread? We now talk of recruitment and synchrony, and he expressed those concepts in the later 1880s, but in 1870 he did not have them.

An Ambiguity Resolved
In Young's extensive review of Jackson's contributions to 'a thoroughgoing sensory-motor view … [of the] cortex and its functions …' he concludes that when 'Jackson's statements on the convolutions and the striatum up to 1870 are brought together and compared … they defy integration into a consistent, unified view'. And a few years later I shared his frustration.[213] We both found Jackson's 1870 statements about the corpora striata to be confusing, because he continued to localize some motor functions and some seizure foci in those subcortical structures, while simultaneously saying that motor representation and seizure foci also exist in the cortices. We had both fallen into the either/or trap. Jackson's apparent ambiguity is resolved by realizing that he meant that those localizations are not mutually exclusive.[214] His hierarchical view of the nervous system was just beginning to take shape in 1870, but even at this early stage he considered the striatum to be at a lower functional level than the cortices—motor movements that are 'represented' in the striatum are represented

---

[212] See Chapter 4.

[213] Young 1970, p.220; Greenblatt 1977, p.430.

[214] Actually, they are. The corticospinal tract runs from the cortical motor strip (area 4) to the spinal cord largely without intermediary, but continuing, connections, and there is no primary motor localization in the striatum. See Definition Section 2 in Chapter 3.

again in the cortices.[215] Working at those problems was part of his obligation to 'Medical Physiology'.

The Perspective and Status of 'Medical Physiology'

In the first part of his 'Study' Jackson dropped a remark that is quite telling with regard to his view of his own scientific enterprise. A young female patient had focal Jacksonian seizures beginning in the right thumb, sometimes arrested by 'tying up' the right hand. At the end of his detailed description of her attacks, Jackson said, 'The foregoing is little more than physiology—medical physiology it is true, but still physiology'.[216] The little phrase 'it is true', after 'medical physiology', implies that 'medical physiology' is of a lower order than some other, higher standard of physiology. In 1870, of course, the privileged standard was laboratory-based, experimental physiology, which was the *sine qua non* of truly 'scientific' work. In the continental world of Claude Bernard, and the school of Johannes Müller,[217] messy clinical data were second class, and Jackson was well aware of this higher standard.[218]

One could nominate Jackson's *Suggestions* of 1863 as his first attempt to improve the 'medical physiology' of the nervous system. In 1865 he used the term 'Medical Physiology' and protested its lower status:

> ... perhaps, strictly speaking, it is incorrect to class the experiments of disease with those performed to ascertain the functions of organs in healthy animals. Vivisection cannot help us much in ascertaining the functions of the corpus striatum, as it is too deeply placed for operation; but this organ is often damaged by rupture of a blood vessel in man.
>
> I think, then, it is convenient to use the name "Medical Physiology" for the line of investigation of which I am now speaking. Our School Physiology and our Medical Physiology do not very well harmonize; and this is, I think, particularly true of the physiology of the corpus striatum ...[219]

A year later, in 1866, Jackson lamented the prospects for scientific Medical Physiology, because of the poor organization of the British medical profession.

> To establish the laws of healthy muscular movements, and of those variations in them which occur in certain altered states of nerve tissue and nervous organs, is a thing of fundamental importance for the progress of the Medical Physiology of the Nervous System. I have no faith that this sort of physiology will make steady progress until the body medical is more highly organised. There is great differentiation in Medical Practice, but not enough unity of aim in cultivators of Medical Science.[220]

---

[215] Jackson began to use the term 're-represented' in 1873; see Jackson 1873k, p.532.

[216] Jackson 1870g, p.173.

[217] See Porter 1997, pp.320–341; and Bynum et al. 2006, pp.113–120. On the 'school' of Müller's numerous students see Otis 2007.

[218] Hagner (2012, pp.245–247) says that the results of Fritsch and Hitzig's experimental results with cortical stimulation tended to force German physiologists back toward some regard for clinical data; on Fritsch and Hitzig see Chapter 7.

[219] Jackson 1865f, p.301; for Jackson's later comments on this passage see Jackson 1873x, pp.181–182. Also in 1865 Jackson noted that he had a 'written scheme' for examining the 'physiology of [the] nervous system' (Jackson 1865c, p.627).

[220] Jackson 1866p, p.254.

Here Jackson was complaining about the effects of the different practice patterns of family doctors and consulting physicians, which leads to loss of follow-up data. This was a frequent theme in his writing. Remember that his first published notice of Broca in 1864 was a letter to the editor of the *British Medical Journal*, asking its readers to look into their records for relevant cases.[221] In 'A study' he made a similar plea.[222] This kind of effort was a significant factor in Jackson's early reputation within the profession. In 1866 Wilks was much more upbeat about the situation. He thought that '... the last few years have added much to our knowledge in this [physiological] direction ...' He listed Jackson and Broadbent among 'The workers in our country in this department ...', i.e., in 'the physiological study of nervous disease'.[223]

In Chapter 2 I referred to Geison's description of 1840–1870 as a period of 'stagnancy' in English physiology.[224] Perhaps it is not entirely coincidental that Jackson's major treatise on 'medical physiology'—his 'Study'—appeared in 1870.[225] In any case, unknown to Jackson at the time, two clinical physiologists in Germany were obtaining experimental data that supported his clinically derived theories. In 1873 those theories provided part of the impetus to one of the most important British contributions to experimental physiology in the nineteenth century.

---

[221] Jackson 1864c, p.572.

[222] Jackson 1870g, p.168: 'I therefore ask those in family practice, who can watch patients longer than a physician can, if they can give records of cases ...'

[223] Wilks 1866, p.154.

[224] Geison 1972 and 1978.

[225] On 'medical physiology' see also Jackson 1873a, p.84.

7

Jackson's Developing Theories of Brain Organization and Ferrier's Experimental Results, 1870–1874

'A study of convulsions', Jackson's iconic paper, was published in an obscure journal, but it was also reprinted as a pamphlet.[1] In *The Lancet* of November 12, 1870, the pamphlet was reviewed by an anonymous writer who concluded that, 'Dr. Hughlings Jackson once and again contributed some valuable additional information relative to the study of nerve diseases'.[2] Unlike the fate of many fundamental contributions, which often have to wait a generation to be widely accepted, Jackson's main ideas were confirmed experimentally in 1870 by the team of Gustav Fritsch (1838–1891) and Eduard Hitzig (1838–1907) in Berlin. However, Jackson referred to the German work only after David Ferrier's (1843–1928) first publication of his confirmatory experiments, which appeared on April 26, 1873.

Fritsch and Hitzig, Jackson, and Ferrier, 1870 to Fall 1873

Fritsch and Hitzig Find Motor Cortex, 1870

In the history of experimental neuroscience, Fritch and Hitzig's 1870 paper 'On the electrical excitability of the cerebrum' is a classic.[3] They showed that low-current 'galvanic' (DC) stimulation of the frontal surface of the dog's brain causes reproducible movements of the animal's face and legs. To explain the many previous failures, they attributed part of their success to the fact that they explored the cortical surface widely, including the frontal areas that are hard to expose. Their findings 'overthrew three theories that had stood since Flourens [in the 1820s]: they established [1] cortical excitability, [2] a role for the cortex in the mechanisms of movements, and [3] cerebral localization'.[4] It was not exactly a case of resurrected phrenology, but they did say that they had found 'The possibility to stimulate narrowly defined groups of muscles ... restricted to very small foci that we shall call centers ["Centra"]'.[5]

Jackson knew nothing of this until 1873, and the ignorance was mutual. 'Jackson's name is conspicuously absent from Fritsch and Hitzig's otherwise thorough review of work leading up to their own', so Young concludes there is 'no evidence that Jackson's ideas played any role in leading [them] ... to conduct their experiments'.[6] They were interested only in the normal

---

[1] A25 in York and Steinberg 2006, p.141.
[2] Jackson 1870h.
[3] Fritsch and Hitzig 1870; the publication is dated April 28, 1870.
[4] Young 1970, p.229; my square brackets.
[5] Young 1970, p.229; 'Centra' is found in Fritsch and Hitzig 1870, p.311. Young (1970, p.224) remarks that 'Fritsch and Hitzig's psychological views neither arose from nor were they compatible with the sensory-motor associationist tradition ... their psychophysiology was part of the tradition which Jackson explicitly rejected'.
[6] Young 1970, p.228, footnote 5; my square brackets. Hagner 2012, p.240, says that, as of 1870, 'Hitzig had been for a few years at least familiar with Jackson's teachings. In 1865, he wrote a review of a clinical textbook by the British

physiology of the brain. Similarly, before 1873 there were very few notices about Fritsch and Hitzig in the British or American press.[7] In sum, there is nothing to indicate that Jackson had any intimation that something so relevant to his own work was brewing on the Continent.

Jackson's Ongoing Work from 1871 to Spring 1873

A brief look at Jackson's bibliography for 1870 and 1871 shows that his usual rate of production abated in those 2 years.[8] Since there was nothing in his personal or professional lives to explain this, I can only speculate that he was catching his intellectual breath after the effort of his 'Study'. In 1872 he started to pick up the pace. He delivered the Oration of the Hunterian Society on February 7[9] and the Hunterian Oration on February 17,[10] both before the Hunterian Society of London. These were separate and distinct lectures, sponsored by the same medical fraternity.[11] In both presentations Jackson talked about 'The physiological aspects of education'.[12] The Oration began with summary statements of Jackson's views on the development and functions of the cerebral hemispheres. In discussing the nature/nurture issue, he cited Spencer's analogy of a society to an organism.[13] In the end he came to the reasonable conclusion that the final product derives from a mixture of both processes. In agreement with his Victorian milieu, he assumed a hierarchical order of the animal kingdom, ascending to the lower races of man and then to the higher races.

> The inherited structural differences of nervous systems involve differences in mind between individuals as vast as their physical dissimilarity. How this may be is suggested to us by the observations on the increasing asymmetry of the two halves of the brain as we pass upwards in the animal kingdom, and upwards in the degree of civilisation of the human race. The great aim of the education of the future should be to detect these inherited differences, and to give ability fair play, so that both in individuals and in society that which is highest in nature may become highest in life.[14]

---

physician John Churchill ...'. However, Hagner gives his citation of Hitzig's review as: 'Hitzig E (1865): Review of John Churchill, clinical lectures and reports by the medical and surgical staff of the London Hospital: London, 1864. *Berliner klinische Wochenschrift* 2: 173–174.' John Churchill was the *publisher* of the *London Hospital Reports*, not an author. Jackson published three papers in the *Reports* in 1864 (J64-08, J64-09, and J64-10). At that time he had not yet begun to work out his ideas about epileptic foci, so Hitzig would not have encountered them. Jackson's theories about foci were partially formed in his 'Study' of 1870 (Jackson 1870g), but Fritsch and Hitzig's (1870, p.332) paper was dated 'den 28. April 1870', and the 'Study' was published later in that year (York and Steinberg 2006, p.60). Hence, I agree with Young that Jackson's ideas had no effect on Hitzig.

[7] Lazar 2009a.
[8] See York and Steinberg 2006, pp.60–63.
[9] Jackson 1872e.
[10] Jackson 1872f.
[11] Woolf 1936. I don't know if at that time it was common for the same person to deliver both lectures. These Orations are not to be confused with the Hunterian Oration at the Royal College of Surgeons or with the series of lectures at the Hunterian Museum; both were larger organizations and carried more prestige.
[12] Only the first lecture carried that title. The lectures were not overtly sequential; the second was not labeled 'continued', and they were published in different journals.
[13] Jackson 1872e, p.180. Jackson gave no citation to Spencer, who discussed societies as organisms in his *First Principles* (Spencer 1867a, pp.316–319).
[14] Jackson 1872f; Jackson conjectured that the Chinese, among others, had been subject to 'premature intellectual development'.

On another subject, in November 1872 Jackson described the clinical findings in an unusual brainstem stroke that has come to be known as 'Jackson's syndrome'.[15] The patients had articulatory deficits. They were originally described without autopsies in 1864, just when Jackson's interest in speech disorders was starting.[16] Since their pathology was described in great detail by Lockhart Clarke in a report of 1872, one could argue that the entity should be the 'Jackson–Clarke syndrome'. In truth, the condition is so uncommon that the reputation of neither man would be appreciably altered by instantiation of such a claim.[17]

David Ferrier's First Experiments, Spring 1873

Even after Jackson learned about Fritsch and Hitzig, the details of their findings had little effect on his thinking, because he saw them through the lens of their presentation by Ferrier. The latter's impact, on the other hand, was immediate and profound. David Ferrier was born in 1843 near Aberdeen, Scotland, where, at the University, he took an M.A. with first-class honors in Classics and Philosophy in 1863. At Aberdeen, he became a 'favourite pupil' of Alexander Bain,[18] who had accepted the principle of cerebral localization at least as early as 1861.[19] In 1864 Ferrier studied at Heidelberg, which was then home to the physicist-physiologist Helmholtz and the experimental psychologist Wilhelm Wundt (1832–1920). Ferrier enrolled in the medical school at Edinburgh in 1865. He was graduated M.B. in 1868, with a host of honors. At Edinburgh he studied with Laycock. In 1870, Ferrier earned the M.D. with a gold-medal thesis on the comparative anatomy of the corpora quadrigemina. In the same year, he moved to London and was briefly Lecturer on Physiology at the Middlesex Hospital Medical School. In 1871 he began his lifelong association with King's College Hospital and Medical School.

Given this background, Ferrier's career in the neurosciences would seem to have been foreordained, and so it was. Soon after his arrival in London in 1870,

> His attention dwelling specially upon the physiology of the nervous system, he had contact with Hughlings-Jackson and with Jackson's views ... on the cerebral mechanism of certain forms of convulsions. In March, 1873, when he was paying a visit to his friend ... James Crichton-Browne [1840–1938], then Director of the West Riding Asylum, Wakefield [Yorkshire], conversation turned upon the excitability under galvanism of part of the cerebral surface of the dog as reported from the Continent by Fritsch and Hitzig. There

[15] Jackson 1872r. 'Garrison and Morton' (Morton 1961, p.397) give 'Jackson's syndrome' its imprimatur and describe it as 'consisting of paralysis of half of the tongue, the same half of the palate, and of one vocal cord'. Jackson described another case in 1886 (Jackson 1886a).

[16] In Jackson 1864i, pp.361–374, Jackson described two similar cases—'Case X' (unilateral): *Paralysis of the right side of the tongue, with wasting. Paralysis of the same side of the palate, and of the right vocal cord ...*'; and 'Case XI' (bilateral): *Sudden paralysis of the tongue on both sides.- difficulty of deglutition, and loss of voice ...*' (Jackson's italics). In Jackson 1872r, he reported Clarke's post-mortem findings on the bilateral Case XI, which turned out to have a unilateral hemorrhage in the left medulla, at the level of the inferior olivary nucleus. This lesion would account for wasting of the ipsilateral (left) tongue, but Jackson admitted that he had no explanation for the tongue's bilateral involvement.

[17] In 1904 William Osler had trouble finding a 'good account' of 'the Hughlings Jackson triad' (see Cushing 1926, p.647). Osler's use of 'triad' refers to 'Jackson's syndrome', as defined above; Osler was *not* referring to the triad of tumor symptoms that Jackson also described (see Chapter 6). Subsequent definitions of 'Jackson's syndrome' have been variable; see Bing 1939, p.99, and Jelliffe and White 1935, p.615.

[18] Sherrington 1928, p.viii.

[19] See Young 1970, p.104.

followed, during the course of the spring and summer of 1873, in the laboratory recently founded at the Asylum ... the memorable experiments with which Ferrier opened his detailed systematic exploration by faradic [AC] stimulation of all parts of the central nervous system in representative types of vertebrate[s] from lowest to highest.[20]

Ferrier's commonalities with Jackson are clear enough, but the dates of their contacts are not. Presumably Ferrier sought out Jackson in London at some time in 1870 or 1871, and in any case before 1873. Given Ferrier's experience in Germany in 1864, we would also like to know when he knew about Fritsch and Hitzig, since he might have been a conduit for such information to Jackson, but there's no clear evidence for Ferrier's knowledge of it until the spring of 1873.

On January 18, 1873, *The Lancet* began to carry a serialized paper by Jackson, 'On the anatomical & physiological localisation of movements in the brain'.[21] It was largely a repetition and occasional refinement of Jackson's positions in 'A study'. At the end of the third paper it says: '(*To be continued*)'.[22] Jackson's text indicated that more was coming, but the series actually stopped after that third installment. A survey of its contents shows that the series' title was a little off the mark. The papers did review many of Jackson's ideas about localization, but the most original parts were about brain organization related to hemispheric and interhemispheric functions. In order to continue the story of Jackson's relationship to Ferrier, I will defer my discussion of this interrupted series to later in this chapter, but it is well to keep in mind that Jackson had these issues in *his* mind when Ferrier's first results appeared.

Ferrier's First Report and Jackson's Initial Reaction

On April 26, 1873, the *British Medical Journal* contained a brief report by Ferrier about his 'Experimental researches in cerebral physiology and pathology'. It was clearly intended to establish priority, albeit after Fritsch and Hitzig.[23] The report began with a note of thanks to Crichton-Browne and his laboratory at the West Riding Asylum, where Ferrier had the opportunity of 'experimenting on over thirty guinea-pigs, rabbits, cats and dogs ...' He neglected to say that his experimental technique involved electrical stimulation of the cortices— probably a sign of hurried authorship.[24] Among twelve 'of the more important conclusions',

---

[20] Sherrington 1928, p.ix; my square brackets. Ferrier started his experiments in March 1873 (Morabito 1996, pp. 72, 75). Sherrington's use of the hyphenated 'Hughlings-Jackson' was archaic in 1928, since the 'saga of the inconsistent hyphen' occurred in the early 1870s (Critchley and Critchley 1998, pp.177–179, 181). In June 1871 Jackson asked the House Governor at the London Hospital to hyphenate his name in order to 'individualise one's self' (Critchley and Critchley 1998, p.178). However, no one was consistent about this, including Jackson. The first use of the hyphenated name that I have found is in a review of a Jackson paper that dates to 1868. The reviewer said, 'Dr. Hughlings-Jackson has done good service ...' (Jackson 1869h), but Jackson's name was not hyphenated in the reviewed article (Jackson 1868w). The hyphenated version is found on the editorial pages of *Brain* from its inception in 1878 to 1886–1887 (vol.9).

[21] Jackson 1873a (January 18), Jackson 1873c (February 1), and Jackson 1873d (February 15). This was 2 months *before* Ferrier began his experiments at West Riding; see next section below.

[22] Jackson 1873d, p.234.

[23] Ferrier 1873a; he felt that his report was 'worthy of a brief preliminary notice, pending the publication of details ... in the West Riding Asylum Reports'.

[24] Lorch (personal communication) points out that cutaneous electrical stimulation was then widely used for diagnostic and therapeutic purposes, so Ferrier could have assumed that his readers would be familiar with it. The National Hospital had an 'electrical room'; see Shorvon and Compston 2019, pp.123–126.

the first three in effect confirmed Jackson's advancing ideas about cortical localization of movements, and the next two referred to Jackson by name:

1. The anterior portions of the cerebral hemisphere[s] are the chief centres of voluntary motion and the active outward manifestation of intelligence.

2. The individual convolutions are separate and distinct centres; and in certain definite groups of convolutions (to some extent indicated by the researches of Fritsch and Hitzig) ... are localised the centres for the various movements ... differences corresponding to the habits of the animal are ... found in the differentiation of the centres.

3. The action of the hemispheres is in general crossed; but certain movements of the mouth, tongue, and neck, are bilaterally co-ordinated from each cerebral hemisphere.

4. The proximate causes of the different epilepsies are, as Dr. Hughlings Jackson supposes, "discharging lesions" of the different centres in the cerebral hemispheres. The affection may be limited artificially to one muscle, or group of muscles, or may be made to involve all the muscles represented in the cerebral hemispheres ... When induced artificially in animals, the affection as a rule first invades the muscles most in voluntary use, in striking harmony with the clinical observations of Dr. Hughlings Jackson.

5. Chorea is of the same nature as epilepsy, dependent on momentary discharging lesions of the individual cerebral centres. In this respect, Dr. Hughlings Jackson's views are again experimentally confirmed.[25]

Note that Ferrier acknowledged Fritsch and Hitzig's contributions 'to some extent', but Jackson's ideas were 'experimentally confirmed'. Note also that Ferrier attributed to Jackson the view that the 'discharging lesions' are located in 'the different centres in the cerebral hemispheres'. In fact, Jackson had not said anything about 'centres' in print. His overlapping and graded view of localization was inimical to strictly delimited, mosaic localization.

Another of Jackson's ideas that Ferrier claimed to have confirmed is in item 5: 'Chorea is of the same nature as epilepsy'. This perturbs the modern neurologist, because the etiologies of seizures and movement disorders are now thought to be different. Nonetheless, Ferrier's conclusion was a natural extension of Jackson's early interest in unilateral phenomena, including hemichorea. As early as 1864 Jackson localized the seat of the mischief in chorea to 'convolutions near the corpus striatum'. By 1868 he was insisting on this view.[26] For both Jackson and Ferrier, their mutual opinion on the etiology of chorea was derived partly from their evolutionary associationism, with its view of the cortices as sensory-motor. Mistakes in words (paraphasias) and choreiform movements are both 'positive' symptoms of higher-order dysfunctions—i.e., higher than the simpler movements of Jacksonian seizures. Therefore the seat of both abnormalities must be cortical.[27]

For Jackson, the most important effect of Ferrier's work was its validation of his effort to create a unified pathophysiology. Two weeks after Ferrier's initial report Jackson published his response in the *British Medical Journal* of May 10, 1873.[28] It began with a reference to Ferrier's brief report of April 26.[29] Jackson said: 'It will be particularly interesting

---

[25] Ferrier 1873a; my square brackets. Despite Ferrier's direct contact with Jackson, he described stimulation of muscles rather than movements in item 4. The remaining seven items were largely conclusions about specific anatomical structures.

[26] See Jackson 1864j, p.459; and Jackson 1868r.

[27] Ferrier said this clearly in 1873b, p.92; see also Jackson 1873k, p.532, footnote at asterisk.

[28] Jackson 1873k.

[29] Ferrier 1873a. In Jackson 1873k, p.531, asterisked footnote in left column, Jackson listed the three papers in his interrupted series (Jackson 1873a, Jackson 1873c, Jackson 1873d) and 'A study' as those to which Ferrier had referred, but Ferrier did not list any citations in 1873a.

to me to know what effects Dr. Ferrier will obtain by faradising the homologous part of a monkey's brain, for he tells me that these animals will shortly be subjected to experiment.'[30] Ferrier announced some of his results in monkeys at a meeting of the British Association on September 19, 1873.[31] In any case, Jackson clearly had prior knowledge of the primate results. Concerning the abrupt suspension of Jackson's series in *The Lancet*, I surmise that the two men were in contact soon after Ferrier began his experiments in March 1873. Jackson was able to go much further in his comments on Ferrier's work than would have been possible if his knowledge of it were restricted to the contents of Ferrier's brief report in the *British Medical Journal*. For example, Jackson said:

> The differences in the external conformation of animals imply differences in the normal functions of their nervous centres ... although this is what one would expect *à priori*, Dr. Ferrier's experiments have the great value of *demonstrating* special differences in different animals ... we have in Dr. Ferrier's researches a starting point for a "Comparative Physiology" of the Convolutions.[32]

Jackson did not expand on that comparative theme in this paper, although it was important for his argument in other papers soon to follow. Instead, he went on to develop another idea that had been similarly lurking in his thoughts for several years: 'The convolutions in the region of the corpus striatum *are* the corpus striatum "raised to a higher power". Each part of the brain in this region re-represents the whole of the movements which have been represented in the corpus striatum ...'[33] Here is another 'first'. The idea of re-representation is inherent in Jackson's brief discussion of localization at the separate levels of the striatum and the cortex in 'A study',[34] but it was not well developed, and the term 're-represents' was not used. Since the concept was central to Jackson's mature view of cerebral organization, it is important to note that he sharpened his definition of the idea in response to Ferrier's experimental findings.

Finally, in a footnote at the end of his paper Jackson invoked Spencer's associationist view of the role of the sense of touch in the development of intelligence.

> The significance of the fact, that the hand is the part in which convulsions, beginning unilaterally, most often start; that the arm suffers first ... in the greater number of motor affections from brain-disease ... will be better realised after reading Herbert Spencer's remarks ... in chap. viii, vol.i, p.359, of his *Psychology* (second edition) ...
>
> He [Spencer] points out ... the significance of the "striking instances which the animal kingdom presents of unusual sagacity co-existing with unusual development of organs, which, by help of complex muscular arrangements, give complex tactual impressions ... the *most far-reaching cognitions, and inferences the most remote from perception*, have their roots in the definitely combined impressions which the *human hands* can receive."[35]

---

[30] Jackson 1873k, p.532.

[31] Ferrier 1873d. The date of September 19, 1873, was given in Ferrier 1873c, p.152, which was published in 1874. The meeting was in Bradford, which is in the West Riding of Yorkshire, so Jackson might have attended.

[32] Jackson 1873k, p.531; Jackson's italics.

[33] Jackson 1873k, p.532; Jackson's italics, my underlining.

[34] See Jackson 1870g, pp. 32, 40.

[35] Jackson 1873k, asterisked footnote on p.533, left column; Jackson's italics, my square brackets. Although Jackson cited 'p.359' in Spencer 1870, his Spencerian quotations are actually found in fragments on pp.358–362.

Spencer's attribution of cognitive primacy to the sense of touch is entirely in keeping with mainline associationism. Bain emphasized the importance of the sense of touch as the source of our conceptions of the extension, weight, and resistance of objects in the environ- ment,[36] and Carpenter thought likewise.[37] Evolutionary associationism figured prominently in Ferrier's next publication about cortical localization.

Ferrier and Jackson in the *West Riding Lunatic Asylum Medical Reports*, Fall 1873

Ferrier's Evidence and Conclusions in the 'West Riding Reports', Fall 1873

As promised, Ferrier published a detailed report of his initial experiments in Crichton- Browne's *West Riding Lunatic Asylum Medical Reports* of 1873.[38] He began with a clear state- ment of his objectives, in the order of their importance.

> The objects I had in view in undertaking the present research were twofold: <u>first</u>, to put to experimental proof the views entertained by Dr. Hughlings Jackson on the pathology of Epilepsy, Chorea, and Hemiplegia, by imitating artificially the 'destroying' and 'discharging lesions' of disease, which his writings have defined and differentiated; and, <u>secondly</u>, to follow up the path which the researches of Fritsch and Hitzig (who have shown the brain to be susceptible to galvanic stimulation) indicated to me as one likely to lead to results of great value in the elucidation of the functions of the cerebral hemispheres, and in the more exact localisation and diagnosis of cerebral disease.[39]

In describing his results, Ferrier expressed surprise at the marked focality of the stimulation sites,[40] if they were found at all. Among other things, he showed that the brains of pigeons are 'apparently insensible to electric stimulation', thus refuting Flourens after more than four decades.[41] Stimulation of the striatum in dogs produced 'pleurosthotonus',[42] but not 'choreic spasms', and stimulation of the thalamus produced no movements.[43] Stimulation of the cere- bellum produced only movements of the eyes.[44] On a comparative note, he found that the 'higher development of the centres for the movements of the mouth in rabbits would be quite in accordance with the habits of the animal, just as we see the higher development of

---

[36] Bain 1855, pp.171–195.

[37] Carpenter 1855, pp. 575–576, 655.

[38] Ferrier 1873b; here Ferrier (p.89, footnote 2) said: 'I have now (June 14) … ' continued some experiments. On December 13, 1873, Jackson (Jackson 1873w) discussed Ferrier 1873b extensively, so he had Ferrier's paper by then. I infer from this that the *Reports* for 1873 probably appeared in the fall (October–November) of that year. For the history of the *Reports* see Viets 1938, and George and Trimble 1992.

[39] Ferrier 1873b, p.30; my underlining. On the technical differences between Ferrier's stimulation parameters and those of Fritsch and Hitzig see Taylor and Gross 2003.

[40] Ferrier 1873b, p.39.

[41] Ferrier 1873b, p.61; on Flourens see Chapter 3.

[42] Ferrier 1873b, p.62. 'Pleurothotonus' (not pleurosthotonus) was 'A variety of tetanus, in which the body is curved laterally by the stronger contractions of the muscles of one side of the body' (Dunglison 1874, p.813). This spelling appears to mean the same as Ferrier's 'pleurosthotonus', based on his description of the animals' postures. Ferrier's 'opisthotonus' is the same as ours, involving severe backward arching of the entire spine.

[43] He approached the basal ganglia and thalami via an interhemispheric, transcallosal route to the lateral and third ventricles (Ferrier 1873b, p.62).

[44] Ferrier 1873b, pp.69, 72.

the centres for the paw in cats, and the tail in dogs'. [45] These comparative data accorded nicely with Ferrier's positions on the issues that really motivated him.

> ... It will be seen that the movements recorded in the above experiments ... are purposive or expressional in character, and such as we should ... attribute to ideation and volition ... we may conclude that the cortical centres are not merely motor but voluntary motor, and concerned with the outward manifestation of intelligence.
>
> The ... question next arises, What is the relation between the convolutions as motor centres, and the parts of the cerebral hemispheres which are subservient to the mental processes ... related to these definite muscular movements? Are the ideational centres situated in the same regions as the corresponding motor centres; or does a high development of certain motor centres indicate only ... a corresponding development of the ideational centres which manifest themselves outwardly through these? [46]

Ferrier favored the idea that 'the ideational centres [are] situated in the same regions as the corresponding motor centres'. He buttressed his argument by quoting the same passage from Spencer that Jackson had quoted in the *British Medical Journal* of May 10, 1873.[47] Reaching further, he said:

> These speculations are suggested by the now tolerably well established fact of loss of speech following destructive lesions of the lower frontal convolutions in the neighborhood of the Island of Reil[48] ... It is a significant fact that the centres for the mouth and tongue in cats and dogs are localised in regions ... which ... I should be inclined to regard as the homologues of the lower frontal and Island of Reil in man. The question, then, is, do lesions in this neighborhood destroy the organic centres of the memory of words, or do they only interrupt the channels whereby these are manifested outwardly as articulate speech? The fact that the speechless patient is likewise unable to write, i.e., in the sense of expressing himself by written symbols ... would seem to indicate that it is not the mere channel for articulate expression of ideas that is interrupted, but that the very centres of word-memory are destroyed.[49]

So Ferrier was suggesting that the 'centres of word-memory' are located in Broca's area, rather than further afield and more diffusely in the cortices. He supported this position with a long quotation from Jackson's 'Study', where Jackson discussed his conclusion that, 'It is *à priori* incredible that a person who cannot speak should be able to write ... [because] ... he cannot revive words voluntarily'.[50] Jackson's blunt prediction is not credible now, because we know that aphasia and agraphia can be dissociated.[51] Given Ferrier's background of philosophical and psychological studies in Aberdeen and Heidelberg, it is no surprise that he was excited by the possibility of correlating behavior with brain structure, even in nonprimate animals. Turning to humans, Ferrier observed that when people are reading,

---

[45] Ferrier 1873b, p.61.

[46] Ferrier 1873b, pp.73; note that this passage appears to attribute conscious volition and intelligence to animals.

[47] Ferrier 1873b, pp.73–74. He quoted Jackson 1873k, footnote on p.533, including the same mistake in page citation.

[48] The 'Island of Reil' is the *insula*, which is infolded peri-sylvian cortex; Broca's area is on its superior-anterior edge.

[49] Ferrier 1873b, p.74.

[50] Ferrier 1873b, pp.74–75; taken from Jackson 1870g, footnote on pp.180–181.

[51] M. Lorch (personal communication).

they make 'movements of the tongue and lips unconsciously'. From that observation, he said he was

> ... inclined to regard the intimate relation subsisting between ideation and the unconscious outward expression of the idea in muscular action as a strong proof of the close local association of the ideational and voluntary motor centres. Hence I should incline to the opinion that the organic centres of word memory are situated in the same convolutions as the centres which preside over the muscles concerned in articulation.[52]

In these speculations Ferrier appeared to be stretching his nonprimate results beyond their warrant. It turns out, however, that the stretch was more in his reporting than in his evidence. In a footnote near the end of his paper he said, 'I have now (June 14) ascertained the position of all these centres in the brain of the monkey, and therefore, by implication, their situation in man'.[53] So his speculations had support from experimental data in primates that was not available to his readers. Moreover, he had Jackson's clinical data. At the end of his paper Ferrier went back to his original objective.

> The pathology of epileptiform convulsions, chorea, and epileptic hemiplegia, receive much light from the foregoing experiments. I regard them as experimental confirmation of the views expressed by Dr. Hughlings Jackson. They are, as it were, an artificial reproduction of the clinical experiments performed by disease, and the conclusions which Dr. Jackson has arrived at from his observations of disease are in all essential particulars confirmed by the above experiments.[54]

Accordingly, in rabbits and cats,

> While moderate stimulation of a centre caused merely the apparently normal excitation of the muscles co-ordinated there, more powerful stimulation excited an epileptiform condition of the same muscles, while diffused irritation of the whole hemisphere ... was sufficient to produce general convulsions, usually, but not always, restricted to the opposite side. In these general convulsions the animal apparently lost consciousness.[55]

In this statement Ferrier's purpose was to confirm Jackson's opinion that the pathophysiology of genuine epilepsy is the same as focal cases, so genuine epilepsy is not a separate entity.[56] Immediately after the above Ferrier continued:

> An abnormally <u>irritable</u> condition of the cerebral centres thus artificially excited was sufficient to cause repeated explosive discharges, on very slight provocation. This abnormal condition, once induced, caused such an epileptic habit that frequently localised exploration of the individual motor centres had to be given up on account of the readiness with which fits occurred ... the similarity between the conditions induced by faradisation, and those caused by the presence of a foreign body pressing on some part of the hemispheres,

---

[52] Ferrier 1873b, p.75.
[53] Ferrier 1873b, p.89, footnote 2.
[54] Ferrier 1873b, p.85.
[55] Ferrier 1873b, p.86.
[56] Later in his paper Ferrier also dismissed the medulla as the purported locus of the initial discharge in generalized seizures; see Ferrier 1873b, p.90.

is manifest. The irritating effect of such a lesion is well characterised by Hughlings Jackson as a 'discharging lesion.'[57]

As we have seen, Jackson also had an early conception of neural hyper-excitability, purportedly derived from hypernutrition. Nonetheless, I think Ferrier's use of the term 'irritable' is original— at least in the sense of physiological 'irritability' applied to the pathophysiology of seizures.[58] Jackson thought that cases of genuine epilepsy have foci that simply can't be found, and Ferrier thought that his own artificial induction of widespread cortical irritability was analogous to the effect of a chronic foreign body that damages and thus destabilizes cortical gray matter.[59] One way to understand the inconsistencies in all of this is to suggest that Jackson and Ferrier were each groping his way toward the later concept of seizure 'threshold'. In any case, Ferrier's discussion of these issues led him toward a related concept that is now widely used.

Early Definitions of the Cortical Motor and Sensory Strips

The 'primary motor cortex'[60] in man is located in the precentral gyrus, which runs from medial to lateral, just in front of the 'rolandic' ('central') sulcus. This deep sulcus separates the frontal and parietal lobes.[61] Most motor stimulation points are in this part of the frontal lobe, but not all. From the beginning, there have been arguments whether the precentral motor cortex is strictly motor or actually sensorimotor.[62] To follow the history accurately, it is essential to keep track of exactly what was described by whom and when. With disturbing frequency, one finds remarks such as 'the British neurologist Hughlings Jackson predicted the pattern in which movements are mapped on the precentral gyrus...'[63] But such statements are not correct.

There is a salient difference between (1) predicting that there will be some kind of somatotopic pattern of motor representation somewhere in cortical tissue, and (2) predicting on which gyrus such representation will be found. Jackson surely achieved the first point, but he did not venture on the second. He simply stated that there are motor functions in some part of the cortices supplied by the middle cerebral arteries, which irrigate most of the precentral gyri, except their medial portions. Furthermore, he knew that the 'motor area' would have to be organized *somatotopically*, in a pattern that explains the different sequences in the various patterns of Jacksonian marches. Moreover, Jackson would have predicted that there should be much overlapping of sites that produce very similar movements, but Ferrier did not address this point.

The initial discovery of the existence of motor cortex in mammals, and its relatively anterior position, was made by Fritsch and Hitzig in 1870. However, their map of cortical points whose stimulation causes reproducible movements in the dog did not show a linear pattern

---

[57] Ferrier 1873b, p.87; my underlining.

[58] Fritsch and Hitzig's (1870) 'Erregbarkeit' in their title is usually translated as 'excitability'; see Bonin 1960, p.73, and Hagner 2012, p.237. Ferrier's 'irritable' implies a longer-lasting state. Nor was Ferrier's meaning in English otherwise in use in this context at the time; see 'Irritability' and 'Irritable' in Dunglison 1874, pp.556–557, where the definition is Hallerian. Albrecht von Haller (1707–1777) ascribed irritability to all living tissue.

[59] Ferrier 1873b, p.86.

[60] Alias 'motor cortex' or 'motor strip'; it is essentially Brodmann's histological area 4.

[61] For the history of the anatomical description of the central sulcus and its adjacent gyri see Meyer 1971, pp.133–141.

[62] For histories of the concept and its controversies within the experimental tradition see Mott 1894, Hitzig 1900, Meyer 1978, Meyer 1982, Boling 2002, and Gross 2007.

[63] Nolte 2002, p.541. A less egregious example is that Jackson 'first described the somatotopic organization of the motor cortex...' (Kandel and Schwartz 1981, p.469). A related statement in the fourth edition of Kandel et al. (2000, p.759), is more nuanced.

along the precentral gyrus.[64] In fact, it is difficult to be sure about the anatomical definition of the central sulcus in dogs, so it is not valid to homologize from the dog's motor cortex to the precentral gyrus in primates.[65] From his work with nonprimate mammals, Ferrier could add only a small mountain of details, including the observation that

> ... even when ... diffused irritation of the whole of the centres was induced ... an order was observable in the course of the spasms ... In the rabbit the convulsions usually begin in the mouth and lips, and in the cat the eyelids and face first, next the shoulder and paw, and lastly the hind leg and tails were thrown successively into convulsions. Here we observe the muscles most in voluntary action are the first to be attacked. The centres for these are situated in the more anterior parts of the brain, and ... these are more excitable and more easily discharged than those situated more posteriorly ... Hence, a general irritation of the whole hemisphere manifests itself primarily in the more excitable parts, and these coincide with the most voluntary centres. But ... when the electrical current was made to traverse other centres ... the convulsions began in the muscles whose centres were there represented, and then spread to the more irritable anterior centres for the eyelids and face. The bearing of these facts on the diagnosis of the exact seat of the discharging lesions in the hemispheres, such as tumours, is evident. When epilepsy begins in the hand ... we have every reason for diagnosing a discharging lesion of some part of the superior frontal convolution of the opposite hemisphere.[1][66]

Three general principles are juxtaposed in this long passage: (1) The first concerns Jackson's theory that there is more cortical tissue representing voluntary movements than there is for less voluntary movements; hence, focal seizures are more likely to originate in neural tissue that represents voluntary movements because there is more of that tissue. Ferrier was confirming this idea, and he was also seeing the same phenomenon that Fritsch and Hitzig saw: more anterior cortical fields are more susceptible to lower currents.[67] This observation can lead to (2), the general principle that different cortical locations can differ in their seizure thresholds, but the concept of seizure threshold was not yet available as such. And (3), the third principle in this passage is in its last two sentences, where we find the first recognizable suggestion of the idea that the primary motor area is located in the precentral gyrus, with somatotopic organization of the motor functions.[68] Ferrier probably had his unpublished primate results in mind when he began to formulate the idea of a motor strip,[69] but he also had Jackson's clinical data.

In the superscript footnote 1 at the end of the above quotation, Ferrier referred to two case reports by Jackson. In the earlier one, Jackson said that in 1869 he had 'published the case of a man who had fits affecting the *right* arm. In this case there was a tumour of the hinder part of the first (uppermost) frontal convolution of the left hemisphere'.[70] Subsequently, in May 1873, Jackson reported that he had seen another patient 'who had literally innumerable fits limited to the right arm ... *Here I correctly predicted disease of the hinder part of the*

---

[64] Fritsch and Hitzig 1870, p.313; see Bonin 1960, p.83, and Wilkins 1992, p.20.

[65] Jenkins 1978, pp.292–293.

[66] Ferrier 1873b, pp.88–89; footnote 1 is Ferrier's.

[67] See Fritsch and Hitzig 1870, translated in Bonin 1960, pp.81–85.

[68] Famously cartooned as the 'homunculus' by Penfield and Rasmussen (1950, p.25). See also Snyder and Whitaker 2013.

[69] Ferrier 1873b, p.89, footnote 2.

[70] Jackson 1869k.

first (upper most) frontal convolution ...'[71] On the basis of his experimental findings, Ferrier declared that the '... diagnosis grounded on clinical facts by Hughlings Jackson has been triumphantly verified'.[72] However, Jackson's diagnosis in the second case was entirely empirical. As he said, he knew where the lesion was located in the first patient, so he was able to predict its location in the second. Jackson was not saying anything further about motor localization in the precentral gyrus, but it is easy to see how a superficial reading of Ferrier's footnote might lead to the impression that Jackson was defining the motor strip.

So what about sensory cortex? In a case report of 1867, Jackson used the term 'march of the sensation' to describe one aspect of a patient's complex focal seizures.[73] Beyond that, however, he did not pursue the sensory idea any further around that time. In 1873 Ferrier saw the possibility of focal cortical localization for sensory functions, analogous to the motor functions that he was observing in mammals and man. In seizure states, he said:

> The psychical [sensory] perversions may be supposed to depend on the same conditions of nerve tissue as lead to explosive muscular action ... it will form a valuable subject of future research ... to determine whether the disorders of perception and volition of the 'petit mal'[74] are ... only abortive stages in the development of the 'grand mal' ... or whether those forms of sensory epilepsy, characterized more especially by temporary (often followed by permanent) symptoms of mental alienation ... are dependent rather on the same abnormal condition of only the posterior parts of the brain, which are more probably connected with these mental processes.[75]

Here Ferrier was broadening the nosology of epilepsy by suggesting the likelihood that its symptoms could include sensory *and* more complex psychical manifestations. His reasoning was Jacksonian. Since he had found anterior cortical areas where motor functions are represented, it seemed plausible that similar posterior areas would be found for sensory functions. Following Jackson and others, he thought that such areas would be posterior to the motor areas, as indeed they are.[76] Furthermore, if such be the case, then Jackson's pathophysiological theory of seizures—confirmed by Ferrier's experiments—would predict that sensory seizures should occur. The above passage is potentially confusing because Ferrier mixed 'psychical perversions', 'petit mal', and 'grand mal'. He was predicting that sensory seizures might be preliminary stages of 'symptoms of mental alienation', so it is not clear that he was thinking of *primary* sensory seizures, involving a sensory march. Nonetheless, Ferrier must be given credit for advancing the semiology and pathophysiology of seizures and epilepsy into sensory tissue.

At the end of his long paper in the *West Riding Reports*, Ferrier reprinted the entire text of his earlier report in the *British Medical Journal*[77] as a form of summary. He said that his results 'explain many hitherto obscure symptoms of cerebral disease, and enable us to localise with greater certainty many forms of cerebral lesion'.[78] Like Jackson, Ferrier's ultimate

---

[71] Jackson 1873k, pp.533; Ferrier italicized Jackson's text.

[72] Ferrier 1873b, p.89; my underlining.

[73] Jackson 1867l, p.330.

[74] The term 'petit mal' was imported from France, where it originated before the nineteenth century; see Temkin 1971, pp.257–258. In the 1870s in Britain and the United States, its meaning was still rather loose compared to our current definition; see Dunglison 1874, p.367.

[75] Ferrier 1873b, pp.91–92; Jackson's parentheses, my square brackets and underlining. There is little about sensory seizures in Temkin 1971, in Eadie and Bladin 2001, or in Friedlander 2001.

[76] See Jackson 1869d, quoted in Chapter 6.

[77] Ferrier 1873a.

[78] Ferrier 1873b, p.95, conclusion '12'.

purposes were clinical, so perhaps that was what caused him to ignore one of the theoretical underpinnings of Jackson's cerebral pathophysiology.

Despite Ferrier's stated intention 'to put to experimental proof the views entertained by Dr. Hughlings Jackson,'[79] he said nothing about Jackson's *xyz* theory. Thereby he started a tradition that has lasted to the present—almost everyone has ignored it.[80] But Ferrier had to know about Jackson's theory, because Jackson discussed it in his 'Study' of 1870,[81] whose contents Ferrier had set out to verify. It would have been possible for Ferrier to investigate the overlapping (ordinal) nature of elicited movements in the course of his experiments, but he admitted at the outset that he was struck by the marked focality of separate stimulation points.[82] From the time of Gall to the present, the pendulum in brain science has swung back and forth between the lumpers and the splitters—more politely known as the holists and the localizers. Here we see one of its oscillations toward the splitters, because Ferrier's conception of cortical motor localization ignored the subtleties of Jackson's *xyz* theory.

Jackson's Papers in the 'West Riding Reports', Fall 1873: Epilepsy, Method, and Evolution

Jackson published two titles later in the same volume of the *West Riding Lunatic Asylum Medical Reports* for 1873.[83] Since he made no reference to Ferrier's paper,[84] there was no explicit relationship between the articles of the two authors in the same volume. Jackson's first article was a review of his previous 'Observations on the localisation of movements in the cerebral hemispheres …'[85] In effect it was an elaborate introduction to the second, with Ferrier's early results very much in mind.

> In this paper … I try to show (1) That convulsions, choreal movements, affections of speech, and other motor symptoms, are not *only* to be thought of as 'symptoms of disease,' but can be considered also as results of experiments made by disease revealing in the rough the functions of cerebral convolutions; (2) To urge that the study of such *motor* symptoms is of direct importance for *mental* physiology; (3) That if we … reduce the very *different* symptoms to their lowest terms … we shall find that there are certain *fundamental* principles common to … symptoms so specially different as 'aphasia,' and a convulsion of one side of the body.[1]
>
> The most important matter … is the study of the localisation of movements on the *double* plan – by comparing the effects of destroying and discharging lesions on the brain of *man*.[86]

---

[79] Ferrier 1873b, p.30.

[80] But see Greenblatt 1988, and York and Steinberg 1994, 1995, and 2006, pp.17–18, 25–27.

[81] Jackson 1870g, pp.190–191.

[82] Ferrier 1873b, p.39.

[83] Jackson 1873x and Jackson 1873y. Actually he published three papers, because his long appendix to the second constituted a third, independent article.

[84] Jackson's first citation of Ferrier 1873b was in a paper dated December 13, 1873 (Jackson 1873w). Ferrier 1873b was not cited in Jackson 1873v, dated November 15, 1873. In Jackson 1873w (p.840), Jackson said (via a reporter), 'Had the experiments of Fritsch, Hitzig, and Ferrier … then appeared, Dr. Hughlings Jackson might have known which convolution to search for minute changes'.

[85] Jackson 1873x.

[86] Jackson 1873x, p.176; Jackson's italics. In his footnote 1 he said that in reviewing his manuscript he had found 'more recapitulation from former papers than I expected'.

Jackson had discussed his comparative methods since at least 1867.[87] In light of Ferrier's results he could compare animal versus human 'experiments', but he insisted that, *'there is no other way* of ascertaining the localisation of movements in the cerebral hemisphere *of man*, than by the study of his convulsive seizures'.[88] He felt that his ideas had been validated by Ferrier, but they were meeting resistance anyway, and he knew why. As he explained:

> To urge that the study of *convulsion* from discharge of *convolutions* is most important for *mental* physiology ... will seem more than strange to those who hold that the convolutions are parts of the 'organ of mind', and are for 'ideas', and that the subjacent 'motor tract' is the only part of the brain for movements ...
>
>   There seems to be an insuperable objection to the notion that the cerebral hemispheres are for movements ... In another paper I hope to show clearly that there is no contradiction in supposing that the convolutions are for ideas and for movements too. I shall try ... to show that *sudden discharges* give *proof* that the sensori-*motor* processes are the *anatomical substrata of ideas.*[89]

These statements follow from positions that Jackson had staked out in his 'Study'.[90] They are based on associationism, as seen in 'sensori-*motor* processes are the *anatomical substrata of ideas*'. In a generic discussion of aphasic defects, he referred to another fundamental principle of associationism: 'The objection that when we speak internally ... there *is no movement* of the articulatory organs, is not of weight. To remember a word is to have a faint excitation of the sensori-motor process of that word.'[91] As already mentioned, a valuable feature of this paper is its evidence concerning how his ideas were being received by his colleagues. He said that some of his ideas had '... received some favor (chiefly that of being disputed) ...'[92] and he defended himself by striking another blow for his intellectual independence.

> It may be remembered in extenuation that my investigations of epilepsies have not been from orthodox points of view. I have not simply repeated accepted doctrines with slight variations and new illustrations. Working on a novel method, I run continual risk of making novel blunders. But in thinking for one's self there are certain kinds of blunders which almost must be made. And it is always easy to avoid appearing to go wrong if one does not go far from the beaten track.[93]

---

[87] Jackson 1867b, p.295; see Chapter 4.

[88] Jackson 1873x, p.181; Jackson's italics. He went on to discuss the issue of 'medical' versus 'physiological' knowledge.

[89] Jackson 1873x, pp.182–183; Jackson's italics.

[90] See Jackson 1870g, pp.183, 189.

[91] Jackson 1873x, p.189; Jackson's italics. Jackson's footnote 1 again referred to Spencer's *Principles of Psychology*: 'Spencer on Memory, &c.' (Spencer 1855, 1 ed., p.359). On the same page there is another reference to Spencer in the form of an old personal communication (see footnote 2 on Jackson's pp.188–189). Later in the paper (p.195) Jackson used 'Physiological Units', with a reference to Spencer's *Principles of Biology* but without a page citation.

[92] Jackson 1873x, p.182; Jackson' parentheses.

[93] Jackson 1873x, p.177.

A Historiographic Breakpoint

Since Jackson's 'novel method' was comparative, up to this point (late 1873) he seldom wrote a substantive paper about one clinical subject without invoking evidence from others. Thus, his second paper in the *West Riding Reports*[94] marks a turning point for my approach to his writings. The paper was focused on its subject (epilepsy) to an extent that no single paper was before it. Therefore, starting in 1873 it is legitimate to follow the development of Jackson's ideas about any one clinical subject without constantly interjecting extended discussions of others. Rather than adhering to absolute chronology, going forward I will analyze single subjects in Jackson's writings over short chunks of months or a few years.

A Revised Method, Fall 1873

Jackson's second paper in the *West Riding Reports* started with a revised edition of his tripartite method.

> In the investigation of Epilepsies, or of any kind of case of nervous disease, we have three lines of investigation. We have –
> 1. To find the Organs damaged (Localisation).
> 2. To find the Functional affection of nerve tissue.
> 3. To find the alteration in Nutrition.
> There is, in brief, (1) Anatomy, (2) Physiology, (3) and Pathology 1 in *each* case.[95]

When Jackson reviewed his manuscript he apparently realized that his argument would be easier to understand if he gave his most recent definition of epilepsy at the beginning, so he added a footnote to explain how his revised method facilitated his expanded definition.

> [1] This division will be clearer if I anticipate the definition to be given [later] ... of an_ Epilepsy – an occasional, sudden, excessive and rapid discharge of grey matter of some *part of the brain*. The functional alteration (No. 2) is plain, for the very existence of repeated paroxysms tells us that there is a 'discharging lesion.' Under Anatomy (No. 1) we try, from a study of the paroxysm, to find where the discharging lesion is – to localise. And under Pathology (No. 3) we try to trace the steps of the abnormal process of nutrition by which the discharging lesion resulted ... [96]

In his effort 'To find the Organs damaged (Localisation)', Jackson's new definition emphasized '*local* discharges of grey matter'.[97] This was a substantive change from his definition of 1870, which said: 'A convulsion ... implies only that there is an occasional, an excessive, and a disorderly discharge of nerve tissue on muscles'.[98] By emphasizing the focality of epileptic discharges in the hemispheres he expanded the nosological boundaries of 'epilepsy' beyond their motor limits.

---

[94] Jackson 1873y.

[95] Jackson 1873y, p.315; Jackson's italics.

[96] Jackson 1873y, p.315; Jackson's parentheses, my underlining. His definition later in the paper (p.331) says (in his italics): '*Epilepsy is the name for occasional, sudden, excessive, rapid, and local discharges of grey matter.*'

[97] See footnote 96 immediately above; Jackson's italics, my underlining.

[98] Jackson 1870g, p.162; my underlining.

... numerous and very different symptoms may be epileptic in my definition of the term. And as any part of the grey matter of the cerebrum may become unstable, there will be all varieties of epilepsy, according to the exact position ... and there will be all degrees according to the degree of instability ... I wish to speak first of cases of limited seizures, or, if the expression be preferred, of <u>partial seizures</u> ... we must not take *degrees* of epilepsies for *varieties* of epilepsies.[99]

This is the first instance when Jackson used the expression 'partial seizures'.[100] His wording implied that the term 'partial' was already in use. He probably had predecessors in this usage, but he thought through its pathophysiological implications, whereas most others simply used the word to indicate semiological and/or nosological distinctions.[101] On the other hand, we've seen that Ferrier used Jackson's pathophysiological reasoning to arrive at an understanding of sensory seizures. Thus, some of the expansion of the nosological boundaries of epilepsy grew out of the exchange between Jackson and Ferrier. Probably the same should be said for Jackson's increasing conviction about the focal etiology of generalized epilepsy.

... a fit which ... *becomes universal* depends on discharge in but *one* hemisphere; for ... each half of the brain represents movements of both sides of the body,[1] but ... it represents the movements of the two sides in different degrees and orders.[102]

The second of Jackson's 'lines of investigation' was 'To find the Functional affection of nerve tissue', which meant pathophysiology.

Let us now consider 'discharging lesions', with a view to a more formal definition of epilepsy in the sense in which I use the term in this paper. It will, however, be convenient to state first <u>what things are not essential to the novel definition</u>.
First ... Whether ... there be a *convulsion* ... matters nothing for the definition ...
Secondly ... the separation into cases where there is and where there is not loss of consciousness, has no *physiological* warrant. It is an <u>arbitrary distinction of psychological parentage</u>. Loss of consciousness ... is not to be spoken of as an epiphenomenon, nor as a complication ... The sensori-motor processes concerned in consciousness are only in degree different from others. They are ... the series evolved out of all other (lower) series.
To lose consciousness is to lose *the use of the most special of all nervous processes* ... If those parts of the brain be first affected by strong discharge where the most special of all nervous processes lie, there will be loss of consciousness *at the outset*. If processes of a subordinate series be discharged, loss of consciousness ... occurs later.[103]

Here Jackson's use of Spencerian evolution assisted his amalgamation of genuine epilepsy with other varieties of the disease. If generalized seizures are fundamentally the same as

---

[99] Jackson 1873y, p.333; Jackson's italics, my underlining. On the next page, Jackson gave examples of six different 'varieties of epilepsy', including 'A sudden and temporary stench in the nose, with transient unconsciousness'.
[100] In the '1981 ILAE classification of epileptic seizures' (Engel and Pedley 2008, vol.1, p.512) 'Partial seizures are those in which ... the first clinical and electroencephalographic changes indicate initial activation of a system ... limited to part of one cerebral hemisphere'.
[101] See Eadie 1999 and 2002.
[102] Jackson 1873y, p.337; Jackson's italics. His footnote 1 refers to his earlier paper of February 15, 1873 (Jackson 1873d), which contained an extensive discussion of contralateral versus bilateral motor representation in the cerebrum—differences between representations in the two hemispheres increase as the organism ascends the evolutionary hierarchy.
[103] Jackson 1873y, pp.330–331; Jackson's italics and parentheses, my underlining.

those without loss of consciousness, then their underlying pathophysiology must be the same, and that was Jackson's position with regard to the metabolic basis of unstable foci. His third 'line of investigation' was 'Pathology', i.e., 'alteration in Nutrition' (metabolism).[104]

> ... the highly unstable nervous matter ... in a 'discharging lesion' ... differs ... [chemically] ... from the comparatively stable grey matter of health ... such that the nervous substance formed is more explosive ... One striking constituent of nervous matter is phosphorus ... My speculation is that in the abnormal nutritive process producing unstable nervous matter the phosphorus ingredient is replaced by its [more explosive] chemical congener, nitrogen.[105]

Jackson's speculation was obviously dependent on the limited knowledge of brain chemistry at the time, so it is crude. In fact, he was right about the importance of phosphorus in all cellular metabolism, as compounds he couldn't know about. Despite his affinity for chemistry, his basic mode of thought was biological.

Jackson's Advancing Evolutionary Analysis of Seizures and Brain Organization, Fall 1873

In his Appendix, 'On Evolution of Nervous Centres',[106] Jackson extended his evolutionary analysis of brain organization. A central concept in this process was 're-representation'. This is the idea that functions mediated ('represented') in lower centers are 're-represented' in higher brain structures. That is, the more elementary functions in the lower structures are recombined in heterogeneous ways in the higher structures. This concept was present in embryonic form in the hierarchical view of the nervous system that Jackson evinced in his 'Study'.[107] However, he did not use the term 're-represents' until it appeared in a paper published on May 10, 1873,[108] 5 or 6 months before the Appendix that we are now discussing. With regard to Spencer's role in Jackson's developing thought, 'compounding' of ideas is an associationist concept that Spencer promulgated, but I have found no evidence that Jackson's use of the words 'representation' and 're-representation' was derived from Spencer.

In his Appendix Jackson dealt first with the problem of correlating experimental data from animals with epileptic phenomena in humans. He cited two animal experiments from the neurophysiology monograph of Charcot's collaborator, E.F. Alfred Vulpian (1826–1887).[109] The first 'case' was 'that of a rat from which the cerebral hemispheres, corpora striata, and a large part of the optic thalami had been removed', and the second was a rabbit treated similarly but sparing the thalami.[110] Part of Jackson's purpose was:

> To consider an objection to the view that the cerebral hemispheres are the seats of epileptic discharges, which is often inferred from the statement (the correctness of which I will

---

[104] Jackson 1873y, p.315.

[105] Jackson 1873y, pp.326–327; my square brackets.

[106] Jackson 1873y, pp.342–349. This was actually Jackson's second appendix to the paper. The first (untitled) concerned Jackson's modification of Broadbent's hypothesis; on the latter see Jackson 1870g, pp.192–193, and my discussion in Chapter 6.

[107] See Jackson 1870g, pp.189–190.

[108] Jackson 1873k, p.532.

[109] Presumably Jackson's citation of Vulpian's 'Physiology of the Nervous System' was actually to Vulpian's 'Leçons sur la Physiologie Générale et Comparée du Systéme Nerveux' (Vulpian 1866), since there was no English translation of Vulpian's book.

[110] Jackson 1873y, p.343; Jackson cited these experiments from Vulpian 1866, pp.666, 680.

admit) that epileptic fits are producible in animals whose cerebral hemispheres have been removed.[111]

Since a rat or a rabbit, mutilated as described by Vulpian, does make adapted movements when noises are made, or cries when pinched, and since a pigeon, similarly mutilated, turns its head after a moving candle, it is plain enough that in the *lower* centres of these animals there are sensori-motor processes for the adjustment of *very general* movements to *very general* impressions. But the inference is not that these very same kinds of impressions and movements are not also represented in the *higher* parts removed. Rather the very same processes are in the higher centres *re-represented* in greater complexity and speciality ... Co-ordination in the higher centres is the co-ordination in the lower 'carried a stage further.'[1][112]

Jackson's footnote 1 contained quotations from Spencer and Vulpian in support of his position. As quoted by Jackson, Spencer said, theoretically: 'it is not improbable that in the course of nerve evolution, centres that were once the highest are supplanted by others in which co-ordination is carried a stage further, and which thereupon become the places of feeling, while the centres before predominant become automatic'.[113] Vulpian said the same from a comparative standpoint, i.e., progressively larger ablations of animals' cerebral hemispheres have less and less observable effect as one goes lower in the evolutionary scale.[114]

Returning to Jackson's main text, the wording of his next paragraph indicates that his conclusion about re-representation was not taken directly from Spencer.

The <u>conclusion I have arrived at</u> from the study of cases of disease is, that the higher centres are evolved *out of* the lower ... The higher centre re-represents more specially the impressions and movements already represented generally in the one below it. The co-ordinations are continually being re-coordinated; for example, those of the pons and medulla are re-coordinated in the cerebrum.[2] There are in the lower centres sensori-motor processes for very *general* purposes ...[115]

And again Jackson offered more support for his argument by quoting Spencer's conception of progressive evolution in footnote 2.[116] Here Jackson again maintained his intellectual autonomy *vis-à-vis* all of his sources, including Spencer. As he matured, the fierceness of his defense moderated, but not his sense of independence *per se*. His usual method was to work toward a theory from his clinical data, and then test it—often by comparing it to Spencer's theories. Jackson's next paragraph was an example, where he invoked his *xyz* theory to support his argument. The theory itself was Jackson's, not Spencer's, although Jackson developed it in consonance with Spencer's theoretical statement that cerebral localization must entail an 'insensible shading off' of functional areas rather than strict, phrenological boundaries.[117]

If such be the plan of structure of nervous organs, we can understand how it is that part of a highly evolved ... part of the brain ... may be wanting, with ... not an obvious loss of

---

[111] Those animals' postures are not epileptic; see Definition Section 8 in Chapter 9.

[112] Jackson 1873y, pp.343–344; Jackson's italics and single quotation marks.

[113] Jackson 1873y, p.344. Jackson cited the quotation from Spencer as 'Spencer, "Psychology," vol. i ch. vi. p. 105 ...' Where Jackson wrote 'nerve evolution', Spencer had said 'nervous'.

[114] Jackson (Jackson 1873y, p.344); he quoted Vulpian 1866, p.677, to this effect.

[115] Jackson 1873y, p.344; Jackson's italics, my underlining.

[116] Jackson 1873y, p.344. The quoted text is from Spencer 1870, vol.1, p.67. It illustrates Bowler's (1988, pp.2–14) point about the progressive nature of Spencerian evolution.

[117] Spencer 1855, p.609; see Chapter 4.

movement or faculty. Or returning to our very rough illustration, many terms[118] may be lacking in the highest ranges of evolution without producing loss of any one power, as of *x*, or of *y*, or of *z*, as each of these will be represented in innumerable other remaining terms... In this way we can understand how... recovery occurs from hemiplegia, notwithstanding that part of the corpus striatum ... is permanently lacking; the rest of the corpus striatum also represents the very same muscles, although made up into somewhat different movements...

The above stated conclusions seem to me to be essentially the same as those deductively arrived at by Spencer ...[119]

And so, Jackson again concluded: 'in the convolutions there is not only elaborate structure, but, as a consequence of this, there is a large quantity ... of explosive material ..',[120] which has the potential to become unstable. From there he expanded an older idea by grounding it in Spencer's evolutionary associationism. With that phylogenetic perspective he was able to rebut an experimental argument against his localization of human seizures in the cortices. Referring to the 'well-known experiments' of Kussmaul and Tenner, in which generalized convulsions were supposedly produced by exsanguination of animals with partial brain ablations,[121] Jackson said:

Their experiments show that removal of all parts in rabbits up to the thalami optici does not exercise any influence upon the production of general convulsions. But I think the speculation I have advanced shows that in less differentiated animals than man discharge of the lower centres would be enough to produce severe universal convulsion ... the condition of the mutilated rat and rabbit ... shows that they have much grey matter left in the lower centres, the centres not removed. For, as stated, very general actions are performed by these mutilated animals.[122]

Clearly Jackson was skeptical about efforts to apply generalizations to man from 'mutilated', lower-order animals. He was convinced that unilateral seizure foci in the hemispheric cortices are responsible for generalized seizures with loss of consciousness.

... the *two* sides of the body are represented in *each* side of the brain. Hence there is convulsion of both sides of the body from discharge of but one hemisphere ... But there are cases in which the convulsion is nearly universal to *begin with*, and nearly equal on both sides. Yet it is significant that the spasm of the two sides is rarely, if ever, absolutely contemporaneous, and rarely, if ever, absolutely equal. The first conspicuous movement in the cases where the fit begins ... least *one-sidely* ... is usually turning of the head and eyes to one side; I suppose the discharge to be of some part of the opposite cerebral hemisphere. I believe these cases differ from those simpler ones just mentioned ... in that the

---

[118] This was apparently Jackson's first use of 'term' for 'units' in his *xyz* theory, although he seemed to assume that he had already defined 'term'. See Chapter 6.

[119] Jackson 1873y, pp.344–345; my underlining. Jackson's reference is to Spencer 1870, vol.1, p.60, where Spencer's statements are the same as Jackson's.

[120] Jackson 1873y, p.346.

[121] Jackson (Jackson 1873y, p.346) cited ' "Syd. Soc. Trans." ... p.69'. The relevant section in Kussmaul and Tenner 1859 *begins* on p.69; for summaries of their work see Temkin 1971, pp.284, 296; and Eadie and Bladin 2001, pp.129–130.

[122] Jackson 1873y, p.346; my underlining.

sensori-motor processes discharged are more highly evolved; the evidence for the last statement is that loss of consciousness is the *first* thing, or it is lost *very soon* after a *most general and vague warning*. [123]

So the bilateral motor phenomena of generalized seizures can be explained by bilateral motor representation in each hemisphere, which functions as a single focus *à la* Broadbent. To deal with loss of consciousness in generalized seizures, Jackson had to define the physiology of normal consciousness. For that he again enlisted Spencer.

'*The seat of consciousness is that nervous centre to which ... the most heterogeneous impressions are brought.*'¹ The statement is not of the most numerous impressions, but most heterogeneous ... To the seat or seats of consciousness impressions of *all orders* are brought, and from it issue motor impulses of all orders. It will perhaps be safer to limit this remark by saying that 'all gradations will exist between wholly unconscious nervous actions and wholly conscious ones' (Spencer).[124]

Spencer thus viewed levels of consciousness on an evolutionary scale of increasing complexity of integration. Jackson finished his appendix with another long quotation from Spencer, which he introduced by saying:

The following quotation from Spencer ... is given here particularly to oppose the notion that the sensori-motor processes concerned in consciousness are fundamentally different from, and as it were tacked upon lower series. Why during the excitation of any set of sensori-motor processes, will, memory, &c., arise is unknown. The nature of the connection betwixt physiology and psychology, is ... an <u>insoluble problem</u>.[125]

We might note that in 1867 Jackson had called 'genuine epilepsy' an 'insoluble problem', [126] but 6 years later he had reached some understanding of it. From that partial resolution, in 1873 he was again led to the mind-brain problem, as a direct consequence of trying to deal with loss of consciousness in 'genuine' epilepsy. In the normal state Spencer said:

... all modes of consciousness can be nothing else than incidents of the correspondence between the organism and its environment; they must be all different sides of, or different phases of, the co-ordinated groups of changes whereby internal relations are adjusted to external relations. Between the reception of certain impressions and the performance of certain appropriate motions, there is some internal connection. If the internal connection is organised, the action is of the reflex order ... and none of the phenomena of consciousness proper exist. If the internal connection is not organised, then the psychical changes which come between the impressions and motions are conscious ones ...¹[127]

---

[123] Jackson 1873y, p.347; Jackson's italics.
[124] Jackson 1873y, p.348; Jackson's italics. In his footnote 1, Jackson cited Spencer 1870, vol.1, p105; the second quotation from Spencer (starting: 'all gradations ...') is actually on p.106.
[125] Jackson 1873y, p.348; my underlining.
[126] Jackson 1867b, p.296; see same quotation in Chapter 4.
[127] Jackson 1873y, p.349. Jackson's footnote 1 cites the source of the Spencerian quotation as 'Spencer's "Psychology". No. 25, p.496 ...' The passage is actually in Spencer 1870, pp.495–496; 'No. 25' refers to fascicle 25, a preprint that Jackson and other subscribers received before publication of the complete volume; see Perrin 1993, p.119.

Spencer and Jackson both conceived of the evolutionary emergence of consciousness as a form of biological adaptation. For Jackson, that perspective also derived from his interest in epilepsy and cerebral localization, reinforced by Ferrier's results. Indeed, it turns out that Jackson had again started to think about brain organization for language at some time in later 1872, after his 'Study' of 1870 but before Ferrier started his experiments.

'The Duality of the Brain': Restarting an Interrupted Train of Thought, 1873–1874

Chronologically, my narrative should now be at the beginning of 1874. However, early in this chapter I suspended my analysis of Jackson's interrupted series of papers of January–February 1873,[128] because Ferrier's initial report had apparently diverted his attention. Now we must go back to the interrupted series. From the very beginning of his writings on aphasia in 1864, Jackson assumed that the fundamental unit of speech is the individual word.[129] By 1868 he had absorbed associationism, so he thought that words are stored and manipulated in the brain as acquired 'arbitrary *motor* signs'. These stored signals are revived and sometimes brought to full consciousness by incoming 'perceptive signs'.[130] The initial revival is 'automatic' (involuntary), so it takes place in the right hemisphere, but only in some pre-cognitive way. Since the essence of conscious (voluntary) thought *and* speech is 'propositionising', the words in random order in the right hemisphere must somehow get to the left to be put in an order that carries meaning.

Despite the partition in the roles of the two hemispheres, Jackson insisted that there is no 'abrupt difference' in their functions.[131] He conceived of will or mind as emerging from this process of organizing words into propositions. Hence, the physical and the psychical are conflated. What Jackson's model did not explain was the mechanism by which words revived in the right hemisphere are selected and transmitted to the left. It is also important to note that in his 1868 paper Jackson had said nothing about aphasic phenomena in relation to this model of normal language processing.

Brain Organization and 'Dissolution' in the Interrupted Series of January–February 1873

The main thrust of Jackson's first paper of 1873 was an explication of his concepts of destroying versus discharging lesions, including the application of those principles to brain lesions associated with aphasia.[132] His ideas about brain organization are scattered within the paper in unconnected paragraphs and footnotes. In an early footnote he drew a direct connection between hemispheric organization and association theory. According to the 'law of similarity',[133] an incoming idea that has been previously encountered will cause a 'revival'

---

[128] Jackson 1873a, Jackson 1873c, Jackson 1873d.
[129] Max Müller theorized that the basic unit is the 'root', i.e., the smallest unit that carries meaning, thought to be derived from an ancestral language; see Radick 2007, p.22.
[130] Jackson 1868u, p.528; Jackson 1868u is discussed in Chapter 5. See also Jackson 1868q, p.358: 'We think by help of words—i.e.,—by acquired arbitrary signs—and these are motor processes.'
[131] Jackson 1868u, p.527.
[132] Jackson 1873a.
[133] See Definition Section 7 in Chapter 5.

of the traces left from the earlier activation. It follows that a 'new' incoming idea must excite greater attention if it is to be recognized as similar or dissimilar to any previously encountered idea.

> ... the nervous system is double; this conclusion runs physiologically parallel with the psychological law that all mental operations consist ... in the double process of tracing relations of likeness and unlikeness ... But the very highest movements—those for words—are *apparently* in single order ... It is because we only consider the *end* of word-processes (speech) and neglect altogether the prior automatic reproduction of words.[134]

On the following page Jackson expanded on this theme:

> Coining the word "verbalising" to include all the modes in which words serve, we see that there are two ... extremes of verbalising: one is the voluntary use of words (speech); the other is the automatic use of words as in receiving speech of others ... For the physiological reality of speech it matters nothing whether the proposition be uttered aloud or to ourselves; it is enough that certain nervous powers be ... excited in definite order: if they be strongly excited, there is external speech; if slightly there is internal speech.[135]

Jackson's neologism 'verbalising' is likely to be confusing to the modern reader, because we use the term to mean speaking aloud, i.e., as a synonym for the actual production of external speech. By contrast, Jackson meant 'verbalising' to refer to any kind of word manipulation in the brain, i.e., within the spectrum of internal speech, whether voluntary or automatic. Then he went on to propose:

> This physiological order will ... be of great use in the investigation of mental disease proper ... After some epileptic or epileptiform seizures, the patient becomes strange or outrageous, and acts queerly or violently. My speculation is, that in those cases he is reduced by the fit to a more automatic mental condition. Thus I have recorded the case of a man ... who walked eight miles in a state like that of somnambulism. He was subject to fits, beginning by a subjective sensation of a disagreeable smell ... Now, just as after a fit of unilateral convulsion a patient is often reduced to a more automatic condition, so far as his *physical* state goes ... so I suppose this patient was reduced to a more automatic condition, so far as his mental state was concerned.*[136]

In the footnote to this passage Jackson put a label on his idea of reduction to a lower level.

> * In cases of slow deterioration of brain ... I fear ... that our more animal, our more instinctive habits and desires are no longer subordinated. There is reduction to a more automatic condition; there is dissolution, using this word as the corresponding opposite of evolution.[137]

---

[134] Jackson 1873a, p.84, footnote at asterisk; Jackson's italics and parentheses. On 'likeness and unlikeness' see Chapters 5 and 7.

[135] Jackson 1873a, p.85; Jackson's parentheses. In Jackson 1878g, p.320, Jackson again said, 'Coining a word ... Verbalising ...'

[136] Jackson 1873a, p.85; Jackson's italics. The previously reported case was in Jackson 1871a, pp.376–377. It had been 'mentioned' in Jackson 1866e, p.660, where the mention was indeed very brief.

[137] Jackson 1873a, p.85; my underlining.

This is the first instance where I have found the word 'dissolution' in Jackson's writings—in January 1873.[138] Its next appearance was in a paper of May 1873. There Jackson brought the term out of its footnoted obscurity and into the main narrative: 'In evolution (development, education, etc.), the progress is from the general to the special. In the opposite process of <u>dissolution</u> the more special parts suffer first.'[139] In neither of Jackson's early references to 'dissolution' is there any mention of Spencer. Nonetheless, it would be difficult to claim that Jackson's use of dissolution was completely original, because Spencer discussed it in lengthy generic terms in his *First Principles* of 1862 and later.[140] It is possible that by 1873 Jackson was so immersed in Spencer's ideas that he had lost sight of the boundaries between his own thoughts and Spencer's, but I doubt it. More likely, he simply assumed a knowledge of Spencer's writings on the part of his readers. In any case, Jackson *was* original in applying dissolution to disorders of the brain.[141]

The concept of retrograde 'dissolution' is one of Jackson's most enduring contributions. In the last paper of the interrupted series he defined the functional consequence of dissolution as loss of inhibition of lower centers by higher ones. Citing 'the increased excitability of a nerve after its division' and 'the increased reflex excitability of the lower segment of the cord when cut off from the brain', he said:

> I believe that the outrageous and violent conduct which occasionally occurs in an epileptic patient who *has lost consciousness* is a fact of the same order – that after *sudden* loss of voluntary power there is an increase of *automatic* action. In hysteria[142] there is loss of voluntary power, and yet there is often excitement. The contradiction disappears if we can establish that the excitement is of lower and more automatic processes from lack of inhibition by the higher and more voluntary.[143]

Indeed, it fit nicely with the sociocultural views of his day, which seemed to reinforce his biological analysis of hemispheric asymmetries.

> ... referring to the *whole nervous system*, we see that *its* highest halves are not *mere* duplicates ... the convolutions of the two hemispheres are not symmetrical. These differences in form imply differences in function ... This is the more significant when we find that the asymmetry becomes greater the higher we go in the animal kingdom, not only from lower to higher animals, but from the lower to the higher races of men. According to Dr. Todd, there is greater asymmetry in the convolutions of intellectual men. We see, then, that the

---

[138] Jackson 1873a, p.85. Critchley and Critchley 1998, p.54, state that Jackson first used 'dissolution' in 1876, but they obviously missed this footnote. Jackson 1873a is not reprinted in Jackson's *Selected Writings* (SW), but Jackson 1873k is in SW vol.1, pp.112–117.

[139] Jackson 1873k, p.532; my underlining.

[140] Spencer 1862/1864, pp.351–352; and Spencer 1867a, pp.518–537.

[141] As Temkin (1971, p.343, footnote 229) pointed out, Jackson acknowledged his predecessors in this line of thought in 1875 (Jackson 1875ll, footnotes on pp.111–112), including 'Dr. Monro', Laycock, Francis Anstie, and Dickson. However, I have not found any citation to Anstie or Dickson before 1875, or to Laycock in this regard. On Francis E. Anstie see R. Smith 1992, p.23. Anstie's *Stimulants and Narcotics* was published in 1864. On J. Thompson Dickson see Eadie 2007d. Anstie and Dickson were concerned with the phenomenon of 'release', which is one major component of Jackson's 'dissolution'. R. Smith (1992, p.23) states that Anstie and Jackson 'reformulated already widespread ways of thinking about human action. Anstie re-expressed a commonplace of Victorian moral understanding, and he was only one among many physicians to do so'.

[142] Dunglison (1874, p.528) defined 'Hysteria' as a 'neurosis', which 'generally occurs in paroxysms', consisting of 'alternate fits of laughing and crying', without loss of consciousness. The latter distinguished it from epilepsy. The 'neuroses' were 'diseases supposed to have their seat in the nervous system' (Dunglison 1874, p.700).

[143] Jackson 1873d, p.233, footnote in left column, continued from p.232; Jackson's italics.

higher in the scale of intellectual life the less of a duplicate are the two halves of the highest and most important divisions of the nervous system.[144]

With respect to his social views, Jackson was a conservative, upper middle class man of his Victorian times, so it is no surprise that ideas about degeneration—including dissolution—sometimes intruded into his 'scientific' thinking. In fact, there is now evidence that human brains *are* more asymmetrical than other animals, including primates,[145] but the evidence does not extend to any differences within the human species. The important historical point concerns the general principle of increasingly hierarchical brain organization in phylogenetically higher species, which Jackson felt had been confirmed by Ferrier's experiments. He could thus go back to a previously interrupted theme with strengthened evidence for his conceptualizations.

'On the Nature of the Duality of the Brain', January 1874

Jackson again took up 'the duality of the brain' in a series of three papers in January 1874.[146] In the one he began at the beginning.

Prior to the researches of Dax and Broca it might have been supposed that the brain was double in function in either of two ways – 1st. That action of both halves was required in any mental operation; 2nd. That either half (indifferently) would serve alone. Neither of these opinions can now be held ... since extensive damage in a certain region of the *left* hemisphere will destroy speech altogether.[147]

The importance of Broca's discovery notwithstanding, Jackson hastened to define the limits of its implications with a caveat that still resonates.

The reader will observe that there is no expression of opinion as to the very exact part of the brain injury of which produces loss of speech. Whilst I believe that the hinder part of the third left frontal convolution is the most often damaged, I do not localise speech in any such small part of the brain. To locate the damage which destroys speech and to locate speech are two different things.[148]

This proclamation shows Jackson's interest in trying to 'locate' speech, i.e., trying to understand its normal anatomy and physiology. To that end he could start with an accepted datum: '*the matter of most significance is that damage to but one hemisphere will make a man speechless. This no physician denies, so far as I know.*'[149] So by 1874 he thought that Broca's

---

[144] Jackson 1873d, p.233, col.2; Jackson's italics. In a part of this passage not quoted here, Jackson still referred to 'the statement of Gratiolet that the left frontal and right sphenoidal [temporal] and occipital convolutions are developed earlier than their fellows', although he had previously acknowledged that this statement by Gratiolet had been discredited; see Chapter 5. I have not found the source of Jackson's reference to Todd regarding cerebral asymmetry. It could be buried in Todd 1847, especially in his section '*Of the brain in different races of mankind*' (pp.665–670) or in his further descriptions of 'The Encephalon'.

[145] See Damasio, A.R. and Geschwind, N. 1984/1997.

[146] Jackson 1874b, Jackson 1874c, Jackson 1874e.

[147] Jackson 1874b, p.19. He accepted Dax's priority in Jackson 1866o, p.606; see Chapter 5.

[148] Jackson 1874b, p.19; my underlining.

[149] Jackson 1874b, p.19; Jackson's italics, my underlining.

contribution was widely accepted in British medicine. Therefore he could take the functional asymmetry of the cerebral hemispheres as a starting point.

> The left half of the brain is that by which we speak, for damage of it makes us speechless; the right is the half by which we receive propositions (*a*).

And in the footnote:

> (*a*) ... betwixt propositionising and receiving a proposition ... The essential difference is not that betwixt the internal and external use of words, for speech may be internal; we can, and constantly are speaking to ourselves. The difference ... corresponds to, the voluntary and automatic use of words.[150]

To use a presentistic comparison, here Jackson was ascribing to the nondominant hemisphere the function that we now localize to Wernicke's area and its surrounding tissue on the dominant side. We call it 'comprehension' in the auditory modality. This is not exactly the same as propositionising, because the latter was proposed by Jackson to include a strong motor element. In accordance with associationism, he would have said that any internal manipulation of words is inherently a motor act. Moreover, he claimed to eschew the psychological side of associationism in physiological inquiry.

> We have, as anatomists and physiologists, to study not ideas, but the material substrata of ideas (anatomy) and the modes and condition of energising these substrata (physiology). Where most would say that the speechless patient has lost the memory of words, I would say that he has lost the anatomical substrata of words (*b*).
>
> The anatomical substratum of a word is a nervous process for a highly special movement of the articulatory series ... Ours is not a psychological inquiry ... We have no direct concern with "ideas," but with more or less complex processes for impressions and movements.[151]

Footnote (*b*) issued a further warning about a likely source of confusion.

> (*b*) Psychology is the elder science; mental operations were studied before the brain was known to be the organ of mind. Hence, however much we may wish to study the anatomy and physiology of the higher parts of the nervous system without psychological bias, we are obliged for lack of others to use words which have psychological implications. The words voluntary and automatic are such words, but they are also used physiologically.[152]

---

[150] Jackson 1874b, p.21. This conceptualization of 'the voluntary and automatic use of words' originated in 1868; see Jackson 1868p, p.238, Jackson 1868u, p.527, and Chapter 5. Jackson's 'internal and external use of words' is not the same fundamental distinction that he had learned from Brown-Séquard, for whom articulatory functions were external and brain processes for language were internal. Neither Brown-Séquard nor Jackson used the nomenclature of 'external' and 'internal' for that distinction; see Chapter 3.

[151] Jackson 1874b, p.21.

[152] Jackson 1874b, p.21. Similar statements were made by J.S. Mill in 1851 (Mill 1851, vol.2, p.423: 'Imperfect as is the science of mind, I do not scruple to affirm, that it is in a considerably more advanced state than the portion of physiology which corresponds to it ...'); and by Cajal in 1911: 'In places where we were bereft of exact anatomico-physiological facts, we have resorted to the teachings of psychology in order to fill certain gaps ...' (DeFelipe and Jones 1988, p.470).

In actual practice, Jackson struggled to heed his own advice about separating the psychological and the physiological. He was seeing the same range of aphasic syndromes that we would see now—from straightforward Broca's to classical Wernicke's—and he knew that they constituted a clinical spectrum,[153] but in January 1874 he did not know about Wernicke.[154] He was trying to understand the clinical phenomena within the framework of his theory about the complementary functions of the two hemispheres. About a Broca's aphasic Jackson said: 'He cannot propositionise internally',[155] and he offered some theoretical details to support this conclusion: 'The speechless man can think ... because he has in automatic forms [in his right hemisphere] all the words he ever had; he will be lame in his thinking, because, not being able to revive words (to speak to himself), he will not be able to register new and complex experience of things.'[156] Jackson actually had precious little clinical data to support his theory about the right hemisphere's role in decoding incoming speech—a deficiency that he acknowledged in subsequent papers.

The 'Doubleness' of Brain Processing of Language, January 1874

The second article in Jackson's series of January 1874 began with his distinction of automatic versus voluntary speech.[157] His examples included a bit of social commentary: 'The Communist Orator did not really make a blunder when he began his oration, "Thank God, I am an atheist", for the expression "Thank God" is used by careless, vulgar people simply as an interjection, there being no thought at all about its primitive meaning.'[158] He quoted Baillarger at length on this distinction,[159] and then he made an uncharacteristic assertion: 'I do not know ... that anyone but myself has advanced any hypothesis as to the duality of word-processes, and the relation of the elements of the dual[ity] to halves of the brain.'[160] This priority claim was actually buried in a long footnote. In his main text, he went on to a generalization.

> I believe that doubleness in the verbalising series is but one instance of doubleness in all the nervous processes of the organism ... I wish to compare the *movements* of words with other classes of movements ... we are not about to compare and contrast mental phenomena with physical phenomena, but physical phenomena underlying certain mental phenomena with other and grosser physical phenomena.[161]

---

[153] See Jackson 1874b, p.19, column 2, footnote (b): 'there are numerous varieties and degrees of defect of speech from different degrees of damage to different parts in the [cortical] region of the corpus striatum'.

[154] Wernicke (1874) described 'sensory' (posterior) aphasia. However, in 1869 Jackson's colleague Bastian had described Wernicke's aphasia and given it some theoretical background; see Tesak and Code 2008, pp.61–62, 81–82; on their pp.225–227 they also point out that the Bastian–Wernicke model excludes any language function in the nondominant hemisphere, whereas both Broca and Jackson postulated some right hemisphere participation.

[155] Jackson 1874b, p.20.

[156] Jackson 1874b, p.20, column 2, footnote (a); Jackson's parentheses, my square brackets. As Jackson said it, this is not correct in modern terms, but examination of patients with complete surgical sections of the corpus callosum shows that there is some language in the 'nondominant' hemisphere (Gazzaniga et al. 1962).

[157] Jackson 1874c, p.41.

[158] Jackson 1874c, p.42.

[159] Jackson 1874c, p.42, column 1, footnote (a).

[160] Jackson 1874c, p.42, column 2, footnote (a); my square brackets.

[161] Jackson 1874c, p.43; Jackson's italics, my underlining.

The key word here is 'underlying', which conceals our difficulties with the relationship of the physical to the mental. Jackson's perspective was uniformitarian: 'I consider it to be erroneous to suppose that the unit of composition of the highest nervous processes is of a kind fundamentally different from that of the lower; it will be a sensori-*motor* process in the highest as well as in the lowest'.[162] To illustrate his point he said that the seemingly single movement of respiration is actually a 'unified double', and,

> Similarly ... if we limit ourselves to the voluntary process of verbalising – to speech – we should have no doubt that there was only a linear series, for the words of a proposition are in linear order. In reality, speech is but the result of an earlier process. Before a proposition is uttered, before voluntary use of words, words must have been automatically revived. The double process in verbalising seems to be linear, because the parts of the two halves of the brain serving in verbalising do not, like the parts of the nervous system superintending respiration, act equally in range ... and together in time.[163]

Jackson explained part of his meaning by applying this idea to precognitive language.

> I believe that the most fundamental law of developmental education of the mind is the continuous reduction of successions to co-existences. Things [such] as voice, automatic use of words, and voluntary use of words, which are developed in successive order, come more and more nearly into simultaneous order; this is one aspect of becoming more and more automatic ... Operations occupying many separate units of time come to occur in fewer or in a single unit of time.[164]

And a subsequent footnote defined the neurology of simultaneous 'co-existences'.

> ... the anterior part of the cerebrum is the chiefly motor region and the posterior the chiefly sensory region of the brain. This is almost equivalent to saying that in the highest ranges of evolution the sensory and motor elements of nervous processes are largely separated geographically; but this does not imply that they do not act together – together in the sense of immediate succession ... for in the simplest reflex action the movement *follows* the impression. But in the highest processes the movement does not ... follow immediately.[165]

One way to understand Jackson's 'doubleness' of brain function is to compare it to our parallel processing. Needless to say, he was not analogizing brains to computers. He simply thought of different processes in voluntary and automatic tracks as two separate 'linear series', i.e., as physiologically simultaneous (or nearly simultaneous) events occurring in separate arrays of connected anatomical structures, with a unified outcome.

Although Jackson did not cite Spencer on 'co-existences', we have to assume that he took it from that source. Spencer discussed 'coexistence' at several points in the first and second editions of his *Psychology*,[166] albeit in highly theoretical terms. Here again Jackson translated

---

[162] Jackson 1874c, p.43, column 2, footnote (*d*); Jackson's italics. A similar statement is found in Jackson's main text on the same page: 'It would be marvellous [*sic*] if the highest nervous processes differed *fundamentally* from the lower.'

[163] Jackson 1874c, p.43; my underlining.

[164] Jackson 1874c, p.43, column 2, footnote (*a*); my square brackets and underlining.

[165] Jackson 1874c, p.44, column 1, where footnote (*d*) is carried over from previous page; Jackson's italics.

[166] Spencer 1855, pp.302–309; and Spencer 1872, pp.271–278. See also citations to Spencer's other discussions of 'Coexistence' in Collins' Index (Collins 1889, p.548).

a generic Spencerian concept into a *neurological* theory that has some specificity. No similar neurological concept is found in Spencer or, to my knowledge, in the writings of Jackson's other contemporaries. Spencer actually paid little attention to the unilaterality of aphasia or to its implications for normal brain function.[167] For Jackson, on the other hand, it was crucial. With his neurological background, he could postulate physiological possibilities where Spencer could not see any. Nonetheless, Jackson continued to quote Spencer extensively, because he needed theoretical support in the absence of clinical data.

> But, it may be asked, How do you know that speech is preceded by the *automatic* reproduction of words? *A priori*, the evidence is strong.
> That automatic action must precede voluntary action is, I submit, certain … [gives motor examples] … Taking a psychological illustration, we note that we desire before we will (*c*).[168]

In footnote (*c*) Jackson quoted Spencer on free will.[169] In another footnote he gave a long quotation from Spencer on mental 'integration' of 'feelings' (sensations) from different sensory modalities as the basis of 'mental actions'.[170] On the neurological side of the mind-brain divide we have seen that he thought about language processing in the automatic and voluntary tracks of the two hemispheres as two different 'linear series'. About this he said: 'In popular language words are said to contain or to be symbols of ideas. In physiological language we say that the highest sensori-motor processes of the word series have organic connections with the sensori-motor processes of other series'.[171] And then he gave a physiological example.

> Just as we have in our brains educated processes for a great number of words, so we have educated processes for a great number of objects. The sensori-motor processes of the former [words] are central processes built out of auditory impressions and consequent articulatory adjustments. (These we may label the <u>audito-articulatory series</u>.) The processes educated in objects are central processes built out of retinal impressions and ocular adjustments. (These we may conveniently call <u>retino-ocular</u>.)[172]

In the underlined phrases of this passage Jackson introduced a nomenclature that is potentially confusing but actually straightforward. The key is to substitute our term 'system' for his 'series'. Then 'audito-articulatory series' becomes the anatomical system that receives oral speech and responds with articulatory words. And the 'retino-ocular series' becomes the

---

[167] The second edition of *The Principles of Psychology* (Spencer 1870/1872) was a closely correlated expansion of Spencer 1855, and the latter pre-dated Broca. In Collins' Index, I do not find listings for 'Aphasia' or 'Aphemia' in Spencer. Collins does list 'Language' (Collins 1889, pp.557–558), but not in any relation to brain structures. Nor is there anything about aphasia or brain asymmetry for language in recent analyses of Spencer (e.g., Smith 1982, Richards 1987, Francis 2007). Spencer had to know about aphasia in the 1860s, because he corresponded about language disorders with Jackson. Also, Spencer's friend Lewes was in direct contact with Jackson and other neurologists who were interested in aphasia (see Chapter 6).

[168] Jackson 1874c, p.43; Jackson's italics, my square brackets.

[169] Spencer 1870, p.500.

[170] Footnote (*a*) on p.44 of Jackson 1874c contains a long quotation that Jackson cited from Spencer 1870, p.187; it is actually on pp.187–188. Jackson's direct quotation is otherwise faithful to Spencer's original text, except for Jackson's omission of many commas.

[171] Jackson 1874c, p.43.

[172] Jackson 1874c, p.44; Jackson's parentheses, my square brackets and underlining. On the 'audito-articulatory series' and the 'retino-ocular' series see below and Fig. 7.1.

visual system, etc. So, Jackson said, 'The next question is, "What are the relations betwixt these two series, the Audito-articulatory and Retino-ocular", the processes for words and [the processes for] images of objects'.[173] And there the second article ended, anticipating the third with that rhetorical question.

The *à priori* 'Doubleness' of Parallel Cognitive Functions, January 1874

Unlike the first two papers in this series, it is relatively easy to follow the argument of Jackson's third paper, because its logic is sequential. At the outset he said:

> We have seen that the speechless patient does understand what we say to him. But we have only traced the process by which he understands so far as the automatic revival of words on the right side of his brain. There must be something further ... for words by themselves have no meaning; they are symbols. But the words revived, next revive in him the images of the things they symbolise ...[174]

Here Jackson was postulating that words received in the right hemisphere ordinarily follow at least two tracks ('series'). In one track, as he had said earlier, they are somehow put into propositional order in the left hemisphere, but they also initiate a separate, parallel process in the right hemisphere, and the latter is still available to the aphasic patient.

> In short, there is intact in the speechless man all the processes he ever had for the Recognition of objects (which is putting ideas of objects ... in propositional order) ... The speechless man has lost speech only. His audito-articulatory series is damaged in one-half of his brain; but his retino-ocular [series] is damaged in neither half. Hence, although he cannot *name* them, he recognises objects, he points out in a picture any object which we name; although he cannot read he recognises handwriting; although he cannot write he can copy writing, and he may be able to play at cards or dominos. In none of these things is speech (the voluntary revival of words) concerned, and thus, *à priori* there is no reason to expect that the speechless man should be unable to perform them. For these things the action of *another* series is required, the series for the Recognition of objects – the series for putting objects in relation to one another, making "propositions of objects." This series we have called "retino-ocular."[175]

This process of revival of images in the retino-ocular series is 'automatic', Jackson said, and automatic processes are 'entirely unconscious': 'There is nothing strange in supposing that there is an unconscious use of words. The hypothesis accords with the law that the more operations are automatic the less are we conscious of them; of the most automatic of the bodily operations we are not conscious at all'.[176] Hence,

> We have concluded that the verbalising (or audito-articulatory series) is double, and now we have to infer ... that the retino-ocular series is double also. But just as we

---

[173] Jackson 1874c, p.44; my square brackets; no question mark at the end in the original.
[174] Jackson 1874e, p.63.
[175] Jackson 1874e, p.63; Jackson's italics, my square brackets. Most Broca's aphasics do have some difficulties with reading and writing, although such deficits are not universal; see Benson and Ardila 1996, pp.194–195, 217–218.
[176] Jackson 1874e, p.64.

did not consider the audito-articulatory series to be in mere duplicate, so we do not consider the retino-ocular series to be in mere duplicate. It must be admitted, however, that the direct evidence in favour of the doubleness of the latter series ... is very vague and fragmentary. But there seems to me to be a strong <u>à priori warrant for the assumption</u> that there is in it a doubleness analogous to that in the audito-articulatory series.[177]

In elaborating further on his neurolinguistic model, Jackson suffered the difficulty that he had warned against—keeping separate the mental and the physical—because part of the evidence for his physiological model was from introspection.

... limiting mental operations to the audito-articulatory and retino-ocular series, the speechless man has thought as far as reviving images go. <u>He has words which can be automatically revived so as to place images of objects in order.</u> Although he has but one side for verbalising – the automatic side – he has, according to my hypothesis, *two* sides for the revival of images, and thus he can still think, can still have certain relations of likeness and unlikeness. No doubt he is lame in his thinking. He will be unable to learn novel and complex things, for he will be unable to keep before himself the results of complex arrangements of things ... he can bring two images into co-existence ... but cannot, without speech organise the connection, if it be one of difficulty.[178]

Since Jackson was not deterred by my critique of his method, he proceeded to define the functional anatomy of his hypothetical, parallel processing model: 'we must consider in which region of the hemisphere the revival of images ... occurs. I believe it is chiefly (*a*) in the hinder part—in the posterior lobe ...'[179] And footnote (*a*) added a caveat:

(*a*) I say "chiefly" because I do not believe in abrupt geographical localisations. Thus, very sudden and very extensive damage to *any part* of the left cerebral hemisphere would produce *some* amount of defect of speech, and I believe that similar damage to any part of the right hemisphere might produce *some* defect of recognition.[180]

To support his idea that '*some* defect of recognition' would result from damage to the right hemisphere, Jackson cited evidence from Lockhart Clarke,[181] Bastian,[182] and 'Rosenthal'.[183]

---

[177] Jackson 1874e, p.64 Jackson's parentheses and italics, my underlining.

[178] Jackson 1874e, p.64; my underlining.

[179] Jackson 1874e, p.64; see Jackson 1869d and Chapter 6. Jackson was here using 'posterior lobe' as a term of convenience, to include the parietal and occipital lobes and perhaps the posterior part of the temporal lobe as well. Dunglison 1874, p.605, under 'Lobe', lists the same five lobes that we now recognize, but he implied that the nomenclature was settled only recently.

[180] Jackson 1874e, p.64; Jackson's italics.

[181] Jackson said: 'Lockhart Clarke has found the intimate structure of the convolutions to differ in the two regions ...'; he gave no citation for Clarke, but see Clarke 1863, p.721, and Chapter 6.

[182] Jackson quoted Bastian on 'The Human Brain, *Macmillan's Magazine*, November, 1865, page 71': 'the evidence in our possession *points to the posterior rather than to the anterior lobes of the cerebrum as those concerned more especially with the highest intellectual operations*' (Jackson's italics).

[183] Jackson quoted Rosenthal without citation: 'In the case of new growths in the posterior lobes the *psychical* disturbances are *incomparably more frequent* than in that of tumours of the anterior or middle lobes' (Jackson's italics). Presumably he was referring to Moriz Rosenthal (1833–1889), Professor of Diseases of the Nervous System at Vienna; see Lesky1976, pp.349–350. Rosenthal's *Klinik der Nervenkrankheiten* was published in 1870; it was translated into French in 1878 and into English in 1879. A statement similar to Jackson's quotation of 'Rosenthal' is found in Rosenthal 1879, vol.1, p.112, but that translation was 5 years after the events we are now discussing.

Summing up his model to this point, he theorized the existence of counter-balancing asymmetries.

> So far we have concluded that the revival of images does not occur in the anterior lobes, and we have brought evidence to show that the posterior lobes are more important than the anterior in intellectual operations. The latter is almost equivalent to saying that the posterior lobes are the parts in which revival of images occurs; for the greater part of our intellectual operations is carried on in images – in eye-derived, or, as we call them, retino-ocular processes ...
>
> I think that the left is the side for the automatic revival of images, and the right the side for their voluntary revival—for Recognition.[184]

In further support of his model Jackson offered references to the (mostly French) neuroana-tomical literature that he had quoted before, and then he said: 'The other evidence is supplied by cases of disease, and I may say at once that it is <u>slight and doubtful</u>.'[185]

This admission was followed immediately by the seamless, almost casual introduction of a methodological strategy that is still part of our thinking.

> ... we must consider how loss of power to revive images voluntarily, that is, recognise, would appear as a symptom – in other words, what would be the obvious result of damage to the retino-ocular series; in other words still, what in the retino-ocular series would cor-respond to loss of speech in the audito-articulatory series. Such a condition would be one of imbecility. The condition of a patient who could recognise nothing, would pass as a gen-eral, not as it really would be, a special mental symptom ...
>
> In a *minor* degree, such a state would be one which the patient or his friends would call "loss of memory." The patient would have *difficulty* in *recognising* things ... not from lack of words, but from a prior inability to revive images ... This again might be looked on as a *general* mental defect, not as a defect really as special as defect of speech.[186]

In this passage Jackson's neurolinguistic model *predicted* the existence of the clinical syn-drome that we call *agnosia*.[187] He did it by figuring out the clinical deficit that should result from damage to his retino-ocular series. Of course, finding such predicted cases was not so easy, and he admitted that 'my facts are very few'.[188] Nonetheless, he was able to offer a broad clinico-anatomical idea that had the potential to lead to a specific localization.

> ... I do think that patients who have that variety of left hemiplegia in which the leg suffers more than the arm have <u>greater mental defects</u> of the kind I speak of than occur in other kinds of hemiplegia on the right or left.

---

[184] Jackson 1874e, p.64.
[185] Jackson 1874e, p.65; my underlining.
[186] Jackson 1874e, p.65.
[187] In broad terms, '*agnosia* indicates lack of recognition ..', with intact primary sensory modalities (vision, hearing, etc.). It has been defined as 'a percept stripped of its meaning' (Benson and Ardila 1996, p.303). In a dis-cussion about anterior–posterior and right–left cerebral localization in 1872, Jackson (1872h) described a patient who had 'general imperception of mind', but that is not the same thing as agnosia. For *our* agnosia Jackson also used 'imperception'; see Jackson 1875n for his first published use of the term. In 1876 (Jackson 1876l, p.437) he said that imperception is 'a defect as special as Aphasia'.
[188] Jackson 1874e, p.65.

It is important to note the effects of plugging of the <u>posterior cerebral artery</u>, which vessel supplies the posterior lobe, and also … sends a branch to the corpora quadrigemina. I have seen but one case of this kind, and … in that case, both posterior cerebral arteries were blocked, and also the right middle cerebral, the case is scarcely worth mentioning as evidence.[189]

This passage represents an early attempt to understand the clinical syndromes of the posterior cerebral arteries, which can include greater weakness of leg than arm. Although specific 'mental defects' can be one of those syndromes, we would not say that their frequency is greater than those that occur in the syndromes of other cerebral arteries. It is also worth noting that only a month later Jackson published an autopsied tumor case which did provide slightly better evidence than his vascular patient.[190] The statement '*(To be continued)*' followed immediately after the above passage, but the series actually ended here, on January 28, 1874.

A Summary of Jackson's Model for the Brain's Parallel Processing of Words and Images, January 1874

Jackson's first attempt to present a neurolinguistic model of speech and language in 1868 was incomplete.[191] As we have just seen, by January 1874 his efforts were more advanced, so at this point it will be helpful to outline his model with a diagram (Fig. 7.1), remembering that *Jackson never published any kind of connectionist diagram*. The era of the 'diagram-makers' had not yet arrived, although it was fast approaching.[192] When it did come, he did not join it. Figure 7.1 is merely my heuristic device.

We can begin by noting Jackson's broad division of the brain into anterior and posterior parts. Probably he meant a division between the frontal lobes anteriorly and the parieto-occipital lobes posteriorly,[193] but he was not explicit about it. In all likelihood his ambiguity was deliberate, because he did not like 'abrupt geographical localisations'.[194] The anterior part of the brain, he said, is largely devoted to motor functions and the posterior part to sensory functions. The basic units of language are words. In his associationist theory they were considered to be motor in nature, because they have the effect of causing revival of pre-existing auditory images. Incoming words in the 'audito-articulatory series' (oral modality) initially have this effect automatically (without consciousness) in the right frontal brain, but only in an unorganized way. In order to carry propositional value, words have to be organized semantically. This process is carried out in the left frontal area, though Jackson did not venture to say how the scrambled words get from the right to the left. He simply assumed the existence of some mechanism of selection and interhemispheric transmission. In the

---

[189] Jackson 1874e, p.65. The corpora quadrigemina are small nuclei in the dorsal brainstem (midbrain). They were known to have some kind of visual function, as were the 'optic thalami', but the visual functions of the occipital cortices were not known. See Carpenter 1855, p.497; and Todd and Bowman 1857, p.312.

[190] Jackson 1874k. The patient had a hemorrhagic tumor deep in the center of the right hemisphere. The actual date of publication is 'Feb. 28'; York and Steinberg 2006, p.72, list it as '24 Feb', which must be a misprint.

[191] Jackson 1868u, discussed in Chapter 5.

[192] See Tesak and Code 2008, pp.67–108.

[193] Jackson would have objected to the false impression of precision that is conveyed by the dashed horizontal line which divides the anterior and posterior parts of the brain in Fig. 7.1. Nonetheless, his concept bears some resemblance to Benson's (1967) division of the aphasias into 'anterior' (nonfluent) and 'posterior' (fluent) types.

[194] Jackson 1874e, p.64.

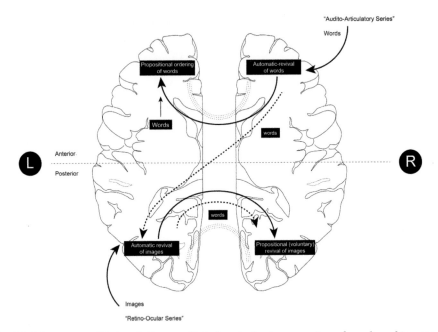

Fig. 7.1 My cartoon of Jackson's theory of interhemispheric processing of words and images. The broken bold lines represent the anterior and posterior extents of the corpus callosum, which Jackson did not specifically mention. He did not specify any interhemispheric pathways. Drawing and illustration by Kendall Lane.

diagram, I've assigned those transfer functions to the corpus callosum, but that is only to try to facilitate our understanding of Jackson's conceptions.[195]

In the above scheme, we would say that the left frontal (anterior) area is dominant for processing words at the conscious (voluntary) level.[196] For reasons of balancing asymmetries, Jackson postulated that the right posterior area is dominant for visual images. They arrive initially in the 'retino-ocular' series at the left posterior part of the brain, where their previously stored counterparts are revived automatically. Propositional ordering of visual images takes place in the right posterior area. In the diagram, there is also a secondary pathway for unsorted words to get to the left posterior brain, where they can cause revival of their corresponding images and thence activation of visual images in the right posterior area.[197]

---

[195] In Fig. 7.1 the broken, bold lines that indicate the anterior and posterior extent of the corpus callosum are meant to show ambiguity about the functional role of the corpus callosum. Carpenter (1855, p.525) said that the fibers of the corpus callosum 'may be traced into the substance of the hemispheres on each side, particularly at their lower part, where their connections are the closest with the Thalami Optici and Corpora Striata'. Todd and Bowman (1857, p.329) said: 'The anatomy of the corpus callosum favours the hypothesis that it is the bond of union to the convoluted surface of the hemispheres, and that it is the medium by which the double organic change is made to correspond with the working of a single mind'. Ferrier (1873b, p.77) specifically nominated the corpus callosum as the 'agency' of interhemispheric transmission. In 1876, Jackson (Jackson 1876v, p.302) said, 'in the scale of animal life ... the corpus callosum is more and more developed the more independent are the movements of the arms'. He implicated the corpus callosum as the pathway for 'lateral' spread of signals from the highest centers, in healthy states and in spread of seizures.

[196] Jackson et al. did not use the terminologies of dominant–nondominant, nor did they think in that way. Their terms were usually just right–left and, by implication, anomalous. Sometimes they used 'leading' as we would use 'dominant'.

[197] Modern experimental and clinical investigations to define the cerebral visual system are usually dated from the work of Hermann Munk (1839–1912) in 1878 to Gordon Holmes (1876–1965) in 1919. See Finger 1994, pp.87–91, and Clarke and O'Malley 1996, pp.537–539.

By looking at the diagram of Jackson's nineteenth-century model with twenty-first-century eyes, we can explore its implications for his developing theories of brain organization. Since there are essentially four quadrants in the model, we might ask what clinical syndromes would be associated with lesions in each quadrant. By 1874 it was established that 'loss of speech' (nonfluent aphasia) is associated with left anterior lesions. Beyond that, however, Jackson's evidence was, as he said, 'à priori', i.e., theoretical. The theory had some power, because Jackson was able to predict the existence of agnosia, even if he hardly had any cases and no convincing autopsies. On the other hand, he made no predictions about syndromes of damage to the right anterior and left posterior areas, which carry out automatic (unconscious) functions. Indeed, it appears that he had not thought about the possibility of predicting clinical deficits of precognitive processing.[198] The difference between our expectations and Jackson's is related to the fact that the idea of a predictive model in brain science was new in the 1870s, although it had been part of the physical sciences.

There is another difficulty in trying to apply this model to clinical situations. In 1874 Jackson thought that extensive destruction of cortical grey matter does not cause clinical deficits,[199] and Ferrier held the same opinion.[200] If one thinks about the model in Fig. 7.1 vis-à-vis the idea of destructive versus irritative lesions, involving negative and positive symptoms, the number of predicted combinations of lesion types and locations becomes absurd. But not to worry. Jackson didn't confront this absurdity, because he didn't think about his model as a source of syndromic predictions. For him it was more broadly a way to relate clinical phenomena to brain organization, at a time when the latter was just beginning to develop its modern form.

---

[198] Harrington 1987 (p.228, italics in original) points out that, 'For Jackson, *only* states of object consciousness could be contemplated or known ...' However, one could still postulate that defective preconscious processing might show up downstream as abnormalities in cognitive language. For the more complete quotation from Harrington see Chapter 8.

[199] Jackson 1874t, p.99: '... disease in the convolutions, so far as it destroys, causes no symptoms'.

[200] See Ferrier 1873b, p.77: 'The fact that extensive lesions, particularly if slowly developed, of the hemispheres on one or other side may exist without causing any obvious loss of voluntary movements, does not to my mind conflict with the positive results ascertained by the direct rousing of the functions of the various centres by means of electrical stimulation.'

8

An Unfinished Book on Epilepsy and Irreplaceable Loss, 1874–1876

After the last of Jackson's three 'duality' papers appeared on January 28, 1874, his next long series of coordinated articles—'On the scientific and empirical investigation of epilepsies'—started on October 14 of the same year. During the intervening 8½ months he published at least 17 other papers.[1] To set the historical stage in this chapter, I will first review some issues about evolution and the brain in Jackson's milieu in the mid-1870s. Then I will look into some of his papers between January and October 1874. From there we will go on to his series about epilepsy, which was intended to be a book, although it was never completed.

Evolution and the (Absent) Brain in British Science and Culture, Early to Mid-1870s

Because Darwin's genius has loomed so large we tend to think that his ideas were always at the center of biological debates soon after publication of *On the Origin of Species* in 1859. However, the relatively modest place of 'Darwinism' in the program of the British Association in 1868 shows that it was not ubiquitous,[2] and Jackson's disregard of Darwin is additional evidence for the same conclusion.[3] It is true, of course, that Darwin added fuel to the cultural fires when he published *The Descent of Man* in 1871 and *The Expression of the Emotions in Man and Animals* in 1872. Thus, by the mid-1870s the debates about Darwinian evolution were fully engaged. Nonetheless, Robert M. Young thought that something was missing.

> When psychophysiology was placed on an experimental basis in the early 1870s by the findings of Fritsch and Hitzig and of Ferrier in their research on cerebral localization, these findings were available for the debate surrounding *The Descent of Man*, but they were not taken up. When they were extended by physiologists and neurologists – especially John Hughlings Jackson – the failure of the evolutionists and anti-evolutionists to exploit them becomes astonishing.[4]

---

[1] See York and Steinberg 2006, pp.71–74; the exact publication dates for Jackson 1874kk and Jackson 1874ll are not known.

[2] See Chapter 5.

[3] See Jacyna 2009, p.3486: 'Jackson's example demonstrates that in the 19th century the theory of evolution was not synonymous with "Darwinism".'

[4] Young 1985, p.64. In the Index to Richards' (1987) thorough study of *Darwin and the Emergence of Evolutionary Theories of Mind and Behavior* there are *no* listings for brain, cerebrum, nervous system, Broca, Jackson, or Ferrier. The brain was not a significant part of the biological debate.

His astonishment notwithstanding, Young has an explanation.

> This is not to say that psychological, physiological, and phrenological issues never got mentioned in the general debate. However, when they did come up, they were isolated from the mainstream of the debate and/or treated polemically. Those who were upholding the traditional picture of the order of nature and society were unwilling to dignify the sciences of mind and brain by debating their findings, when their whole position required them to deny that man's mind lay within the domain of science.[5]

This is another way of saying that the debates about Darwinian evolution and the physiological functions of the brain were carried out in different domains of discourse, involving different sets of data. The Darwinian issues were couched in terms of comparative anatomy, not physiology, and at the beginning there were other considerations. Regarding the problem of mind as a physiological function of brain, Jacyna says:

> Darwin excluded such speculations from the first edition of the *Origin of Species* largely for strategic and prudential reasons. He realized that the thesis that species were not fixed ... was sufficiently contentious without being mixed with the potentially incendiary claim that the human mind was in essence no different from the mental powers manifested by the lower animals and that all thought derived from the properties of the evolving brain.[6]

In later editions of the *Origin*, 'The concomitant evolution of brain and intellect is simply taken for granted'. Even so, in 1871, 'Darwin acknowledged that "little is known about the functions of the brain"'.[7] While he maintained some interest in things neurological, Darwin's engagement with neuroscience was not highly sophisticated.[8] Although he was an expert comparative anatomist, for the second edition of *The Descent* in 1874 Darwin recruited Huxley to write a ten-page 'Note on the Resemblances and Differences in the Structure and the Development of the Brain in Man and Apes'.[9] Huxley's contribution was entirely concerned with comparative neuroanatomy.[10] It said nothing about physiology. In neither *The Descent* nor *The Emotions* is there is any reference to Jackson.[11] The participants in the different domains were reading some of the same literature, but they were thinking about it differently. In truth, the physiological data were not well established.

To understand Jackson's relationship to the British scientific community in the mid-1870s, it is helpful to remember that the brain science of the time developed along two tracks, whose beginnings were separated by a decade: (1) clinico-pathological data on aphasia in the 1860s, and (2) experimental cerebral localization in animals in the 1870s. Broca began his work in 1861, and Jackson brought it to British attention in 1864. In the 1870s the cerebral

---

[5] Young 1985, p.65.

[6] Jacyna 2009, p.3483.

[7] Jacyna 2009, p.3483.

[8] This is my interpretation of Jacyna 2009, p.3484, and Lorch and Hellal 2010, p.152.

[9] Darwin 1874/1901, pp.309–318.

[10] On the ultimately minor affair of the hippocampus minor see Wilson 1996, Smith 1997, and Owen et al. 2009. Jackson never commented on this short blind alley in the history of brain science.

[11] See Barrett et al. 1987, p.526, and Barrett et al. 1986, p.242; I searched for 'Jackson' and 'Hughlings Jackson' in both. Nor is there any reference to 'Jackson, J.H.' or to 'J. Hughlings Jackson' in Darwin's extensive correspondence; see Darwin 1994, p.669, and *Darwin Correspondence Project* (www.darwinproject.ac.uk, accessed March 21, 2017). In 1873 Max Müller used Jackson's distinction between emotional and propositional language to support the conservative position by arguing that animals do not have real language; see Radick 2000, pp.66–67, and Radick 2007, p.62.

basis of language was quite befuddled, especially with regard to the puzzling phenomenon of hemispheric dominance. In the realm of experimental localization, Fritsch and Hitzig's pioneering experiments of 1870 were confirmed and brought to British attention by Ferrier, starting in 1873. However, the experimental work was not widely accepted until the early 1880s.[12] In sum, during the 1870s the human language data were entirely clinical and profoundly unsettled, while the experimental animal data on localization were preliminary at best. Since both tracks were part of the vexing issue of cerebral localization—remember phrenology!—they were commonly conflated, adding to the confusion. Even so, Jackson's enterprise was flourishing.

A Miscellany of Subjects and a Consistent Theme, February–October 1874

For Jackson's developing ideas about brain function and its disorders, 1874 was one of those fruitful years when many different ideas bubbled to the surface. Aside from the two series on 'duality' and 'investigation of epilepsies', throughout 1874 he published several other papers about a potpourri of subjects, including brain tumors,[13] hemiplegia, Ménière's disease, syphilis, and 'drunkenness'. Hemiplegia, of course, had been a longstanding interest. On May 2, 1874, a writer for *The Lancet* reported from the London Hospital, 'On a case of recovery from hemiplegia (Under the care of Dr. Hughlings Jackson.)'.[14] The patient was a 30-year-old woman with 'a loud presystolic murmur' (presumably rheumatic) and sudden onset of severe right hemiparesis, but little facial involvement and no aphasia. She was markedly improved after 3 weeks.

> From her age, and from the presence of valvular disease of the heart, the diagnosis of plugging of some branch of the left middle cerebral artery was warranted … the part of the motor tract destroyed is still wanting. He [Jackson] does not conclude in such a case … that recovery follows because circulation is re-established by collateral anastomosis; according to Cohnheim the cerebral arteries are "terminal arteries." Nor does he think that recovery follows because the plug is absorbed; arterial plugs are absorbed; but is there proof that they are absorbed soon enough to prevent permanent local softening? He believes that recovery is to be explained on the <u>Principle of Compensation</u> … the corpus striatum is a mass of little corpora striata. When a small part of the organ is destroyed, the undamaged remainder "takes on" the duty of the part destroyed … recovery from hemiplegia will occur [even] when a considerable part of the corpus striatum has been permanently destroyed …[15]

---

[12] The turning point toward wide acceptance of Ferrier's work is traditionally attributed to Charcot's remarks at the International Medical Congress in London in 1881; see Mac Cormac 1881, vol.1, p.237; also Chapter 10.

[13] 'A series of cases illustrative of cerebral pathology. Cases of intracranial tumour' in the *Medical Times and Gazette*. The series began on November 16, 1872, and continued to May 1, 1875. The papers in the tumor series were: Jackson 1872o, Jackson 1872p, Jackson 1872q, Jackson 1872s, Jackson 1872t, Jackson 1873f, Jackson 1873g, Jackson 1873j, Jackson 1873m, Jackson 1874a, Jackson 1874d, Jackson 1874f, Jackson 1874k, Jackson 1874v, Jackson 1874z, Jackson 1874bb, Jackson 1875g. A total of 16 autopsied cases were presented, with primary interest in diagnostic efforts before death by history and examination, including ophthalmoscopy. There was no analysis of clinical deterioration in terms of dissolution.

[14] Jackson 1874o.

[15] Jackson 1874g, p.619; my square brackets and underlining. On recovery with large permanent lesions see Jackson 1874kk. Julius Cohnheim published *Untersuchungen ueber die embolischen Processe* (*Investigations of the Embolic Process*), Berlin: A. Hirschwald, in 1872; it contained material 'on the relation of the terminal arteries to embolic processes' (Garrison 1929, p.573).

This is the place where Jackson formally christened his 'Principle of Compensation', which he derived from his *xyz* theory.[16] He had explained that derivation in 1873, without giving the theory a name.[17] It is also important to notice Jackson's remarks about the corpus striatum. Despite his attribution of Jacksonian seizures to cortical tissue in his 'Study' of 1870, here in 1874 he was still thinking about the corpus striatum as the most rostral site of the destructive lesion in hemiplegia. Indeed, he still did not think that cortical lesions cause negative symptoms, although they could be responsible for positive symptoms such as seizures.[18] And other postictal phenomena were even more interesting.

> * ... The after effects of strong epileptic discharges deserve careful consideration ... in epileptic mania, and in so-called "masked" epilepsy, the highest nervous processes are put *hors de combat* by a strong nervous discharge ... the raving in epileptic mania is not owing to the epileptic discharge; it begins when that discharge is over, and results from uncontrolled action of processes more automatic than those temporarily paralysed by the discharge.[19]

On the same theme of disrupted hierarchical brain organization, in May 1874 Jackson wrote an unsigned, two-part editorial for the *British Medical Journal* (*BMJ*) on the subject of 'The comparative study of drunkenness'.[20] In the original editorial piece on intoxication, dated November 8, 1873, the editor (not Jackson) had drawn 'attention to the far too common mistake which the police make in treating certain cases of apoplexy as if the sufferers were drunk. We pointed out that apoplexy, even when caused by so gross a lesion as intracranial haemorrhage, does not always imitate the comatose stage of intoxication, but sometimes the stage of uproariousness'.[21] With this introduction, he went on to apply his idea of dissolution to the problem, but 'dissolution' had a pseudonym.

> We wish now to speak of the importance of making a comparative study of the results of what we shall call "Reduction" ... and especially to speak of the mode of action of alcohol taken in intoxicating, but not comatising, doses. A sudden intracranial hemorrhage, a certain kind of epileptic seizure, a large quantity of spirits, are severally very different things; but each of them reduces the subject *to a more automatic condition*. The general doctrine ... is one which has been recently applied to the explanation of acute and temporary insanity after epileptic attacks and of insanity in general.[22]

Of course, it was Jackson himself who had 'recently applied' his theory of 'Reduction' (dissolution) to these problems. Presumably he labeled it 'Reduction' to preserve his anonymity,

---

[16] See Greenblatt 1988, and York and Steinberg 1995.

[17] Jackson 1873y, pp.344–345; Jackson said that he 'put forward' the 'Principle', without the name in Jackson 1867i. In Jackson 1875a, p.xiv, he said that he had stated 'what I now call the Principle or Hypothesis of Compensation as regards chorea' in Jackson 1868r; indeed, in Jackson 1868r, pp.301–302, the principle is there, albeit vague, but the word is not.

[18] Jackson 1874t, p.99; see also Jackson 1874kk.

[19] Jackson 1874u, p.237, footnote at asterisk; Jackson's italics. Jackson liked the expression '*hors de combat*', meaning 'out of action' or 'disabled'. In 1881 (Jackson 1881s, p.400, footnote (*b*)), when he used *hors de combat*, he explained, 'I avoid the expression "loss of function," because I believe that elaborate psychical states cease not only during loss of function ... but during very excessive function also ...'

[20] Jackson 1874p and Jackson 1874q. York and Steinberg (2006, p.73) state that Jackson claimed authorship of these two editorials in J81-08. The wording and conceptualizations could only be Jackson's. About his relationship to the editor of the *BMJ*, Ernest Hart, see Chapter 9.

[21] Jackson 1874p, p.652. This quotation is Jackson's summary of the original editorial of November 8, 1873. Nothing about the original suggests that Jackson was its author.

[22] Jackson 1874p, p.652; Jackson's italics. In J74-35, p.498, he used 'reduction or dissolution'.

but I doubt that such a ruse would have been successful. In any case, the basic idea involved increased automatic action by release from control of higher levels. He credited Laycock, Bernard, and Francis Anstie (1833–1874) with earlier versions of the same idea, and then he said:

> Let us now illustrate the general doctrine of Reduction to a more Automatic Condition of Mind by the particular case of Drunkenness ... The processes most affected by this poison are the very highest processes. More or less of them are ... paralysed by the alcohol; and ... it is not to their excitement that the drunkards silly behaviour or violent conduct is due ... the silly behaviour or violent conduct is due to uncontrolled action (uninhibited action) of lower processes ... Similarly, the mental symptoms in a case of epileptic mania are not ... the [direct] result of the discharge ... The discharge has put the highest processes *hors de combat*; the raving occurs when the discharge is over ...[23]

To support his view, Jackson quoted a well-known author, Thomas De Quincey (1785–1859), who 'says that the expression "disguised in liquor" is erroneous. He remarks that most men are disguised by sobriety, and exceedingly disguised'.[24] Jackson then described 'three arbitrary degrees' of reduction in the postictal state, which could also be applied to alcoholic intoxication. In the first, 'the mental automatism is of a high kind'. In 'the second degree, the reduction is deeper, the "mental automatism" tends to be an exhibition of the lower or more animal faculties ... there is epileptic mania'. And in the third degree, 'the automatism is no longer mental, but physical; there is coma ... Coma, in this view, is a degree of reduction lower than mania.' Referring to De Quincey, Jackson said that the specific 'mental automatism' in drunkenness will depend on the 'temperament' of the patient.[25]

In the second part of Jackson's editorial he developed this theme of individual propensities by discussing the factors of (1) immaturity in children's brains, (2) heredity, and (3) suddenness of onset of the reduction. Then he applied all of this to dreams.

> Here may be mentioned a qualification of the statement that obscene dreams partly show the character of the dreamer. They may result from ... certain excentric [*sic*] irritations and physiological processes.
>
> Starting from ... so common a condition of the brain as that in dreams, we submit ... that an external impression, acting on a person who is reduced, developes [*sic*] subjective states of mind, which, *because he is reduced* ... cannot be corrected by objective states. Dreaming is a physiological insanity; and insanity, says Comte, "is definable as that state of mind in which subjective impressions are stronger than objective judgments."[26]

At the conjunction of dreams and physiology is the problem of consciousness. Although Jackson had previously expressed some thoughts about the insanities,[27] here, in May 1874, is where his analysis began in depth. Using his comparative method, he applied dissolution to both dreaming and insanity. At the end of his editorial he proposed that,

---

[23] Jackson 1874p, p.652; Jackson's italics and parentheses, my square brackets.
[24] Jackson 1874p, p.653. De Quincey was the author of *Confessions of an English Opium-eater*, first published in book form in 1822; 'disguised in liquor' is found in De Quincey 2003, p.46.
[25] Jackson 1874p, p.653.
[26] Jackson 1874q, p.685; Jackson's italics, my square brackets. He gave no citation for the quotation from Auguste Comte (1798–1857), the French philosopher of positivism.
[27] Jackson 1866m.

'consideration of the several factors we have mentioned in the causation of automatism supplies … a basis for the scientific classification of insanity'.[28] Continuing his comparison, he addressed the problem again in a 'Clinical lecture on a case of hemiplegia', published in July 1874,[29] and he concluded: 'I do not locate consciousness so geographically as I try to do the representation of the limbs and face. Consciousness will be lost in any "grave" lesion of the brain on either side.'[30] Now these are materialistic statements. Some years earlier they would have been culturally problematic—and they actually were at the time.[31] But Jackson made no apologies in 1874. Still, he was not without opposition. We get a sense of this from a review of Jackson's lecture on hemiplegia by W. Bathurst Woodman (1836–1877), Jackson's colleague at the London Hospital. Woodman was sympathetic to Jackson's enterprise but,

> It is possible that some of the opponents of all attempts to localise nervous actions in definite regions of the brain are swayed by conscientious motive, which we must respect. They fear lest 'giving a local habitation and a name' to special functions of the nervous system should end in a crass materialism. In this we think they err, for surely an instrument is no less an instrument, merely because it is complex …[32]

At the same time, Woodman indicated that there were some who questioned Jackson's entire approach. Referring to Jackson's large corpus of publications, Woodman retorted:

> Enough has been said to show that his reasoning is justified … It is no longer possible to sneer at this sort of teaching as transcendental … Nature is not to be bound down by our narrow nosologies, and the cramped notions of our text-books. Yet amidst all the apparent confusion and disorder of disease, there is a method, a divine cosmos, which is discoverable only by the most painstaking observation on the one hand, and a logical use of the imagination on the other. Neither singly can suffice.[33]

It would be helpful to know what Woodman meant by 'transcendental'. 'Metaphysical' comes to mind.[34] Probably some people objected to Jackson's deprecation of nosology. On the other hand, at the same time Jackson was gaining recognition from an eminent supporter, Charcot. In April 1874 Jackson published two papers about 'Charcot and others on auditory vertigo (Ménière's disease)'.[35] They contain Jackson's first published notice of Charcot as someone special. Jackson said: 'Several important articles have recently appeared on … Ménière's disease; the most recent and one of the most able is by Charcot. This physician's great knowledge

---

[28] Jackson 1874q, p.686.

[29] Jackson 1874s and Jackson 1874t. The clinical case that forms the basis of the presentation was published on June 20, 1874 (Jackson 1874r), a month before publication of the lecture itself. The tone of the lecture indicates that it was originally given for medical students.

[30] Jackson 1874t, p.101.

[31] At the British Association in Belfast, August 24, 1874, Huxley (1874) stirred up a hornet's nest by discussing the 'hypothesis that animals are automata', only 5 days after Tyndall (1874) had stirred up even bigger hornets by claiming the primacy of cultural authority for science over theology; see Huxley 1900, vol.1, pp.412–415. On Tyndall see Lightman 2017.

[32] Jackson 1874x, p.649; this review was written by Woodman, not by Jackson.

[33] Jackson 1874x, p.650.

[34] In 1876 Lyttleton Forbes Winslow used 'transcendental' in criticizing everything about Jackson 1875a (listed as pamphlet A30 by York and Steinberg 2006, p.141). Winslow's editorial (Jackson 1876q) is listed as a 'Third person review' by York and Steinberg 2006, p.85.

[35] Jackson 1874l and Jackson 1874m.

of nervous diseases and remarkable power of original research, enable him to give any such subject wide and yet precise bearings'.[36]

Charcot reached the height of his fame in the early 1880s,[37] but Jackson had already known about him for many years. Theirs was a very mutual admiration society. It is likely that they met more than once—certainly at the International Medical Congress in London in 1881,[38] and probably earlier.[39] Charcot's examining room in Paris was 'rather lugubrious'. 'On the walls there were several engravings by Raphael and by Rubens and a large portrait with a dedication from the English neurologist John Hughlings Jackson.'[40] Thus, the two primary founders of modern neurology recognized each other's genius by the 1870s.[41] Their bilateral esteem was based on their mutual understanding that each was working at the level of fundamentals. Charcot particularly recognized Jackson's contribution to our knowledge of seizures and epilepsy,[42] which Jackson expanded in an extensive series of papers.

The First Three Chapters of an Unfinished Book, 'On the Scientific and Empirical Investigation of Epilepsies', October–December 1874

On October 14, 1874, the *Medical Press and Circular* (*MPC*) carried the first in a long series of articles with the title 'On the scientific and empirical investigation of epilepsies'. They continued for more than 2 years, until December 13, 1876. Viewed broadly, they were a major link in Jackson's process of integrating Ferrier's results into his own conceptions. The series was long because 'This and subsequent chapters to be published in this journal are the introductory chapters of a forthcoming work on Epilepsy.'[43] He explained that he had

> ... for several years delayed the execution of this work; but the recent brilliant researches of Ferrier encourage me in the belief that a connected account of the work I have done on epilepsies may be acceptable ...
>
> The value of Ferrier's researches as contributions to the anatomy and physiology of the nervous system could scarcely be overrated. But very naturally to me, a physician, their greatest value seems to be for the help they afford for the methodical investigation of that most inhuman of all diseases, epilepsy. It is a matter of great satisfaction to me to find that my views have passed well through the ordeal.[44]

Jackson's use of 'ordeal' implies the feeling that he was under siege. Since Ferrier's experimental results were more than just medical physiology, he wanted to believe that the siege had been partially lifted. Still, the idea of 'genuine' epilepsy would not go away. At the same

---

[36] Jackson 1874l, p.238. Ménière's 'disease' was and is attributed to abnormality of the inner ear. Its exact pathophysiology is still not understood; see Kandel et al. 2000, pp.807–808.

[37] See Goetz et al. 1995, pp.217–235.

[38] See Goetz et al. 1995, p.220.

[39] See Hierons 1993.

[40] Guillain 1959, p.52; I have no information about the provenance or date of the portrait.

[41] Goetz et al. (1995, p.122) say: 'Charcot ... frequently cited Hughlings Jackson's works in his lectures ...', and they give a citation from Charcot dated 1872. Charcot's lectures in the 1870s, containing references to Jackson, were translated into English in 1881 (Charcot 1881 (1962), pp.286, 291).

[42] See Chapter 9.

[43] Jackson 1874y, p.325.

[44] Jackson 1874aa, pp.351–352.

time, of course, he took pride in the very method that was under attack. This was exhibited in his *apologia* for writing yet another book on epilepsy. He acknowledged that his papers on epilepsy had been written in 'scattered volumes' and sometimes under misleading titles, but, he said, 'This has been the result of my way of investigating. I have studied epilepsy and epileptiform seizures on a novel method, and have written on it from widely different points of view'.[45]

Jackson's 'novel method' was his comparative approach. His faith in the method depended on his conviction that it was 'scientific', in contrast to nosology, which was dominant in medical thought and teaching. Starting in the 1860s he had railed against nosology's monopoly, but now he was ready to make a major concession. It was evident in his title for his promised book, 'Scientific and Empirical Investigation of Epilepsies', where 'Empirical' was in second place.

> ... I do not now object to Clinical Entities for practical purposes. I now admit that they are absolutely necessary. But I object just as strongly as ever I did to the claims of those investigations to be considered Scientific whose aim is only to determine whether a case be or resemble one of 'genuine epilepsy'. Such investigations are very valuable, but they are Empirical only.[46]

Since this statement represented a significant change in Jackson's thinking, he explained himself by acknowledging that he had '... modified my opinion so far as to hold that we require two kinds of classification. I believe that I have been much influenced in this matter by Dr. Moxon ...' In 1870, Jackson's friend, Walter Moxon, had written a paper that dealt with the problems of classification.[47] Moxon had recommended that '... we must keep in view the distinction between a science nomenclature and an art nomenclature'. An art, he said, 'must borrow from the nomenclature of the sciences which it rests upon such names only as are useful for its practical purposes',[48] and it was clear that Moxon considered medicine to be primarily an art. Since the rise of modern scientific medicine can be dated to approximately 1870,[49] it is not surprising that prominent practitioners at that time would still consider medicine to be *primarily* an art, even if it 'rests upon' science.[50]

Jackson's book was intended to bring together his previous work, but a historiographical problem arises from the fact that the serialized papers were published over a 2-year period, 1874–1876. During this same time, of course, Jackson was thinking and publishing about other problems. Any new ideas in those concurrent papers could have had some impact on the book chapters that were published after them. Hence it would be chronologically illegitimate to analyze the entire book seriatim, without knowing what new thoughts Jackson had developed simultaneously. My approach to this problem will be to analyze the book's

---

[45] Jackson 1874y, p.325.

[46] Jackson 1874y, p.327, footnote (*a*).

[47] Moxon's (1870) paper was written in response to the publication of the *Nomenclature of Diseases* by the Royal College of Physicians in 1869 (Moxon 1870, p.483). Moxon felt that it was inappropriately skewed toward pathological anatomy rather than practical clinical use. On the history of the *Nomenclature* see Cooke 1972, pp.38–40.

[48] Moxon 1870, p.482; Jackson quoted these passages in Jackson 1874hh, p.475.

[49] See Temkin 1973, p.191.

[50] In a paper of 1878 Jackson said (Jackson 1878g, footnote 1, pp.315–316): 'See Moxon, On the Necessity for a Clinical Nomenclature of Disease ... In this paper Moxon shows conclusively the necessity of keeping the clinical, or what is ... called empirical ... and scientific studies of disease distinct. After reading this paper, my eyes were opened to the confusion which results from mixing the two kinds of study. It is particularly important to have both an empirical arrangement and a scientific classification.'

chapters in 'clusters'. In Table 8.1 it will be seen that there are generally intervals of several months between the four clusters. Within each cluster I will review the articles in chronological order, with discussion of Jackson's other papers interposed between clusters.

Epilepsy and the Mind-Brain Problem, October 1874

Despite Jackson's belief that his ideas had been experimentally verified by Ferrier, genuine epilepsy remained tenaciously entrenched in medical thinking—as it would for the remainder of the century.[51] He was getting impatient about it, because he had been promulgating his ideas for a decade. In his second installment he introduced the theories that he had derived from evolutionary associationism, including hierarchical re-representation, dissolution, and compensation.[52] However, his primary concern was to find the reason for genuine epilepsy's stranglehold on his colleagues.

> Epilepsy, like Aphasia, has been studied with a Psychological habit of mind, and, as I think this way of studying such a disease is unfruitful, I have to point out in detail the vast difference there is betwixt Psychology and the Anatomy and Physiology of the Nervous System. The confusion of the two ... is really one of the great hindrances to the acceptance of the view that the convolutions (parts of the "organ of mind") represent movements. The notion seems to be that the "organ of mind" being for "ideation," cannot contain processes representing movements.[53]

In the last sentence Jackson encapsulated his contemporaries' view of the cortices. The fundamental problem, he thought, was the intransigence of the mind-brain conundrum, which leads to confused thinking. Accordingly, if the underlying problem was an unhelpful interpretation of the mind-brain relation, he needed to offer an alternative, and he had one.

> Admitting, as the whole educated world now does, that all mental states have parallel physical states, I think our direct concern as physiologists and physicians is with the latter only. Hence, I should not use such expressions as that hemiplegia is "owing to loss of volition," or that a person did not speak *because* he had lost the "memory of words" ... our concern, as physicians, is with the anatomical substrata of ideas and emotions ... the expressions objected to refer only to the material basis of mind. To give a material explanation of mental states, admitting its correctness as far as it goes, is not to give an anatomical explanation.[54]

Jackson's further discussion of this last point was based on his ideas about 'sensori-motor processes', but he added a clarification: 'A reader may perhaps suppose that I imagine processes for impressions and movements to become in the highest centres so fine that they

---

[51] See Eadie and Bladin 2010, p.209. In 1875 (Jackson 1875ll, p.108) Jackson lamented, 'my opinions as to the nature of epilepsy are accepted by very few physicians'.

[52] Chapter I, Part II (Jackson 1874cc).

[53] Jackson 1874cc, p.348; Jackson's quotation marks. In Jackson 1873y, p.348, Jackson called 'the connection betwixt physiology and psychology ... an insoluble problem'.

[54] Jackson 1874aa, p.348; Jackson's quotation marks and italics, my underlining. Jackson's 'whole educated world' actually referred to the inhabitants of his professional and intellectual milieus in London and to a few individuals outside of the Metropolis. See Young 1970, p.233, where he shows that Jackson could not have been including the French- and German-speaking worlds.

Table 8.1 *Epilepsy Book 1874–1876*: published only as a series of papers, 'On the scientific and empirical investigation of epilepsies' in the *MPC*. The chapters are numbered with Jackson's Roman numerals, and the chapter titles (in quotation marks) are his. The far right column shows the citation for each installment in Jackson's bibliography. See text for explanation of Clusters.

Cluster 1 – October 14, 1874, to December 16, 1874

1874

I – Part I – 'Introductory'	Oct. 14	Jackson 1874y
Part II – 'Summary'	Oct. 21	Jackson 1874aa
II – 'Definition'	Nov. 4	Jackson 1874ee
- continued	Nov. 11	Jackson 1874ff
III – 'Classification and methods'	Dec. 2	Jackson 1874hh
- continued	Dec. 9	Jackson 1874ii
- 'concluded'	Dec. 16	Jackson 1874jj

Cluster 2 – April 26, 1875, to May 19, 1875

1875

IV – 'General remarks on the causes of epilepsy'	Apr. 28[a]	Jackson 1875f
V – 'Physiology of epilepsy'	May 12	Jackson 1875i
- continued	May 19	Jackson 1875l

Cluster 3 – October 20, 1875, to April 19, 1876

VI – 'The pathology of epilepsies'[b]	Oct. 20	Jackson 1875hh
VI – 'The pathology of epilepsies' (continued)	Nov. 3	Jackson 1875jj
- 'The pathology of epilepsies' (continued)	Dec. 15	Jackson 1875kk

1876

VI – 'The pathology of epilepsies' (continued)	Jan. 26	Jackson 1876d
VII – 'Anatomy'	Feb. 16	Jackson 1876e
- continued	Mar. 1	Jackson 1876g
- continued	Apr. 19	Jackson 1876k
(Mrs. Jackson died May 23, 1876.)		

Cluster 4 – June 14, 1876, to December 13, 1876

VIII – 'Recapitulation – The Method Exemplified'	June 14	Jackson 1876n
IX – 'Unilaterally beginning Convulsion'	Aug. 23	Jackson 1876o
- 'Unilaterally beginning Convulsion' (continued)	Sep. 6	Jackson 1876p
X – 'Sequence of Spasm unilaterally beginning in convulsions'	Dec. 13	Jackson 1876r

---

[a] York and Steinberg 2006, p.77, list this date as '26 Apr 75', but the date on the article is 'April 28, 1875'.
[b] The first part of the chapter on 'THE PATHOLOGY OF EPILEPSIES' (J75-32) was actually published with the number and title 'CHAPTER V. (*continued from Vol.XVIII., N.S., p.421.*)', but in the next installment (Jackson 1875jj, p.351, footnote (*a*)), Jackson said, 'The heading of the last instalment [*sic*], p.312 [actually p.313], should have been Chapter VI., not V.'

"fine away" into mental states. I do not. To show what I really think, let me quote the words of Herbert Spencer ...'[55] This was followed by two Spencerian quotations. First: 'Though accumulated observations and experiments have led us by a very indirect series of inferences to the belief that mind and nervous action are the subjective and objective phaces [*sic*] of the same thing, we remain utterly incapable of seeing and even of imagining, how the two are related.'[56]

And second: 'See, then, our predicament. We can think of Matter only in terms of Mind. We can think of Mind only in terms of Matter. When we have pushed our explorations of the first to the uttermost limit, we are referred to the second for a final answer; and when we have got the final answer of the second, we are referred back to the first ...'[57]

Now exactly how Jackson reasoned from Spencer's metaphysical speculations to his own unambiguous statement that 'all mental states have parallel physical states' is not clear. I would argue that he saw these things as he did because, as a physician, he felt an imperative to get on with the practical demands of clinical medicine.[58] Sometimes a word that implies a theoretical position has practical implications. In Jackson's case, 'parallel' was such a word. 'Psychophysical parallelism' had been part of associationism since Hartley.[59] In contrast to interactionism, parallelism assumes constant separation between the mental and the physical. They simply run along together on separate, 'parallel' tracks.[60] With interactionism, the problem is to decide what interacts with which, when, etc. Parallelism obviated those difficulties.

> ... the psychophysical parallelism of the Spencer–Jackson–Ferrier view eliminates all these complex issues by precluding interaction and even the discussion of psychological faculties in a physiological context ... The philosophical assumptions of the Germans' [Fritsch and Hitzig's] view were anathema to the Englishmen, whose parallelism allowed them the luxury of ontological agnosticism while they got on with their work.[61]

After Jackson's conversion to associationism in the 1860s he adhered increasingly to the logic of parallelism. In 1874 he first expressed it clearly by using the word 'parallel'.[62] Thence he set out on the path that ultimately led to his 'doctrine of concomitance', which was his version of parallelism. Here, in 1874, is where he began to explore that path in depth.

> How from or during the energising of sensori-motor processes or of the highest of them, there arise mental states, is not our concern ... it is of no importance, for this investigation, what view of the connection of mind and matter we take. If any reader supposes mind to

---

[55] Jackson 1874aa, p.348; Jackson's quotation marks.
[56] Jackson 1874aa, p.348. The quotation is from Spencer 1870, p.140, where the spelling is 'faces'.
[57] Jackson 1874aa, p.348; the quotation is from Spencer 1870, p.627.
[58] Commenting on the meaning of 'practical', Jackson said, '... I think some people have the notion that to take a materialistic view is to take a "practical" view ... under this supposed "practical" guise work has been done on the old-fashioned system ... [which] spoke of an immaterial mind. The very same method in a new dress still speaks of a brain as if it were a solid mind, governing and acting on the body, and not as if it were simply the most developed part of the nervous system ...' (Jackson 1874aa, pp.348–349; Jackson's quotation marks, my square brackets). Other Jacksonian scholars have also remarked on the 'practical' aspects of Jackson's psychophysical parallelism; see Young 1970, p.233, and York and Steinberg 2006, p.21.
[59] See Young 1970, p.96; also Daston 1982, pp.100–103.
[60] See Young 1970, pp.232–233.
[61] Young 1970, p.233; my square brackets.
[62] Jackson 1874aa, p.348.

be a function of matter (thought, let us say a secretion of brain), I would simply say to him that one does not concern ones self with that "function" in an anatomical and physiological inquiry, but with another function – viz., the energising of cells and fibres representing peripheral impressions and adjusted movements.[63]

Jackson emphasized that there is a substantial motor component in 'sensori-motor', but it tends to be ignored because 'The word "sensation" is often confusedly applied both to a physical state and to the mental state which occurs along with it ...'[64] The truth, he said, is that,

> Although I have, for convenience, spoken separately of afferent and efferent processes, and, if I may so speak of afferent and efferent centres, both are concerned together on the anatomical and physiological side of "ideation." The former are evidently concerned in acquiring ideas of the dynamical or secondary qualities of objects, the latter in *acquiring* ideas of statical or primary [qualities].[65]

After extensive discussion of this point, Jackson went back to his book's primary subject, epilepsy. In reference to the preceding, he said: 'Remarks like these are foreign to the subject of epilepsy as that disease is usually studied, but not foreign to my view of it ... I believe epileptic paroxysms result from discharges of parts of the organ of mind, from discharge of parts containing anatomical substrata of ideas, into which substrata the element movement necessarily enters.'[66] Here he was following the associationist premise that 'ideas' are the contents of consciousness. This assumption was combined with his evolutionary outlook to offer a hierarchical view of the pathophysiology of 'Loss of Consciousness'.

> In order to obtain a realistic view of the symptom, Loss of Consciousness, I have to speak in detail of the Evolution of the higher nervous centres out of the lower ... The highest centres are those which form the anatomical substrata of consciousness ... They represent over again ... the very same impressions and movements which the lower, and through them the lowest, centres represent. They represent the whole Organism.[67]

With his adaptive, evolutionary view of consciousness Jackson continued his battle against genuine epilepsy, starting with those epileptic cases in which

> ... loss of consciousness is the first event in the seizure (cases without a "warning"). Now these are the cases in which the discharge begins in the very highest centres ... which commonly go by the name of true or idiopathic epilepsy. To say of a paroxysm of epilepsy that it begins with loss of consciousness is a symptomatic expression; to say that the discharge begins in the very highest processes is the anatomico-physiological expression corresponding to it.[68]

---

[63] Jackson 1874aa, p.348.
[64] Jackson 1874aa, p.349; Jackson's quotation marks (double in original). To support this statement, Jackson cited 'Mill's Logic, vol.ii., p.43'. I can find no similar statement in Mill 1851, vol.2, p.43, or in Mill 1872, vol.2, p.43.
[65] Jackson 1874aa, p.349; Jackson's quotation marks and italics, my square brackets.
[66] Jackson 1874aa, p.349.
[67] Jackson 1874aa, p.349. Jackson began to see loss of consciousness as loss of the highest (re-representative) centers in 1873 (Jackson 1873y), so this part of his book was an expansion of that insight.
[68] Jackson 1874aa, p.349.

Jackson also had to contend with some recent experimental results that seemed to support the old idea that the brainstem is the site of the mischief in genuine seizures.[69] For this he enlisted his evolutionary view of the nervous systems of animals.

> Taken with the principle of evolution, the principle of compensation [*xyz* theory] accounts ... for the fact that fits, <u>declared to be like the epileptic fits of man</u> ... can result in lower animals from discharge of the pons variolii and medulla oblongata ... In man re-representation or evolution is carried many stages further than in the brute: Man has the large cerebral hemisphere; the brute the large pons and medulla.[70]

The underlined clause shows Jackson's skepticism about analogizing from induced seizures in animals to human epilepsy. His skepticism followed logically from 'the principle of evolution', because the nervous systems in animals are not evolved as far as man's, so the manifestations of their abnormalities are likely to be different. On this topic, this is as far as Jackson would go. From there he changed the subject to his 'principle of Dissolution', which he followed in an unexpected direction.

'Epileptic Mania' and 'the Insanities' as Separate Entities, October 1874

In this part of his narrative Jackson drew a direct comparison between postictal 'epileptic mania' and its apparent counterpart in psychiatric disease. He referred to 'what was implicitly stated of Evolution ... that there is a continuous transition from the lowest centres ... to the anatomical substrata of consciousness ...' Thus it follows that 'The insane man has lost the use of ... the most special of all nervous processes ... he has, indeed, defect of consciousness'.[71] In both cases—postictal and psychiatric—the principle of dissolution is applicable.

> ... we can ... by taking note of the experiments of disease, show stages of lowering of adjustment as consequences of different depths of Dissolution of the higher centres. Such lowering of adjustment ... is equivalent to saying that the organism is reduced to a more automatic condition. On this way of putting it ... The question is – '<u>How is the Organism adjusted to its Environment?</u>'[72]

And Jackson's answer to his rhetorical question was that

> ... there are, after different degrees of epileptic discharges beginning in the highest centres ... *all* degrees of lowering of adjustment (*a*) of the organism to its environment. Starting from ... only slight confusion of thought, we can trace all gradations to deepest coma ... There is indeed sometimes a loss of all adjustment, which is death.
>
>   The condition of things in <u>Insanity differs only in degree</u> from that in epileptic mania. The ordinary insane patient has *defect* of consciousness, analogous to the *loss* of

---

[69] Among his opponents was Brown-Séquard; see Temkin 1971, pp.279–285, and Eadie and Bladin 2001, pp.131–137.

[70] Jackson 1874aa, p.350; my square brackets and underlining.

[71] Jackson 1874aa, p.350.

[72] Jackson 1874aa, p.350; my underlining.

consciousness of the epileptic maniac; the "symptoms" of insanity are due to quasi-healthy actions of more automatic processes, as are also those of the epileptic maniac.[73]

In the underlined phrase Jackson made a statement that he soon had to qualify, because there are differences between the delirium of the insane and postictal delirium. Nonetheless, this passage represents an advance in his thinking. Earlier in this chapter we saw that he began to apply his principle of dissolution to the phenomena of 'drunkenness' in May 1874, when he also extended his ideas to dreaming and insanity. Here, in October 1874, he began his in-depth analysis of mental disease within his pathophysiological framework.

In the nineteenth century, both epilepsy and insanity were commonly thought to be hereditary.[74] Without denying the possibility of some hereditary element, Jackson's revised tripartite method gave him a biological point of view.

> Two things which should ... be considered separately, are often considered together under Heredity ... under Pathology ... there is hereditary transmission (1) of a tendency to diseases of Tissues ... there is (2) transmission of imperfect Organs. The "facts" of these hereditary transmissions are not ... evidence that there is inherited a tendency to particular *diseases* or *symptoms*, such as chorea, epilepsy, insanity, &c....[75]

To illustrate 'diseases of Tissues', he gave the example of hemiplegia with genuine epilepsy. The hemiplegia *per se* is not hereditary. It is due to disease in 'arterial' (vascular) tissue in the brain, not to disease in 'nervous' tissue. Equally to the point, insofar as genuine epilepsy was classified as one of the neuroses, by definition,

> The Neuroses[76] ... are mostly <u>supposed</u> to be hereditary ... [but] I draw attention to the significant fact that *the pathology of these diseases, which are supposed to be pre-eminently hereditary, is ... unknown.* Under pathology ... in nearly all cases of "nervous" diseases or symptoms of which the pathology *is* known, morbid anatomy declares that the changes begin in non-nervous tissues ... my impression is that this will be found to be the case with epilepsy and the allied neuroses.[77]

We can infer from Jackson's use of 'supposed' that he was skeptical about the pervasive hereditary ideas and about the data supporting them.[78] The above passage claims that the underlying pathology in 'epilepsy and the allied neuroses' is not in the patients' neural tissues but in other intertwined tissues. In contrast, he postulated that the basic abnormality in mental disease is defective *development* of the brain.

> A man does not, according to my hypothesis, inherit insanity of any kind. The man whose insanity is said to have been transmitted is ... a person who inherits an imperfect nervous system, not imperfect in its tissues, but in relative development of its higher and lower

---

[73] Jackson 1874aa, pp.350–351; Jackson's italics, my underlining. In footnote (a) Jackson quoted a passage from Spencer's *Psychology* (1870, pp.495–496), which I have quoted in Chapter 7.

[74] On heredity and degeneracy in epilepsy see Temkin 1971, pp.260–264, 348, 365–370.

[75] Jackson 1874aa, p.351; Jackson's italics and quotation marks.

[76] The 'neuroses' were 'diseases supposed to have their seat in the nervous system' (Dunglison 1874, p.700), but without demonstrated pathology.

[77] Jackson 1874aa, p.351; Jackson's italics and quotation marks, my square brackets and underlining.

[78] In the sentence just before this passage, Jackson also complained about other '"facts" brought forward as proof of inheritance of *nervous* diseases ...'.

centres ... the higher, and metaphorically speaking, *controlling centres* are in him imperfectly developed ... psychologically speaking, the latest faculties acquired by the race are in him ill-developed ... the lower centres and corresponding lower faculties are in comparison over-developed ...

Such a man is more liable than another man to become insane ...[79]

In sum, according to Jackson in 1874 the etiology of epilepsy—and probably the other 'neuroses'—is disease of the non-neural tissue in the brain, which in turn injures or destroys the neural tissue. For this, of course, he had substantial clinical and autopsy data, though without histology. On the other hand, he proposed that the abnormality in psychiatric disease is defective ontogenesis of the higher brain structures, perhaps with over-development of the lower centers. To support this idea about insanity Jackson had only the observation of differing clinical manifestations in the two separate nosological entities.

> Insanity and such diseases as epilepsy and chorea are not fairly comparable. The active symptoms of insanity are not directly due to the disease of the brain or of any other part of the nervous system, as [are] ... chorea, convulsion, and spasm... The "symptoms" of insanity are due to the action of lower centres of the brain, which centres are healthy except for exaggerated action, consequent on loss or defect of the highest and controlling centres, the parts really diseased.[80]

This passage encapsulates Jackson's scientific and nosological separation of epilepsy from the other neuroses, including insanity. Such separation was necessary if the underlying pathogenesis of epilepsy were to be understood as *sui generis*. So far, then, Jackson's plan for his book was clear. In Part I of Chapter I ('Introductory') he declared his intention to incorporate the phenomena of genuine epilepsy into the larger nosological category of epilepsy. In Part II of the first chapter ('Summary')[81] he laid out his basic principles of analysis, which were largely associationistic. With that background, he went on to his Chapter II ('Definition').

Refining the Definition of Normal and Abnormal Discharges, November 1874

Chapter II began with a unifying definition: 'Epileptic discharges are occasional, abrupt, and excessive discharges of parts of the cerebral hemisphere (paroxysmal discharges).'[82] A year earlier he had given essentially the same definition twice, with slightly different wordings. The only noticeable difference now is the fact that in 1873 he had localized the site of the discharge to 'some *part* of the brain' or to gray matter,[83] whereas here in 1874 he said specifically, 'the cerebral hemisphere'. This was an outright rejection of the brainstem as the site of any

---

[79] Jackson 1874aa, p.351; Jackson's italics.
[80] Jackson 1874aa, p.351; Jackson's quotation marks, my square brackets.
[81] In the actual publication of Jackson 1874aa, the article is labeled 'Lecture I. Part II ... ', but I take this to be a mistake; it should have been 'Chapter I'.
[82] Jackson 1874dd, p.389.
[83] In Jackson 1873y, Jackson gave two definitions. The first (on p.315, Jackson's italics) said, 'Epilepsy—an occasional, sudden, excessive and rapid discharge of grey matter of some *part* of the brain'. The second (p.331, in Jackson's italics), '*Epilepsy is the name for occasional, sudden, excessive, rapid, and local discharges of grey matter*'.

epileptic focus.[84] By implication, Jackson was also turning away from the corpus striatum as a site of epileptic discharge, because he said little about it. He had found Ferrier's stimulation results to be thoroughly convincing about the cortices. It is also true that Ferrier tried to stimulate the striatum directly and got no conclusive response.[85] In the event, Jackson's opening definition was for 'Epileptic discharges', not epilepsy.

> We have, so far as is practicable, to study epilepsies as departures from healthy states. We must, then, give a <u>brief sketch of healthy nervous discharges</u> ...
>
> Where there is grey matter ... discharge occurs during healthy functional exercise ... If I move my arm there is of necessity an expenditure of force ... [thus,] there is in every movement a discharge of a part [of the brain] where movements are coordinated.[86]

Jackson's conception of the 'anatomical unit' through which discharges travel was sensori-motor—and modern.

> The anatomical unit of a nervous organ is not a cell or a fibre, or a compound of both ... The anatomical unit is a sensori-motor process. It is not an afferent (sensory) process only, nor a motor process only, but these two put in a particular relation by cells of grey matter ... The anatomical unit represents ... a peripheral impression associated with a muscular adjustment. The peripheral impression may be either on the surface of the body, or in its interior ... The surface impressions vary from those most general of mere contact of ordinary objects ... to those so special as retinal impressions. The impressions from the interior ... are from muscles, viscera, &c.[87]

Having thus defined the 'anatomy' of normal neural units, Jackson turned to their 'physiology', i.e., to 'their conditions of discharge'. His argument was uniformitarian.

> There are discharges of the highest sensori-motor processes when we think, just as there are of lower processes when we walk ... There are central discharges when I speak internally, just as there are when I speak aloud. That in the former there are no outward effects makes no essential difference; there is a central discharge in both cases, and of the same series of processes ... in the spreading ... of the discharge ... it is stronger and spreads from the centre first excited, to lower centres and to the muscles when I speak aloud.[88]

---

[84] See Eadie and Bladin 2010, pp.214–215.

[85] Ferrier 1873b, p.66. None of this caused Jackson to dethrone the striatum as the rostral end of the motor system: see Jackson 1874t, p.100, Jackson 1874ff, p.409, and Jackson 1874kk.

[86] Jackson 1874ee, p.389; my underlining and square brackets.

[87] Jackson 1874ee, p.390; Jackson's parentheses. In a footnote shortly after this passage Jackson articulated a fundamental of psychophysiology, i.e., there must be a delay in any response that entails the higher centers. This follows from his conception of re-representation by units in the higher centers: 'In the ordinary reflex action the movement follows the afferent incitation with, no or with little, delay. In the highest centres ... the movement will not be immediate ... there is in the highest centres wide geographical separation, and thus probably delay' (Jackson 1874ee, p.390).

[88] Jackson 1874ee, p.390. Later on the same page, Jackson used the word 'mentation'. In a footnote he said, 'The word Mentation ... was, I believe, introduced by Mr. Metcalfe Johnson'. Jackson again attributed the term to Johnson in J78-07, p.307. Presumably this was Surgeon-Major Metcalfe Johnson (1823–1902), who frequently contributed articles to the medical press, including 'Cerebral and ganglionic disorders of mentation' (see obituary: [Johnson] 1902).

Connecting all of this to associationist analysis, Jackson said that another characteristic of normal discharge is the concept that in the normal state there are 'vivid ideas and faint ideas'.[89]

> When we actually see and *recognise* external objects, we have *vivid* visual ideas. There is then strong excitation of the retina, thence to the highest centres in the cerebrum, and back to the ocular muscles ... When we have faint visual ideas, (Think of objects when they are absent – "recollect" them, &c.) there is slight or nascent excitation (discharge) of higher centres ...[90]

It follows that 'the epileptic discharge ... is an excessive discharge. Not only is it very much more excessive than the discharges which occur when we have faint mental states, but it is very much more excessive than those occurring in vivid mental states ...'[91] Continuing the same theme, Jackson applied the associationist idea of strong and weak visual impressions to tactual and other systems, including 'the so-called centre for "memory of words" on the left side of the brain ...'[92] In a footnote to this passage, we get a sense of how Ferrier had affected Jackson's perception of his own situation: 'Until very recently I have been alone in that opinion [about the motor substrata of words] ... I am very glad, therefore, to find that Ferrier has quite independently reached a conclusion essentially similar'.[93] Now we might question whether Ferrier's results were obtained in a state of complete independence from Jackson,[94] but Jackson perceived them in that spirit. Clearly he felt less 'alone' after Ferrier's reports. Hence, he felt justified in continuing to pursue his unified theory of epilepsy, which needed boundaries.

> ... all abnormal nervous discharges are not epileptic ... There is ... an almost continuous stream of discharges in tetanus, and there are rapidly succeeding discharges in chorea. The epileptic discharge comes on with more or less suddenness. The paroxysm is violent, and it is soon over.
> Briefly, the epileptic discharge differs from the other kinds of abnormal discharges ... in being paroxysmal.[95]

Our current definition of epilepsy still stresses its paroxysmal nature, which is a necessary, albeit insufficient part of the definition. Another Jacksonian concept that is still with us is the idea that some parts of the hemispheric cortices are more susceptible to instability than

---

[89] Jackson 1874ee, p.390.

[90] Jackson 1874ee, p.391; Jackson's italics and parentheses. He also said: 'If we *recognise* an object, the very highest centres must be engaged; for Recognition is, in common with Classification, a modified form of reasoning (Spencer's "Psychology", vol. ii, p.127).'

[91] Jackson 1874ee, p.391. Later in the same paragraph Jackson used one of his famously colorful expressions to describe motor seizures, in this case as applied to the extraocular muscles: 'There often occurs also, as part of a larger fit, that <u>clotted mass of movements</u> of the ocular muscles which we call spasm ...' (my underlining). At the end of the same paragraph he used another, less-quoted description of the same phenomenon, saying that the discharge 'jams innumerable ocular movements into one stiff struggle'.

[92] Jackson 1874ee, p.391.

[93] Jackson 1874ee, p.391, (a); my square brackets.

[94] Did Ferrier set out to *test* Jackson's theories or to *confirm* them, or both? Ferrier (1873b, p.30) said that his purpose was 'first, to put to experimental proof the views entertained by Dr. Hughlings Jackson'.

[95] Jackson 1874ee, p.391.

others.[96] Jackson thought that this is true of all cortex within the distribution of the middle cerebral artery.

> ... any part of the nervous system which contains grey matter may become unstable, and may discharge abnormally ... however ... some parts of the nervous system are very much more liable to become diseased than other parts, and in the brain the region in the district of the middle cerebral artery suffers more often than other cerebral regions. Further, it is not certain that abrupt and paroxysmal discharges result from disease of the lower parts of the Nervous System in Man.[97]

To complete the first part of his Chapter II, Jackson gave many examples of 'epilepsies' within his pathophysiological definition: 'strong smell in the nose', and 'coloured vision ... other initial symptoms of an attack of migraine are all epilepsies'.[98] So, in general, 'Since ... any part of the cerebral hemisphere may become the seat of a discharging lesion, there will be all kinds of phenomena produced; and since there are supposed to be all degrees in the extent of the discharging lesion, the symptoms will vary in degree as well as in kind'.[99] One of the symptoms that most interested him was 'epileptic mania'.

The Pathophysiology of 'Epileptic Mania', November 1874

In the second part of his Chapter II Jackson again took up this subject. His text gives us some insight into an important change in his conception of the pathophysiology of epilepsy, which had occurred some years earlier.

> Epileptic Mania is usually ... spoken of as if it were owing to an *epileptic* discharge ... In agreement with this opinion ... I used to suppose that [it] directly resulted from such discharges as those which produce other paroxysms ... I have for some years thought otherwise. There are discharges in epileptic mania, and they are abnormal, and they are of the organ of mind, but they are not epileptic ...[100]

In accordance with the logic of dissolution, Jackson was claiming that the discharges responsible for mania are normal discharges in lower centers, which are uncontrolled but not actually epileptic. For this conclusion he had a further point—about unobserved seizures.

> I have several reasons for change of opinion. There is in most cases of epileptic mania clear evidence that ... the maniacal action is post-epileptic rather than epileptic. There are, however, cases in which there is ... no outward sign ... before the maniacal action begins, as

---

[96] For explanations of 'seizure threshold' see Engel 2013, pp.157–158, 162, 186.

[97] Jackson 1874ee, p.392. We think of the frontal and anterior temporal lobes as more prone to seizures. They are only partly irrigated by the middle cerebral arteries.

[98] Jackson 1874ee, p.392. Jackson was a migraineur; see [Jackson, J.H.] 1935. If migrainous phenomena are epileptic, then by his own definition Jackson was an epileptic! To my knowledge he never commented on this.

[99] Jackson 1874ee, p.392.

[100] Jackson 1874ff, p.409; Jackson's italics, my square brackets.

in cases of so-called masked epilepsy. I do not … adopt the accepted explanation of these cases – that they "replace" an epileptic fit. I think the evidence is in favour of another hypothesis … a slight and unobserved fit.[101]

To explain the condition *after* the paroxysm, Jackson offered the 'simpler' case of post-epileptic (Todd's) paralysis following unilateral seizures.

… after the discharge is over, there is, if the discharge has been unusually excessive, hemiplegia. This is … a sign to us that the corpus striatum has been put *hors de combat* by the violent discharge. We venture from these cases on the generalisation that '*Strong Epileptic Discharges Paralyse the Nervous Centre (or much of it) in which they Begin or through which they Spread*'.[102]

In applying this generalization 'to the cases where the discharge begins in the highest series', Jackson offered some guidance: 'My opinion is that the mania is the result of over-action (morbidly increased discharge, but not epileptic discharge) of the processes just below those which have been put *hors de combat*.'[103] The meaning here is that 'processes just below' are not necessarily below the cortex. That is, they need not be fully subcortical or in the brainstem. Immediately following this passage he quoted Bernard and Anstie to support his idea that in mania there is 'over-action of lower centres from the mere removal of the higher centres',[104] but then he extended the meaning of mania. Up to this point, he had generally used it to describe raving or other violent behavior. Now he included under this rubric 'cases of elaborate mental automatism after very slight epileptic discharges'.

… a man subject to epileptic attacks is found unconscious in the kitchen, mixing cocoa in a dirty gallipot (intended for the cat's food) with a mustard spoon. This was a very elaborate action, and that it was only a caricature of a normal action is plain, because it had just before been agreed on that his sister-in-law, who was on a visit, should have cocoa for her supper.[105]

In twentieth-century terminology this patient had 'temporal lobe epilepsy' (aka psychomotor seizures, complex partial seizures) in addition to his 'slight attacks (*petit mal*) and severe attacks (*grand mal*).'[106] Here again Jackson was refining his conception of epilepsy, in this case by defining the physiological difference between (1) discharge in normal cortical tissue that would elicit normal, complex behavior, and (2) release of that behavior from higher centers. With regard to the 'cocoa-mixing affair', he said, 'An epileptic discharge could not produce actions so elaborate as [this kind of] maniacal action'.[107] Our current view, based on EEG monitoring, holds that there *is* epileptic discharge during

---

[101] Jackson 1874ff, p.409; Jackson's parentheses and quotation marks.
[102] Jackson 1874ff, p.409; Jackson's italics, parentheses, and quotation marks.
[103] Jackson 1874ff, p.409; Jackson's italics and parentheses.
[104] Jackson 1874ff, p.410.
[105] Jackson 1874ff, p.410. 'Unconscious' here means *altered* consciousness. A gallipot is a small glazed clay pot. In 1888 Jackson admitted that he had failed to mention here that this episode was preceded by a 'dreamy state' in the patient; see Jackson 1888e, p.188; also Temkin 1971, p.344.
[106] Jackson 1874ff, p.410.
[107] Jackson 1874ff, p.410; my square brackets.

automatisms. But Jackson didn't have EEG. He was simply following the logic of his definition, which described the epileptic discharge as 'occasional, abrupt, and excessive', i.e., 'paroxysmal'.[108]

In summarizing his view of the epileptic discharge, Jackson said that it 'is a <u>very local</u> discharge ... of some highly unstable part of the cerebral (*a*) hemisphere ...'.[109] And his footnote (*a*) added emphatic specificity: 'I wish particularly to mention now that I think *universal* convulsion with which there is loss of consciousness at or about the onset ... depends on discharge of parts in <u>one cerebral hemisphere</u>.'[110] Now one could claim that the idea of the unifocal etiology of all genuine seizures was present in the theory of epilepsy's origin in the brainstem, but Jackson was radical in his claim about 'one cerebral hemisphere'. Either way, any theory of a unifocal etiology necessarily includes the assumption that what starts in one place causes symptoms beyond the initial site by affecting other parts of the nervous system.

Consciousness and the Spread of the Discharge, November 1874

Shortly after his statement about the cortical unifocality of epileptic seizures Jackson again attacked his old nemesis, the nosological distinction between genuine and epileptiform seizures. In the process he commented on the spread of normal and abnormal discharges. The idea that something spreads in the brain during epileptic attacks had been supported by Brown-Séquard's vasoconstriction theory. Although Jackson had abandoned that idea in the 1860s, most of his colleagues had not.

> The accepted position is that two different and distinct parts (the medulla oblongata and the cerebral hemisphere) are concerned in the epileptic paroxysm ... The discharge, of course, spreads through lower centres ...
>
> The accepted view assumes two different processes – (1) a *discharge* of the medulla oblongata, and (2) a *contraction of the arteries* of the brain. Correspondingly there are ... two essentially different states – (1) passive, in the cerebral hemisphere, and (2) active, in the medulla oblongata. I think there is but *one* process in the paroxysm, an active one – that is, a discharge beginning in the highest processes of the cerebral hemisphere.[111]

Left unspecified was the physiological explanation of how the discharge propagates from one neural element to the next. Everyone simply agreed that propagation happens somehow, vertically and horizontally.[112] What Jackson did say about the phenomenon of the spreading discharge concerned its location, strength, rapidity, and distance.

> ... whether consciousness be lost or not in an epilepsy ... or whether it be lost first of all or later in the paroxysm, depends on the seat of the discharging lesion, and on how far

[108] Jackson 1874ee, p.389.

[109] Jackson 1874ff, p.410; my underlining.

[110] Jackson 1874ff, p.410; Jackson's italics, my underlining.

[111] Jackson 1874jj, p.519, footnote (*a*); Jackson's italics.

[112] Neural signals can propagate vertically (up or down the neuraxis from the focus) and/or horizontally (into adjacent neural tissue which is at the same level as the focus). In a footnote to a later chapter of his book (Jackson 1875f, p.353) Jackson described vertical and horizontal propagation. He further stated that 'Co-ordination' in 'Time' is mediated by sudden arterial contraction, which determines horizontal spread. See also J76-22, pp.301–302, where he used 'laterally' and 'downwards'.

the discharge spreads. If those parts of the brain where the most special of all nervous processes lie, be *first* affected by the epileptic discharge, there is loss of consciousness first of all. If the discharge be slight there may be ... loss of consciousness only. This is so in very slight cases of *petit mal*. If strong, the discharge spreads from these very highest centres to lower centres ... and ... The discharge widens as it spreads lower, and rapidly reaches the lower centres and their muscles. There is loss of consciousness followed by convulsion.[113]

Here Jackson recognized a difficulty that affected all sides of the debate: 'although medical men speak *clinically* of loss of consciousness as if there were a well-defined entity called consciousness, there is probably not amongst educated persons any such belief. We must for Clinical purposes have arbitrary standards (definitions by type).'[114] Part of his advancing definition of 'loss of consciousness' included *alteration* of consciousness, which obviously is much broader than complete loss *per se*.[115]

It must be admitted that the two-fold use, the empirical and scientific, of terms leads to apparent contradiction in some of our medical phrases. Thus it is said 'the patient was confused but quite conscious'. To be confused is to have defect of consciousness. Again, loss of consciousness is sometimes spoken of as being synonymous with coma.[116]

To address the confusion about confusion, Jackson heeded the promise of his book's title by elaborating on the problem of empirical versus scientific methods of investigation.

On Scientific and Empirical Nosologies, December 1874

Jackson's Chapter III was titled 'On classification and on methods of investigation'.[117] It began with a reference to the Moxon paper that we have already discussed.[118] To support his view Jackson quoted extensively from J.S. Mill (who quoted Comte), Bain (who quoted Whewell), and Spencer (who quoted himself).[119] In this process he liked to use the analogy of the gardener versus the botanist, this time with an interesting twist.

The gardener arranges his plants as they are fit for food, for ornament, &c.... His object is the direct application of knowledge to utilitarian purposes ... The other kind of classification ... is rather for the better organization of existing knowledge ... its principles are Methodical guides to further investigation ...

The difference here is plain, because the gardener and the botanist are different persons. But in our profession, the same person has to Classify for the organisation and advancement of his knowledge, and to make an Arrangement for direct utilitarian purposes of daily life.[120]

---

113 Jackson 1874ff, p.411; Jackson's italics.
114 Jackson 1874ff, p.411; Jackson's italics.
115 See Posner et al. 2007, pp.5–9, about alteration as loss of consciousness.
116 Jackson 1874ff, p.411; Jackson's quotation marks, my underlining. There is still much confusion about 'confusion'; see Posner et al. 2007, pp.183–184.
117 Chapter III includes the last three articles in Cluster 1: Jackson 1874hh, Jackson 1874ii, Jackson 1874jj.
118 Moxon 1870; see above in this Chapter 8.
119 Jackson 1874hh, pp.475–476.
120 Jackson 1874hh, p.476; my underlining.

One of the 'utilitarian purposes' that Jackson acknowledged was the necessity of an empirical arrangement for reasoning to a diagnosis by the process of elimination.[121] Thus compelled by Moxon, and by his own dialectic, he said:

> I admit two classifications to the Empirical Classification, or rather Arrangement of Varieties of Epilepsies, and of Epileptiform Convulsions would be –
> EMPIRICAL ARRANGEMENT.
>   A. Epilepsy Proper.
> (1) Vertigo.
> (2) Petit mal
> (3) Grand mal.
>   B. Epileptiform, or Epileptoid.
> (1) Convulsions beginning unilaterally.
> (2) Unilateral Dysesthesia (migraine)
> (3) Epileptiform Amaurosis.
>   &c.[122]

Despite his professed acceptance of the need for a practical nosology, Jackson used the verb 'admit' as if he were making a concession, and the '&c.' at the end indicates that he did not want to continue such a listing. His real interest was on the scientific side.

The '*Four Variables*' of Insanity Applied to Mania, Epileptic and Insane, December 1874

To advance his understanding of the various forms of insanity,[123] including those associated with epilepsy, Jackson used his comparative method: 'when I come to speak at length on epileptic mania, I shall have to speak generally of insanity. It is a part of my subject, for epileptic mania is acute temporary insanity'.[124] To remind his readers about his way of thinking, he repeated a caveat from his first chapter:

> I must ... urge strongly that we are to rid ourselves as much as possible of psychological bias in what is an anatomical and physiological inquiry. I do not mean that we have no concern at all with psychology. On the contrary, it is perfectly obvious that it is impossible for us to *begin* to study the anatomical *substrata* of mind without prior psychological analysis ...
>   But ... our concern with states of mind is indirect. We start with the <u>assumption that all mental states have material bases</u>, and our direct concern in such an inquiry as this is with the latter only.[125]

---

[121] Jackson 1874hh, p.478.
[122] Jackson 1874jj, p.519.
[123] Dunglison 1874, p.546, defined 'Insanity' as including 'all the varieties of unsound mind,—Mania, Melancholia, Moral Insanity, Dementia, and Idiocy'.
[124] Jackson 1874ii, p.497.
[125] Jackson 1874hh, p.476; Jackson's italics, my underlining.

Now the 'assumption that all mental states have material bases' would seem to be inconsistent with the 'parallel' part of Jackson's earlier statement that 'all mental states have parallel physical states'.[126] So, Dr. Jackson, which position are you going to espouse, straight materialism or parallelism? At this stage of his development he was using both. In the same paragraph where he wrote 'all mental states' he also said, 'To give a material explanation of mental states, admitting its correctness as far as it goes, is not to give an anatomical explanation'.[127] The implication is that old-fashioned materialism is correct as a working 'assumption', but it is ultimately insufficient because it does not take adequate account of current and projected scientific knowledge.

> ... what we here call the Scientific Investigation of Insanity is really an experimental investigation of Mind; and in this regard the slightest departures from a person's standard of mental health are to be studied, and not only the cases of patients who require to be kept in asylums ... the more special (the more nearly normal) the mental automatism after an epileptic discharge is, the easier it is understood. The cocoa-mixing automatism is a more valuable experiment on mind than is a case of epileptic mania.[128]

This call for a 'Scientific Investigation of Insanity' has a manifesto-like quality that echoes Jackson's proclamations in the 1860s about the comparative study of hemiplegia, aphasia, and unilateral seizures.[129] And why not? His comparative approach had served him well. As a guide to carrying out his new program he said: 'Insanity is a Function of four Variables'.

> The varieties of insanity would be explained (1) by the depth of the reduction or dissolution; (2) by the rapidity of the reduction; (3) by the kind of brain in which the reduction occurs; and (4) by the influence of external circumstances and internal bodily states on the patient ... These factors will vary in relative amount infinitely.[130]

This passage is important because it prefigures the title of a well-known paper that Jackson published two decades later, 'The factors of insanities'.[131] In that paper of 1894 he discussed the same four 'factors', so this place in his unfinished epilepsy book is where he first began to formulate his thoughts on the subject. Note that his study of the 'varieties of insanity' took root from his interest in the clinical manifestations of epilepsy, when he began to investigate insanity by applying the first of his four factors to its analysis.

> ... in an anatomico-physiological inquiry the question is not the psychological one – Is consciousness displayed? But, How is the organism adjusted to its environment? We have to trace all degrees of defective adjustment corresponding to different depths of dissolution. In the cocoa-mixing affair the adjustment was almost as special as is normal; in

---

126 Jackson 1874aa, p.348.
127 Jackson 1874hh, p.476; my underlining.
128 Jackson 1874ii, p.498. The 'cocoa-mixing automatism' in Jackson 1874ff, p.410, is discussed in the section 'The Pathophysiology of "Epileptic Mania", November 1874' in this chapter.
129 Jackson 1864h.
130 Jackson 1874ii, p.498.
131 Jackson 1894j.

mania where the dissolution is deeper it is far more general; and in deepest coma the adjustment is of the most general character compatible with life.[132]

Here Jackson took his example from an epileptic phenomenon, and his second factor could also be used to distinguish epileptic insanity from other insanities.

Epileptic mania is acute temporary insanity, but in insanity ordinarily so-called there is clinically an essentially similar double state. There is *defect* of consciousness analogous to *loss* of consciousness, and there is slightly increased automatic action analogous to the raving. The difference in degree depends ... on the second Variable ... on the difference in the rapidity with which the dissolution is effected (control removed). Dissolution is effected with extreme rapidity by an epileptic discharge, whereas in insanity ordinarily so-called the morbid process removing or impairing control is usually very slow indeed.[133]

Taking the analysis of the dissolution further,

The [insane] patient who has a delusion has it for the same reason that the dreamer has delusions. There is in each loss of ability to correct automatically arising mental states ... by objective states, because, since the processes serving in the latter are implicated, clear objective states are not possible ... The nervous processes implicated are those which form the anatomical substrate of consciousness, or, otherwise expressed, those by which the organism, *as a whole*, is adjusted to its environment. There is in [ordinary] insanity a less special ... adjustment.[134]

Jackson's discussion of adaptation is incomplete. It was not taken to its full conclusion, which would be that a reduced level of adjustment to the environment is dangerous or even fatal. He had acknowledged this disturbing implication in an earlier chapter,[135] but generally it lingered just below the surface. At the end of Chapter III he struck a hopeful note about the prospects for his Scientific Investigation.

The researches of Hitzig and Ferrier will help this investigation to an extent difficult to over-estimate; for I most willingly admit that the method I uphold has made very little way. From their researches we shall learn where to look for the minute changes which constitute the discharging lesions in different epilepsies. Whatever interpretation may be put on their facts, there is no doubt ... that irritation of different parts of the surface of the brain leads to different classes of movements.[136]

At this point Jackson put aside further questions about the details of hemispheric localization. In his next two chapters he pursued more fundamental issues about the nature of those 'minute changes which constitute the discharging lesions ...'.[137]

---

[132] Jackson 1874ii, p.498; my underlining.
[133] Jackson 1874ii, p.498; Jackson's italics and parentheses, my underlining.
[134] Jackson 1874ii, p.498; Jackson's italics, my square brackets.
[135] Jackson 1874aa, p.351: 'There is indeed sometimes a loss of all adjustment, which is death.'
[136] Jackson 1874jj, p.520; my underlining.
[137] This next section covers Cluster 2 of Jackson's book chapters (Table 8.1). It includes his Chapter IV (Jackson 1875f) and most of V (Jackson 1875i, and Jackson 1875l, which latter is continued into Cluster 3 as Jackson 1875hh).

Chapters IV and V of an Unfinished Book, April–May 1875

Method, 'Causes', and the Pathophysiology of Epilepsy, April 1875

Chapter IV was titled 'GENERAL REMARKS ON THE CAUSES OF EPILEPSIES', where 'causes' was more or less synonymous with 'etiology'. However, Jackson might have objected to 'etiology', because it would fail to separate the different components of his tripartite method.

> … we have to study the Anatomy, the Physiology, (*b*) and the Pathology of Epilepsies, or rather of each epilepsy … It is an <u>anatomical inquiry</u> to search for the seat of the lesions. It is a <u>physiological inquiry</u> to note how the function of nervous matter is affected. It is a <u>pathological inquiry</u> to trace the morbid nutritive processes [abnormal metabolism] by which local changes of instability are brought about.[138]

In his next paragraph he explained what he was really looking for.

> The above shows … how we use the word Cause. We must use it, however, not in a threefold, but in a fourfold sense. The fourth group of so-called causes is for the conditions which determine individual paroxysms, but more particularly the first paroxysm in a case … for the present we speak only of Causes with reference to the three lines of investigation – Organ, Function, Nutrition. The word cause is frequently used by medical men for any one of the three.[139]

More than anything else, Jackson wanted to understand the abnormal processes of cellular instability at the chemical and physiological levels—that was his holy grail. In retrospect we can see that there were insurmountable obstacles. Investigative techniques at the cellular level were not available, and this was a place where the absence of the neuron theory frustrated his search for the 'cause' of epileptic discharges. For any individual patient, he said: 'When we … [consider] … mobile affections [motor seizures] resulting from nervous discharges in epilepsies, we cannot accomplish this threefold classification. We can often only be certain of the second—the nature of the Functional affection.'[140] That is, in the living patient he could know only the likely existence of an unstable focus somewhere, but he had little chance of finding its location.

The Pathophysiology and Histology of the 'Minute Changes' in the Seizure Focus, May 1875

In the opening paragraphs of Jackson's Chapter V ('PHYSIOLOGY OF EPILEPSY') Jackson repeated his conception of neurophysiology, which 'has to do … with the conditions for and modes of activity (discharge) of arrangements of nerve cells and fibres'. The word

---

[138] Jackson 1875f, p.354; my underlining and square brackets. Footnote '(*b*)' says: 'Of course we mean by Physiology in this application abnormal function …' So 'Physiology' actually means *patho*physiology.

[139] Jackson 1875f, p.354.

[140] Jackson 1875f, p.355; my square brackets.

'Physiological', he said, 'is used for the two *abnormalities* in this healthy function of nerve tissue —viz., for loss of its function and for over-function ...'[141] He wanted to explain the mechanism by which destructive lesions and discharging lesions can account for 'loss ... of function and for over-function'. But first he clarified his use of 'functional'.

> ... I do not use the word 'functional' in senses in which it is frequently used. The word Functional is sometimes used as the name for 'minute' changes, or for those the existence of which we can only infer because nervous symptoms are present, but which we do not expect to discover *post mortem* ... the changes ... are so slight that they do not involve actual alterations of structure. It is thus a term for the neuroses. The <u>neuroses</u> are often spoken of as "<u>functional diseases</u>." This is ... an inconvenient way of using the word. The real meaning in this application is little more than that the morbid changes in the nervous organs are as yet undiscovered.[142]

Furthermore:

> The term functional is often used more loosely still ... when a patient has a transient and imperfect paralysis ... the internal changes on which it depends may be declared to be functional, *i.e.*, in the sense of slight change, *simply because the external symptom presented was a slight and transitory one.* There are several reasons why this error should be pointed out ... The slightness and transientness of a paralytic symptom depend on the slight *extent* of lesions of nervous organs, not on slight *degree* of change.[143]

The importance of these considerations is their relevance to 'Recoverability'.

> ... transientness of paralysis cannot be taken as evidence that nervous *structure* has not been permanently destroyed ...
>   That parts of the cerebral hemisphere may be destroyed when there are no obvious or striking symptoms has long been well known. But it is so of the motor tract also.[144]

To explain such phenomena, Jackson invoked his Principle of Compensation, elaborating its relevance in terms of loss or hyperactivity of function. Then he rather abruptly shifted gears to neurohistology. In the mid-1870s the basics were only a little different than they had been *circa* 1860.[145] According to Jackson in May 1875:

> There are ganglion cells and nerve fibres. The [healthy] cells store up force and discharge. The [healthy] nerve fibres carry the current, and provoke discharge ... there are notable differences in the blood supply of grey and white matter – differences in their vascular condition corresponding to differences in their function[s] ... this separation of duty is to

---

[141] Jackson 1875i, p.397; Jackson's italics. Immediately after these passages Jackson explained that he used the adjectival form of 'physiology' ('Physiological') very much as we use it clinically today—to indicate that a symptom is of 'organic' rather than psychogenic origin.

[142] Jackson 1875i, p.398; Jackson's italics, my underlining.

[143] Jackson 1875i, p.398; Jackson's italics.

[144] Jackson 1875i, p.398, Jackson's italics. He still considered the motor tract to end rostrally in the corpus striatum; see Jackson 1875i, p.399, footnote (*a*) in column 2.

[145] See Definition Section 1 in Chapter 3; also Shepherd 1991, pp.25–66.

some extent artificial, for the cell is not only a mass of "explosive" matter, but also a connecting link betwixt nerves ... [i.e.] a conductor of nerve force.[146]

In saying that the cells are 'a connecting link betwixt nerves', Jackson was recognizing a role for the cells that he had not previously mentioned. And immediately after the above passage he used a new term for 'fibres'.

As Spencer says, the 'centres in which molecular motion is liberated are also the centres in which it is coordinated'.[147] Similarly, as the axis cylinder of the nerve is composed of matter similar to that of the cell, we may suppose that it also stores up and expends force. It must ... be admitted that instability of the axis cylinders of fibres will produce some over-function, and that destruction of the cells will produce some loss of function. But it is not likely that instability of the axis cylinder [alone] would produce such excessive discharges as occur in convulsion, chorea, and neuralgia ...[148]

Here Jackson was recanting his older notion that 'fibres' could discharge separately from cells. His problem in the last sentence of this passage would not exist with the neuron theory, because all 'fibres' are now known to be parts of cells, including 'axis cylinders' (axons). That term is a translation of the German *Achsencylinder*, which was first introduced in 1839.[149] The axon carries efferent signals away from the neuronal cell body. However, to Jackson's generation the 'axis cylinder' appeared to be either a type of fiber or a structure within some fibers. Its connection to the cell was not established, and its strictly efferent function was not known. Jackson's acceptance of the new term ('axis cylinder') is interesting,[150] but it did not change his conception of how normal neural tissue functions and dysfunctions. That had changed in his 'Study' of 1870. Before then, he now said, he had made a 'great blunder'.[151]

The *xyz* Theory Corrects a 'Great Blunder', May 1875

With the tone of a *mea culpa*, Jackson declared, 'I confess that I used to consider the two functional states of nerve tissue to be degrees of but one condition. I now see that this was a great blunder; they are diametrically opposite states.' Furthermore, he declared, 'A satisfactory explanation can be given of the co-existence of palsy and spasm – I mean of parts permanently paralysed, being subject to occasional spasm.' Part of his explanation depended on his long-standing view: 'That the corpus striatum does not ... represent the *muscles* of the face, arm, and leg, but *movements* of these parts in which movements the muscles serve in all degrees and combinations; speaking metaphorically, it represents, not notes, but chords.'[152]

---

[146] Jackson 1875i, p.399; my square brackets.
[147] This exact Spencerian quotation is found in Spencer 1870, p.67. A similar statement is also found in Spencer 1870, p.46.
[148] Jackson 1875i, p.399; my underlining and square brackets.
[149] See Shepherd 1991, p.19: 'work on nerve fibers ... appeared in the dissertation of ... J.F. Rosenthal in 1839. Here was introduced the term *Achsencylinder* ("axis cylinder"), which was to become the prevalent mode of referring to the long fibers of the nervous system for the rest of the nineteenth century, until replaced around 1900 by "axon".'
[150] As Jackson said, the original source of his acquaintance with this term was Spencer. In his *Principles of Psychology* Spencer (1870, pp.49–52) used 'axis cylinder' in the midst of a lengthy discussion of 'The grey substance and the white substance ...'.
[151] Jackson 1875i, p.399.
[152] Jackson 1875i, p.399; Jackson's italics.

In the 1860s he had thought that partial damage to any piece of brain tissue is responsible for seizures, *and* he thought that complete destruction of the same tissue causes paralysis. However, his *xyz* theory showed that adjacent pieces of tissue can be responsible for the two different phenomena.

> Suppose the corpus striatum be divided into three parts from front to back, A B C. Symbolising the parts of the external [muscular] region as $x\, y$ and z, we say that A represents them as $x^3\, y^2\, z$, B as $x^2\, y^3\, z$, C as $x\, y^2\, z^3$ ... Each third represents the whole region, but represents it differently... From destruction of a third there is only weakening, because the remaining two-thirds represent the same muscles, although they represent different movements of them...
>
>   ... From partial destruction of the centre there is not "paralysis of parts" of the region, but "partial paralysis" throughout the region. We infer, then, that each of the three divisions A B C [in the corpus striatum] contains movements for the whole region ... We thus understand that loss of function of a certain number of these units may be causing partial palsy of the face, arm, and leg, whilst occasional discharge of other unstable units may cause ... [seizures] of the very same external parts.[153]

This reasoning, using the *xyz* theory, goes back to Jackson's 'Study' of 1870. Now, in 1875, his use of capital letters was different, and the subscript multipliers of 1870 were superscript, but the meaning had not changed.[154] In the same way, he offered a new speculation. Referring to the above passage, he said:

> We supposed ... the corpus striatum to be divided into three parts, each third representing muscles of the face, arm, and leg ... So we may suppose that the muscles of the face, arm, and leg ... are all represented in each of nine places in the next range of evolution – that is, in the convolutions ... Suppose that a patient should [l]ose from a certain sized lesion of the lower centre (corpus striatum) one-third of the power he should have over the muscles of the face, arm, and leg, he would on the principle of evolution lose only one-ninth of his power over these muscles if a lesion of the same size occurred in our next stage of evolution – that is, in convolutions evolved out of the corpus striatum.[155]

Jackson cited 'the principle of evolution' to support his idea of *squaring* the amount of tissue in a lower center, in order to approximate the amount in the higher.[156] He did not try to represent such squaring in the symbolism of his *xyz* theory, and on the next page he characterized his geometric multiplication as 'quite arbitrary' and meant only for illustration.[157] But then he went on to further speculation. If the amount of tissue that is evolved out of the 'First centre' is squared at the next, 'second' level, then 'the third centre will represent eighty-one different movements, and so on'.[158] Thus, Jackson's evolutionary *xyz* theory was an integral

---

[153] Jackson 1875i, pp.399–400; Jackson's italics (in *x, y, z*), my square brackets.

[154] See Jackson 1870g, pp.190–191; discussed in Chapter 6.

[155] Jackson 1875l, p.420. Before this passage (on p.419) Jackson tried to account for the irregular periodicity of seizures by invoking Paget's theory of waves of nutrition (quoted 'from Baker's edition (seventh) of Dr. Kirkes' "Physiology" (p.141)', but Paget's only evidence was the regular periodicity of the heartbeat.

[156] Jackson 1875l, p.420.

[157] Jackson 1875l, p.421, footnote (*a*).

[158] Jackson 1875l, p.421. This last clause, about 'the third centre', is the first place where Jackson said anything about a third level of representation, an idea that eventually became central to his conception of the brain's hierarchical organization.

part of his thinking when he began to interpret his clinical data about focal seizures in light of the new experimental results from cortical stimulation.

An Interregnum Between Chapters V and VI, May 1875–January 1876

A Series of Brain Tumors, 'Bearing on the Experiments of Hitzig and Ferrier', May 1875–January 1876

The last part of Chapter V in Jackson's epilepsy book came out in May 1875, and the beginning of his Chapter VI appeared in October 1875. During the 5 months' interregnum he published a series of case reports that were not part of the book: 'Cases of partial convulsion from organic disease of the brain, bearing on the experiments of Hitzig and Ferrier'.[159] In fact, the series had actually begun under a different title in 1872,[160] before Jackson knew about Fritsch and Hitzig and a year before Ferrier's initial experiments. This 'old' series of November 1872–May 1875 consisted of 16 cases of tumors in various locations. Since Jackson considered the 'new' series ('Hitzig and Ferrier') to be a continuation, the first case in the new series was labelled 'Case 17'.[161]

Because the tumors were usually large by the time of death, precise localization of seizure foci was difficult. An exception in the old series was Jackson's Case 2, who died of pulmonary tuberculosis. His seizures began in the left thumb. A tubercle the size of a 'hazel-nut' was found 'in the hinder part of the third right frontal convolution'.[162] About this apparent confirmation of his theories, Jackson said at the time (1872), 'I have never found disease so very local in any other case of convulsion beginning unilaterally'.[163] However, he did not then conclude that 'the hinder part of the third right frontal convolution' is a center for thumb movements. Rather, 'such observations ... will lead us to a knowledge of the particular movements represented in particular regions of the brain, and ... to a knowledge of the order in time in which movements are therein represented ... they will lead us to a knowledge of *fundamental* principles of localisation'.[164] Indeed, '*fundamental* principles' were his real interest. In the preface to his new series, 'bearing on the experiments of Hitzig and Ferrier', Jackson said:

> I now publish ... more cases of convulsion from cerebral tumour which are the clinical counterparts of the valuable experiments of Hitzig and Ferrier. Such cases of disease may

---

[159] The series started on May 29, 1875, and continued through January 1, 1876, including: Jackson 1875o, Jackson 1875p, Jackson 1875u, Jackson 1875x, Jackson 1875cc, Jackson 1875ee, and Jackson 1876a. Thus, the series occurred largely between Cluster 2 and Cluster 3.

The revised title of Jackson's new series of tumor cases said 'Hitzig and Ferrier', not 'Fritsch and Hitzig and Ferrier', and not 'Ferrier' alone. In 1874 Ferrier tried to publish his results in the *Philosophical Transactions of the Royal Society*, but the reviewers felt that he had not given sufficient credit to Fritsch and Hitzig, and the ever truculent Hitzig weighed in. One of the three reviewers (Michael Foster) feared that the outcome would be 'unfavourable to English Science'. As a result, the *Transactions* published only a three-page summary of Ferrier's results in 1874 (see Millett 1998, pp.293–294), although the Royal Society did publish Ferrier's extensive reports in 1875 (Ferrier 1875a, 1875b, 1875c). I think the consistency of Jackson's references to 'Hitzig and Ferrier' is explained by his usual deference to the priority claims of others *and* by his attention to these events. He continued this usage into the 1880s; see Jackson 1881z, p.54, and Jackson 1884g, p.703.

[160] 'A series of cases illustrative of cerebral pathology. Cases of intracranial tumour.' A list of the articles is provided in this chapter in footnote 13.

[161] Jackson 1875p.

[162] Jackson 1872q, p.597. In Jackson's Case 5 (Jackson 1873f, p.224), 'a lump of about the volume of three walnuts' was pulled out from 'the junction of the parietal and frontal lobes'; but there was also widespread softening of the brain.

[163] Jackson 1872q, p.597.

[164] Jackson 1872q, p.597; Jackson's italics.

be looked upon as experiments on the brain; but they are very coarse experiments ... For this reason <u>I have very little to say on the exact relation of the particular convulsive movements to the seat of disease</u>. Yet the experiments of disease ... are of great value as illustrating the *order* of representation of movements – that is, their relation to one another (sequence of spasm).[165]

Throughout his presentations of these tumor cases Jackson adhered to the underlined message. He gave the details of the cases and left the reader to decide their localizations. In one instance he did give some examples of trying to work out the localization of movements from focal seizures, citing papers by Ferrier and by William R. Gowers (1845–1915).[166] But what he emphasized was the strength of the evidence for the general principle of localizing motor functions in the hemispheric cortices. In the process he made several statements that might be interpreted as priority claims, but they actually had a flavor of frustration, as in 'I-told-you-so'.

> For more than ten years I have held that convolutions represent movements ... this notion had become in my mind almost automatic ... in every paper written during and since 1866, whether on chorea, convulsions, or on the physiology of language, I have *always* written on the assumption that the cerebral hemisphere is made up of processes representing impressions and movements. It seems to me to be a necessary implication of the doctrine of Nervous Evolution as this is stated by Spencer.[167]

Although this is historically correct as far as it goes, one could argue that Jackson was being disingenuous, because he decided that *all* seizures are of cortical origin *only* after he learned about Ferrier's results. In any case, Jackson took his usual pains to acknowledge his (and Ferrier's) opponents, citing the 'counter experiments' of several authors, 'Dupuy, Carville, Duret, and Burdon-Sanderson'.[168] After quoting passages from his own papers of 1866, 1868, and 1870,[169] he expressed his true feelings.

> Those who have read the quotations above ... will not accuse me of affectation when I say that I was surprised that anyone hesitated to accept the conclusions of the recent experiments. My own opinion is that the prevalent confusion of Psychology with the Anatomy and Physiology of the Nervous System is much to blame for the incredulity ... I hold that the anatomical substrata of ideas are sensori-motor processes ... I beg the reader to take note that <u>this is not an after-thought</u>. I do not write this because Hitzig and Ferrier find ... movements ... by electrical excitation of certain parts of the cerebral cortex. I believed that movements ... must be represented in the cerebral hemispheres before their experiments were begun.[170]

---

[165] Jackson 1875o, p.578; Jackson's italics and parentheses, my underlining.

[166] Jackson cited Ferrier 1874c and Gowers 1874. In 1870 Gowers was the first Medical Registrar appointed to the National Hospital. In 1872 he became Honorary Assistant Physician (see Scott et al. 2012, pp.93–94), and he soon became one of Jackson's most important, if somewhat prickly colleagues. His home base was at the nearby University College Hospital.

[167] Jackson 1875o, p.578; Jackson's italics.

[168] Jackson 1875o, p.579; see Millett 1998, p.292. Ferrier's response was in Ferrier 1874b and in Ferrier 1876, pp.132–137. In Lewes' disparaging review of Ferrier 1876, Lewes (1876, p.73, etc.) complained that Ferrier did not consider the opinions of his opponents.

[169] He cited/quoted Jackson 1866f, p.661; Jackson 1866p; Jackson 1868u, p.526; and Jackson 1870f.

[170] Jackson 1875o, p.579; my underlining.

Jackson's thinking changed over time as follows. In 1866, having embraced associationism, he accepted the theory that there are sensori-*motor* functions in the hemispheric cortices. However, this was not integrated into his clinical thinking until his 'Study' of 1870. In that classic paper he worked out an explanation of how motor seizures could result from discharge in gray matter (the *xyz* theory), while he retained the corpus striatum as the rostral end of the motor tract. When he learned about Ferrier's results in 1873–1874, he decided that *all* types of seizures must originate in the cortices, even those that begin with generalization. To understand the relationship between Jackson's localizing efforts and Ferrier's— and its impact on developments in epilepsy—we need to go back to some of Ferrier's earlier statements.

Ferrier, Jackson, and the (Sensori-)Motor Strip, 1874–1875

In 1874–1875 identification of the motor strip was not simply a matter of finding another piece of the cortical puzzle. It was the *only* known piece.[171] Aphasia notwithstanding, the rest of the cortices was *terra incognita*. Part of what drew Jackson and Ferrier together was the clinical imperative—the urgency of the duty to care for patients. Both Ferrier and Jackson understood that the ability to localize lesions would be a great boon. In Chapter 11 we will see that knowledge of the motor strip was crucial to the establishment of modern brain surgery. Indeed, Ferrier was eager to work with monkeys because he felt that their relationship to humans was close enough to warrant anatomical homologies from primates to people. His cortical stimulation experiments on monkeys began in the latter part of 1873.[172] By March 1874 he could say that:

> Generally, it may be stated that the centres for the movements of the limbs are situated in the convolutions bounding the fissure of Rolando, viz., the ascending parietal convolution with its postero-parietal termination as far back as the parieto-occipital fissure, the ascending frontal, and posterior termination of the superior frontal convolution. Centres for individual movements of the limbs, hands, and feet are differentiated in these convolutions ...[173]

Ferrier had found motor stimulation points on both sides of the rolandic sulcus, including the post-rolandic gyrus, which we now consider to be for somatic sensation, more or less. At this stage he had no information about cortical representation of sensation. What bothers us now was not bothering Ferrier. He was simply trying to establish monkey-to-human motor homologies. He couldn't experiment with irritative lesions in humans,[174] but he could try to homologize from his results in monkeys to the irritative and destructive lesions of disease in humans. In the *West Riding Reports* of 1874,[175] he described five patients from that hospital. They had various combinations of dementia, aphasia, and seizures. At their autopsies the

---

[171] For some of the earlier history of the motor strip see Chapter 7.
[172] See Ferrier 1873c, p.152, and Ferrier 1873d. The latter predates Ferrier 1873c, but I discovered it only in 2017.
[173] Ferrier 1874a, p.230; my underlining.
[174] This was actually done and quickly published in April 1874 by an American, Roberts Bartholow (Bartholow 1874), who equally quickly earned transatlantic opprobrium; see Morgan 1982. Ferrier mentioned Bartholow in Ferrier 1874c, p.45, and in Ferrier 1876, pp.296–297.
[175] Ferrier 1874c.

locations of the patients' large hemispheric lesions were consistent with his monkey data, and there were no significant lesions in the brainstems, but the lesions were much too large to warrant any precise localization. Nonetheless, Ferrier repeated his peri-rolandic localizing statements of earlier in the year, with even more detail about the localization of movements of each limb on specific gyri.[176] He also commented extensively on the meaning of his findings for understanding aphasia.[177]

In May 1875 Ferrier delivered the prestigious Croonian lecture at the Royal Society of London, titled 'Experiments on the Brain of Monkeys (Second Series)'.[178] Unlike the stimulation technique in his other experiments, here Ferrier described a series of 25 *ablative* experiments, involving lesions throughout the hemispheres. In his conclusions he said:

> Destruction of the grey matter of the <u>convolutions bounding the fissure of Rolando</u> causes paralysis of voluntary motion on the opposite side of the body; while lesions circumscribed to special areas in these convolutions, previously localized by the author, cause paralysis of voluntary motion, limited to the muscular actions excited by electrical stimulation of the same parts.[179]

Thus the ablative experiments strengthened Ferrier's conclusions from cortical stimulation. In doing this work he had adhered to Jackson's precept to conduct the 'study of the localisation of movements on the *double* plan – by comparing the effects of destroying and discharging lesions on the brain of *man*'.[180] All of this was background to Jackson's report of the first case (Case 17) in his new series ('Hitzig and Ferrier'), which was published in the *Medical Times and Gazette* of June 5, 1875.[181] That event was part of the historical process of identifying the motor strip in man. Table 8.2 outlines the chronologies of Jackson's reports of his Cases 15 and 17. It continues my narrative, because the details are otherwise impossible to follow—too many dates to remember. From Ferrier's perspective in 1873 I have already discussed these cases in Chapter 7. Table 8.2 is concerned with their reporting and interpretation by Jackson to 1875.

Clearly Jackson was at pains to show that he had made a straightforward, empirical correlation between the two cases, without reference to 'physiological knowledge'. Presumably that meant knowledge of cerebral localization—so what changed between May 1873 and June 1875? In 1873 he could have raised the possibility that the 'arm area' is in the tumor's location in the frontal lobe in Case 17, but he didn't. His full acceptance of Ferrier's findings in primates came slowly, so without Ferrier's demonstrations of stable motor points in the primate cortex he would have been justified in writing off the similar localizations in Cases 15 and 17 as mere coincidence.

---

176 Ferrier 1874c, pp.49–50

177 Ferrier 1874c, pp.54–60. Earlier in 1874 (Ferrier 1874a, p.230) he said: 'At the posterior termination of the inferior frontal convolution and corresponding part of the ascending frontal are the centres for various movements of the mouth and tongue. This is the homologue of "Broca's convolution".'

178 Ferrier 1875b and 1875c. There is some confusion about the date of the lecture. A February date is given in Clarke 1971, p.594, but the publication says, 'Read May 13, 1875'. This Croonian Lecture is not to be confused with the lecture series of the same name at the Royal College of Physicians, which Ferrier gave in 1890; see Chapter 12.

179 Ferrier 1875b, p.431; my underlining.

180 Jackson 1873x, p.176; Jackson's italics.

181 Jackson 1875p.

Table 8.2 Chronologies of Jackson's reports of his Cases 15 and 17 in his two linked series on 'tumors' ('old' series) and the 'Experiments of Hitzig and Ferrier' ('new' series).

Case 15 (in 'old' series)—

September 1, 1869—in a 'Report of a case of disease of one lobe of the [left] cerebrum, and of both lobes of the cerebellum' Jackson described a man who had focal seizures in the right hand without further spread. At autopsy: 'There was a nodule ... situated in the hinder part of the superior frontal convolution ... about a cubic inch in size.' Similar lesions were found in each lobe of the cerebellum. In his discussion, Jackson's emphasis was on the absence of cerebellar signs. [a]

October 24, 1874—full report of the above case in the tumor series, labeled 'Case 15', but without any comments on hemispheric localization. [b]

Case 17 (in 'new' series)—

May 10, 1873—at the end of Jackson's first published reference to Ferrier's initial report of his stimulation experiments, Jackson reported a patient 'who had literally innumerable fits limited to the right arm ... The spasm passed down the arm except in the later fits, then it passed up ... Here I correctly predicted disease of the hinder part of the first (uppermost) frontal convolution—not from physiological knowledge, but because of what I found in the other case [Case 15] ...' [c]

June 5, 1875—Jackson published 'Case 17 ... Convulsions nearly always Limited to the Right Arm – Tumour of the Hindermost Part of the Uppermost Frontal Convolution on the Left Side'. In this full report Jackson again pointed out that he had: 'predicted the seat of the disease correctly; but I did this empirically. There were very frequent convulsions limited to one arm, and as I had seen another case (Case 15 in this series) very like it, I predicted tumour of the same region'. [d]

---

[a] Jackson 1869k; my square brackets.
[b] Jackson 1874bb.

[c] Jackson 1873k, p.533; my square brackets and underlining. The patient was first seen by Jackson in November 1872; she died February 20, 1873.

[d] Jackson 1875p, p.606; Jackson's italics and parentheses, my underlining. In our terms, the '*Hindermost Part of the Uppermost Frontal Convolution*' is the superficial paramedian part of primary motor cortex, i.e., the arm area of the motor strip.

Jackson introduced his report of Case 18 by saying: 'In the following case I diagnosed tumour of the hinder part of the first (uppermost) frontal convolution; the disease was much more extensive ...'[182] In his abstract he described a man who had '*Right-sided fits, most of them limited to the Right Arm – Subsequently Hemiplegia – Double Optic Neuritis – Tumours of Left Cerebral Hemisphere*'.[183] At Gowers' post-mortem '*Examination of the Brain*' there were 'several growths' of various sizes, all on the left.[184] One of them was 'beneath the posterior extremity of the superior frontal convolution ...'[185] Although the details of the patient's seizures and the locations of the tumors were fully described, nowhere in Jackson's discussions of his Cases 15, 17, or 18 did he actually try to correlate the location of the patients' tumors with Ferrier's motor localizations.[186] He seemed to be putting the cases out there for anyone else who might want to try to work out the correlations. In Case 18 there could

---

[182] Jackson 1875u, p.660.
[183] Jackson 1875u, p.660; Jackson's italics.
[184] Jackson 1875u, p.661; my square brackets. Because of their multiplicity and the absence of a 'capsule', the most likely pathological diagnosis would be metastases from an unknown primary, but that is highly speculative. Low-grade infection is a lesser possibility.
[185] Jackson 1875u, p.661.
[186] This statement applies also to the last three cases in: Case 19 (Jackson 1875cc), Case 20 (Jackson 1875ee), and Case 21 (Jackson 1876a). At the end of Jackson 1876a it said, '(*To be continued*)', but it wasn't.

have been a correlation of the right arm seizures to the small lesion in the posterior superior frontal gyrus, but that was not mentioned.[187] Part of the explanation for his lack of interest in detailed correlation with Ferrier's data may be found in his usual conservatism, but there was also another factor.

Jackson's unifying conception of all epilepsies included the idea of local foci of hyperirritable tissue, which might consist of only 'minute changes'. In Case 18 there are two gross lesions that could have been causing those changes. But large tumors have large surface areas touching the brain, and there was no way to know exactly where the irritative lesion was located within the large area of brain tissue that surrounded the tumors. Nonetheless, it was Jackson who first proposed that mass lesions can be indirectly responsible for seizures because they damage adjacent brain tissue and thus make it irritable. Recall: 'The lump does not discharge.'[188] This was a subject that he could not take any further, nor did he seem to be interested. His real interests were in the larger principles of localization and in the operational difficulties of the mind-brain relation.

Absorbing Ferrier: A Pamphlet on Localization and an Editorial on 'Psychology', Fall 1875

Jackson's epilepsy book was the primary vehicle for his absorption of Ferrier's results into his own thinking. The process took three and a half years, measuring from Ferrier's first reports in mid-1873 to the final chapters of the epilepsy book in December 1876. In addition to the book, he used other venues for the same effort. In the Fall of 1875, during the 8-month interregnum between his Chapters V and VI, Jackson published two titles that served in this process.[189] They appeared to be on different subjects, but he intended them to be complementary.

The first of the two pieces was a privately printed pamphlet, titled 'On the localisation of movements in the brain'.[190] It appeared in August or September, 1875. In it Jackson reprinted his three installments with that title from January to February 1873.[191] In the pamphlet, the reprints were preceded by his 47-page 'Preface ... 1875'. He admitted that 'This Preface ... is now larger than the paper it precedes. Moreover, it is itself in substance a reprint; much of it has appeared in some papers on Epilepsy, published in the *Medical Press and Circular*.'[192] The tone of his Preface was rather polemical. From this I surmise that the pamphlet venue was not considered to be as much in the public domain as a paper in a journal, but neither was it entirely private. In the contents of the papers of 1873, as reprinted in 1875, the only major change was his insertion of section headings, which gave the reprint a sense of organization that was not found in the original.

---

[187] Probably Jackson had some pre-publication knowledge of Ferrier's results, but it is hard to know exactly how much. The details of the monkey experiments were not published until Ferrier's Croonian Lectures in May 1875 (Ferrier 1875c), and Ferrier's explicit efforts to draw homologies of localization from primate to man were published in 1876 (Ferrier 1876, pp.296–314). However, the last three cases in Jackson's 'new' series were published in September 1875 (Jackson 1875cc and Jackson 1875ee) and January 1876 (Jackson 1876a), when the data in the Croonian lecture were apparently available.

[188] Jackson 1870g, p.188.

[189] Jackson 1875a and [Jackson] 1875b.

[190] Jackson 1875a. In [Jackson] 1875b, dated September 25, Jackson 1875a was referred to as 'recently ... presented'.

[191] Jackson 1873a, Jackson 1873c, Jackson 1873d.

[192] Jackson 1875a, p.i.

At the beginning of his pamphlet Jackson repeated a priority claim when he said: 'In this Preface I shall show that I have for more than ten years, and before the experiments of Hitzig and Ferrier were made, held that convolutions contain nervous arrangements representing movements.'[193] About the 'ten years'—going back to the mid-1860s—we might need to give him some benefit of the doubt; but certainly his claim is valid from the later 1860s, remembering that he retained the striatum as the rostral end of the *direct* motor tract. At first glance this quoted sentence would appear to contradict Jackson's statement of 1864, in which he eschewed concerns about priority.[194] However, here in 1875, at age 40, it is likely that he had his legacy in mind, meaning that he was making an ordinary historical priority claim. But it's more complex than that.

We have seen that Jackson prized his intellectual independence, and that did not change in 1875. Indeed, the advent of Ferrier's experimental results made his sense of independence even more important to him. He proclaimed his method of clinical investigation—disease as experiment—to have its own independent weight, quite apart from the results of animal experimentation. In Jackson's mind, Ferrier's data could confirm his theories only if the two data sets were truly independent and of equal value, especially since Ferrier had specifically stated that he was testing Jackson's theories.

The second major piece in the interregnum of 1875–1876 was published in September and October, 1875. It was a four-part, unsigned editorial in the *British Medical Journal*, titled 'Psychology and the nervous system'.[195] Although it was anonymous in theory, it could have been written only by Jackson. The text said that the material in the editorial 'has recently been presented in a pamphlet, of which this article is in great part a summary'.[196] In truth, the putative anonymity of this editorial was specious, because the identity of the author would have been transparent to anyone who knew this literature.

Beyond the factor of independence, there was also a feeling of frustration in Jackson's tone. By his reckoning, most of his colleagues continued to deny the whole idea of motor centers in the hemispheric cortices. It had taken him three and a half years of careful reflection to fully absorb Ferrier, but after he had done that he could not understand why everyone else had not come to the same irresistible conclusion. In the first two sentences of his editorial Jackson said: 'Some of those who are sceptical as to there being representation of movements in the cerebral hemispheres seem to us to altogether overlook several kinds of evidence in favour of it.'[197] And later he said:

> The best reasons for the belief that the convolutions represent movements are the facts of the experiments of disease – for example, partial convulsive seizures from disease in the cerebrum – and more especially the experiments, properly so called, of Hitzig and Ferrier … It is not … because we underrate them, that we bring forward other evidence. The argument in the following is … entirely in harmony with the conclusion Hitzig and Ferrier draw from their experiments, that convolutions are centres for movements. But, as their

---

[193] Jackson 1875a, p.ii; this was a repetition of Jackson 1875o, p.578.

[194] Jackson 1864j, p.389.

[195] [Jackson] 1875b. Not listed in York and Steinberg 2006. The first three installments are labeled parts 'I', 'II', and 'III'; the fourth (pp.499–500, not so labeled), apparently also written by Jackson, was in response to a reader's letter to the editor. Jones 1972, p.306, states that Bastian attributed this editorial to Jackson in *Brain* 10:107–109, 1887, but I find no such statement in those pages of Bastian's paper. However, in Jackson 1881h, p.330, Jackson said, 'In earlier papers I used the term "Reduced to a More Automatic Condition".' He used the same expression in Jackson 1874p, p.652, and throughout Jackson 1874p and Jackson 1874q.

[196] [Jackson] 1875b, p.400.

[197] [Jackson] 1875b, p.400.

facts are not considered by very many to be conclusive, we shall advance a different kind of evidence.[198]

Jackson's 'different kind of evidence' amounted to discussions of the mind-brain conundrum in relation to the issue of motor representation in the cortices. What he meant by 'Psychology' was any kind of activity on the mental side of that contraposition.

> A common popular doctrine is this. Up to the corpus striatum ... we have to do with the co-ordination of impressions and movements. When we come to the convolutions, we have to do with psychology. We believe this, which seems so clear, is only the clearness of shallowness ... Psychology, dealing with mental states, is one thing. The anatomy and physiology of the nervous system are quite other things ...[199]

In the pamphlet Jackson complained about the 'prevalent confusion of Psychology with the Physiology of the Nervous System ...*', and he put his full critique in a footnote.

> * The expression "Physiology of Mind" is, strictly speaking, a very erroneous one, and is itself an example of the confusion spoken of ... Neural Physiology is concerned only with the varying conditions of anatomical arrangements of nerve cells and fibres ... Yet the expression is now almost universally used by medical men, and it is hopeless to try to displace it. I am not answerable for it ... the term Psychology and its derivatives, are constantly used when speaking of the functions of the highest parts of the nervous system; they are used when dealing with those diseases of the *brain* which are attended by mental symptoms. There are such expressions as "Psychological Medicine," "Mental Pathology," &c. I use the term "Physiology of the Mind" because, as far as I know, *all* medical men use it.[200]

From Jackson's lamentations we get a sense of how most people were thinking—or not thinking—about these problems: 'So far as we know, the anatomical study of the substrata of states of mind has met with little favour at the hands of medical men. Centres for ideas are spoken of, but nothing is said of the anatomical constitution of these centres ... '201 In other words, most of Jackson's contemporaries were adhering to the common theories of the time, without giving them much thought. But occasionally there was a vocal critic. Such was 'Chas. M. Crombie', of Aberdeen, a Scot who appears to have been of the 'common sense' persuasion.202 The *BMJ* of October 16, 1875, contained a letter to the editor from Crombie.203 Referring to Part I of Jackson's editorial, he asked: 'Why is the ... article ... so puzzling?' Then Crombie raised issues apparently intended to reduce Jackson's arguments to absurdity.

> ... if the nature of the connection between mental states and physical states be ... irrelevant to this doctrine [parallelism], and ... is in itself an insoluble problem, why is so

---

198 [Jackson] 1875b, p.400.
199 [Jackson] 1875b, p.400.
200 Jackson 1875a, pp.xxix–xxx; Jackson's italics.
201 [Jackson] 1875b, p.433.
202 The 'Scottish Common Sense Philosophy' was a form of radical empiricism that originated in Aberdeen in the eighteenth century; see Olson 2004, pp.161–165.
203 Crombie 1875.

much perplexing discussion devoted to it? Perplexing, indeed, it is to be told that "there is no *more* difficulty as to the connection between physical states and mental states, if the physical states are ... nervous arrangements for the co-ordinations of movements and impressions; because the problem is an insoluble one, whatever the physical states may be." If one makes up one's mind that a problem is insoluble, does it therefore follow that all difficulty connected therewith is for ever abolished all the world over, as well as in our own cranium?[204]

Jackson's reply to Crombie was published in the *BMJ* of October 16, 1875.[205] In effect, it was 'Part IV' of his three-part editorial. He began with an *ad hominem* rejoinder:

> Our critic no doubt overlooked the number under the heading "Psychology and the Nervous System," or he would have inferred that what he was criticising was only the first instalment [*sic*] of an article. The evidence which he supposes the writer to have forgotten is given in Nos. 2 and 3. We will reply to his criticisms, however, as carefully as we can. We see no contradiction in the statement that a problem is insoluble, and that it is a problem in metaphysics.[206]

Among Jackson's counter-points, the last one was a bit of a putdown.

> We are sorry to find ... that another expression, "experiments of disease," is considered misleading. It may be understood, Dr. Crombie seems to think, to imply that an inanimate agency is an experimenter. It never occurred to us as possible ... that any one could take the expression other than metaphorically, especially as in the sentence containing it we use the expression "the experiments, *properly so called*, of Hitzig and Ferrier."[207]

The bottom line in Jackson's pamphlet and in his editorial was his clinical perspective.

> I do not concern myself with mental states at all, except indirectly in seeking their anatomical substrata. I do not trouble myself about the mode of connection between mind and matter. It is enough to assume a parallelism.‡ That along with excitations or discharges of nervous arrangements in the cerebrum, mental states occur, I ... admit; but how this is I do not inquire ... so far as clinical medicine is concerned, I do not care.[208]

Some of this cavalier attitude was just rhetorical, of course. Jackson certainly did concern himself with mental states, and he cared a great deal about the 'connection between mind and matter'. Both concerns were to come up again soon, but at the beginning of the next chapter he turned to another fundamental problem in epileptogenesis—its pathophysiology.

---

[204]   Crombie 1875; italics in Jackson's original ([Jackson] 1875b, p.400), my square brackets.

[205]   [Jackson] 1875b, pp.499–500. The same issue of the *BMJ* (p.496) also contains an unsigned editorial comment about 'Dr. Ferrier's Researches'. It could have been written by Jackson, or under his direction, since it contains references to the experiments of Dupuy and Burdon-Sanderson, who are also cited in J75-13, p.579.

[206]   [Jackson] 1875b, p.499; my square brackets.

[207]   [Jackson] 1875b, p.500; Jackson's italics here are not in his original ([Jackson] 1875b, p.400).

[208]   [Jackson] 1875a, pp.xxviii–xxix; my underlining. The footnote at '‡' is a quotation from 'Professor Clifford, *Fortnightly Review*, Dec., 1874, p.278', who espoused parallelism.

Chapters VI and VII of an Unfinished Book, October
1875–May 1876

The last part of Jackson's Chapter V had been published in May 1875, and the first install-ment of his Chapter VI appeared 5 months later, in October.[209]

'The Pathology of Epilepsies', October 1875–January 1876

Recall now that Jackson defined 'pathology' as disturbance of 'nutrition', where the latter is roughly synonymous with our 'metabolism'. Within that meaning he again defined the basic problem: How to understand the epileptic focus as a site of 'local over-nutrition of grey matter ... From what pathological process does the *local* instability result? This ... is equally a question for those who consider ... that epilepsy depends on instability ... of the medulla oblongata.'[210]

His disinterest in the specific details of localization was amply exhibited in his plan for Chapter VI: 'In this chapter ... it is a matter of secondary moment ... so far as broad prin-ciples are concerned, *where* the unstable grey matter may be ... By what pathological pro-cess does grey matter anywhere become unstable?'[211] Regarding his effort to advance this principle, he again expressed frustration. His words were even tinged with an accusation of sloppy thinking by some of his medical brethren.

> I confess I find it difficult to make the distinction betwixt the physiology and the pathology of cases of nervous disease clear to many people ... A visible ... alteration in the nervous system, is sometimes spoken of as a "cause" of convulsion. The rudest part of a pathological process ... which only *leads* to instability is spoken of as "the disease" ... And it seems to many easy to "understand" that a tumour on the left side of the brain can "cause" convul-sion of the opposite side of the body, but when nothing is *discovered* post-mortem they are not convinced that any local disease exists. This is not always owing to carefulness from *scientific* scepticism, for the strangest "causes" of such seizures are easily admitted, such as fright, dyspepsia, anxiety ...[212]

Turning to his basic principles, Jackson extrapolated further.

> A little thought would show two things – 1st, that local symptoms of necessity imply local disease; and 2nd, that the state of nervous organs or tissues on which a discharge directly depends (the "discharging lesion") is not likely to be easily discovered; for the discharge in convulsion is only an excessive exaggeration of the normal function of the cells and fibres. What we should have to discover is the difference betwixt cells which discharge excessively and those which discharge normally – not a likely thing to be easily discovered.[213]

---

[209] The first part of Jackson's Chapter VI was mistakenly labelled 'Chapter V' in Jackson 1875hh, but Jackson corrected this error in Jackson 1875jj, p.351, footnote (*a*).

[210] Jackson 1875hh, p.313; Jackson's italics.

[211] Jackson 1875hh, p.314.

[212] Jackson 1875hh, p.314; Jackson's italics.

[213] Jackson 1875hh, p.314; Jackson's parentheses. To support his position, Jackson (Jackson 1875hh, p.314) quoted from Kussmaul and Tenner 1859, pp.86, 97, and 107, including their statement (p.87) that 'it is only micro-scopic alterations of the brain that can be the cause of epileptic affections'. On Kussmaul and Tenner see Chapter 7.

In the last sentence of this passage Jackson astutely predicted a persisting challenge. From the histological knowledge of his time he observed that in gray matter the cells have much better arterial irrigation than the fibers, and so 'when both the cell and the fibre are subjected to the same conditions of altered vascularity, the cell will be more affected than the fibre'.[214] The question then follows, 'How is the nutrition of the nerve-cell so altered that there results a mere exaltation of its normal function? ... I confess that in most cases we cannot tell how this increased nutrition is brought about',[215] but he pursued the inquiry by asking three questions:

> (1) What is the *general* nature of the altered nutrition of the nerve cell? (2) In what tissues that make up a nervous organ does the pathological process begin which leads to this over-nutrition; does it begin in the nerve tissue or in some subordinate tissue? (3) How do the changes beginning in tissues of nervous organs lead to the increased nutrition of the nerve cells?[216]

By '*general* nature' in his first question, Jackson really meant *chemical*. Here he expanded on his earlier ideas about the relative roles of nitrogen and phosphorus in 'unstable' tissue.[217] Despite his affinity for chemistry, Jackson's greater emphasis—and more useful insight—was in his answer to question (2). In his Chapter V, he had already said that 'whilst loss and excess of function depend on abnormalities of nerve tissue, the pathological process by which those abnormalities are caused *begin* in the non-nervous elements of nervous organs'.[218] Accordingly, the next installment in Jackson's Chapter VI was devoted to the 'several materials which make up nervous organs', and to their different susceptibilities to disease.

> ... the ingredients of a nervous organ are only in part nervous ... Besides nerve fibres and cells ... there are arteries, capillaries, veins, and some connective tissue ...
>
> Nervous organs, like all other organs, are made up of materials which exist in different combination in other parts of the body. The non-nervous elements are those which are usually attacked first; the nervous elements suffer secondarily. There are, indeed, very few 'diseases of the nervous system' if by that expression pathological processes *beginning in nervous tissue* be meant.[219]

From the proposition that the 'non-nervous elements' are 'attacked first', Jackson tried to understand the problem of epileptogenesis at the cellular level.

> In what tissue of a nervous organ does the pathological process begin which leads to instability of cells? This is the question in each case of epilepsy ... we are far from being able to say how the change ... leads to instability of the nervous tissue. Thus, in a convulsion "caused by" syphiloma [gumma] of the brain, we know that the change constituting syphiloma begins in the connective tissue. But how the syphiloma formed by that growth

---

[214] Jackson 1875jj, p.355.

[215] Jackson 1875jj, p.356.

[216] Jackson 1875jj, p.356. The three questions in this passage correspond roughly to the three parts of Jackson's revised method; see Jackson 1873y, p.315, and Chapter 7.

[217] Jackson 1875jj, pp.356–358.

[218] Jackson 1875i, p.398; Jackson's italics.

[219] Jackson 1875kk, p.487; Jackson's italics. On the next page he quoted his earlier paper (Jackson 1864h, p.153), showing that he had understood and taught this point in 1864.

of connective tissue acts on the grey matter about it ("irritates it") so as to produce changes of instability we know not ...[220]

Jackson was asking these questions before the twentieth century's knowledge of cellular biochemistry and physiology was available, and he could only take an evolutionary approach.

Some tissues in an organ are more liable to *become* diseased than are the other ingredients of the same organ when all are subjected to apparently the same evil influences. This statement is in accordance with what Beale says ... "The connective tissues, fibrous tissues, capillaries, arteries, and veins ... [are] ... involved before the nerve elements are attacked, *and of these the lowest as regards function suffer before those which are concerned in the most exalted nervous actions. (a)*"[221]

In footnote (*a*) Jackson offered more details about his theory of a hierarchy of susceptibility to disease among 'non-nervous' tissues.

(*a*) This is a very striking remark [by Beale], and the principle involved in it is of great practical importance. I therefore give the following further quotation from Beale's work ...

" ... different forms of ... [protoplasm]²²²... in all parts of the organism suffer *in inflammation* in different degrees and in different *order*. Generally those which are of least importance, and which ... are lowest in the scale, are the first to suffer ...."[223]

Further on Jackson quoted Beale's list of the order in which different tissues are usually affected, the last being 'nerve elements', and then Beale remarked: 'The living matter concerned in mental operations is that which is last formed, and is probably the highest condition which living matter has yet assumed'.²²⁴ Since Jackson liked to think in evolutionary hierarchies, it is easy to understand that he found a kindred spirit in Lionel S. Beale (1828–1906), at least in those matters quoted above. Beale was a prominent physician at King's College Hospital. His 'reputation derived primarily from his practical books on the microscope and from his vocal opposition to the mechanistic interpretation of life'.²²⁵ In a word, he was an anti-Darwinian *vitalist*, remembering that natural selection *per se* was widely opposed, or just ignored, when evolution was otherwise widely accepted.²²⁶

We would like to know what Jackson thought about Beale's vitalism, but there is nothing in his published writings to help us. In any case, it would be absurd to think that Jackson was unaware of Beale's reputation. Most likely, Jackson was simply not interested in the issue. As he did with Spencer, Jackson took what was useful from Beale and ignored the rest. In

---

²²⁰ Jackson 1875kk, p.487; Jackson's parentheses, my square brackets.
²²¹ Jackson 1875kk, p.487; Jackson's italics, which are not in Beale's original (Beale 1870, p.152); my square brackets. Jackson's earliest mention of Lionel Beale was in 1869 (Jackson 1869m, p.481, footnote (d)). He also quoted Beale's complaint about the 'soft rickety tissues of some of our weak, flabby, over-fed, town-bred, highly precocious children ...' (Jackson 1875jj, p.356).
²²² Beale's term was 'germinal matter', by which he meant a concept of tissue components 'essentially equivalent to protoplasm' (Geison 1970, p.540).
²²³ Jackson 1875kk, p.487; Jackson's italics, my square brackets.
²²⁴ Jackson 1875kk, pp.487–488; quoted from Beale 1870, pp.152–153. Jackson said it was from Beale's p.154; but Jackson's transcription of Beale's text is otherwise accurate.
²²⁵ Geison 1970, p.540; see also Pye-Smith 1907.
²²⁶ See Bowler 1988, pp.2–14, and Chapter 2.

any case, the issue of vitalism *per se* would have been largely peripheral to Jackson's quest to understand the 'pathology' of epilepsy.

In the last installment of Chapter VI, Jackson began by asking, '*How do changes beginning in non-nervous elements damage nervous tissue so as to cause "discharging lesion"?*'[227] Acknowledging that his idea about '*non-nervous elements*' was 'but an hypothesis', he offered two examples.

> The pathological processes which lead to . . . grey matter instability are no doubt numerous. I can only speak with some degree of confidence of two processes which I believe to start in the non-nervous elements of nervous organs.
>   1. Occlusion of vessels (embolism and thrombosis).
>   2. The 'irritation' of coarse disease.[228]

Jackson began his discussion of 'Occlusion of vessels' by saying: 'The reader will bear in mind that we are seeking the causes of instability, not the cause of some clinical entity. Thus the remarks apply to the <u>production of changes of instability in general</u>.'[229] Embolism and thrombosis had been given their modern definitions by the German pathologist Rudolf Virchow (1821–1902) and his student Julius Cohnheim (1839–1884), in the 1840s and 1850s.[230] In mid-century Britain, the discussions were centered on embolism. Thrombosis got less attention, as evidenced by its relative absence in Jackson's writings to this point.[231] Given the prevalence of rheumatic and other cardiac diseases, embolism was encountered more frequently.

Understanding vascular disease was central to Jackson's ideas about epileptogenesis, because he thought that a consequence of acute cerebrovascular occlusion was hypernutrition. That is, the nutrients in the acutely stagnant blood were thought to leak into the nearby tissues, where hypernutrition could be a cause of cellular instability: 'From such a morbid stagnation of blood as embolism . . . we should expect a greater quantity of nutrition, but one . . . of worse quality. I suppose a tissue of more nitrogenous and less phosphorised composition.'[232] Jackson's thoughts about hypernutrition and its molecular basis were clearly speculative, as he acknowledged. However, he did have clinical and pathological data to support a different idea.

Brown-Séquard's Troublesome Guinea Pigs, December 1875

Throughout class-conscious Victorian society there was constant apprehension about 'degeneration' in general and about 'degenerative' diseases in particular, especially when the higher classes gazed warily at the lower ones.[233] Jackson's political and social views were largely in sync with those of his own upper middle class,[234] but he had a dissenting theory

---

[227] Jackson 1876d, p.63; Jackson's italics.
[228] Jackson 1876d, p.63; Jackson's parentheses.
[229] Jackson 1876d, p.63; my underlining.
[230] See Schiller 1970, and Storey and Pols 2010, pp.405–410.
[231] This statement is only relative; see Jackson 1875kk, p.488.
[232] Jackson 1876d, p.64.
[233] See Shorvon 2011, pp.1036–1037, on the relation between concepts of societal and epileptic degeneration; also Temkin 1971, pp.260–264, 348, 364–370, and Eyler 1992.
[234] See Hutchinson 1911, p.1553. For a scathing comment by Jackson about the lower classes and their beer see Jackson 1866q, p.243.

about the mechanism of hereditary transmission, especially for syphilis. He thought that apparently hereditary diseases of the nervous system are actually inherited weaknesses in vascular and connective tissues.[235] In general, he said: 'I do not ... believe that nervous diseases or symptoms are transmitted. I believe that a person is born with (1) a tendency to changes in systems of tissue, and (2) that an inferior brain is transmitted.'[236] But there was a persisting threat to his argument.

Starting in 1856–1857, Brown-Séquard had reported a series of experiments, largely on guinea pigs, in which he partially severed the spinal cords and then produced 'epileptiform' phenomena by facial irritation. From this he concluded that epileptic seizures in man originate in the brainstem.[237] When Jackson discussed the distinction between epileptic mania and insanity in his Chapter I, he seemed to put aside the difficulty that: 'at present I have no satisfactory answer to the objection ... that epilepsy artificially induced in guinea-pigs (Brown-Séquard) is hereditary.'[238] That was in October 1874. In December 1875 he conceded:

> ... there is one fact against the doctrine I here put forward which is a very powerful one. I am trying to show that *diseases* like epilepsy are not hereditary. But Brown-Séquard finds that epilepsy artificially produced in guinea-pigs is hereditary. I most willingly admit that this is a most damaging fact to my hypothesis ...[239]

To this day neither the motor nor the 'hereditary' aspects of Brown-Séquard's experiments are understood by modern neuroscience. Some analogies have been drawn between the motor phenomena and Sherrington's scratch reflex, but even that explanation is not fully satisfactory.[240] Although Jackson seemed to predict dire consequences if Brown-Séquard were to prevail, I get the sense that he thought there was a major weakness in Brown-Séquard's interpretation. Probably it was related to the guinea pig's lower evolutionary rank.[241] He didn't want to insult his old friend, so he got around the problematic guinea pigs by acknowledging their existence and then ignoring them. He simply went on to the conclusion of his argument: 'Whilst expressing my opinion (which is only an hypothesis, *as is the opinion to the contrary*) that epilepsy ... is not hereditary *as a nervous* disease, I am not denying that it may be hereditary in the indirect way ...'[242] This passage was literally Jackson's last word on the subject to this point.[243] It completed his Chapter VI, on 'The pathology of epilepsy'. In the next chapter he turned to a different subject.

---

[235] See Jackson 1874aa, p.351.

[236] Jackson 1875kk, p.488. In a footnote ('a') Jackson again discussed his similar view on the inheritance of insanity; see my discussion of that view in this chapter. Later in his main text he added: 'I confess I think it will turn out that the pathology of the neuroses is in most cases owing to arterial disease' (Jackson 1875kk, p.489).

[237] For citations to Brown-Séquard's reports see Temkin 1971, p.405, items 170–173. For further on his experiments see Temkin 1971, p.281; Aminoff 1993, pp.148–154; Koehler 1994; and Aminoff 2011, pp 189–193.

[238] Jackson 1874aa, p.351.

[239] Jackson 1875kk, p.489; Jackson's italics. On Lamarckian heredity in Brown-Séquard's 'epileptic' guinea pigs see Aminoff 2011, pp.192–193.

[240] See Aminoff 2011, pp.189–193.

[241] This was stated explicitly in Jackson 1886b, p.6.

[242] Jackson 1875kk, p.489; Jackson's italics and parentheses.

[243] The guinea pigs came up again in 1886; see Jackson 1886b and Chapter 11.

'Anatomy' and the Mind-Brain Relation, January and February 1876

Jackson's Chapter VII is titled 'Anatomy', but the first two (of three) installments were actually concerned with his evolving thoughts about the mind-brain relation and with other issues about consciousness. His ideas were developed in the context of Spencer's associationism, and with important references to Lewes. In his introduction he said:

> Anatomy is concerned with the Statics [mechanical dynamics] of the Nervous System. The Nervous System is a representing system. A knowledge of the anatomy of any section of it is a knowledge of the parts of the body which that section represents and of the degree of complexity with which it represents those parts. Now the only things it can represent are Impressions and Movements.[244]

The last sentence, about impressions and movements, is pure associationism. In his subsequent text Jackson repeated material that we have already reviewed, about representation and re-representation.[245] Concerning the definition of 'Anatomy', he said, it 'applies to those centres which are in activity whilst we have mental states quite as much as it applies to the lower centres, during energising of which centres there is <u>commonly supposed</u> to be no attendant mental state. (*a*)'[246] And again the most interesting comment is in the footnote.

> (*a*) I say "as commonly supposed," but it seems to me more and more evident that we must accept Lewes's doctrine – that a "Sensibility" attends energising of all centres ... [H]owever ... there is nothing ... to imply that when the nervous centres have reached an exceeding complexity of structure any kind of physical states *becomes* any kind of mental states, but simply that as centres become exceedingly complex a mental state *attends activity of them* – is parallel with their activity. This is the <u>most commonly received doctrine</u>. Mr. Lewes, on the contrary, thinks "that the <u>neural process</u> and the feeling are one and the same process under different aspects."[247]

This passage contains important clues to Jackson's thoughts about the mind-brain relation, so it will be parsed with regard to: (1) Lewes' definition of 'Sensibility', and (2) Lewes' meaning in the clause that Jackson quoted about the 'neural process'. To begin, Lewes' definition of 'Sensibility' had been given in 1860.

> Sensibility is the inherent property of the ganglionic tissue forming the grey matter of the nerve-centres. This property is stimulated into activity by the Neurility of the nerves ... the nerve does not transmit ... [an] ... irritation, it has its own Neurility excited, and *this*

---

[244] Jackson 1876e, p.129; my square brackets.

[245] Jackson did insert something new when he said, 'all efferent nerves do not provoke movements, some stop movements, are inhibitory. The inhibition of movements is represented in nervous centres' (Jackson 1876e, p.129). This was a first for Jackson, though not for European physiology. Central inhibition was well recognized by Ivan Sechenov in the 1860s, and Ferrier was familiar with Sechenov's work; see Ferrier 1876, p.18. On Sechenov and inhibition see R. Smith 1992, pp.94–112; and on Ferrier see R. Smith 1992, pp.117–120. Jackson had used 'inhibition' in 1873 in the sense of release, i.e., 'lack of inhibition' (Jackson 1873d, p.233), but here he clearly meant an active physiological process, not just release.

[246] Jackson 1876e, p.130; my underlining.

[247] Jackson 1876e, p.130; my square brackets. Here again Jackson exhibited his London-centric tendency when he used 'commonly' as if his environment in London were normative for the entire world. Doubtless this assumption was shared by most of his audience.

awakens the Sensibility of the centre – when the nerve goes to a centre; when it goes to a muscle it awakens Contractility.[248]

The meaning of 'Contractility' is obvious, and 'Neurility' refers to a nerve's basic function of conducting a signal, so 'Sensibility' refers to grey matter's property of interpreting an afferent signal and potentially creating a response. And Lewes added later: 'we are not ... to suppose, as the dominant doctrine does, that, unless a train of thought be excited, no sensation at all has been excited. [Conscious] Sensation is simply the active state of Sensibility, which is the property of ganglionic [gray matter] tissue.'[249] The 'dominant doctrine', of course, was associationism, whose psychophysical parallelism countenanced the existence of two separate 'substances', i.e., mental states and physical states. In contrast, Lewes was a 'dual-aspect identity theorist'.[250] His position was displayed in the second volume of his *Problems of Life and Mind*, published in 1875, which was the source of Jackson's short quotation from Lewes about 'the neural process'. In full context, Lewes had said:

Motion we know and feeling we know; but we know them as utterly different ...
   That the *passage* of a motion into a sensation is unthinkable and that by no intelligible process can we follow the transformation, I admit; but I do not admit that there is any such transformation. When I am told that a nervous excitation is *transformed* into a sensation on reaching the brain, I ask ... On what evidence is this fact asserted? ... there is no evidence at all for such a transformation; all the evidence points to the very different fact that the neural process and the feeling are one and the same process viewed under different aspects. Viewed from the physical or objective side, it is a neural process; viewed from the psychological or subjective side it is a sentient process.[251]

Now what we want to know is whether Jackson was a dual-aspect identity theorist in 1876, or did he still adhere to strict psychophysical parallelism? The manner in which he quoted Lewes about 'the neural process' would seem to indicate that he was leaning toward Lewes' position, but he skirted the mind-brain issue by concentrating on the utility of Lewes' concept of 'sensibility'.[252] Two weeks earlier he had discussed the physical changes in the nervous system that occur when we have experiences.

(*a*) What the exact nature of the structural modification may be we do not know. Huxley ("On the Hypothesis that Animals are Automata ...") says: – "Physiology is at present incompetent to say anything positively about the matter or to go further than the expression of the high probability that every molecular change which gives rise to a state of consciousness leaves a more or less persistent structural modification, through which the same

---

[248] Lewes 1860, p.20; my square brackets. In his *Suggestions* (Jackson 1863a, p.9) Jackson said: 'I should hold, too, as Lewes does, that there are various kinds of sensibility, and that sensations from the viscera, &c., are constantly registering themselves in their own proper centres.' Later in the *Suggestions* (p.26) Jackson cited Lewes again on 'sensibility'.

[249] Lewes 1860, p.59; my square brackets.

[250] C.U.M. Smith 1989, p.56. On Lewes and the 'hard problem' see Price 2014; also Reed 1997, pp.154–157.

[251] Lewes 1875, pp.409–411; italics in original, my underlining. Also quoted fully by C.U.M. Smith 1989, p.51.

[252] In Jackson 1876g (p.173, footnote (*a*) in column 2) he said: 'The term 'sensation' is very awkward ... it is meant that there is a contribution to a state of sub-consciousness, bordering on consciousness. Lewes' doctrine that Sensibility attends activity of all nervous centres would save us from the awkwardness of using expressions which are strictly equivalent to the contradiction of "unconscious sensations".'

molecular change may be regenerated by other agencies than the cause which first produced it."[253]

In Jackson's quotation from Huxley, Huxley was simply saying what others had been postulating throughout the associationist tradition—that sensory experiences must leave physical traces in the brain. For Jackson, what was new was Huxley. Recall that in 1863 Jackson published his *Suggestions*, which was based on a theory of Richard Owen, who was Huxley's conservative arch-rival in the early debates about Darwinian evolution.[254] Even in 1876, Jackson's boycott of Darwin continued. Despite many references to 'consciousness' in Darwin's *Expression of the Emotions* of 1872,[255] Jackson rarely cited Darwin in print,[256] and he quoted Huxley sparingly. Although it is not surprising that Jackson knew Huxley's essay on animals as automata, it is noteworthy that by the mid-1870s he would publish a quotation from it. On the related nature–nurture issue, Jackson followed Spencer.

> Everybody believes that our ideas are acquired by experience, or rather, that experience is an essential factor. This is admitted by those who hold that we have innate forms of thought, whether they admit the Spencerian doctrine that our forms of thought are inherited experiences of things or believe that they are <u>innate</u> in the old sense of the word ... ideas are acquired during the correspondences betwixt the organism and its environment – the innate forms are then developed and filled up. The sensori-motor arrangements we have been speaking of constitute the inherited mechanism by which these correspondences can be effected; the mechanism itself being perfected during the process.[257]

Then Jackson turned to the sensori-motor 'units of the substrata of consciousness'.

> ... they represent the tissues (including the skin as a *tissue*), the viscera, the intestines, heart, arteries, &c. – that is to say, they receive afferent nerves concerned in systemic (Lewes) or organic ... (Bain) sensations, and they send out fibres for the corresponding organic or systemic movements. That these are represented in the very highest nervous arrangements disease shows. And we should infer such representation *à priori* from the constant accompaniment of intellectual by emotional states.[258]

This passage is evidence—as if any were needed—that Jackson was trying to ground his speculations in clinical realities. The motivation for his concern with representation of the viscera in the highest level of the cortices was his need to explain seizures with initial auras of visceral sensations. In developing this theme he offered a dynamic understanding of the neurology of consciousness as a distributed system that is constantly in shifting equilibrium.

> In speaking so far of the substrata of consciousness we have ignored the fact that they are in several parts of the cerebrum ...

---

[253] Jackson 1876e, footnote (*a*) in column 2 of p.130; Jackson cited Huxley's essay from the '*Fortnightly Review*, Nov., 1874, p.563'. This passage is also found in the reprinting of Huxley's essay in Huxley 1904, pp.215–216, which I have used. Huxley's address was originally delivered to the British Association, Belfast, in August 1874.

[254] See Chapter 3.

[255] Darwin 1872. In the concordance to the *Emotions* (Barrett et al. 1986, p.92) 'consciousness' is listed 22 times.

[256] See Chapter 2.

[257] Jackson 1876e, p.130; my underlining. By 'innate in the old sense of the word' Jackson apparently meant inborn but not necessarily inherited; see Dunglison 1873, p.545.

[258] Jackson 1876e, p.131; Jackson's italics and parentheses.

Consciousness is not a constant unvarying independent entity. Consciousness arises during activity of some of those of our highest nervous arrangements by which the correspondence of the organism with its environment is being effected. Our present consciousness is our now mental state ... As this correspondence is continually changing, the nervous arrangements concerned are continually different.[259]

This dynamic view of the neurological basis of consciousness was not part of classical association theory, but it can be understood as Jackson's extension of that tradition.[260] We have already seen a similarly dynamic conception in his ideas about the complementarity of hemispheric functions in language processing. In his next installment he drew directly on his previous writings about the duality of brain functions.[261]

Object and Subject Consciousness and the Dualities of Brain Function, March 1876

In this difficult part of his Chapter VII, Jackson expanded the neurology of 'object' and 'subject consciousness' well beyond anything he had inherited from Bain and Spencer.[262] He was trying to work out the neurological bases of these precognitive[263] and cognitive functions, because he wanted the information to serve in localizing the onset of seizures that begin with disturbances of consciousness.[264] Accordingly, there were three new elements in this installment: (1) his definition of 'object' and 'subject consciousness', (2) how those two different aspects of consciousness fit into his theories about the duality of hemispheric processing for all precognitive and cognitive functions, and (3) how these 'localizations' might be used to understand the onset of seizures.[265]

Briefly stated, for Jackson object consciousness is ordinary consciousness of the external environment, and subject consciousness is precognitive processing of attention to the self, i.e., to internal states, including thought. In evolutionary perspective both are forms of adjustment to the environment, because the body that contains the brain is part of the brain's environment. However, because subject consciousness is preconscious in Jackson's conception, Harrington explains that some confusion was almost guaranteed.

In calling the two "halves" of thought *subject* and *object* consciousness, Jackson was making use of terms with a long, respectable history in British mental philosophy ... subject consciousness corresponded to introspection, or contemplation of the self and its thoughts,

---

[259] Jackson 1876e, p.131.

[260] On the mental side, C.U.M. Smith (1982, p.69) has observed that for Spencer, 'consciousness was an activity, a perpetual movement from one "state" to another "state" ...'

[261] Jackson cited Jackson 1874c and '&c.', which latter means Jackson 1874e.

[262] For a helpful exposition of this section see Harrington 1987, pp.226–234. A limitation of her analysis is her mixing of Jackson's statements from the 1860s, 1870s, and 1880s. This is inconsistent with my method of reading Jackson's papers chronologically. Nonetheless, in 1893 Jackson (Jackson 1893b, p.206) said: 'We must not say that, whilst speaking aloud ('external speech') is an objective process, speaking to oneself ('internal speech') is a subjective process; both are objective ...', thus validating Harrington.

[263] I will use the terms 'precognitive' and 'preconscious', which Jackson never used, to include all of the various words and meanings that he attributed to 'subject-conscious'.

[264] See Jackson 1876e, p.131: 'There is as certainly a localisation in some part of the nervous system of arrangements concerned in each particular state of consciousness as there is a localisation of movements of the hand, or of the face, or of the foot.'

[265] See closing paragraph of Jackson 1876e, p.131.

while object consciousness corresponded to contemplation of objects recognized as distinct from the self; i.e., consciousness directed outward. This ... is *not* what Jackson meant by subject and object consciousness ... and his unfortunate choice of such familiar nineteenth-century expressions practically invited misunderstanding of his views. For Jackson, *only* states of object consciousness could be contemplated or known ...[266]

Jackson thus postulated that *all* incoming signals arrive first in precognitive, subject consciousness, including afferents from internal states, which would have been thought of as objective when that term was used in its standard way as defined above by Harrington. So the problem was Jackson's conception of subject consciousness, which he thought was never fully cognitive: 'Subject-consciousness is not commonly spoken of as consciousness; it is a sub-consciousness bordering on unconsciousness.'[267] He did see a difficulty, but it was not Harrington's. Rather, he objected to the persistence of the faculty psychology in scientific discourse, because he felt that psychological categories (faculties) are out of place in physiological analyses. His conception, he said, was:

> ... not parallel to the view popularly taken that we have a consciousness apart from, and as it were served by quasi-independent faculties of "volition," "memory," &c.... On the contrary, these so-called faculties are only different sides of constantly varying states of object consciousness which *arise out of prior states of sub-consciousness or unconsciousness* ... It is supposed that there is a constant play betwixt the two – an unceasing rhythm.[268]

Jackson then gave a long quotation from Spencer, which shows that Spencer's psychological view of consciousness was also dynamic.[269] In this respect Spencer's contribution clearly preceded Jackson's. Jackson also quoted Bain on object and subject consciousness. Taken together, he said: 'This division into substrata of object and substrata of subject consciousness appears to me to correspond anatomico-physiologically with the psychological distinctions betwixt subject and object made by Spencer and with that by Bain betwixt (*a*) Object and Subject-consciousness.'[270]

In contrast to Bain and Spencer, Jackson's neurological background allowed him to postulate *brain mechanisms* for the instantiation of his physiological ideas. He gave his own biological explanation of the dynamism of consciousness, which harked back to his earlier ideas about the duality of the brain: 'the substrata of consciousness are double, as we might infer from the physical duality and separateness of the highest nervous centers'.[271] Afferent signals from the environment arrive first in the neural apparatus of subject consciousness.

> Subject-consciousness is first in all mentation. This half of the double substrata is made up of nervous arrangements representing the parts of the whole organism in relation to one

---

[266] Harrington 1987, p.228; italics in original. On this page Harrington gives a passage from Jackson '(1876a, [Jackson 1876g] p.73)', which is actually found on p.173. For Jackson's self-declared usage of 'subjective' and 'objective' in 1880 see Jackson 1880j, p.196, and Chapter 9.

[267] Jackson 1876g, p.173; footnote '(*a*)' in column 1.

[268] Jackson 1876g, p.174; Jackson's italics.

[269] Jackson 1876g, p.174; Jackson quoted from Spencer's *Psychology* (1872, p.438).

[270] Jackson 1876g, p.174. In footnote (*a*) in column 2 Jackson gave several quotations from Bain's ' "Emotions and Will", 3rd ed., p.575, *et seq.*'.

[271] Jackson 1876g, p.173.

another ... By this half of the substrata impressions from the environment are received; it is the passive half; the chiefly sensory half.[272]

With regard to normal function:

> The activity of the substrata of subject-consciousness in health is not affected by what is commonly called full consciousness. They form the anatomical side of what is a continued under-consciousness (persistence of consciousness) and are those most concerned in the wide bodily states which are the physical side of emotions. (*a*) These substrata are in constant slight action ... They rise in activity before [the beginning] of those nervous arrangements which constitute the second half of the double ...[273]

Then, by an unspecified process, some of the contents of subject consciousness are transmitted to the neural mechanisms ('substrata') of object consciousness.

> The second half of the substrata of consciousness represents the physical side of object consciousness – consciousness commonly so-called. Nervous arrangements represent parts of the body in the order from the most special and voluntary movements and sensations to the most automatic and general movements and sensations. So that these like the [substrata of subject consciousness] represent the whole organism ... they represent the body in the order of its power of reacting on the environment, not in its possibilities of being acted on. This is the chiefly movement half. Movement here comes first.[274]

About the entire scheme Jackson said: 'the noteworthy thing is that in the highest parts of the nervous system the two halves of the double unit are not *mere* duplicates as they are in the lower centres. One half acts before the other, and acts differently.'[275] This reference to asymmetrical action of the two cerebral hemispheres raises the issue of hemispheric dominance, which in turn brings up the neural basis of language. After the above, Jackson gave citations to his 'Duality' papers of 1874,[276] about the neurology of language. Then he referred to the interconnections of language and consciousness.

> ... to speak is to be conscious in words; to perceive is to be conscious in objects. But such full consciousness arises out of, and is posterior [subsequent] to, the corresponding under-consciousness called subject consciousness. For example, the automatic and unconscious (or sub-conscious) reproduction of words and images precedes ... that reproduction of them which is attended by full consciousness.[277]

---

[272] Jackson 1876g, p.173.
[273] Jackson 1876g, p.174; my square brackets. Footnote (*a*) says: '*Emotion* is the most general feeling; we are always in some state of feeling ... What are commonly called emotions ... are variations of this constant state ... there are variations of feeling from those forming part of subject-consciousness only to those rising into object-consciousness; there is in this ascending series of mental states diminishing consciousness of the organism and increasing consciousness of the environment.'
[274] Jackson 1876g, p.174; my square brackets.
[275] Jackson 1876g, p.174; Jackson's italics.
[276] Jackson 1874b, Jackson 1874c, and Jackson 1874e.
[277] Jackson 1876g, p.174; Jackson's parentheses, my square brackets.

Here Jackson was using his physiological theory of language processing to explain his conception of the neural substrata of subject and object consciousness. The latter was based on his model of the brain's processing of language, as I cartooned it in Fig. 7.1. In Fig. 8.1 I have cartooned Jackson's narrative description of his ideas about subject and object consciousness. Again, the localizations are Jackson's, as far as they go, but responsibility for converting them to a diagram is mine.

In Figs 7.1 and 8.1 Jackson gave warrant for the division of the hemispheres into anterior-motor and posterior-sensory regions. However, he did not specify the anatomy of interhemispheric connections—hence my use of interrupted lines for the borders of the corpus callosum. Both diagrams assume the dominance of the left hemisphere for cognitive motor functions. In Fig. 8.1 there are only two arrows to indicate directions of flow of information *in the brain*, because he gave no license for any others.

In Jackson's language model (Fig. 7.1) incoming words are first received preconsciously in the right anterior motor region. Thence by some unspecified mechanism they are organized into propositional (syntactic) order in the left anterior region. Analogously, in Fig. 8.1, precognitive information from the external world is considered to be in the motor modality, so it would enter the right frontal (motor) area for subject consciousness, whereas the signals from the internal environment would initially go to the left posterior area. This would be consistent with the flow of information in Fig. 7.1, where incoming words (motor by definition) are initially received in the right frontal area, and images, being sensory, are received in the left posterior area. However, Jackson actually conceived of these functions in a spectrum, which is not represented in Fig. 8.1.

> ... the substrata of consciousness are double, as we might infer from the physical duality and separateness of the highest nervous centres. The <u>more correct expression</u> is that there

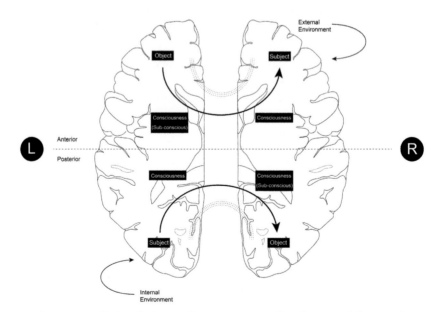

Fig. 8.1 My cartoon of Jackson's theory of representation of localization of <u>object and subject</u> consciousness. See text for explanation.

Drawing of illustration by Kendall Lane.

are <u>two extremes</u>. At the one extreme the substrata serve in Subject-consciousness, at the other extreme in Object-consciousness.[278]

This spectral view was part of the dynamism of Jackson's ideas about normal interhemispheric function.

> Although we speak of the correspondence betwixt the organism and the environment, what occurs anatomically and physiologically is a rhythm betwixt the two sides of the brain (or betwixt two differing units of one side); one representing the organism as it is acted on in this or that part, the other as reacting on this or that thing in the environment ... the only difference betwixt seeing [a] brick and thinking of it is a difference of degree. To perceive a thing is ... to refer it to the environment; we do this just as certainly when we think of the brick as when we see it. The former is commonly called an idea, the latter a perception. But an idea is only a faint external perception, and an external perception is only a vivid idea.[279]

In the last sentence Jackson was exhibiting his associationist *bona fides*. Using his example of a brick in relation to Fig. 8.1, the faint idea of a brick would arise in the left posterior (sensory) region of the brain, with or without any external stimulus to excite it. In contrast, the vivid (motor) idea of seeing an actual brick would arise from visual afferent signals entering the right frontal region. Either type of subject consciousness could rise to object consciousness, albeit in different brain regions and despite the reality that it is the same brick in states of both preconscious and conscious experience. Now, to use a twenty-first-century expression, something here doesn't compute—there would seem to be the possibility of two clashing centers for object consciousness and no obvious way to resolve the conflict. But not to worry. This was as far as Jackson tried to push his conception of the neural substrata of subject and object consciousness. In the last part of his book's Chapter VII, he made use of those distinctions when he turned to the problem of localizing seizures that have early onsets of altered consciousness.

Abnormalities of Consciousness and the Localization of Seizures, March and April 1876

Jackson began this analysis by pointing out that different ideas (in the associationist sense of 'ideas') must have differently located substrata, and seizures can originate in any of this tissue.

> A convulsion from disease of the brain is a *brutal* development of the [normal] function of the substrata of some ideas ... the discharging lesions in epilepsy are not only local, but their discharges being very strong, [they] lead to excessive developments of the functions of the part of the brain which they happen to involve ...[280]

---

[278] Jackson 1876g, p.173; my underlining.
[279] Jackson 1876g, p.175; my square brackets and underlining.
[280] Jackson 1876g, p.175; Jackson's italics, my square brackets and underlining. He was using 'brutal' in the evolutionary sense of primitive.

This was his strategy for integrating genuine epilepsy into his unified pathophysiological framework. He wanted to show that seizures with early disturbances of consciousness are often caused by focal discharges, which accounts for the clinically focal but subtle onsets that are seen in many generalized cases.

> We begin with sensations. The left posterior lobe is the lobe where the substrata represent sensations in the order from the most general (systemic) to the most special (sight); the right posterior lobe where sensations are represented in the reverse order ... Hence a fit beginning by coloured vision I think most often depends on a discharge beginning in the right posterior [Objective] lobe, whereas discharge beginning in the left posterior [Subjective] lobe should most often produce first such brutal development of sensation as that feeling referred to the epigastrium by many epileptics ...
>
> I do not pretend to know that there are these particular local differences in representation. I am only certain that there are the several kinds of fits, and thus that the discharges must be differently seated.[281]

Having thus established some principles of function of the posterior lobes, he went on to the same task for the (motor) anterior lobes, which was less problematic because motor phenomena are easier to observe.

> We now speak of the *first* effects of epileptic discharge of the anterior lobes. They are chiefly turning of the eyes and head; if the head and eyes turn to the left, there will be discharge of the right cerebral hemisphere, if to the right, of the left cerebral hemisphere. Vertigo in epileptics is on its physical side a motor symptom; even when unattended by outward movements it implies nascent movement of certain parts of the body, and this depends on slighter epileptic discharge of those parts of the anterior lobe than those discharges that actually make them move ...[282]

Although Jackson's conjecture about vertigo was indeed speculative, his observations about head and eye turning were right on. We still attribute such turning to contralateral frontal foci. More to the point, Jackson was showing that a brief but readily observable clinical phenomenon often precedes the onset of many generalized seizures. Thus, many purportedly genuine seizures were shown to have focal sites of origin in the hemispheres. Jackson's polemic against a separate nosology for genuine epilepsy continued into the last installment of his Chapter VII, where he repeated a basic principle and a persisting complaint.

> The first thing we do in the scientific investigation of a case of epilepsy is, as in a case of palsy, to localise the lesion – to seek the organ damaged. In no case of nervous disease of any kind is there any *rational* clue to the seat of the internal lesion other than that furnished by observing the external symptoms. The principle ... is not fully acted on in practice. It is carried to its logical conclusion in cases of paralysis of muscles, but not in cases of mobile

---

[281] Jackson 1876g, pp.175–176; Jackson's parentheses, my square brackets.
[282] Jackson 1876g, p.176; Jackson's italics. There he also said: 'There *is* stoppage of the pulse at the onset of some paroxysms of epilepsy ...' This recalls his *Suggestions* (Jackson 1863a, pp.43–44; see my Chapter 3), where he had said that: 'many seizures called epilepsy depend on sudden and total stoppage of the heart ...' In 1863 this had been a causal statement. In 1876 he was claiming only that epileptic discharges can cause slowing or standstill, not vice versa.

affection of muscles, chorea, convulsion, &c.... there is little, if any, attempt made to note the regions affected in cases of chorea and convulsion.[283]

Following his own logic, Jackson also said: 'a so-called aura is not a fit of a different kind from one which goes on to universal convulsion. It is an aborted paroxysm'. Therefore, instead 'of aura or warning, we shall use the expression <u>first symptom</u>, including in that both what the patient can tell us and what we see'.[284] To avoid the work of careful observation, he said, would be futile, because 'To deny that partial external symptoms imply internal local lesions is to deny that there is any kind of local organisation in the nervous system. If local external symptoms do not imply corresponding local internal lesions, it is ... sheer nonsense to attempt studying the localisation of nervous disease at all'.[285] Since 'sheer nonsense' meant reduction to absurdity, he could not accept it. This existential statement was published on April 19, 1876.

Irreplaceable Loss, May 1876

After a short illness, Mrs. Jackson died on May 23, 1876, childless and only 39 years of age. She was buried at Highgate Cemetery, London, on May 26.[286] As with so many mysteries about her, we have few details, but one detail can be certified. It has generally been said that the cause of her death was 'cerebral septic thrombo-phlebitis', or something similar.[287] On her death certificate (Fig. 8.2) the cause of death is indeed 'Thrombosis/of Cerebral vessels/ Effusion/2 weeks/P.M. Certified by Samuel Wilks MD'. 'P.M.' usually means 'post mortem', but the meaning of the '2 weeks' is not clear—it could mean 2 weeks of illness. Wilks was Jackson's longtime friend and an expert in neurological autopsies.[288] Since he said 'vessels', not arteries or veins, probably he saw thrombosis in both, and presumably they were on the hemispheric surfaces, likely near the midline. 'Effusion' means there was a fluid collection over the surface of the hemispheres. One can easily imagine that Jackson would have felt uncomfortable about an autopsy, and yet duty-bound to authorize it.

Adding to Jackson's distress, his younger colleague, James Taylor, said that in her illness Mrs. Jackson suffered 'with local [Jacksonian] convulsion of the type ... with which his name is now inseparably connected'.[289] I believe this to be accurate. Taylor (1859–1946) would have had to obtain the information from someone who was present in 1876, and that is very likely, since he would have known such people. The question arises, of course, why an apparently healthy woman of her age developed such a devastating illness. It has been said she was pregnant,[290] and that would make some sense. Cerebral venous thrombosis is a known complication of pregnancy. Nonetheless, there is no reliable information about pregnancy in Mrs. Jackson.

What is overwhelmingly attested is the enduring depth of her husband's grief. Many of these testimonies are cited in the Critchleys' biography,[291] so I will not repeat most of them.

---

283   Jackson 1876k, p.313; Jackson's italics, my underlining.
284   Jackson 1876k, pp.315–316; my underlining.
285   Jackson 1876k, p.315.
286   Critchley and Critchley 1998, p.173; I could not find an obituary in *The Times* of London.
287   See e.g. Critchley and Critchley 1998, p.173.
288   See Hutchinson 1911, p.1552; on Wilks see Pearce 2009a and 2009b.
289   Taylor 1925, p.15; my square brackets.
290   Critchley and Critchley, p.173, cite Huhn 1965 (p.5) about her seizures and pregnancy, but they note that Huhn gives no source for either statement.
291   Critchley and Critchley, pp.173–175.

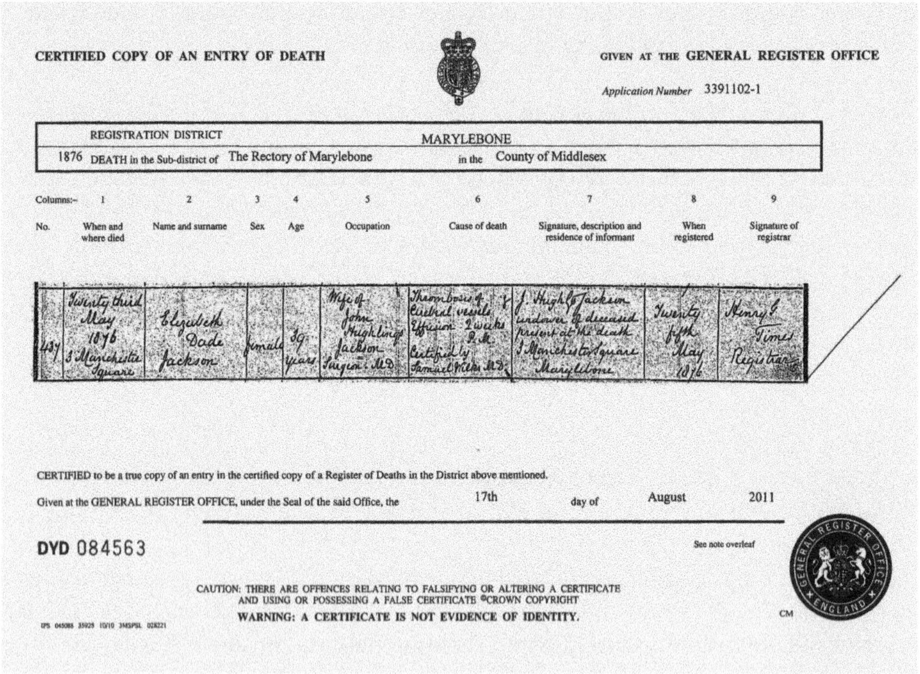

Fig. 8.2 Mrs. Jackson's death certificate, registered 'Twenty fifth May 25 1876'. This is a 'Certified copy of an entry of death given at the General Registry ... 17 August 2011'. Application number 3391102-1.

(© Crown copyright.)

However, one of the most poignant—and probably most accurate—is found in Hutchinson's 'Recollections' of Jackson. Among those to whom Jackson was attached, said Hutchinson, 'First ... was, of course, the lady whom he ultimately married. Mrs. Hughlings Jackson, a most accomplished woman, was his first cousin, and had been his associate from childhood. Jackson was always keenly conscious of the debt which he owed to her in the development of his character, and her loss was to him unspeakably great.'[292] In the next chapter there will be more to say about Mrs. Jackson's influence on him. For now I will consider some immediate effects of her loss.

Diminished Productivity and Originality

Given the sudden death of his soul mate, a reasonable question is how much that loss affected Jackson's intellectual life and his rate of publication. With regard to the latter, a survey of his papers for the remainder of 1876 (after May) indicates some slowing but no abrupt cessation.[293] He published three more chapters for his epilepsy book, plus four shorter pieces and a longer article for the *West Riding Reports*.[294] In 1877, the number began to go down,[295] and

---

[292]   Hutchinson 1911, p.1553.
[293]   See York and Steinberg 2006, pp.85–86.
[294]   Assuming that Jackson 1876v was published after May 1876.
[295]   The number of 23 separate citations for 1877 in York and Steinberg's *Catalogue* (2006, pp.87–89) is artificially high, because four different journals carried abstracts or full reports of Jackson's lecture on 'Ophthalmology

in 1878 his total publications for the year were only eight. All of this is by comparison to the years 1873–1875, when the numbers averaged 33 per year.[296] Of course, one might argue that no mortal could keep up Jackson's pace of 1873–1875 indefinitely. It is likely that he would have slowed down even if Mrs. Jackson had remained alive. As usual, however, numbers alone do not tell the whole story.

When his wife died Jackson was 41. He had been producing an immense body of original thought for 13 years, since 1863. This kind of productivity requires substantial periods of intense concentration. Moreover, in the course of those years the complexity of his ideas increased significantly, so presumably the required intensity also increased. For Jackson this meant pursuing the logic of his theories into previously unexplored territory. An example would be his writings about subject and object consciousness. We will see shortly that for some years after 1876 this kind of originality was diminished. He tended to follow out the theories that he had already created by applying them to a variety of clinical problems. In the next chapter we will look at his progress in trying to convert his colleagues to his way of analyzing neurological disease. First, however, I will complete my discussion of the remaining chapters in his unfinished epilepsy book, and we must also attend to some of Jackson's other papers of 1876.

The 'Final' Chapters of an Unfinished Book,
June–December 1876

The preceding remarks about Jackson's diminished originality are not meant to imply that he lost it entirely, and I certainly do not mean that he never got it back. Some of his papers from the 1880s are among the most often cited in his entire corpus. Although there is only a little that is truly new in the last three chapters of his epilepsy book, there are some points of interest in the last two (Chapters IX and X).[297]

'Unilaterally Beginning Convulsion' and 'Sequence of Spasm',
August–December 1876

Jackson's Chapter IX began with restatement of a principle that had ample clinical support. Regarding unilateral seizures: 'in hemiplegia and in these convulsions the parts which suffer first and most are those which have the most varied uses...' And now this 'Law of Dissolution' had experimental confirmation in 'Ferrier's independent researches [which] confirm the general principle regarding the modes of onset of these convulsions so far as experiments on lower animals can be supposed to be comparable with the experiments [of] disease... on man. (The parts which have the most varied uses will not be the same in each animal.)'[298]

in its relation to general medicine' (York and Steinberg 2006, pp.88–89); 13 of the 23 were reports for that one lecture, often as installments.

[296] See York and Steinberg 2006, pp.67–82.

[297] Jackson's Chapter VIII (Jackson 1876n) was titled 'Recapitulation—The Method Exemplified'. It is a recap of his revised tripartite method as applied to epilepsy (see Jackson 1873y, p.315, and Jackson 1875f, p.354, discussed respectively in Chapters 7 and 8). I have placed it in Cluster 4 on the basis of its publication date, June 14, 1876, just 3 weeks after Mrs. Jackson's death. Jackson may have written it before she fell ill, but that would not affect its place in the order of his thoughts.

[298] Jackson 1876o, p.145; Jackson's parentheses, my square brackets.

Ferrier was keen to find detailed homologies of cortical representation between monkeys and man,[299] but Jackson was more cautious. A significant limitation on monkey-to-man homologies was Ferrier's finding that different proportions of cortex are devoted to movements that are specific to different species, e.g., thumb/hand representation in monkeys is proportionately less than in man.[300] Here Jackson also made an interesting claim about cerebral histology: 'So far as there is a degree of independence of movement, so far must there be a degree of separateness of representation of that movement by (a) distinct cells in the nervous centres.'[301]

> (a) ... the highest centres (anterior and posterior lobes) have [the] smallest cells. Hitzig and Ferrier's points of excitation, that is to say, the subordinate motor centres have many very large cells ... of the subordinate centres, those which represent movements in small muscles (eyes, face, and hands) will have cells comparatively small – smaller than the cells superintending movements of the large muscles of the limbs, but not so small as the cells of the very highest centres ... it is probable that instability of numerous small cells will produce currents of greater "intensity" than instability of the same quantity of grey matter in [a] few large cells ... when small and large cells are subjected to the same abnormal nutrition the small cells sooner become unstable.[302]

Jackson's remark about 'very large cells' can only be a reference to the work of Vladimir Betz (1834–1894). In 1874 he described large, pyramidal-shaped cells that are found only in primary motor cortex, which is the area where Hitzig and Ferrier were stimulating. These unique neurons are now called 'Betz cells'. The original paper of 1874 was in German,[303] but within a year it was abstracted in English.[304] Jackson would have found the abstract to his liking, because it was another vote for his anterior-motor, posterior-sensory conception of the brain. However, where Jackson said 'subordinate motor centres', we would say 'primary motor cortex', remembering that our conception would include the corticospinal tract, which Jackson did not yet have. At the beginning of his Chapter IX he said that 'unilaterally beginning' convulsions are 'the results of Discharging Lesions beginning in subordinate nervous centres – viz., in the convolutions which are near to the corpus striatum ...'[305] For Jackson, our 'primary' motor cortex is inferior in the hierarchical sense, compared to the cortical fields that are at greater distances from the corpora striata. On the other hand, the area where Betz cells are found is 'superior' to the striatum, which is still the most rostral part of the motor tracts *per se*.

---

[299] See Ferrier 1876, pp.296–314.

[300] Jackson 1876o, pp.145–146.

[301] Jackson 1876o, p.146; my underlining.

[302] Jackson 1876o, p.146, column 2; Jackson's parentheses, my square brackets and underlining. I don't know where Jackson got his information about small cells in 1876; Lockhart Clarke would be one suspect. In 1881 Jackson cited the 'masterly researches of Bevan Lewis', who showed 'that those parts of Hitzig and Ferrier's region which especially represent small muscles have most small cells ...', presumably referring to Lewis 1878. In 1890 (Jackson 1890e, p.770, footnote 26) Jackson said: 'My attention was first directed to this subject on reading Spencer's *Biology*, where he expounds his theory of growth.'

[303] See Kushchayev et al. 2012, pp.290–293.

[304] Betz 1875.

[305] Jackson 1876o, p.145. Per my Definition Section 1 (Neuroanatomy), I am using 'corpus striatum' (singular), 'striatum' (singular), and 'corpora striata' (plural) as synonymous for stylistic purposes, unless a side is specified.

The March of Unilateral Seizures and the Frustration of the Second Side, December 1876

With this mindset about the striatum, Jackson made another effort to reconcile Broadbent's hypothesis with the more recent findings of the neuroanatomists. Broadbent had originally proposed that there is bilateral and *equal* representation of less voluntary muscles on each side of the brain, presumably in the striatum.[306] In 1869 Jackson modified this conception by proposing that there is asymmetry of representation in the striatum, with contralateral movements more strongly represented.[307] And in 1873, using the example of a lesion of the left striatum, he had said: 'whilst wishing to prove that movements of the left side of the body *are* represented on the left side of the brain, I also wish to prove that they are less represented therein than are the movements of the right side'.

> … there is proof that fibres pass from the left corpus striatum down into the left side of the cord, as well as into the right side; there are "direct" as well as "decussating" fibres … After old lesions of the left corpus striatum there is Wallerian wasting of nerve-fibres, traceable from the seat of disease not only down into the *right* side of the cord, but also into the left.[308]

About unilateral seizures that spread to the second side asymmetrically, Jackson had previously speculated: 'it is … most reasonable to conclude that the non-crossing fibres are for the movements of the muscles of the left face, arm and leg, although perhaps chiefly for those of the left side of the trunk'.[309] That was in 1873. In the last chapter of his epilepsy book he continued his discussion of the underlying anatomical arrangements, which he felt supported the general principle of Broadbent's hypothesis. His focus was on the 'non-decussating fibres'.

> In saying … that the unilateral muscles of both sides have … a representation on each side of the brain … we did not imply that they are represented alike. We suggested that the representation becomes more unequal and more different the higher the class of animal … the less bilateral and synchronous became [*sic*] the movements of the limbs of the two sides of the body …[310]

For this assertion about the differences between ipsilateral and contralateral fiber tracts Jackson had new support from contemporary neuroscience.

> There is strong *à priori* warrant for the assumption that the movements of the second side are represented in different order from those of the first side, and therefore that in epileptic

---

[306] Broadbent 1866; see Chapter 4.

[307] Jackson 1869c, p.345; see Chapters 5 and 6. In his 'Study' Jackson (Jackson 1870g, pp.192–193) pursued a similar argument about Broadbent.

[308] Jackson 1873d, p.233. Jackson gave no citation for his (correct) information about the fiber tracts in the cord, or for 'Wallerian wasting'. The latter was described by Augustus Waller (1816–1870) in 1850–1851, when he was practicing in London; see Clarke and O'Malley 1996, pp.70–74, and Sykes 2000. It refers to what happens when a nerve's axon is cut. The nerve distal to the cut degenerates. The proximal segment dies back to the cell body, but it can sometimes send out a new axon. The phenomenon can be used to trace nerve pathways in the brain and spinal cord; see Sanes and Jessell 2000, pp.1108–1109. Wallerian degeneration cannot be fully understood without the neuron doctrine, which Waller did not have; see Shepherd 1991, pp.114–117. Thus, when Jackson and his contemporaries saw lesions in the striatum, they thought that degeneration of fibers distally was from cells *or* from fibers in the striatum. The cell bodies are actually in the motor cortex.

[309] Jackson 1873d, p.233.

[310] Jackson 1876r, p.476; my square brackets.

discharges of the centres representing them, the spasms will present a different sequence ... in the descending atrophy ... whilst the wasting is of the fibres in the lateral column of the side opposite the half of the brain (motor tract) injured – that on the same half is in the anterior column. Thus the inference is ... that the two sets of fibres are for different kinds of movements of the two sides.[311]

With this anatomical background, the theme of the last part of Jackson's Chapter X was an attempt to understand the pathophysiology of the spread of the march to the 'second' side, i.e., to the movements that are innervated from the same side of the brain as the epileptic focus: 'We have to note the sequence of spasm in the several parts of this second side. There are few observations ... on this matter.'[312] To his frustration, this exhortation was as far as he could go. Even today, most textbook descriptions of Jacksonian seizures state that when seizures spread to the second side they quickly become generalized, especially if they are 'versive', i.e., if they involve turning of the eyes and head.[313] So the consistent patterns of spread on the first side—which Jackson had analyzed so brilliantly—do not exist on the second side.

Why Was the Epilepsy Book Not Completed?

It is perhaps appropriate that Chapter X ended with an unfinished quest. At the end it said, in the usual way: '(*To be continued*)',[314] but it wasn't. Jackson apparently had plans for more chapters, because he had mentioned the title of one of them.[315] So the question arises, what stopped him from completing the book? The first and most obvious cause is the death of his wife, but another potential factor is hesitancy on the part of a publisher. If he had a publisher, we don't know who it was, but strong suspicion falls on the publisher of the *Medical Press and Circular* (*MPC*), where the existing installments were published. From 1866 to 1931 Albert Alfred Tindall (1841–1931) was the energetic publisher, business manager, and editor of the *MPC*. In 1870 he bought the London branch of the French publishing firm Baillière, which became Baillière, Tindall & Cox.[316] I think it is reasonable to speculate that Jackson had some kind of agreement with Tindall, formal or informal. And the plot thickens. In 1876 the *MPC* faced its first libel suit. It was tame by our standards, but quite upsetting to the defendants.[317] So, probably a distracted author had a distracted publisher. Putting everything

---

[311] Jackson 1876r, p.476; Jackson's italics, my underlining. Jackson did not give a source for this new knowledge. Ferrier 1876, p.4, said: 'The anterior [ventral] columns are regarded more as commissural connections between the motor nerves and adjacent segments ..', which is not what Jackson was saying. Ghez and Krakauer 2000, pp.669–672 state that the anterior corticospinal tracts innervate axial muscles, so Jackson was correct.

[312] Jackson 1876r, p.476. In 1873 (Jackson 1873d, p.234) Jackson had expressed frustration that there were 'no useful observations of the order of spreading of spasm on the [ipsilateral] left side'. In late 1876 (actually early 1877) he gave a further discussion of this problem; see Jackson 1876v, pp.291–294.

[313] See Kotagal and Lüders 2008, p.522.

[314] Jackson 1876r, p.478; Jackson's italics.

[315] Jackson 1876p, p.187: 'We should here speak of aphasia attending epileptic discharges of the centres for speech; but it is convenient to consider it when discussing the After-Effects of strong Epileptic Discharges.'

[316] Rowlette 1939, pp.83–88; see also the summary in online University of Reading Special Collections, Archive of Baillière, Tindall & Cox. Accessed 5/24/2012 via www.reading.ac.uk/special-collections/collections/sc-bailliere.aspx. Jackson and Tindall shared similar, liberal views on the admission of women to medical schools; see Rowlette 1939, pp.89–90. In 1881 Tindall apparently tried again to induce Jackson to produce a book; see Chapter 10.

[317] Rowlette 1939, p.92.

together, I conclude that he simply got tired of the book project. Indeed, he was tired and unhappy altogether.

Papers Outside of Jackson's Epilepsy Book, March 1876–Early 1877

Before this overly long chapter can be finished we must consider some of the papers that Jackson published outside of his epilepsy book in 1876 and a little beyond. Most of the material is related to epilepsy, which leads to further issues about brain organization.

'Mental Automatisms' and 'Dreamy States', December 1876

In late 1875 Jackson proposed the term *'mental automatism'* to label the kinds of complex behaviors that we would call 'behavioral' rather than 'mental'.[318] The title of that paper was 'On temporary mental disorders after epileptic paroxysms',[319] which is important because of the 'after'. It shows Jackson's ideas about the pathophysiology of all complex behaviors related to seizures—he did not think they could be ictal. In March 1876, a medical reporter heard him describe a patient who exhibited such behaviors. About this case, said the reporter, Jackson 'thinks it … likely that there was a slight and transient seizure before the automatic actions began'. Moreover, *'He believes that the slighter the fit, the more elaborate the mental automatism, the more it is influenced or guided by external circumstances occurring just before, during, or after the paroxysm'.*[320]

Later, in December 1876, a reporter recorded Jackson's description of a boy who 'suddenly went up to a stranger and said, "You've got my mother's saucepan".'

> Dr. Hughlings-Jackson supposes that this was not the first symptom of a fit, but the after-effect of a very slight fit. He believes all elaborate paroxysmal mental states occurring in epileptics … are post-paroxysmal. His hypothesis is that there is first an epileptic discharge, which *exhausts* more or less of the highest centres. This temporary exhaustion is a negative physical condition, and its corresponding mental condition is negative – viz., defect or loss of consciousness. The positive and elaborate mental symptoms occur during over-activity of the <u>next lower nervous arrangements</u> … "from," as Dr. Dickson Thompson puts it, "loss of control." Dr. Hughlings-Jackson adopts Dr. Dickson Thompson's hypothesis as regards the indirect causation of all elaborate mental states in all cases …[321]

---

[318] Jackson 1875ll, p.110; Jackson's italics.

[319] Jackson 1875ll. We do not know exactly when in the year 1875 this volume was published, but I agree with York and Steinberg (2006, p.82), who make the reasonable assumption that it was later in the year, or maybe in early 1876.

[320] Jackson 1876j; Jackson's italics.

[321] Jackson 1876u, p.702; Jackson's italics, my underlining. The text goes on to say that Jackson 'does not adopt his [Thompson's] hypothesis in explanation of the epileptic paroxysm'. Thompson's theory of epileptogenesis invoked cerebral anemia due to vasomotor spasm; see Eadie 2007d, pp.25–29.

Jackson then tried to explain how the postictal phenomena are the products of release *within* the highest centers.

> ... the slighter the fit, the more elaborate and the more "purposive" [are] the post-epileptic actions. The slighter the fit, the slighter the discharge; and thus the less the temporary exhaustion it causes of the very highest nervous arrangements ... it follows that the less the highest centres are affected, the more complex are the nervous arrangements left "uncontrolled;" and consequently the more complex is the mental automatism possible from their over-activity.[322]

The key to understanding Jackson's argument here is in the underlined phrase in the quotation above: '<u>next lower nervous arrangements</u>'.[323] It is ambiguous, but that very ambiguity includes the possibility that he was not necessarily talking about the next 'level' down as being cortex near the striatum (the middle level). He was assuming the existence of hierarchical levels *within* the 'highest centres'. If we approach Jackson's insistence on the postictal origin of complex behaviors in this way, it makes more sense. Cortex that is well away from the striatum may be 'inferior' to other cortex at an even greater distance, and the former's brief release could result in very complex behaviors. One of the behaviors that Jackson discussed within this conceptual framework was the 'dreamy state'. From his first use of this term it is clear to me that it originally came from a patient.

> It is not very uncommon for epileptics to have vague and yet exceedingly elaborate mental states at the onset of epileptic seizures, or rather ... just after the very earliest part of the discharge ... The ... so-called intellectual aura, is always the same or essentially the same in each case. "Old scenes revert." I feel in some strange place (a boy expressed it – "in a strange country"). "<u>A dreamy state</u>." ... Some healthy people occasionally have the *feeling* that they had seen something exactly like what they were then seeing, although *at the same time they believe* that they could not possibly have seen it before ... An educated patient has called the condition one of "double consciousness," which ... is a perfectly accurate account. There is ... diminished object-consciousness, with increased subject-consciousness ...[324]

Among the many words that such patients have used, 'dreamy state' caught the fancy of Jackson and many other neurologists. Then and since, there has been general agreement that the term includes *déjà vu, jamais vu*, 'intellectual' sensations, and other complex behaviors, with or without overt alterations of consciousness.[325] In Jackson's maturing conceptualization the physical correlate of such behaviors was in a very high level of the cerebrum.

---

[322] Jackson 1876u, p.702; my square brackets.

[323] Jackson 1876u, p.702.

[324] Jackson 1876u, p.702; Jackson's italics and parentheses, my underlining. The proper title of this item is given in York and Steinberg 2007, p.86, as 'Notes on cases of disease of the nervous system'. In Jackson's *Selected Writings*, vol.1, pp.274–275, the note on 'Intellectual Warnings of Epileptic Seizures' is reprinted as if it were an independent item with that title. Just before this passage, Jackson referred to 'the second of two important cases of epilepsy reported by Dr. Joseph Coats ...' of Glasgow (Coats 1876); the patient exhibited several varieties of complex, 'intellectual' behavior. Coats (1846–1899) gave a good summary of Jackson's ideas.

[325] See Temkin 1971, pp.344–346; and Lardreau 2011. A person who is overwhelmed by the feeling that he has seen something before, which he has, is experiencing *déjà vu* (already seen). If the patient feels that he has never experienced it, when he actually has, it is *jamais vu* (never seen). Hogan and Kaiboriboon (2003) ascribe more of Jackson's larger insights to his analysis of 'dreamy state' than is valid, because they have not considered the chronology.

Three Levels, 'Re-re-representation', Integration, and 'Lateral' Spread, 1876–1877

In early 1877 Jackson published an extensive review article, 'On epilepsies and on the after effects of epileptic discharges. (Todd and Robertson's hypothesis.)'[326] His reference to Todd and Alexander Robertson (1834–1908) was his apparently belated acknowledgment of their separate and earlier publications on the idea of postictal exhaustion of brain tissue.[327] Much of the article repeated themes from the last chapters of his epilepsy book, but some of its elaborations were significant, especially with regard to his evolving ideas about the dynamics of 'levels' in the brain. About 'the effects of epileptic discharge of motor elements of the substrata of consciousness', he said:

> The very highest motor centres are supposed to be evolved out of the subordinate or middle centres in Hitzig and Ferrier's Region, and perhaps out of still lower centres by <u>fibres not passing through the central ganglia of the brain</u>. Thus the highest centres differ from the middle centres only as the latter differ from their lower centres, (corpus striatum, &c....); the principle of difference being in each case a re-representation of the very same external parts, in more special and complex ways...[328]

In this passage Jackson limited his descriptions to the motor side, and this is the first place where he clearly defined his three levels as corresponding to: (1) 'highest' cortex (higher in evolution than primary motor cortex), (2) 'middle' cortex (primary motor cortex, i.e., 'Hitzig and Ferrier's Region'), and (3) 'lower' ('corpus striatum, &c....'). From there he explained the functional relationships among the levels: 'The corpus striatum represents movements of both sides of the body; these are re-represented in the middle cerebral motor centres; and they are <u>re-re-represented</u> in the highest cerebral motor centres – motor division of substrata of consciousness.'[329]

This was Jackson's first published use of the phrase 're-re-represented', and it is clear that he was using it to refer to the highest of the three levels. He was consistent about this usage for the rest of his life.[330] Later he asked a rhetorical question about the dynamics of integration

---

[326] Jackson 1876v, which appeared in the *West Riding Reports* for 1876 (vol.6). Internal evidence shows that the article and the journal were actually published in early 1877. In a footnote on pp.287–288, Jackson referred to an article by Charcot in ' "Revue Mensuelle de Medicine et de Chirurgie", January 1877, p.4 ...', where Charcot had cited Jackson. At the end of his article (1876z, p.309) Jackson said: 'the argument is incomplete. The remainder of the Paper will, if my engagements permit, be printed for private circulation ...'. This was 8 months after his wife's death. There is nothing in York and Steinberg's (2006, pp.140–150) appendices to indicate that the 'private' reprint was ever produced.

[327] In late 1876 (Jackson 1876u, p.702) Jackson said that he had 'recently found' Todd's statement. In a footnote at the beginning of Jackson 1876v (p.266), he said: 'I fully acknowledge the priority of Todd and Alexander Robertson ... Thus I may proceed ... in my own way.' In Jackson 1876u, p.702, he cited Todd in the Lumleian Lectures of 1849 and Robertson in the *Edinburgh Medical Journal* 1869. Jackson's supposedly late reference to Todd's exhaustion theory is puzzling. In his 'Study' of 1870 (Jackson 1870g, pp.169–171) he had included a section on 'the epileptic hemiplegia of Dr. Todd', which, he said, 'is doubtless the result of "overwork" of the nerve fibres which pass from the part discharged to the muscles convulsed. The nerves and the muscles require time to recover from the effects of the sudden and excessive discharge.' On Todd see Lyons 1998, pp.20–22; on Robertson see Eadie 2015a, pp.295–298; also Chapter 4.

[328] Jackson 1876v, p.297; Jackson's parentheses, my underlining. The phrase 'fibres not passing through the central ganglia of the brain' could be a speculation about the corticospinal tract, i.e., fibers running directly from 'Hitzig and Ferrier's [cortical] Region' to the spinal cord, without any connection in the striatum. However, there is the alternative possibility that such fibers might originate in nuclei ('ganglia') below the striatum.

[329] Jackson 1876v, p.298; my underlining.

[330] In 1898 (Jackson 1898a, p.83, footnote 24) he said: 'by re-re-represent I mean that the highest motor centres represent over again what the middle motor centres (re-representative centres) have represented ...'

in the highest level: 'why is consciousness lost when there is a discharging lesion of but *one* part of *one side* of the brain?'[331] The answer speaks to his theories about increasing integration in ascending levels.

> Currents developed by discharging lesions will pass 'laterally' as well as 'down-wards' – will pass to associated centres of the same rank ... as well as to lower centres.
>
> The higher the centre the more numerous different impressions and movements it represents ... increasing nervous differentiation is attended ... by more complete integration; the higher the centre, the more 'lateral' connexions betwixt the nervous arrangements of the same hemisphere and of the two hemispheres. It is evident *à priori* that the highest centres must be more integrated than the lower; their ['the highest centres'] unity is chiefly the unity of co-operations; the unity of lower centres is more the unity of undifferentiation. Hence the units of the very highest centres ... will have most interconnexions. We see ... in the scale of animal life that the corpus callosum is more ... developed the more independent are the movements of the arms; in the bird whose arms (wings) act equally in range and together in time there is no corpus callosum.[332]

With this conception of intra- and interhemispheric integration, Jackson was able to explain how a focal lesion can cause widespread disruption of cortical function and thus account for the alteration or loss of consciousness that appears to be the initial clinical event in some seizures.

> ... the currents from a discharge in but one of the divisions of the highest nervous centres ... will not only pass 'downwards' but will pass 'laterally' to other divisions of the highest centres with which the centre discharged is in physiological connexion; thus the loss of consciousness from a local discharge is accounted for; the currents developed will affect the brain widely. In some cases (*le petit mal*) of epileptic discharge of the very highest centres the 'lateral' currents are chief; there is thoroughly complete loss of consciousness with little visible peripheral change'; that is to say, little evidence of currents passing downwards ...[333]

A Complaint about Consciousness and the Faculty Psychology, 1876–1877

In the last pages of his review Jackson turned to larger issues about the whole idea of consciousness. Again in rhetorical mode he asked:

> ... what is it for a patient to be comatose? ... we must distinguish betwixt psychical and physical. First ... for the psychical side of the condition. To be comatose is only a greater degree or greater depth of loss of consciousness, as this is only a greater degree of that slight defect permitting only slight confusion of thought (defect of consciousness). What are the

---

[331] Jackson 1876v, p.301.
[332] Jackson 1876v, pp.301–302; Jackson's parentheses, my square brackets. The corpus callosum is found only in placental mammals.
[333] Jackson 1876v, pp.301–302; Jackson's parentheses.

physical states corresponding to these psychical losses? Of course there must be negative states of nervous centres in these cases, as certainly as there are positive states during degrees of consciousness.[334]

And the positive states are in constant flux.

> There is no such [single] entity as consciousness; in health we are from moment to moment differently conscious. Consciousness varies in kind and degree according as the parts of the brain in activity are different, and according to the degree of their activity; and it varies in depth. Object-consciousness is continually changing and varying; subject consciousness is comparatively persistent and unvarying.[335]

Earlier, in 1874, Jackson had made similar remarks about the nonentity of consciousness.[336] Although he claimed to eschew 'metaphysics', he had to deal with it in his effort to convince his audience that it had no place in scientific discussions.

> ... the most psychological of psychologists supposes mind to be independent of organization [of matter]. This view ... only differs from that of those medical psychologists who speak of an immaterial mind influencing the body, in that the mind is considered to be solid. Those who take this view are not materialists in effect, nor psychologists either, but a little of both. On this view the centres for consciousness are not 'evolved out of,' but 'placed upon,' lower centres and 'govern' them autocratically. There is no practical difference in a medical enquiry betwixt this view and that of those psychologists who speak of will, memory, &c. as 'faculties' existing apart from physical organisation. On this metaphysico-materialistic view ... the centres for consciousness are not centres for receiving impressions and giving out impulses for movements, but centres which 'play upon' lower centres for movements autocratically.[337]

So who were the objects of Jackson's anti-metaphysical scorn, 'the most psychological of psychologists'? His expression referred to anyone who continued to use the nomenclature of 'faculties', with or without its attendant theories of brain organization. Broca and most of his French colleagues were among them, but we get no hint about that from Jackson. He was contrasting his sensori-motor approach to 'the explanation actually given by some [people] of the effects of removal of the cerebral hemispheres in certain lower animals ...', i.e., that 'It removes the animal's mind but does not affect his movements'. About this he observed: 'The explanation here combated is a metaphysical one. It is a very common thing in medical writings to meet with pure metaphysics put forward as if they were something highly practical.'[338] On that trenchant note we turn to a new chapter—in this book and in Jackson's life. His personal world and the larger Victorian world were changing.

---

[334] Jackson 1876v, p.305.
[335] Jackson 1876v, p.305; my square brackets.
[336] Jackson 1874gg, p.411.
[337] Jackson 1876v, pp.306–307; my square brackets. The political analogy continued.
[338] Jackson 1876v, p.307.

9

Extending a Paradigm and Consolidating a Reputation, 1877–1879

By the mid-to-late 1870s, Jackson's pathophysiological framework was developed to the point where he used it routinely to analyze neurological problems. At the same time, his standing in his professional community was increasing, so his ideas got attention, positive and negative. In some ways, his paradigm was also in tune with the times, socially and scientifically.[1]

The Cultural and Scientific Background in the Later 1870s

Some Aspects of Victorian Culture and Jackson's Relationship to it in the Later 1870s

For Victorian Britain the 1870s were transitional between the optimistic outlook of the 'age of equipoise' in the 1850s and the fashionable 'decadence' of the *fin de siècle*, roughly 1880–1900. In our own computer age we tend to underestimate the equally life-changing effects of the steam engine and the telegraph in that earlier time.[2] By the 1870s those technologies were well developed, but automobiles were primitive at best. Into the early twentieth century horses were much more reliable for local transportation. At the same time, major changes were occurring in the cultural aspects of Victorian life, driven in part by a sense of uneasiness about growing materialism. Concern about it ran through Victorian society increasingly over the nineteenth century. Secularization was simultaneously advancing and taking its toll.

In the decade and a half between the early 1860s and the later 1870s, the climate of opinion among educated Victorians changed in significant ways, including their views of evolution. Essentially, the liberals/evolutionists got the upper hand, more or less, especially when evolution's adherents tended to downplay Darwinian natural selection. These

---

[1] In current American culture, the popular notion of a 'paradigm' is simply a new way of thinking about something, but there is more to it. In 1962 Thomas Kuhn (1922–1996) introduced 'paradigm' to mean a theoretical and practical model that is accepted and used by the community of its practitioners; see Kuhn 1996, pp.10–11, 18–19. By the later 1870s Jackson's model was widely utilized by his 'community', centered at Queen Square. Thus (as pointed out by Marjorie Lorch, personal communication), because of the requirement for a like-minded community it is not legitimate to use Kuhn's 'paradigm' in reference to Jackson's model before the later 1870s. Legions of commentators on Kuhn have debated the relativistic implications of 'community', as if the beliefs of the community were the only reality. That's not what Kuhn meant and it's not what I mean. Ignoring the issue of what constitutes a scientific 'revolution', I find some of Kuhn's terminology to be heuristically useful. Within a paradigm, 'normal science' refers to the process of working out the consequences of the paradigm; see Kuhn 1996, pp.5–6, 23–24. When the explanatory limits of the paradigm are over-stretched, there is a 'paradigm change'. Kuhn did not use 'paradigm shift' in his writings.

[2] For the effects of the railroads see Newsome 1997, pp.27–39. On the effects of the telegraph see Morus 2000, p.455; he 'focuses on the increasingly common metaphor linking the telegraph network and the nervous system' in the nineteenth century.

circumstances moderated Jackson's innate conservatism, which he maintained in a relative way. That is, as the surrounding society gradually became more liberal and more secular, Jackson moved with it, but his position within the spectrum of his environment probably remained constant.

An apposite example is Jackson's relationship to Huxley. The latter's pugnacious reputation as 'Darwin's bulldog' gradually quieted down in the 1870s, and his place among the respectable intelligentsia became widely accepted. When Jackson was young, he had a distinct preference to cite authors who had highly authoritative and relatively conservative credentials. His *Suggestions* of 1863 was based on the theories of Huxley's arch-rival, Richard Owen. Indeed, we can wonder how the agnostic Spencer would not have been perceived as too radical in mid-Victorian Britain, but it didn't seem to be disabling. Spencer's writings were widely discussed. As we saw in Chapter 8, by 1876 Jackson was willing to quote Huxley on the potentially controversial subject of animals as automata, albeit in a footnote.[3] Thus, Jackson's evolving agnosticism about mind-and-brain was not particularly remarkable in his secularizing milieu. On the other hand, his position on one issue of the day was definitely to the left of center.

It would appear that Mrs. Jackson had an impact on his attitude toward the place of women. He was inclined toward equality when that subject was very much on the Victorians' minds.[4]

In his editorial on drunkenness of 1874, Jackson remarked: 'What Spencer says of women, but which we may suppose really applies to the inferior persons of either sex, applies in a still greater degree to the savage drunkard.'[5] In July 1876 Jackson did not sign a nearly unanimous statement by the Medical Council of the London Hospital Medical College, which opposed the admission of women. It is not clear whether he objected or he was simply absent,[6] but if he was absent it was probably deliberate.

Jackson's Place in Victorian Society in the 1870s

The Critchleys state that Mrs. Jackson was attended in her final illness by Sir William Jenner (1815–1898),[7] who was then Physician-in-Ordinary to the Queen and to Edward, the Prince of Wales. In 1861 he had attended Albert, the Prince Consort, during his fatal episode of typhoid. It was said of Jenner that 'at the height of his powers, [he] was the undisputed leader of his profession …'[8] In short, Mrs. Jackson was apparently attended by one of the Queen's doctors. That alone tells us that her husband was practicing among the upper echelons of

---

[3] Jackson 1876e, footnote (*a*) in column 2 of p.130.

[4] In the *British Medical Journal*, immediately after Jackson's first editorial on drunkenness (Jackson 1874p), the next, unsigned editorial (pp.653–654) is on the subject of 'The education of women'. The writer opposed a move by the University of London to refuse 'to examine women for the higher degrees of the University …'

[5] Jackson 1874p, p.53; Jackson gave no citation to Spencer. The latter's treatment of women is in his *Principles of Sociology*, 1 ed., 1876, which was issued in prepublication fascicles from June 1874 to December 1876 (Perrin 1993, p.121), so Jackson could not have seen those by May 1874. Francis 2007, pp.69–77, discusses 'Spencer's feminist politics', which in his (and others') opinion were inconsistent and sometimes paradoxical.

[6] See Clark-Kennedy 1963, vol.2, p.78. Ellis 1986, p.43, implies that Jackson refused to sign, and that seems likely. The separate London School of Medicine for Women was opened in 1874; see Porter 1997, pp.356–358.

[7] Critchley and Critchley 1998, p.173; no source is given for this statement. Jackson and Jenner had been acquainted since at least 1863; see Jackson 1863b, p.11.

[8] Brown (Munk's Roll) 1955, p.68; my square brackets. Jenner was a signatory to the Testimonial that supported Jackson's application for appointment to the London Hospital in 1864 (Jackson 1863b); see also Andermann 1997, pp.476–479.

bourgeois Victorian society. Although he was not a public intellectual, he was interacting regularly with the English intelligentsia.[9] Much later, in 1930, Crichton-Browne recalled:

> ...I never met George Eliot, but missed my opportunities of doing so. Several times during 1876 and 1877, Hughlings Jackson and Clifford Allbutt asked me to accompany them to the Sunday afternoon reception at North Bank and be introduced to her, but these were busy times with me, on Sundays as well as week-days, and I never succeeded in reaching a shrine at which I should gladly have knelt and worshipped for a little.[10]

Polite Victorian society looked askance at Eliot's and Lewes' domestic arrangement,[11] but Jackson went to The Priory anyway, perhaps to assuage loneliness. Two years after his wife died, he suffered a reminder of his wife's loss when Lewes passed away on November 30, 1878. In a note dated December 8, Jackson wrote to George Eliot, who referred to herself as 'Mrs Lewes'.[12]

> Dear Mrs Lewes
>
> I must send you one word of sympathy. I feel most keenly for you. I know well what such a loss is. I shall miss him very much. He always good naturedly encouraged me. I hope you have yet much happiness to come.
>   With respect and esteem I am, dear Mrs Lewes
>
> Faithfully yours
J. Hughlings Jackson[13]

Aside from its poignancy, what is noteworthy about this letter is the fact was it was preserved among her papers by 'Mrs Lewes'. She must have received a blizzard of sympathetic messages, but the saving of this one is evidence of a personal relationship. Such connections are important to recognize, because many commentators on Jackson have asserted that he became a recluse after his wife's death.[14] *Au contraire*, a recluse withdraws from society, and Jackson did no such thing. I do have the impression that when Mrs. Jackson was alive they did not do a lot of socializing, and in his long widowhood Jackson did exhibit some eccentricities.

Unconventional Sociability: After Irreplaceable Loss in 1876

When Jackson's brother Thomas and family paid a visit some years after Mrs. Jackson was gone, his niece recalled that Jackson 'would not countenance a woman housekeeper after

---

[9]   On one occasion in 1873, Lewes 'Dined with Spencer, Huxley, Tyndall, Hughlings Jackson, and Fiske' (Kitchel 1933, p.268). Raitiere 2012, pp.160–172, provides extensive evidence for Jackson's close personal friendship with Lewes.

[10]   Critchton-Browne 1930, p.277. In the next paragraph Critchton-Browne discussed Allbutt as the model for Dr. Lydgate in George Eliot's *Middlemarch*.

[11]   See Chapter 6.

[12]   Price 2014, p.106.

[13]   ALS manuscript in George Eliot papers at Yale Collection of American Literature, Beinecke Rare Book and Manuscript Library, Yale University. Jackson's handwriting is hard to decipher; my fellow Jacksonophile, George York, has concurred in my transcription of this letter.

[14]   Critchley and Critchley (1998, p.174) state that: 'After his wife's death, Jackson lapsed into a semi-cloistered, reclusive existence.' In his last years Jackson did become reclusive, but that was decades later.

his wife's death. The four of us were asked to sit along one side of the dining table.'[15] In fact, Jackson was somewhat sociable in his widowhood—in his own hesitant way. That way was explained by Jackson's younger colleague at Queen Square, Farquhar Buzzard (1871–1945), whose father, Thomas Buzzard (1831–1919), was also Jackson's colleague on the staff of the National Hospital. The younger Buzzard recalled:

> Dr. and Mrs. Jackson had formed an intimate friendship with my parents, and from the date of her death until the death of my mother 25 years later he was a constant, almost daily visitor to our house … The ritual … admitted of no variation without running the risk of frightening him away. He was, in regard to social amenities, intensely shy and completely embarrassed by anything approaching effusiveness or affectation of manner. We would generally be at luncheon; the door would open and Jackson would appear; no one would rise; he would pull a chair up to the table, exchange a few remarks, perhaps tell a humorous story with only a twinkle of the eye disturbing the solemnity of his features, and after five, perhaps ten, minutes he would mumble something about remembering an engagement and leave the room. No one must see him off the premises, but very often he would ask one of us children, generally my sister, to go for a ride. In that case the child in question would jump up and prepare for the outing in the shortest possible time so that he should not be kept waiting.[16]

The recollections of Jackson by Farquhar Buzzard's sister and others attest to Jackson's fondness for children.[17] In 1871 the Jacksons took one of Hutchinson's sons with them on a carriage excursion to the Lake District.[18] Since we know that Jackson sought solace in later years by trying to recapture memories of earlier times with his wife,[19] we can imagine that in the company of children he may have been envisioning what it would have been like for him and his wife to have had their own. In any case, the existence of these stories obviates the claims that Jackson became reclusive soon after his wife's death. Recluses don't take other people's children for carriage rides. Even in the months and years immediately after she died, Jackson attended professional meetings regularly, and he continued to publish, although at a reduced rate for a few years. Still, in the midst of his vigorous professional life Hughlings Jackson 'was a solitary soul for the last 35 years of his life after his wife's death'.[20]

---

[15] Critchley and Critchley 1998, p.174. The recollections of the niece were recorded when she was 80. Jackson's will left legacies of 'one hundred pounds free of legacy duty' to 'each of the [two female] servants who were formerly in my employment ..', so he apparently did have female servants at some time after his wife's death.

[16] Buzzard 1934, pp.909–910. The Critchleys (1998, p.174) state that at some time after Mrs. Jackson's death 'Jackson met Mrs. Farquhar Buzzard on the street'. Jackson's hostess actually would have been Farquhar Buzzard's mother, Mrs. Thomas Buzzard. She had to issue the invitation three times before he finally accepted.

[17] Critchley and Critchley, p.175.

[18] Hutchinson's son, 'J. Hutchinson', wrote to James Taylor on July 3, 1925: 'One recollection I shall always treasure, when I was a schoolboy … about 1871 Dr & Mrs J called for me in their carriage tour and took me into the Lake district. Mrs Jackson's quiet grace & kindness left a permanent impression on me.' This is from an ALS letter in my personal possession, on letterhead, '1, Park Crescent, Portland Place, w.1'.

[19] See Crichton-Browne 1926, pp.84–85, which is quoted extensively in Chapter 11. See also Critchley and Critchley, p.172.

[20] Harris 1935, p.133.

Jackson's Standing Among His Colleagues, and the Founding of *Brain*, Middle to Late 1870s

In a starched society such as Jackson's, it can be difficult for the historian to assess a person's real reputation, especially with regard to negative opinions. For Jackson in the middle 1870s we find reviews and editorials that were usually positive. In October 1875, *The Lancet* published a synopsis of a lecture that Jackson apparently gave at the London Hospital. The reviewer said:

> We commend to the careful study of our readers the lecture "On Softening of the Brain," by Dr. J. Hughlings Jackson ... The precision of thought and language, the strict adherence to what is justified by clinical and pathological observation, which forms always such a valuable part of Dr. Jackson's treatment of a question, are very noticeable in this communication.[21]

A bumper crop of editorials and reviews appeared in 1876. Most were positive, more or less. One was largely positive, but the anonymous author complained about Jackson's style and his excessive 'scrupulosity' in crediting others.[22] However, the reviewer admitted that 'when a critic is reduced to find fault with style i[t] is often the best proof of the excellence of the substance'.[23] On the other hand, Jackson did not escape the animus that Lyttleton Forbes Winslow (1844–1913) [24] usually poured on everyone, including the entire associationist tradition. Reviewing Jackson's pamphlet of 1875, he said that he (Winslow) had created his own 'epitome' of it, from which the pamphlet had 'been divested of the transcendental language which that school, of which the ardour and originality of Dr. Hughlings Jackson legitimately constitute him the leader ...'[25] In fact, Winslow had correctly identified Jackson's propensity for highly theoretical reasoning, but his tone was so polemical that it is hard to credit the entire piece.[26]

It was approximately in the next year, 1877, when Charcot paid a truly meaningful compliment to Jackson. He gave the name 'Jacksonian epilepsy' to the unilateral seizure pattern characterized by a motor march. In doing this Charcot knew full well about Bravais' priority for description, but he recognized the importance of Jackson's explanation of the pathophysiology, and Jackson also acknowledged Bravais.[27] On the other hand, in April 1877 the editor of the *British Medical Journal* (*BMJ*) complained about the tepid British reception of Ferrier's new book, *The Functions of the Brain* (1876), in contrast to its reception in France.

---

[21] Jackson 1875gg, p.497 (October 2); Jackson's lecture was published as Jackson 1875dd (September 4).

[22] Jackson 1876c, which is a review of Jackson's pamphlet of 1875 (Jackson 1875a).

[23] Jackson 1876c, p.44; my square brackets.

[24] Son of Forbes Benignus Winslow (1810–1874), who wrote Winslow 1860 and founded the *Journal of Psychological Medicine and Mental Pathology*.

[25] Jackson 1876q, p.150, which is actually Winslow's review of Jackson 1875a.

[26] In his obituary (Winslow 1913) it was said of Lyttleton Forbes Winslow that he was 'a leading authority on insanity ... His opinion on any case that happened to interest the public was apparently highly valued by some newspapers, but with his own profession it carried less weight'.

[27] See Critchley and Critchley 1998, p.65; also Guillain 1959, p.124, Temkin 1971, pp.305–306, and Goetz et al. 1995, p.125. Bravais' contribution is explained in Chapter 4. Jackson acknowledged Charcot's earlier citation of Bravais in a footnote to Jackson 1876v (p.288); he also mentioned Bravais in Jackson 1879c, p.34, and many other times. Stephen Paget (1919, p.101) apparently referred to Jackson himself when he said, 'Against his [Jackson's] will, the name of "Jacksonian epilepsy" had been given to these cases. He resented this phrase: it asserted more than it could prove: he preferred the phrase: "the Jacksonian attack".' I have never seen any other direct reference to Jackson's opinion about this.

Up to the present time, that splendid monograph ... has been more fruitful of results in the hands of foreign than of British physicians. Ferrier and Hughlings Jackson have furnished the bases for a new departure in the study of cerebral disease, but their works have hardly yet filtered into the hands of our working practitioners and clinicians; abroad, on the other hand, their results are being absorbed and applied at the bedside and in the deadhouse with the greatest activity. In France especially, Charcot and the whole school of young physicians whom he inspires, are daily adding new series of facts to complete the study of cerebral localisation.[28]

I am inclined to attribute some of the editor's pessimism to English self-flagellation and to his penchant for complaining in general. On the other hand, the editor was correct about Jackson's widening international reputation. In April 1878, while in America, Brown-Séquard referred to 'My pupil and assistant in London who has become a very eminent man since, Dr. J. Hughlings Jackson ...'[29] Brown-Séquard would have carried this opinion with him to Paris in August 1878, when he was appointed to the chair of medicine at the Collège de France. Brown-Séquard and Jackson sometimes disagreed on their views of brain function,[30] but they retained their deep respect for each other. Despite Jackson's perception that his ideas were 'making very little way',[31] his ideas were gaining ground very nicely, thank you. While he did not have everyone's assent to his theories, or even their comprehension, he did have everyone's earnest respect. In 1878 he received the first Marshall Hall Prize from the Royal Medical and Chirurgical Society of London, in recognition of his work on aphasia, epilepsy, and ophthalmoscopy.[32]

Jackson's standing was further enhanced in 1878, when he played a major role in the founding of *Brain: A Journal of Neurology*. To this day, *Brain* competes with a small number of its peers for the conjectural title of the world's most prestigious journal of neurology and neuroscience. It was the first in its field in any language.[33] Unfortunately, we have no original records about the founding, so I can offer no details about Jackson's participation.[34] However, we do know that *Brain* was the direct successor to the *West Riding Asylum Reports*, which ceased publication in 1876.[35] *Brain* was started as an independent entity under the editorship of J.C. Bucknill, Crichton-Browne, Ferrier, and Jackson. Presumably they all provided financial backing. The first number appeared in April 1878, including an article on aphasia by Jackson.[36] Initially Crichton-Browne did most of the editorial work, until 'A. De Watteville came to assist the harassed Editors in 1880 ... '[37] The founding of *Brain* certainly brought additional recognition to Jackson, but by that point in his career he probably gave as much as he got.

[28] 'Cerebral Localisation', April 7, 1877, vol.1, pp.432–433. The correct title of Ferrier's monograph is *The Functions of the Brain*, not *Localisation of the Functions of the Brain*, as it was cited in the editorial. The Editor of the *BMJ* was Ernest Hart (see below in this chapter) who probably wrote the piece.

[29] Brown-Séquard 1878, p.11.

[30] See Koehler 1996.

[31] Jackson 1874jj, p.520.

[32] Hunting 2002, p.117. The actual prize consisted of 'a little over £83'.

[33] See Jellinek 2005, pp.429–430; *Brain* was first by one year.

[34] No records of *Brain*'s founding and operations are extant for its first 25 years (personal communication with Professor Alastair Compston, Editor of *Brain*, October 2011).

[35] Critchley and Critchley 1998, p.157.

[36] Jackson 1878g.

[37] Critchley and Critchley 1998, p.157.

One of the other factors in Jackson's widening reputation was Ferrier's publication of his comprehensive monograph, *The Functions of the Brain*, in 1876. As already explained, it summarized Ferrier's experimental work of 1873–1876 and much of the world's literature on its subject. The book was dedicated:

> To
>
> DR HUGHLINGS JACKSON
> who from a clinical and pathological standpoint
> anticipated many of the more important results of recent
> experimental investigation into the functions
> of the cerebral hemispheres
> This Work is Dedicated
> as a mark of the author's esteem and admiration

Probably Ferrier's book was a significant factor in Jackson's election to the Fellowship of the Royal Society of London on June 6, 1878, when he was 43.[38] The key point is that Ferrier was elected F.R.S. on June 1, 1876,[39] at age 33, 2 years before Jackson and before *The Functions of the Brain* was published.[40] Since Ferrier's results constituted the experimental proof for Jackson's theories, it seems likely that Ferrier and others would have campaigned for Jackson's election. Ferrier's work was emblematic of a reviving experimental current in the British biomedical sciences in the 1870s.

Biomedical Science and Neuroscience in the 1870s

As I discussed in Chapter 3, the year 1870 is a rough marker for the beginning of modern scientific medicine, which was increasingly based in the experimental laboratory.[41] Therefore the decade of the 1860s was transitional.[42] For the general and medical publics, the most spectacular part of the new scientific medicine was microbiology, which had its beginnings in the 1860s, in the work of Louis Pasteur, Robert Koch, and Joseph Lister.[43] In the 1870s the ascendency of the experimental laboratory was strongest in the German-speaking countries. This growing predominance caused some tension with the practitioners of the older, clinico-pathological method of the Parisian school, which also was widely employed in Britain. The Parisian method's correlative approach was certainly scientific, but its examination of organs and tissues was in the gross, without use of the microscope.[44] Charcot escaped most of this criticism because his clinico-anatomical method required the microscope to follow fiber tracts and to examine small structures.[45] Like Jackson, Charcot also had a strong physiological bent.

Jackson's work in the 1860s and 1870s was a significant factor in the revival of English physiology from its 'stagnancy' in the prior decades,[46] particularly because of his influence

---

[38] List of Fellows of the Royal Society 1660–2007, at www.royalsociety.org, accessed July 4, 2012. Critchley and Critchley 1998, p.40, say 'at the early age of 53', but obviously that's a 'typo'. About this honor, Hutchinson (1911, p.1554) said of Jackson: 'That he had gained his F.R.S. in early life always gave him very great pleasure.'

[39] See footnote 38 above.

[40] Ferrier's Preface is dated '*October* 1876'.

[41] See Temkin 1973, p.191; also Chapter 6.

[42] See Poynter 1968, pp.1–43; and Geison 1972, pp.13–47.

[43] See Bynum et al. 2006, pp.123–132, 155–160.

[44] See Bynum et al. 2006, pp.47, 69–77.

[45] See Goetz et al. p.56.

[46] Geison 1972; see also Geison 1978, pp.13–47.

on Ferrier. Although most of the British physiologists of the time had medical training, the increasing professionalization of the field led to a further separation of experimental science from clinical practice in the day-to-day work of the different professions. Jackson had perceived and lamented this trend in the 1860s, but its technological force was irresistible.[47]

Of course, Jackson's work also benefitted from the growing volume of experimental data. The most obvious examples were the information provided by Fritsch and Hitzig and by Ferrier. In Chapter 8 we saw other instances of such benefits in Jackson's discussion of decussating versus non-decussating fibers in the motor tract, and also in his use of Betz' discovery of giant cells in primary motor cortex.[48] In 1852 Ludwig Türck had used Wallerian degeneration to describe the motor tract, but he thought that it originated in the basal ganglia. In 1876 Paul Flechsig began his myelogenetic studies which eventually established the cortical origin of the motor (corticospinal) tract.[49] However, those studies were only beginning in 1876, so they had no immediate effect on Jackson. Nonetheless, the increasing strength of his own clinical data gave Jackson the confidence to apply them to some medical aspects of societal problems.

Epilepsy in Society, and the Clinical Physiology of the Cerebellum, March–April 1877

An Editorial on Epilepsy: Claiming Cultural Authority for Neurology, March–April 1877

On March 31 and April 7, 1877—10 months after his wife's death—Jackson published a two-part, unsigned editorial in the *BMJ*: 'On unconscious and automatic actions after epileptic fits'.[50] It is reminiscent of his editorial in the same journal in 1874, when his purpose was to educate the constabulary to avoid confusing cases of intracranial disaster with drunkenness.[51] The instigation for the editorial in 1877 was 'A recent case of homicide by an epileptic'.[52] Apparently an innocent citizen was killed by a 'bystander with a [fireplace] poker'.[53] Jackson said 'that case has been settled to the satisfaction of the profession, on the report of Dr. Risdon Bennett and Dr. Crichton-Browne, if not to the satisfaction of the public …'.[54] Accordingly, he proposed to 'consider the question of responsibility of epileptics'.

> When any one is killed or savagely treated, the public naturally thinks … that the perpetrator ought to be punished … The scientific explanations given by medical men of

---

[47] See Hagner 2012.

[48] Jackson 1873d, p.233.

[49] Clarke and O'Malley 1996, pp.284–290; also Finger 1994, p.201.

[50] Jackson 1877f, Jackson 1877h; Jackson claimed authorship in Jackson 1881h, p.330, footnote (b).

[51] Jackson 1874p, Jackson 1874q, discussed in Chapter 8. In his piece of 1877 (Jackson 1877f, p.394) Jackson quoted his editorial of 1874. In 1877 he used the term 'Dissolution', which he had not used in 1874, as well as 'reduction', which he almost never used otherwise. His editorial of 1875 ([Jackson] 1875b) concerned a scientific issue, not a societal problem.

[52] Jackson 1877f, p.393.

[53] Jackson 1877f, p.395; my square brackets. It is not clear that the patient with a poker was the same as the case that instigated Jackson's editorial. Despite searches in *The Times* of London, and many other sources, I have not yet (October 2012) identified anything further about this case. On December 18, 1876, *The Times* reported a 'Murder in Pimlico', but the weapon was a gun, and apparently there was a clear motive of robbery. An impulsive act with a poker would be more consistent with a postictal state.

[54] Jackson 1877f, p.393. In 1877 James Risdon Bennett (1809–1891) was President of the Royal College of Physicians; see Brown 1955, pp.45–46. In 1877 Crichton-Browne was 'Lord Chancellor's Visitor in Lunacy'; see Jellinek 2005, p.429.

motiveless crimes are heard with impatience ... The common sense ... view of the cases lead[s] to the ready-to-hand explanation that the crimes arise from the innate depravity of the human heart ... The medical inquirer recognizes "innate depravity of the human heart," although he may not use such an expression ... he can pity the criminal who inherits his depravity. Society, in protecting itself, must do no injustice. Scientific jurists are bound to listen to what careful students of nervous disorders have said on the mental state of certain quasi-criminals.[55]

The last sentence is a call for the primacy of professional expertise. The concept of 'cultural authority' was explained in Chapter 2 by saying that a society's acceptance of knowledge claims depends on the degree of authority which that society accords to the author(s) of the claims.[56] By the later 1870s the claims of the British biomedical community were gaining increased recognition, and Jackson's editorial provided further support. In reference to the 'innate depravity' of 'Primitive Man', Jackson recommended 'what Herbert Spencer has written ... in the first volume of his Principles of Sociology'.[57] He also had high praise for the work of Jules Falret (1824–1902), who had a keen interest in automatisms.[58] The rest of the first part of the editorial was an explanation of Jackson's views on the pathophysiology of postictal automatisms. He emphasized the importance of often-overlooked, relatively minor seizures originating in higher levels of the brain. They can be critical to knowing that a patient/criminal has actually suffered a seizure, because, 'What we wish to show is, that *exceedingly elaborate actions may be done by epileptics when unconscious after their fits*.'[59] Moreover,

The slighter the fit, the more elaborate is the mental automatism. This is the equivalent to the statement ... that the affection [depth] of consciousness and the mental automatism vary inversely ... [here he mentioned the cocoa-mixing case] ... The slighter and more transitory the fit, the more easily it is overlooked, and thus the case may be judged ... by the suddenly occurring actions only, which are often ... when the fit is slight, exceedingly complex and purposive-looking. And unfortunately, even in our own profession there are many who do not attach enough importance to the slight seizures.[60]

The bulk of part II of the editorial was a repetition of several earlier case reports, intended to convince the *BMJ*'s physician-readers by presenting clinical data that they would find persuasive. Among the cases that Jackson discussed was the 'cocoa-mixing affair', which he described in more detail than in his original description in 1874.[61] About it he said: 'Yet it is possible for us to recognise the likeness of the cocoa-mixing automatism to an outburst of fury ending in murder, and at the same time to rate very highly their unlikeness.'[62]

---

[55] Jackson 1877f, p.393; my square brackets. For Jackson's views about the legal status of aphasics see Lorch 2012, p.75.

[56] See Turner 1993; for comments on Turner see Dawson and Lightman 2014, pp.14–15.

[57] Jackson 1877f, p.393. Spencer discussed 'Primitive Man' briefly in his *Psychology* and extensively in his *Sociology*; for page citations see the Index in Collins 1889, p.564.

[58] Jackson 1877f, p.393. On Falret see Temkin 1971, pp.316–321. There were earlier references to Falret in Jackson 1871, p.431, and in the epilepsy book (Jackson 1876k, pp.313–314).

[59] Jackson 1877f, p.394; Jackson's italics. Jackson was using '*unconscious*' to mean an altered state of consciousness, not coma.

[60] Jackson 1877f, p.395; my square brackets.

[61] Jackson 1877h, p.431; the original report is in Jackson 1874ff, p.410. It is discussed in Chapter 8.

[62] Jackson 1877h, p.431.

Regarding the subtlety of this distinction, Jackson took a dim view of people of 'average intelligence' who see only details and not larger principles.

> As George Eliot has said (we quote from memory), the average intelligence is ready to admit that, under most circumstances, the radii of a circle tend to be equal; but thinks that geometry may be carried too far. And so, whilst admitting that there is a tendency in epileptics to act grotesguely [*sic*] when unconscious, yet the principle founded on such actions, that an epileptic just after his paroxysm is irresponsible for what he does, is "carrying the thing too far."[63]

Shortly after this denigration of 'average intelligence' Jackson showed his more compassionate side: 'There are few things more touching than the simple expression of an epileptic, " 'If I could only get rid of these fits!" It rouses one's indignation that these calamitous persons should be occasionally treated as criminals.'[64] His indignation stemmed partly from his faith in science. Politically, as Hutchinson has told us, Jackson was quite conservative,[65] but professionally, with regard to the primacy of scientific data, he was among the expanding numbers of those in the medical community who were claiming cultural authority. Socially, he could be simultaneously disdainful of the habits of ordinary lower-class people, and yet fierce in defense of their basic human rights. When proud British society did injustices to its citizens because it ignored the results of established science, he was incensed. *Noblesse oblige!*

Now the question arises, how did the *BMJ* become the conduit for Jackson's expression of his indignation in 1874 and 1877? Guest editorials are ordinarily requested by the editor, and there is no reason to think that it was otherwise with Jackson and the *BMJ*. This conclusion brings us to a short diversion about the *BMJ*'s contentious but highly successful editor at the time, Ernest Hart (1835–1898). He was a dedicated reformer, i.e., generally on the 'liberal' side of social and scientific issues. When he first took over the editorship in 1866, the more liberal and aggressive *The Lancet* was well ahead of the *BMJ* in terms of circulation and prestige.[66] By the early 1870s Hart's *BMJ* had surpassed *The Lancet* in both respects, so Jackson was declaring his opinions in the leading British medical weekly of the time.[67] Part of Hart's formula was an emphasis on publishing original work, which would have appealed to Jackson. Although we know little about their relationship, there must have been mutual respect and ready communication between Jackson and Hart. For now, to keep with the chronology of Jackson's publications, I will turn back to his neuroscience—to some of his ideas about a still-mysterious structure.

---

[63] Jackson 1877h, p.431; I have not tried to find Jackson's source in Eliot's writings.

[64] Jackson 1877h, p.432.

[65] Hutchinson 1911, p.1553.

[66] Several historians have 'demonstrated the presence of radical scientific communities among London medical men' in the early and middle nineteenth century (Turner 1993, p.117). The founding editor of *The Lancet* (in 1823) was Thomas Wakely (1795–1862), a pugnacious reformer; see Bynum and Wilson 1992, pp.36–38; and Loudon and Loudon 1992, pp.65–66.

[67] Little [1933], pp.213–215; and Bartrip 1990, and 1992, pp.134–139.

Jackson's Physiology and Pathophysiology of the Cerebellum, 1869 to March–April 1877

The cerebellum has been torturing its investigators for a very long time—at least since the Alexandrian anatomists, Herophilus and Erasistratus, in Egypt in the fourth century BCE.[68] Following the work of Flourens in the 1820s, there was general agreement that the cerebellum is involved in motor coordination,[69] although Gall thought that it is the sexual organ of the brain.[70] By the mid-century, when Jackson entered medicine, further investigation had confirmed the idea of motor coordination, but little more had been added.[71] On the clinical side, no one knew how to diagnose cerebellar disease. The cerebellum certainly tortured Jackson, who struggled to understand it.[72] He began to develop his ideas about it in 1869. However, I am only now introducing his cerebellar work, as of 1877, because that is when he began to integrate his speculations about the cerebellum into his larger paradigm. So now it is necessary to go back to 1869 and summarize his thoughts up to 1877.

In September 1869 Jackson published a 'Report of a case of disease of one lobe of the cerebrum, and of both lobes of the cerebellum'.[73] He said then that he 'did not diagnose disease of the cerebellum ... Since no one knows what symptoms result from simple *destruction* of large parts of the cerebellum, we cannot make a diagnosis in the scientific sense of the word'.[74] Now we have seen that when Jackson made similar remarks about the unsatisfactory status of some problem, it often meant that he was preparing to take up the challenge. A month after the report was published, its continuation came out in October 1869, titled simply 'The functions of the cerebellum'. There he said that Brown-Séquard had denied any role for the cerebellum in maintaining truncal stability or coordination of 'symmetrical movements'.[75]

To 'harmonise the seemingly contradictory views on the cerebellum', Jackson referred to his previous papers about the graded and overlapping nature of cerebral localization.[76] Then he gave a long quotation from Spencer, the essence of which was Spencer's a priori 'hypothesis' that 'the *cerebellum* is an organ of ... co-ordination in *space*; while the cerebrum is an organ of ... coordination in *time* ...' Because the outer layers of the cerebellum were laid down later in evolution, Spencer said, 'it is inferable that the superficial parts may be sliced off with the least appreciable effects on the actions, and that the effects on the actions will become conspicuous in proportion as the slices destroy the parts nearer to the lower centres ...'[77] It's not clear that this harmonized anything, but at the end of this paper Jackson

---

[68] On the ancients see Rocca 2003, pp.39, 83, and his Index. For cerebellar research from the Renaissance to the early nineteenth century see Neuberger 1981, pp.259–282.

[69] Clarke and O'Malley 1996, pp.632–661. After Flourens, 'there were no further major advances in cerebellar physiology until the last decade of the nineteenth century' (Clarke and Jacyna 1987, p.302). McHenry (1969, p.193) says: 'Sherrington (1900) wrote that Flourens' interpretation of the phenomenon that cerebellar injury causes incoordination formally introduced into physiology the idea of nervous coordination.'

[70] Macklis and Macklis 1992.

[71] Clarke and Jacyna 1987, pp.285–302; also Finger 1994, pp.212–213. Under 'Cerebellum', Dunglison's *Dictionary* of 1874 (pp.195–196) mentioned 'the instinct of reproduction' as 'not proved'; by others, it said, the organ was regarded 'as the coördinator and regulator of the movements'.

[72] A recent assessment (Stein 1989, p.159) concludes that 'Hughlings Jackson never really came to terms with the cerebellum ...'

[73] Jackson 1869k.

[74] Jackson 1869k, p.126; Jackson's italics.

[75] Jackson 1869l, pp.138–139.

[76] Jackson 1867h and Jackson 1867i.

[77] Jackson 1869l; Jackson's italics, my square brackets. Here in 1869 he was quoting Spencer 1870, p.61, accurately because he had fascicles of Spencer 1870 in 1869. Spencer was right. Neurosurgeons have long known that removal of the lateral third of either cerebellar hemisphere results in limited clinical effect, but invasion of the deep cerebellar nuclei causes truncal ataxia.

expressed hope for the day 'When the general disturbance which results from disease of the cerebrum and cerebellum respectively have been carefully worked out …'[78] Since Jackson already had a way to understand localization in the cerebrum—the *xyz* theory—that was a natural starting point for his assault on the cerebellum. The entire cerebrum, he said,

> … consists of units, each one of which represents movements of the whole of the so-called voluntary muscles of the two sides of the body, although … each unit will represent a different grouping of them … If this hypothesis be accepted for the cerebrum, we may fairly infer that a fundamentally similar plan obtains in the cerebellum, and thus we may understand how it is that no symptoms result, although large parts of the cerebellum be destroyed.[79]

In Jackson's 'Study' of 1870 there was nothing about the cerebellum, but he returned to the problem in 1871,[80] when he was beginning to see a clinical pattern. A 5-year-old boy had a 'Tumour of the middle lobe of the cerebellum'. During life, 'The chief symptoms … were – (1) enlargement of the head, (2) double optic neuritis, and (3) reeling gait, followed by permanent rigidity of the legs and paroxysms of convulsions somewhat like those of tetanus'. The tumor had 'pressed on the corpora quadrigemina and on the veins of Galen', and the lateral ventricles were 'greatly dilated'.[81] Nowadays we would not consider the 'convulsions' in the legs to be epileptic seizures. They would be understood as *decerebrate posturing*, due to the tumor pressing on the midbrain. With the introduction of this term it is necessary to be clear about the differences among three kinds of motor phenomena that are clinically similar and easily confused with each other.

Definition Section 8—Three Clinical Entities with Similar Motor Phenomena

Epileptic motor seizures—including Jacksonian and *grand mal* types. The movements may be *clonic* (largely flexion) and/or *tonic* (largely extension). Jackson established that the basic pathophysiology involves a focus of unstable neurons, thought to be almost always cortical, though not necessarily *neo*cortical.

Motor posturing—*due to lateral and/or downward (caudal)* herniation *of the cerebrum* (brain shifts) caused by enlarging intracranial masses. *Clonic posturing* of the arms and/or legs can look very much like motor seizures (Fig. 9.1, upper), and the same is true for *tonic posturing* (Fig. 9.1, lower).

Motor posturing—*in severe cases of* tetanus *(lockjaw)*. When the disease is severe, patients may go into opisthotonic postures (Fig. 9.2), which can look like *grand mal* seizures. The muscular spasm is actually an effect of the toxin of *Clostridium tetani*, which grows in damaged soft tissue. The toxin enters the nervous system via peripheral nerves and blocks the release of inhibitory neurotransmitters in the central nervous system.

---

[78] Jackson 1869l, p.147.

[79] Jackson 1869l, p.140.

[80] Jackson 1871g is an abstract of a case that was reported at the British Medical Association in August in Plymouth. A full report was given in Jackson 1871j (November), where Jackson thanked 'Mr. Stephen Mackenzie' (1844–1909), who was then a registrar at the London; see [Mackenzie, S.] 1909 and [Mackenzie, S.] 2019.

[81] Jackson 1871g. In Jackson 1872l, Jackson attributed the hydrocephalus to 'pressure on the veins of Galen', rather than to the direct effect of the tumor on the midbrain and aqueduct.

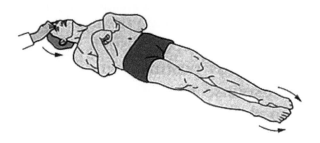

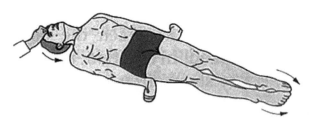

Fig. 9.1 Examples of decorticate motor posture (bilateral flexion of arms in upper figure) and decerebrate motor posture (bilateral extension of arms in lower figure). From Posner et al. 2007, p.73, Figs 2-10B (upper) and 2-10C (lower).

(Reproduced with permission from Saper, C. Brain stem modulation of sensation, movement, and consciousness. Chapter 45 in: Kandel, ER, Schwartz, JH, Jessel, TM. Principles of Neural Science. 4th ed. McGraw-Hill, New York, 2000, pp. 871–909. By permission of McGraw-Hill.)

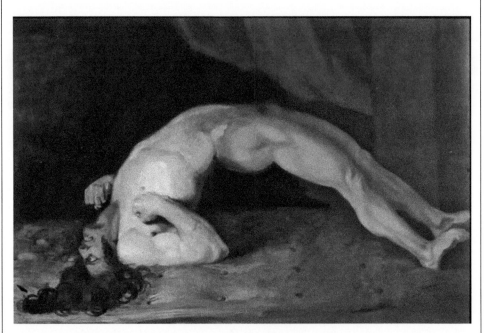

Fig. 9.2 From 'Opisthotonus (Tetanus)' by Charles Bell 1809.

Both kinds of posturing can be misinterpreted clinically as epileptic seizures. Jackson and his contemporaries did not know about brain herniations—our current understanding began in the 1920s.[82] Although Jackson thought the motor phenomena of tetanus might be epileptic, he could postulate a difference in the discharge: 'all abnormal nervous discharges are not epileptic … There is … an almost continuous stream of discharges in tetanus, and there are rapidly succeeding discharges in chorea', so 'the epileptic discharge differs from the other kinds of abnormal discharges … in being paroxysmal'.[83] He used the term 'convulsions somewhat like those of tetanus', which implies that he suspected some pathophysiological difference between epileptic seizures and the posturing of tetanus, but he could not define it any further.

A few months later Jackson published a report of a 5-year-old boy who was found to have a midline cerebellar tumour, probably a tubercle. It was 'about the size of a billiard ball'. In his initial remarks Jackson pledged that he would not use the case as

> … a text for remarks on the functions of the cerebellum. This is the fifth case of disease of the cerebellum which I have had under my observation since January [1871]. The symptoms in these five cases were so different, that I am less inclined than ever … to make <u>general remarks on cerebellar disease</u>.[84]

At the end of the report Jackson said: 'The diagnosis in this case was not difficult', and he repeated his tripartite symptomatology. Then he used his comparative method to analyze the child's decerebrate/opisthotonic posturing,[85] which he differentiated from epileptic seizures.

> It is important to contrast this seizure with those which are more often seen from tumour of the cerebrum. In these <u>cerebellar convulsions</u>, the spasm was chiefly tonic. In cerebral convulsion, it is chiefly clonic. In this case the convulsion affected most the bilateral muscles of the trunk and the legs; whilst in cerebral convulsion the unilateral muscles are most affected, and the arms are more affected than the legs. In the kind of spasm, and in its regional distribution, it <u>resembled</u> rather <u>tetanus</u> than epileptiform convulsions.[86]

In the last sentence Jackson was not sure about the 'epileptiform' nature of the 'cerebellar convulsions'. However, the bacteriological aetiology of tetanus had yet to be worked out in the 1880s. Before then tetanus was thought to be 'functional', i.e., idiopathic, although its connection to open flesh wounds was well known.[87] And despite his proclaimed reluctance to make 'general remarks on cerebellar disease', he could not pass up the opportunity.

> The cerebellum seems to represent the muscles of the body in an order the reverse of that in which they are represented in the cerebrum. The current view is, that the cerebellum co-ordinates more especially those movements which serve in locomotion and other

---

[82] See Meyer 1920, Wilson 1920, Kernohan and Wolfman 1929, Jefferson 1938.

[83] Jackson 1874ee, p.391. This passage is also quoted in Chapter 8. In 1873, Jackson said (Jackson 1873y, p.321, footnote 1): 'The functional change of nerve tissue in epilepsies, in chorea, and in tetanus also, is supposed to be the same.'

[84] Jackson 1871j (November 4, 1871), p.529; my square brackets and underlining.

[85] See Definition Section 8 in this chapter; also Posner et al. 2007, pp.73–75.

[86] Jackson 1871j, p.529; my underlining.

[87] See e.g. Flint 1868, pp.727–730, and Billroth 1878, pp.68–73.

quasi-automatic processes; whereas the cerebrum co-ordinates more especially the movements which serve in voluntary operations.[88]

Two years later, in 1873, Jackson specified some of those 'other quasi-automatic processes'. They included movements of the eyes. Extrapolating from his *xyz* theory, he offered an 'inference'. Since 'The cerebrum contains processes of eye and tactual movements for seeing objects; the cerebellum, we may suppose, contains processes of eye and locomotor movements for <u>estimation of distance</u>'.[89] It is important to note the exact publication date of this passage, which was February 15, 1873, because it predates Ferrier's experiments, which began in March 1873.[90] Although we know that Jackson was in touch with Ferrier in that year, anything that Jackson wrote before March 1873 could not have been influenced by Ferrier's work.

So the idea that the cerebellum functions to estimate distance by controlling eye movements was Jackson's first statement about it—in February 1873. In the same paper he first paid attention to movements of the eyes in seizures and in other conditions.[91] His approach to the problem was based on Bain's biological version of association theory.

> Just as there is an association of lateral movements of the eyes with movements of our tactual organs for ideas of objects, so we may suppose that there will be associations of ocular movements of convergence and divergence ... with those movements of the spine, legs, and arms in locomotion, represented in the cerebellum, for ideas of distance; hence the importance of studying particular ocular deviations in association with accompanying disorder of movement.[92]

In Ferrier's first brief report, dated April 26, 1873, he said simply, 'The cerebellum is the co-ordinating centre for the muscles of the eyeball'.[93] This was based largely on his experiments in rabbits.[94] When he had extended his experiments to monkeys he said: 'The cerebellum is shown to have <u>a function which has never been allotted to it</u>, viz. To be a coordinating centre for the muscles of the eyeballs'.[95] Now this is interesting. In the underlined clause Ferrier was claiming priority for an idea that Jackson had published a few months earlier. Of course, Ferrier had experimental data that Jackson didn't have, but that's not necessarily crucial to priority of the *idea*. I conclude that Ferrier was not aware of Jackson's statements about the cerebellum. After all, one of Ferrier's stated purposes was to test Jackson's theories. If he had been conscious of Jackson's speculations about the cerebellum, I think he would have acknowledged them.[96]

---

[88] Jackson 1871j, p.529.

[89] Jackson 1873d, p.234; my underlining.

[90] Ferrier first visited Crichton-Browne at West Riding in March 1873. His initial experiments were conducted 'in the spring and summer of 1873' (Sherrington 1928, p.ix).

[91] There is nothing about epileptic ocular deviation in Jackson's 'Study' of 1870.

[92] Jackson 1873d, p.234.

[93] Ferrier 1873a (April 26).

[94] Ferrier 1873b, pp.69, 72.

[95] Ferrier 1873c, p.155; my underlining.

[96] In the event, Ferrier (1874a, p.231) simply went on to say that his monkey experiments had confirmed his previous views 'as to the relation of this organ [the cerebellum] to coordination of the optic axes, and the maintenance of body equilibrium'.

And now we get to 1877—to Jackson's 'Remarks on rigidity of [chronic] hemiplegia'—which was published on April 5, 1877.[97] By then his unified paradigm could encompass new data as it came along, in this case about the cerebellum.

> ... the rigidity in hemiplegia is not owing to the cerebral lesion nor to the <u>lateral sclerosis</u> ... Whilst the primary cerebral lesion can account for the paralytic element – the negative condition, it cannot ... account for the tonic condition of the muscles – the positive element. Negative states of the nervous centres cannot *cause* positive states of muscles, they may *permit* them. [Jackson']s <u>speculation</u> is that the rigidity is owing to the unantagonised influence of the cerebellum ... [negative states] are tonic ... [positive states] clonic ... Thus, in walking the cerebellum preserves the equilibrium of the body, tends to "stiffen" all the muscles. The changing movements of walking are the result of cerebral discharges overcoming in a particular and orderly way the otherwise continuous cerebellar influence. This is what is meant by a "<u>co-operation of antagonism</u> ...'[98]

Jackson's conception of the relative roles of the cerebrum and the cerebellum is largely the reverse of our current view, which holds that the cerebellum smooths out the movements initiated by the cerebrum.[99] Nonetheless, in the broader perspective Jackson's style of thought is essentially the same as ours, and he was not completely unique in this. His real contribution was not simply this kind of physiological thinking—it had been done by others. Rather, his role was to unify the physiological with the pathological, as he said, 'on a large scale'.

> When, however, the influence of the cerebrum is permanently taken off by disease ... the cerebellar influence is no longer antagonised; there is unimpeded cerebellar influx, and hence rigidity of the muscles which in health the cerebrum chiefly innervates ...
>
> The above hypothesis is ... only an application <u>on a large scale</u> of Thompson Dickson's Principle of Loss of Control, a principle applicable to all nervous centres, as is ... the physiological Principle of Antagonism. In healthy operations the two principles are displayed; did not centres "resist" one another there could be no independence of operation ... On the other hand, if some centres could not overcome the resistance of others – discharge them by their discharges – there would be no association of operations ... and if there were not some order of "resistances" and of "dischargeabilities" there would be no orderly co-operation.[100]

The maturation of Jackson's increasingly sophisticated physiological thinking continued into the 1890s. At this juncture we have followed the growth of his thought through April 1877, and we will now see that his interest in ophthalmology presented an opportunity to extend his integrating efforts.

---

[97] Jackson 1877g.
[98] Jackson 1877g; Jackson's italics, my square brackets and underlining. 'Lateral sclerosis' refers to Wallerian degeneration in the motor tract of the cord; 'co-operation of antagonism' is redolent of Sherrington's 'reciprocal innervation'; see Sherrington 1940 p.256, footnote 3; and Finger 2000, pp.226–227.
[99] See Ghez and Thach 2000, p.832.
[100] Jackson 1877g; my underlining. On Thompson Dickson see Eadie 2007d.

An Oration on Neuro-Ophthalmology, May–June 1877

In the Spring of 1877 Jackson gave 'An address on ophthalmology in its relation to general medicine', which was 'The Annual Oration delivered before the Medical Society of London*'.[101] Jackson became a Fellow of the Society in 1868. He was President in 1887.[102] Before we discuss the substance of his Oration I will offer some background about the place of the Society in the city's medical scene.

The Medical Society of London and Its Annual Oration

In the century from 1750 to 1850, at least ten local medical societies were founded in London.[103] In general, their purpose was to facilitate communication among practitioners in specific districts within the extended geography of the rapidly expanding city. Among the local societies—excluding the much older, royally chartered Colleges—the Medical Society of London is the oldest continuously operating entity. It was founded in 1773. So the Society was arguably one of the more prestigious among the many local societies in London. Accordingly, the level of prestige of its annual Oration was at a similar level—a distinct honor as Jackson perceived it.[104] His Oration was published or abstracted by four journals, including *the Lancet* and the *BMJ*.[105] The latter serialized the entire address, plus extra paragraphs, in nine-and-a-half packed pages.[106] Neither the *BMJ* nor the other journals routinely published all of London's major medical lectures, no matter how prestigious, so Hart must have thought that Jackson's lecture was worth its space in the *BMJ*.

The live audience for Jackson's Oration would have been the membership of the Society, which included many family doctors and general medical consultants, as well as surgeons, other practitioners, and possibly some laymen. Some ladies might have been present as well. In truth, a more accurate title for his presentation would have been 'Ophthalmology in its Relation to Neurology'. It was a thorough review of the state of neuro-ophthalmology. At the outset he said: 'The subject I have taken up for this address is one which interests me more deeply than any other ... I think it the luckiest thing in my medical life, that I began the scientific study of my profession at an ophthalmic hospital.'[107] From his subsequent remarks it is clear that he valued the training in precision of thought that is required in neuro-ophthalmology.[108] Since ophthalmic surgeons had been making good progress by exercise

---

[101] I do not know the exact date of Jackson's delivery. Currently the Society holds its Annual Oration in the second week of May. This Oration is not to be confused with the Society's annual Lettsomian Lecture, generally delivered in March, which Jackson never gave. For explanation of the asterisk see below in this section.

[102] See Chapter 6, and Hunting 2003, p.326.

[103] See Bailey 1895, pp.24–26, 100.

[104] See Jackson 1877j, p.575. In the late eighteenth century 'the "honour" was not always relished' (Hunting 2003, p.20).

[105] In the *BMJ*, May 12–June 30 (Jackson 1877j, Jackson 1877n, Jackson 1877p, Jackson 1877r, Jackson 1877v); in *The Lancet*, May 12 (Jackson 1877k); in the *Medical Examiner*, May 10–June 28 (Jackson 1877i, Jackson 1877m, Jackson 1877o, Jackson 1877q, Jackson 1877s, Jackson 1877u); and in the *Medical Times and Gazette*, May 12 (Jackson 1877l). See York and Steinberg 2006, pp.88–89.

[106] In the *BMJ* (Jackson 1877j, p.575) an asterisked footnote says, '* This report contains many paragraphs omitted in the delivery of the address'. No such notation is found in the other journals, so either Jackson gave the extra material only to Hart or the others didn't publish the extras—more likely the former.

[107] Jackson 1877j, p.575; on Jackson's affiliation with Moorfields Eye Hospital see Chapter 2.

[108] In reference to medical students, Jackson said (1877j, p575): 'I do not know of any kind of work better fitted for correcting loose habits of observation and careless thinking than a study of palsies of ocular motor nerves.' It's still true!

of such precision, Jackson felt that they represented a model for specialization, which was strongly resisted in many quarters.[109] The problem, as Jackson saw it, was not specialization *per se*—he was doing it himself—but rather its improper use: 'There is no harm in studying a special subject; the harm is in doing any kind of work with a narrow aim and with a narrow mind.' In his Spencerian view,

> As scientific medical research goes on, there is greater specialisation of investigation, just as, in the development of society, there is that continually increasing specialisation, called division of labour. This being so, all the more need is there ... [for] ... greater integration, just as along with division of labour there is need for co-operation of labourers.[110]

Some Contents of Jackson's Oration on Neuro-Ophthalmology, May–June 1877

Three Clinical Concepts

In his first lecture Jackson used three pathological terms that were widely employed at the time: 'cerebral congestion', 'cerebral œdema', and 'overwork' of the brain.[111] He was least convinced about 'cerebral congestion', but he incorporated all three into his thinking. With the ophthalmoscope, he said,

> ... we can *see* the effects of overwork in producing a morbid state ... The facts stated seem to me important also as bearing on one way in which congestion of the brain results. As <u>overwork</u> of the eye causes <u>congestion</u> and <u>œdema</u> of the optic disc, so overwork of the brain causes congestion and even possibly œdema of the brain. I believe it produces arterial fatigue, and thus loss of arterial tonus ... Congestion of the brain, although frequently spoken of, is very difficult to prove even *post mortem*. Wilks and Moxon ... do not deny the existence of congestion of the brain as a fatal disease ... the conclusion that overwork of the brain produces cerebral congestion by arterial fatigue has been reached by Niemeyer.[112]

To understand how Jackson and his contemporaries were using two of those terms we can look at their definitions in Dunglison's *Dictionary* of 1874. 'Congestion' was defined as 'Accumulation of blood in an organ ... It may arise either from an extraordinary flow of blood by the arteries, or from a difficulty in return of blood to the heart by the veins.'[113] Jackson's understanding of the vasomotor nerves (found only in arteries, not in veins) is a prerequisite to his remark about 'loss of arterial tonus'. Despite his skepticism about congestion, he used the idea in connection with 'Œdema cerebri'. This latter Dunglison defined as 'A condition of the cerebral pulp, in which there is an infiltration of serous fluid into it, so that it appears more moist or watery than common; and, when sliced or pressed, small drops

---

[109] See Weisz 2006, pp.26–43; and Casper 2014, pp.13–28 and throughout.

[110] Jackson 1877j, p.575; my square brackets. 'Division of labour' was a central theme in Spencer's thought; see Collins 1889, pp.86, 528–529, and M.W. Taylor 2007, pp.60, 97, 100.

[111] Only 'cerebral oedema' still survives in the twenty-first century, and it is much better defined.

[112] Jackson 1877j, p.576; Jackson's italics, my underlining. No citation is given for Wilks, Moxon, or Niemeyer, but see Niemeyer 1876, p.153.

[113] Dunglison 1873, p.246. For the history of cerebral congestion see Behrman 1982 and Román 1987.

of water are seen to ooze out.'[114]Jackson was indicating that cerebral congestion can lead to cerebral edema, and both could be dangerous.

Dunglison gave no listing for 'overwork', but we can reconstruct some of its meaning by looking outside the Oration—at the example of a consultation that Lewes brought to Jackson. In a letter to a friend dated May 4, 1877, Lewes wrote:

> ... about Mad. Mario I yesterday went to consult Hughlings Jackson ... he insists that galvanism or any other local application is quite useless: "There is but one prescription – absolute rest."
>
>   In case Mad. Mario MUST write and can't dictate, let her by all means use the left and not the right hand; but rest for the brain is the main point. Urge upon her the fact that a short interval of rest now may save her from a very long forced rest in a little while.[115]

'Mad. Mario' was Jessie White Mario (1832–1906), an associate of the Italian nationalist, Giuseppe Garibaldi, and an advocate for the Italian poor. In 1877 she published *La Miseria in Napoli* (*The Poor of Naples*), a strenuous project that might have been thought to be responsible for what 'appeared to be a nervous ailment'.[116] In any case, Jackson's advice to rest was similar to the prescription that would have been given by most of his colleagues.[117] More specifically, it was consistent with the idea of a 'rest cure', championed by his friend Silas Weir Mitchell (1829–1914) of Philadelphia.[118] Jackson probably would have seen Mitchell's first brief paper on the subject in 1873,[119] and he certainly would have known about Mitchell's more extensive discussion in 1875,[120] because Mitchell was in London and in contact with Jackson in 1875.[121]

Vertigo as an Epileptic Motor Dysfunction

The subject of part II of Jackson's Oration was 'vertigo'. Then and now, this term refers to a patient's sensation of spinning, either of the patient himself (subjective vertigo) or of the surrounding environment (objective vertigo), the latter with the patient feeling stationary.[122]

---

[114] Dunglison 1873, p.714.

[115] Haight 1955, vol.6, p.367. It seems that Lewes consulted Jackson with the patient *in absentia*. The letter was addressed to Lewes' friend 'Barbara', i.e., Mme. Eugène Bodichon. Mme. Mario accepted Mme. Bodichon's invitation to recuperate in Cornwall, but Bodichon soon fell ill, and their roles were reversed; see Daniels 1972, p.112. Lewes' casual naming of 'Hughlings Jackson', rather than 'Dr. Hughlings Jackson', supports Raitiere's view (and mine) that by 1877 Jackson was quite intimate with Lewes and potentially with Eliot's entire circle; see Raitiere 2012, p.161, which cites Crichton-Browne 1930, pp.277–278.

[116] Daniels 1972, p.112.

[117] In 1873 (Jackson 1873y, pp.327–328) Jackson ascribed 'nervous debility' to a combination of hypochondriasis and 'nervous tissue [that] is over-nourished in quantity, and yet so imperfectly nourished in quality that is it explosive...'

[118] Mitchell's therapeutic rest cure was not directly related to the diagnostic entity of 'neurasthenia', as used by the American George Beard in the 1880s; for a perspective on the latter see Harrington 2008, pp.142–144. Mitchell's ideas are explained in Walter 1970, pp.127–140. Jackson did not use 'neurasthenia'; it is not listed in the Index of his *Selected Writings* (Jackson 1931–1932).

[119] Mitchell 1873.

[120] Mitchell 1876. Mitchell's paper was published as the installment for April 1875 in Sequin's *American Clinical Lectures*. It emphasized the role of rest as only part of a treatment regimen that is individualized for each patient.

[121] In a reporter's review of Jackson's comments about chorea (Jackson 1875ii, p.483, published October 23) 'Dr. Weir Mitchell, who is now in London, informs Dr. Hughlings-Jackson that chorea is comparatively rare in negroes ...' In 1877 Jackson (Jackson 1877f, p.394) said of Mitchell, 'Everything this physician writes is of the best ...' Mitchell dedicated his *Lectures on Diseases of the Nervous System* (Mitchell 1881; quoted in Walter 1970, p.138) to Jackson, 'with warm personal regard, and in grateful acknowledgement of his services to the science of medicine'.

[122] Compare Dunglison 1874, p.1100, and Weiner et al. 2010, pp.415–416.

Likewise then and now, 'vertigo' was sometimes used loosely to mean severe dizziness. Dunglison's dictionary (1874) gave the definition of subjective/objective spinning, and then said: 'Vertigo is dependent upon the condition of the brain as affected by the circulation, and often announces an attack of apoplexy or epilepsy.'[123]

Presently 'vertigo' is used only grudgingly in epileptology, because the differential diagnosis of vestibular (peripheral/end-organ) versus cortical origin is still difficult.[124] In the 1870s 'vertigo' (and the French *vertiges*) referred to a symptom that was associated with epilepsy.[125]

> As to <u>epileptic vertigo</u>, the demonstration that vertigo is a motor symptom ... helps to show a real relationship betwixt epileptic vertigo and convulsion; it shows that epileptic vertigo is not only clinically but physiologically, a minor degree of convulsion ... note the distinction between a mental state and a nervous state. There is no relationship whatever possible betwixt epileptic vertigo, considered ... as a defect of loss of consciousness, and convulsion; but there is one betwixt convulsion of the eyes, or discharge of the ocular motor centres (the physical side of epileptic vertigo), and general convulsion.[126]

Evidence from Prosper Ménière (1799–1862) and Élie de Cyon (1842–1912), among others, would eventually lead to localization of vertigo in the inner ear,[127] but in 1877 Jackson still thought about it as epileptic. In his conception, vertigo and convulsion shared the same basic pathophysiology, and 'ocular vertigo' shared with epileptic vertigo the commonality of being a motor phenomenon, because ocular vertigo referred to the vertiginous sensations caused by paralysis of the extraocular muscles. Beyond that, 'The facts of ocular vertigo ... help to show that ideas arise, not only during energising of sensory centres, which every body [*sic*] admits, but during energising of motor centres, which scarcely any body [*sic*] seems inclined to believe ...'[128] Jackson's frustration went back to his adoption of Bain's position regarding the motor aspect of cerebral functions, which he had applied to language.[129] To support his contention about 'the inseparable connection of motor activity with sensory activity in ideation', he said:

> Weir Mitchell has independently reached the same conclusion as Bain ... his facts have been explained by the hypothesis that the ideal movements were simply owing to the patient's imagination ... Physiologically, the imaginative explanation is of the same value as the explanation given of the inability of some aphasics to speak, viz., that they do not speak because they have lost the memory of words; these explanations are not physiological, they are attempts to explain physical conditions by psychical conditions; in reality they explain nothing.[130]

---

[123] Dunglison 1874, p.1100. On vertigo and epilepsy see Temkin 1971, pp.318–320, 322–325; also Eadie 2002, pp.1258–1260.

[124] See Bazil 2008, p.2780.

[125] See Eadie and Bladin 2001, p.57, where Delasiauve's (1854) definition of epileptic '*vertiges*' is related to 'today's complex partial seizures'. See also Bladin 1998.

[126] Jackson 1877n, pp.605–606; Jackson's parentheses, my underlining.

[127] See Hawkins and Schacht 2008, pp.R30–R34, R43–R48; also Stevenson and Guthrie 1949, pp.57–59. Jackson discussed Ménière's disease in Jackson 1875z, pp.213–214, where he ignored the possibility that his case with syphilitic disease of the temporal bone might have been explained by disease of the inner ear. For a sketch of Cyon see Feinsod 2012.

[128] Jackson 1877n, p.606; my square brackets.

[129] See Chapter 4.

[130] Jackson 1877n, p.606.

'Co-ordination' as Jacksonian Integration

For Jackson the explanation of language disorders—and everything else neurological—would have to be within the physical realm of sensory and motor processes, which must be integrated for the organism to adapt to its environment. To designate this process, Jackson used the term 'co-ordination', albeit with some hesitation. Its meaning for him was close to our Sherringtonian usage of 'integration'.[131] According to Jackson, coordination is inherent in the system, involving hierarchical and parallel processing. Concerning 'disorders of co-ordination in general', he said: '... the principal is that, when a centre discharges and when one route for the current is stopped, the current ... overflows in other channels, in those for associated movements'.[132] To illustrate he gave an example from Charcot's 'master', G.B.A. Duchenne de Boulogne (1806–1875).[133] As Jackson interpreted Duchenne,

> When the flexors are atrophied, an effort to shut the hand is considerable; and then ... a very intense nervous current reaches the extensors, giving rise to exaggerated extension – not to the desired closure, which is, of course, impossible ...
>
> The principal of double effects in paralysis must be considered in all cases of disorder of co-ordination ... To call ... any ... symptom a disorder of co-ordination is to speak with conventional correctness, but the word co-ordination has such misleading implication that it is scarcely safe to use it. It is frequently used metaphysically, it being implied that there is such a thing as a faculty of co-ordination residing in this or that centre, and that the centre has nothing to do with movements except to regulate them autocratically.[134]

In effect, Jackson was accusing some of his contemporaries of thinking phrenologically, as if there were a localized center for a 'faculty of co-ordination'.[135] In his view, sensory-motor 'co-ordination' is a function of the entire brain, which consists of roughly defined centers, each with overlapping boundaries.

> I have long believed that ocular, and indeed all other movements, are represented in the cerebral convolutions: if they be not, the occurrence of convulsion from disease of them [convolutions] is unintelligible; without admitting such a constitution of <u>ideational</u>

---

131 See Greenblatt 1974, and Greenblatt 1999, pp.379–382.

132 Jackson 1877p, p.672.

133 On Duchenne see Goetz et al. 1995, p.58.

134 Jackson 1877p, p.673. Jackson gave no citation for Duchenne. Referring to sometime after 1861, Allbutt (in Rolleston 1929, p.16) said about Duchenne: 'One of his visits [to England] was made on the importunity of Hughlings Jackson, [Thomas] Buzzard, G.H. Lewes, [W.T.] Gairdner, and myself; Duchenne was to give a demonstration before a gang of us neurologists.' And again, Rolleston (p.18) quoted another statement from Allbutt: 'We got Duchenne over to London one summer, when I gathered my friends Lockhart Clarke, G.H. Lewes, Hughlings Jackson, W.T. Gairdner, and others to meet him.' These two statements are not dated, and it is not clear whether they represent one episode or two—probably one—but they would appear to refer to the later 1860s or early 1870s; Duchenne died in 1875.

135 In Jackson 1878e Jackson said, 'there is no faculty of co-ordination over and above a representation of impressions and movements ...' He made a similar statement in 1880 (Jackson 1880a, p.123). In fact, there was no such center in phrenology; it would have involved motor functions in the cortex, which were not condoned. Nor did Gall accept the existence of the *sensorium commune* (common sensorium) (see Ackerknect and Vallois 1956, p.15); on the *sensorium commune* see Clarke and Jacyna 1987, pp.105–106, 117, 215–216; and Smith et al. 2012, pp.76–77, 81, 85, 88. In Jackson's time, the *sensorium commune* was defined (Dunglison 1874, p.942) as: 'The common centre of sensations. By many it is considered to be represented by the optic thalami, the corpora striata, and the ganglionic nuclei of the nerves of the different senses.' 'Optic thalami' was the term for 'thalami'; see Dunglison 1874, p.1030.

centres, and certainly unless ocular movements are therein represented, what is called the physiology of mind is, I think, an impossible science.[136]

So what did Jackson mean by 'ideational centres'? I think he was using 'ideational' as an adjectival form of 'ideas' in associationism, where ideas are the fundamental units of analysis. Ferrier's data served to extend this position by providing examples of multiple sites of representation for the same or similar movements.

> We see from the experiments of disease, and very evidently from Ferrier's experiments, that the ocular muscles are represented far apart in each of the two great divisions of the nervous system – in the corpus striatum and in the hinder parts of the superior and middle frontal convolutions, and also in the crus cerebelli and cerebellum. There are cerebral and cerebellar movements of the eyes.[137]

Paralysis from Destructive Cortical Lesions

On the motor side, it was Ferrier's work that finally drove Jackson to accept the increasing evidence that destruction of cortex, as well as corpus striatum, can cause paralysis.

> At one time I did not believe that destruction of parts of the cortex produced local paralysis, but Ferrier's experiments on monkeys go contrary to this opinion. It has been recently found by Charcot and others, exactly in confirmation of Ferrier's experiments on monkeys, that from destructive lesions of parts of the cortex there occur limited palsies, as of the face, of the arm; and as Charcot finds *post mortem* wasting of fibres "descending" from the parts of the cortex destroyed, the cases must, I think, be admitted as conclusive.[138]

But observe that what is 'conclusive' is only the evidence for the effects of destructive lesions. Jackson said nothing about the potential anatomical inference that the rostral end of the motor tract might be in the cortex rather than in the striatum. On the other hand, he had much to say about representation of vision in the cortex.

Ferrier's 'Mistake' about Cortical Representation of Vision

In part IV of his Oration Jackson moved on to the vexed problem of cortical representation of retinal images. As usual, he was trying to unify the pathophysiology of many abnormal states. To do this, one has to know where specific physiological functions are located in normal anatomical structures. In the case of vision, the situation was not satisfactory. He knew that in a patient whose single lesion causes both hemiplegia and visual abnormality, the abnormality should be a homonymous hemianopia,[139] but the only experimental data at the time came from Ferrier's experiments. Later it turned out that Ferrier's interpretation of his data was wrong when he concluded that visual images are represented in the angular gyri

---

[136] Jackson 1877p, p.673; my square brackets and underlining.

[137] Jackson 1877p, p.674. The last sentence in this quotation is grossly correct, but it is much more complicated than Jackson imagined (see Goldberg 2000, p.796).

[138] Jackson 1877p, pp.673–674; Jackson's italics and quotation marks. Note that he first announced his conversion here, in a lecture whose title would not suggest this subject (the Oration). A year later, he repeated his announcement while reporting a case of 'temporary hemiplegia after localised epileptiform convulsion' (Jackson 1878f). For Charcot's contribution to understanding the motor tract see Goetz et al. 1995, pp.100–108, 120–127.

[139] 'Homonymous hemianopia' refers to a defect of vision in the same visual field (left or right) of both eyes, implying a lesion in one lateral geniculate nucleus (in the thalamus), or in the optic radiation fibers of one side, or in unilateral visual cortex.

of the parietal lobes.[140] In 1877 neither Jackson nor anyone else knew that it was a mistake, but Jackson had his suspicions.[141] In part III of his Oration, published on June 2, 1877, he had seemed to accept Ferrier's localization of 'retinal expansions' in the 'visual centre – the angular gyrus'.[142] A week later he again tried to bring together the pathophysiologies of migraine and destructive lesions when each involves visual symptoms, and his opinion appears to have changed.

> Ferrier's experiments, if not decisive, supply the only physiological evidence ... as to the cerebral locality where retinal impressions are specially represented. It is true that, in monkeys, he finds that extirpation of the angular gyrus is followed, not by hemianopia, but by loss of sight of the opposite eye; his conclusions are endorsed by Charcot from clinical evidence. Hence I freely admit that there is a want of harmony betwixt present clinical investigations and physiological experiments.[143]

The reasons for the 'want of harmony' were basically two: (1) We now know that the primary visual cortex is in the medial occipital lobes (Brodmann's area 17). It receives retinal inputs via the lateral geniculate bodies in the thalami. Although Ferrier was doing some ablative and stimulation experiments in that posterior part of the brain, his monkeys and other animals did not exhibit any clear visual deficits, such as hemianopia,[144] perhaps due in part to species differences. And (2), more to the point, destruction of the angular gyrus can produce visual deficits that would have been impossible for Ferrier to understand, because his testing methods were only observational. The monkeys had no training before they were lesioned. The behavioral abnormalities that they did exhibit make sense now, because we know about cortically mediated visual neglect, which was probably among the symptoms that Ferrier was observing.[145] In any case, there is no animal model for the visual phenomena of migraine in humans.

The Pathophysiology of Migraine

Migraine is one of the most common neurological conditions with major visual components. It has intrigued physicians since ancient times, perhaps because so many of us suffer from it, including Jackson.[146] Since at least 1874, and probably earlier, Jackson had thought of migraine as a form of epilepsy, because it appeared to involve a discharging, positive lesion.[147] In 1876 he had said:

> I believe cases of Migraine to be epilepsies (sensory epilepsies). Dr. Latham thinks the paroxysm in Migraine to be owing to arterial contraction in the region of the posterior cerebral artery; Dr. Lieving [sic] that there is a 'nerve storm' traversing the optic thalamus and other centres. I think the sensory symptoms of the paroxysm are owing to a 'discharging

---

[140] See Glickstein 1985, and Fishman 1995.
[141] In 1875a, pp.xli and xlvi–xlviii, Jackson denied any cerebral representation of direct retinal input, but he did correctly allow defects of perception (visual agnosias) to be cortical.
[142] Jackson 1877p, p.673.
[143] Jackson 1877r, p.703.
[144] See Ferrier 1876, pp.192–198.
[145] See Glickstein 1985.
[146] On Jackson's migraine see [Jackson, J.H.] 1935; also Chapter 8. Eadie 2012, Chapters 4, 5, and 6, provides an authoritative history of migraine.
[147] Jackson 1874jj, p.519.

lesion' of <u>convolutions evolved out of the optic thalamus</u>, i.e., of 'sensory middle centres' analogous to the 'motor middle centres' …[148]

In his Oration of 1877 Jackson had repeated his assertion about 'convolutions evolved out of the optic thalamus' with different wording: 'It seems to me that all clinical evidence points to the <u>region of the optic thalamus</u> as the seat of the discharging lesion in cases of migraine with visual phenomena.'[149] The change shows his sensitivity to the ontogenetic implications of 'evolved out of' versus 'region of'. The former could imply that in the course of evolution the convolutions connected to the thalami had evolved directly from them, for which there was no information. On the other hand, Jackson often used 'in the region of' to mean that a lower structure in the brain's hierarchy (the thalamus) is connected to a more highly evolved one (the cortex). In general, his solution for such difficulties was to seek 'more *post mortem* evidence', especially about Ferrier's localization of cortical visual function, and about the other sensations of 'smell, sight, hearing or taste'.[150] These were among the themes that he followed in the next 3 years.

Another Historiographic Breakpoint, *circa* 1878

In Chapter 7 I declared 'A historiographic breakpoint'. Starting in 1873, I said, 'it is legitimate to follow the development of Jackson's ideas about any one clinical subject without *constantly* interjecting extended discussions of others'. This change in strategy followed on the observation that a major Jacksonian paper of that year was quite strictly focused on epilepsy,[151] with less attention than usual to his comparative method. For his papers of 1878–1880, and beyond, we are now at a similar juncture. By 1878, Jackson's pathophysiological framework was sufficiently comprehensive so that week-to-week or month-to-month exposition is not always required. Analysis of this period is better served by following one topic over a few years, and then going back to follow others. The themes that I will analyze in this way in this chapter are:

- Cerebellum/tetanus/seizures
- Aphasia/language
- Epilepsy and the motor system
- Psychology and the nervous system (parallelism)[152]

From this point forward most of the important developments in Jackson's thought were presented in formal addresses or similar treatises, but not always—it will still be important to mind the footnotes!

---

[148] Jackson 1876v, p.296, footnote; Jackson's parentheses, my square brackets and underlining. Here again Jackson insinuated an early remark about a basic concept in his use of 'middle centres', which forecasts his later idea of three levels. 'Lieving' should be 'Liveing'. On Latham and Liveing see Eadie 2012, pp.134–136; Eadie 2012, pp.150–153, discusses 'Migraine and Epilepsy', including Jackson's views.

[149] Jackson 1877r, p.703; my underlining.

[150] Jackson 1877r, p.703; Jackson's italics.

[151] Jackson 1873y.

[152] Not listed here are ophthalmology/ophthalmoscopy, which were among Jackson's major interests in 1879–1880 (see Jackson 1879l, Jackson 1879m, Jackson 1879n, Jackson 1880i, Jackson 1880o and Jackson 1880p). They are not analyzed in my narrative because those papers were largely technical, i.e., without anything truly original about neurological issues.

The Cerebellum, Tetanus, and Seizures, 1878–1880

We are now picking up Jackson's ideas about the cerebellum where we left them in the spring of 1877, before his Oration on ophthalmology.[153] In several papers of 1878 and 1880, he extended his analysis of cerebellar function and dysfunction. In the first paper of 1878 he proposed to explain the tremor and rigidity of 'paralysis agitans' (Parkinson's disease) in accordance with the principles that he had laid out a year earlier.[154] About the rigidity of ordinary hemiplegia, he said,

> … the condition is duplex … there is a negative condition, "cerebral paralysis," due to the destructive lesion of the corpus striatum, and a positive condition, "cerebellar rigidity," due to increased cerebellar influx. The hypothesis starts with the assumption that the spinal centres receive impulses from both the cerebrum and cerebellum, which impulses in health interfere with one another (inhibit one another).[155]

Jackson's 'hypothesis' about the 'spinal centres' could bring to mind Sherrington's concept of the 'final common pathway',[156] but that idea requires knowledge of the lower motor neuron (anterior horn cell), and Jackson did not have the neuron theory in 1878.[157] In truth, he was not especially interested in the spinal cord. His attention was on the functional organization of the brain. Applying his pathophysiological reasoning to Parkinson's disease, he said: 'The regional distribution of this motor affection points unmistakably to the cerebrum (whether of the motor tract or cerebrum proper is not said), as the seat of the morbid anatomy. It is essentially hemiplegic; although very commonly it *becomes* two-sided.'[158] Contrasting focal epileptic seizures with the unilateral tremor of Parkinson's, Jackson observed:

> … most of the spasm in ordinary epileptiform seizures … [is] … positive clonic cerebral spasm … On the supposition that the cerebral influence is taken away altogether, we may explain the rigidity [of hemiplegia]. Tremor, at least rhythmical tremor, is a minor degree of tonic spasm … Thus the tremor of paralysis agitans differs from the rigidity of hemiplegia, not fundamentally, but in degree; in the former [tremor] the cerebral influx is diminished; in the latter [rigidity] it is taken off altogether …[159]

In summary, Jackson proposed that the role of the cerebellum in Parkinson's disease could be understood as an exaggeration of its normal function, due to deteriorating cerebral control.

---

[153] This section summarizes Jackson 1878a, Jackson 1878d, Jackson 1878e, Jackson 1878h, Jackson 1880a, Jackson 1880b, Jackson 1880g, Jackson 1880h, and Jackson 1881z. Jackson 1880a, Jackson 1880b, and Jackson 1881z are all the same lecture, which was 'Read before the Medical Society of London, Jan.12th, 1880' (Jackson 1880a, p.122). Jackson 1881z is listed in Jackson's titles for 1881 by York and Steinberg (2006, p.100) because the *Proceedings* of the Society were not published until 1881. I have not discussed Jackson 1880g and Jackson 1880h because they were largely based on the cerebellar papers that preceded them, without any further originality. Jackson's basic approach in Jackson 1880g and Jackson 1880h was to compare the known pathophysiologies of hemiplegia and unilateral seizures with analogous clinical phenomena in cerebellar disease.

[154] Jackson 1878a, p.266, referring to Jackson 1877g.

[155] Jackson 1878a, p.266; Jackson's parentheses.

[156] See Clarke and O'Malley 1996, pp.370, 375–377; Sherrington used 'final common path' *circa* 1904 or earlier.

[157] See Chapters 3 and 5. It was known that damage to the anterior horn of the spinal cord is associated with motor deficits; see Jackson 1880a, p.123.

[158] Jackson 1878a, p.266; Jackson's italics and parentheses. Beginning in the very late nineteenth century, research on Parkinson's focused on the substantia nigra; see Lanska 2010, p.507; also McHenry 1969, pp.409–410.

[159] Jackson 1878a, p.267; my square brackets.

(1) In health the cerebellar influx is fully antagonised; in (2) the early stages of paralysis agitans it is intermittently antagonised – the movement constituting each single tremor occurring betwixt the cerebral impulses; in (3) late stages it is not antagonised at all, and there is such a stream of cerebellar impulses that rigidity occurs. We have cerebral paresis with cerebellar tremor; later, cerebral paralysis with cerebellar rigidity.[160]

From this conception of cerebellar function and dysfunction, Jackson went on to suggest that the cerebellar 'seizures' in tetanus originate from the middle lobe, because tumors are found there in patients who have similar seizures. Pursuing his comparative method, he remarked on

... the resemblance and differences of the commonest variety of cerebral convulsions beginning unilaterally (in one hand) and the paroxysms of surgical tetanus ... In the former [cerebral convulsions] the discharge is unquestionably of some part of one cerebral hemisphere; it is suggested that in the latter [tetanus] it is of some part of the (middle lobe) of the cerebellum.[161]

So Jackson was proposing that seizures can arise from the disinhibited cerebellum. However,

Showing that tetanus is an "inverted" cerebral convulsion would not prove it to be owing to cerebellar discharge. Dr. Hughlings-Jackson has ... never seen anything like a tetanus-seizure from disease of any part of the cerebrum, with one exception. On the other hand, he has reported cases of tumour of the middle lobe of the cerebellum in which seizures practically identical with "surgical tetanus" were noted ...[162]

We can see now that Jackson's difficulty here was partly due to the limitations of neurological knowledge at the time.[163] *The muscle spasms of tetanus are not epileptic.* They are due to the action of the tetanus toxin, which disinhibits motor neurons in the spinal cord. Another piece of unavailable knowledge was probably represented by his 'exceptional case', which 'was that of a boy ... [who had] ... a vast cerebral tumour of the left side of the brain ... The tetanus-like seizures only occurred on the day of the lad's death ...'[164] Probably this patient died due to 'transtentorial herniation', which is a form of pathological brain shift. In this process the medial temporal lobe (uncus) is pushed further medially to compress the midbrain by the mass lateral to it. This phenomenon produces clonic (flexor) and tonic (extensor) posturing movements of the arms and legs. The movements can look like generalized motor seizures *or* tetanus, but transtentorial herniation was understood only in the 1920s.[165] Indeed, Jackson suspected that there was more to the problem than just cerebellar discharge.

---

[160] Jackson 1878a, p.267; Jackson's parentheses. A recent review finds a role for the cerebellum in Parkinson's, but not the driving force that Jackson postulated; see Wu and Hallett 2013.

[161] Jackson 1878d, p.484; Jackson's parentheses, my square brackets. He used 'surgical tetanus' rather than 'traumatic tetanus' (Dunglison 1874, p.1029), which, either way, requires surgical debridement. See also Flint 1868, pp.727–730, and Billroth 1878, pp.68–73.

[162] Jackson 1878d, p.485.

[163] See this chapter, Definition Section 8.

[164] Jackson 1878d, p.485. In January 1880 (Jackson 1881z, p.54) Jackson again used '*Tetanus-like seizures*', indicating his uncertainty about the epileptic pathogenesis of tetanic posturing.

[165] Meyer 1920 and Kernohan and Wolfman 1929. In 1920 Kinnier Wilson analogized 'tonic fits' to decerebrate rigidity and in effect denied the existence of 'so called cerebellar fits'.

Dr. Hughlings-Jackson has himself drawn attention to some objections which may be taken against the opinion he entertains – that the tumour of the middle lobe of the cerebellum … caused the tetanus-like paroxysms … In such cases the subjacent medulla oblongata may have been compressed or otherwise altered. Again, the tumour may have affected the adjacent corpora quadrigemina (they are deformed by pressure in some cases). The latter is important, as Ferrier has produced tetanus-like states from faradisation of these bodies, but not from faradisation of the cerebellum.[166]

The underlined phrase about 'the opinion he entertains' shows that Jackson knew his conception of cerebellar function was largely theoretical. Retrospectively, his statements about the corpora quadrigemina were prescient, but two decades early. In the 1890s Sherrington described the effects of sectioning the brainstem through the midbrain of cats, which was done between the upper and lower mammillary bodies (of the corpora quadrigemina) and through the underlying (ventral) midbrain. This physiological preparation produces extensor posturing of all four limbs, which Sherrington called 'decerebrate rigidity'.[167]

Now we get back to the neurology of the cerebellum in 1878, when Jackson described a case of 'Tetanus-like seizures with double optic neuritis – no autopsy'. The patient was a 3-year-old boy whose 'autopsy was not permitted by the boy's friends'.[168] In trying to understand this case, Jackson discussed two possible etiologies, which were not mutually exclusive. One was the idea of seizures induced by instability of cerebellar tissue. In this regard he referred to a letter to the editor of the *Medical Times and Gazette*, published on November 2, 1878, 'from Dr. [James] Ross, expressing his opinion that the paroxysms of tetanus are owing to a cerebellar cortical discharge'.[169] Second was the theory of disinhibition caused by the mechanical disruption of motor tracts: 'Since the corpora quadrigemina are close upon the middle lobe [of the cerebellum], they might be squeezed by a tumour there placed, but it remains that a tumour anywhere in the encephalon may cause optic neuritis.'[170] Nonetheless,

A further thing which Dr. Hughlings-Jackson believes to point to disease of the middle lobe of the cerebellum was the occurrence of tetanus-like seizures. By "tetanus-like" is not meant the tetany of Trousseau, but resembling ordinary surgical tetanus. He does not think such seizures point necessarily to *tumour* of that part (to secondary changes in grey matter induced by the tumour), although he thinks they did in this case.[171]

Jackson's first paper of 1880 continued his analysis of the cerebellum and its disorders. It was mainly concerned with the semiology of intracranial disease versus localizing signs that point specifically to the cerebellum.

---

[166] Jackson 1878d, p.485; Jackson's parentheses, my underlining.

[167] See Clarke and O'Malley 1996, pp.370–375; Sherrington 1940 reprints several of his writings on the subject. Although the laboratory phenomenon of decerebrate rigidity is clearly relevant to the posturing caused by transtentorial herniation in humans, the correlation is not straightforward; see Posner et al. 2007, p.74.

[168] Jackson 1878h, p.596.

[169] Jackson 1878h, p.596; my square brackets. Ross (1837–1892) was in Manchester, where he 'rapidly won fame as a neurologist'. His biographical sketch (Brown 1955, p.290) says he 'was an unostentatious and lovable man with an endearing absentmindedness caused by his preoccupation with philosophical problems'.

[170] Jackson 1878h, p.596; my square brackets. In 1880 Jackson made a similar statement (J80-01, p.123): 'Tumour under the tentorium probably produces more disturbance by pressure than cerebral tumours do.' This too was prescient but incomplete.

[171] Jackson 1878h, p.596; Jackson's italics. The 'tetany of Trousseau' is a paroxysmal, tetanus-like posturing of the limbs (see Dunglison 1874, p.1028) that is associated with abnormalities of calcium metabolism. On Trousseau's description of it see Pearce 2002, pp.127–128.

There are three motor symptoms which may occur with tumour of the cerebellum; they have their analogues in cerebral disease. (*a*) Reeling. (*b*) A certain persisting rigidity. (*c*) Tetanus-like paroxysms. Reeling, I think, is, or at least depends on, a cerebellar paralysis, the analogue of the hemiplegia [in] a cerebral paralysis; persistent rigidity is the analogue of the well-known rigidity in hemiplegia and the tetanus-like seizures of unilaterally beginning convulsive seizures from cerebral cortical disease.[172]

Jackson's concern to find analogues of cerebral symptoms in the cerebellum originated from his effort to find somatotopy there. Since he had been so successful in predicting the principles underlying Ferrier's somatotropic findings in the cerebrum, he hoped to achieve something similar for the cerebellum.

Hitzig and Ferrier have convinced most [medical] people that some parts of the cerebral cortex represent movements, and Charcot, by a very different kind of evidence, clinical and pathological, has confirmed their opinions. I have long wished to ascertain if the cerebellum cannot be broken up into regions, each representing especially, some movements of the body.[173]

To achieve this Jackson proposed to use the same comparative method that he had applied to the cerebral cortices: 'We have to study all degrees of locomotion, from getting up [from lying down or sitting] to swift running, with the aim of ascertaining *the order* in which movements of different parts of the body are represented in the cerebellum.'[174] However, he recognized that he was trying to analyze segmental movements of the spine, and that is very difficult. Moreover, it has turned out (so far in the twenty-first century) that there is no straightforward pattern of motor somatotopy in the cerebellum.[175] After these papers on the cerebellum in 1880, his subsequent efforts to understand it were intermittent and not really conclusive.[176] Now we will go back to 1878 and rejoin his work on a different subject—our erstwhile friend, aphasia.

A Treatise on Method and Aphasia, 1878–1879

In the first and second volumes of *Brain*, Jackson published a long treatise in three installments, 'On affections of speech from disease of the brain'.[177] This was his first major treatment of aphasia since his 'duality' papers of January 1874.[178] Throughout the paper there are two related themes: (1) 'duality', which refers to his ideas about the brain's organization for cognitive and precognitive functions in health; and (2) the clinical semiology of

---

[172] Jackson 1880a, p.123; my square brackets.
[173] Jackson 1880a, p.123; my square brackets.
[174] Jackson 1880a, p.123; Jackson's italics, my square brackets.
[175] See Mottolese et al. 2013.
[176] Jackson 1881z and Jackson 1890a contain remarks on the cerebellum. See also Critchley and Critchley 1998, pp.83–89, Chapter 11 ('The Cerebellum').
[177] This section summarizes Jackson 1878g, Jackson 1879o, Jackson 1879t, and Jackson 1880e. The last was 'Abstracted from *Brain* by Mr. James Sully'. Its three-page summary of Jackson's entire treatise is succinct, and I am grateful for it. Although Jackson did not use the word 'aphasia' in his title, he did use it in his text, and he acknowledged its wide acceptance (Jackson 1878g, p.311): 'It is too late, I fear, to displace the word aphasia.' In his next paper, 'On aphasia, with left hemiplegia' (Jackson 1880f), he wrestled with cases of anomalous dominance, but he did not reach any generalizations.
[178] Jackson 1874b, Jackson 1874c, Jackson 1874e; see Chapter 7.

language disorders. His goal was to explain the semiology by reference to the duality. In the process he extended his exploration of psychophysical parallelism, which was part of his method.[179] His first installment began with extensive comments about conceptual and methodological issues.

On Method, October 1878

At the outset Jackson emphasized the distinction between 'morphology' and 'anatomy'.

> The morphology of a centre deals with its shape, with its "geographical" position, with the sizes and shapes of its constituent elements. A knowledge of the anatomy of a centre is a knowledge of the parts of the body represented in it, and of the ways in which these parts are therein represented.[180]

Two years earlier, in Chapter VII of his epilepsy book, Jackson had disparaged pure morphology, saying that only functional anatomy can rise into physiology. In the process of explaining this hierarchy, he evinced his ideas about the histological basis of learning and memory. The 'facts of morphology', he had said in 1876,

> ... are facts as to the course of fibres and arrangements of cells disclosed by microscopical examination. The latter is not Minute Anatomy, but Minute Morphology; and however minute it becomes it does not turn into physiology. It is only when the shapes of cells and course of fibres, &c., are shown to be subservient to the reception or conduction of particular impressions and to the development of related movements that morphology ceases or rises into anatomy.[181]

Getting back to 1878, his thoughts about anatomy and physiology led to a larger methodological discussion of the nature of '*medical* inquiry'.

> A method which is founded on classifications which are partly anatomical and physiological, and partly psychological, confuses the real issues. These mixed classifications lead to the use of such expressions as that an *idea* of a word produces an articulatory *movement*; whereas a psychical state, an "idea of a word" ... cannot produce an articulatory movement, a physical state. On any view whatever as to the relation of mental states and nervous states such expressions are not warrantable [*sic*] in a *medical* inquiry.[182]

Notice the emphasis on '*medical* inquiry'. He did not say 'scientific' or 'physiological'. Had he decided that medical and physiological inquiries are fundamentally different? Is 'medical' not 'scientific'? Is it more or less than 'scientific', or just different? Is it different than physiological investigation because it involves disease or dissolution? Some evidence for the latter is found in a footnote a few pages on, where he was discussing dissolution.

---

[179] Jackson first used 'concomitance' in print in 1881 (Jackson 1881l, p.69), but he formally christened his version of psychophysical parallelism as his 'doctrine of Concomitance' in his Croonian Lectures of 1884 (Jackson 1884g, p.706).

[180] Jackson 1878g, p.305.

[181] Jackson 1876e, p.130, footnote (b) in column 1.

[182] Jackson 1878g, p.306; Jackson's italics, my square brackets.

Here I must acknowledge my great indebtedness to Spencer. The facts ... seem to me to be illustrations from actual cases of disease, of conclusions he has arrived at deductively in his *Psychology*. It is not affirmed that we have the exact opposite of Evolution from the ... brutal doing of disease; the proper opposite is seen in healthy senescense [*sic*] ... But from disease there is ... the corresponding opposite of Evolution.[183]

Jackson's discussion of his method was deliberately intermingled with his evolving ideas about psychophysical parallelism. He knew that including the latter in his writing risked confusion, at least in lesser minds, but he persisted.

We cannot go right on with the psychology, nor with the anatomy, nor with the pathology of our subject. We must consider now one and now the other, endeavouring to trace a correspondence betwixt them.

I do not believe it to be possible for any one to write methodically on these cases of disease of the nervous system without considering them in relation to other kinds of nervous disease; nor to be desirable in a medical writer if it were possible.[184]

And later, on the same theme Jackson gave an exhortation that might be a motto for all of the neurosciences: 'I shall make frequent references to other classes of nervous disease. The subject is already complex without these excursions, but <u>we must face the complexity</u>.'[185] As promised, he faced it head-on.

Memory or any other psychical state arises *during* not *from* – if "from" implies continuity of a psychical state with a physical state – functioning of nervous arrangements ... is a purely physical thing – [it is] a discharge of nervous elements representing some impressions and movements ... we must not classify on a mixed method of anatomy, physiology, and psychology ...[186]

Jackson's caveat has been heard before. However, his ideas about classification had evolved during the preceding few years. In the mid-1870s he had accepted the need for empirical classifications, as well as scientific ones, but he had privileged the scientific. In 1878 he was trying to be more egalitarian.

Divisions [1] and Arrangements are easy, Distinctions and Classifications are difficult. But in the study of a very complex matter, we must first divide and then distinguish ... Harm comes, not from dividing and arranging, but ... from taking provisional divisions to be real distinctions, and putting forward elaborate arrangements ... as being

---

183   Jackson 1878g, p.309, footnote 1. On the same theme see Jackson 1879t, p.325, footnote 1.
184   Jackson 1878g, pp.306–307.
185   Jackson 1878g, p.309; my underlining. The next sentence continued, 'Dr. Curnow has well said (*Medical Times and Gazette*, Nov.29, p.616), "The tendency to appear exact by disregarding the complexity of the factors is the old failing in our medical history". John Curnow, M.D., F.R.C.P. (1846–1902), was chair of anatomy at King's College; see Brown 1955, pp.255–256. Later Jackson also said (Jackson 1888c, p.61): 'What all of us dislike is an explanation of difficult problems, the complex. We may easily err in taking the subjective confusion produced in us to be in the objective thing contemplated, which is really only very complex.'
186   Jackson 1878g, p.313; Jackson's italics, my square brackets. His extension of this principle seemed to lead him toward a form of biological panpsychism, when he said (Jackson 1878g, p.314, footnote 1): 'I ... believe, as Lewes does, that in so far as we are physically alive, we are psychically alive; that some psychical state attends every condition of every part of the organism. This is, at any rate, a convenient hypothesis in the study of diseases of the nervous system.'

classifications. In other words, we shall ... consider our subject empirically, and afterwards scientifically ...[187]

Since this is a concession to the heuristic priority of an empirical classification, it appears that Jackson's opinion had changed, but not about fundamentals. Before he began to create typologies of aphasic semiology he issued a warning that still resonates: there is no such real thing as an 'entity' of aphasia. There are only individual cases whose differing symptoms depend on the specifics of a lesion's location, size, and rapidity.[188] Attempts at arrangement and classification are legitimate, but they are merely devices.

A Clinical Classification of the Semiology of Aphasia, October 1878–October 1879

Concerning 'affections of speech', Jackson proposed:

> Let us divide [it] roughly into three degrees: (1) *Defect of Speech*. – The patient has a full vocabulary, but makes mistakes in words ... (2) *Loss of Speech*. – the patient is practically speechless and his pantomime is impaired. (3) *Loss of Language*. – Besides being speechless, he has altogether lost pantomime, and emotional language is deeply involved.[189]

Note that all three of these categories are related to output, i.e., the motor side of language. It is not feasible to map Jackson's categories exactly on to more recent connectionist classifications of aphasia types, because the latter includes comprehension, i.e., the sensory side of language.[190] Readers who are accustomed to Geschwind's twentieth-century connectionist paradigm may want to understand Jackson's categories in those terms,[191] especially given the fact of Wernicke's contribution in 1874.[192] We might say that '(1) *Defect of Speech*' describes anomic aphasics, and '(2) *Loss of Speech*' describes anterior/Broca's aphasics, more or less, but '(3) *Loss of Language*' simply refers to loss of *all* language output, not to (sensory-side) comprehension. Jackson assumed that language comprehension was a function of the whole brain (see Fig. 7.1). For heuristic reasons he chose to begin his analysis with the second type, '*Loss of Speech*', and he never did give a thorough analysis of the first and third types in this paper. '*Loss of Speech*', on the other hand, was subjected to a detailed application of his positive versus negative distinction, starting with 'The Patient's Negative Condition'.[193]

'(1) *He does not speak ...*' A simple utterance is not 'of high speech value ...'[194]

---

[187] Jackson 1878g, p.310. In footnote 1 there is a quotation from Coleridge, who quoted Locke. For this Jackson cited: '*Westminster Review* (art. Locke) January 1877 ...' There is no evidence that Jackson read either author directly. He repeated the same theme in Jackson 1878g, p.315, saying: 'This is the plan adopted in every work on the practice of medicine with regard to all diseases.'

[188] Jackson 1878g, p.314.

[189] Jackson 1878g, p.314; Jackson's italics, my square brackets.

[190] Marjorie Lorch (personal communication) points out that Jackson was focused on degrees of impairment of fluency. He was not especially interested in language comprehension.

[191] Geschwind 1965.

[192] Wernicke 1874. Jackson eventually learned about Wernicke, probably from Bastian; see Chapter 12.

[193] Jackson 1878g, pp.316–319. To create this summary I have extracted sentences from these four pages, hence the quotation marks within the indented block.

[194] For '(2)', in Jackson 1878g, p.317, a footnote explains: 'speech of high value ... is new speech, not necessarily new words and possibly not new combinations of words; propositions symbolising relations of images new to the speaker ...'

'(2) *He cannot write*; that is to say, he cannot express himself in writing. This is called Agraphia (William Ogle)... he cannot speak internally... The speechless patient does not write because he has no propositions to write...'[195]

'(3) In most cases the speechless patient *cannot read at all*...'[196]

'(4) His power of making signs is impaired (pantomimic propositionising).'

In contrast to these absent functions, Jackson said that a typical patient with loss of speech will commonly exhibit a number of positive symptoms, including speech comprehension.[197]

'(1) He can understand what we say or read to him ... although Speechless, the patient is not Wordless. The hypothesis is that words are in duplicate; and that the nervous arrangements for words used in speech lie chiefly in the left half of the brain; that the nervous arrangements for words used in understanding speech ... lie in the right also[198] ... When from disease in the left half of the brain speech is lost altogether, the patient understands all we say to him, at least on matters simple to him.'

'(2) His articulatory organs move apparently well in eating, drinking, swallowing, and also in ... recurring utterances...'

'(3) His vocal organs act apparently well; he may be able to sing.'

'(4) His emotional language is apparently unaffected.'

Our current connectionist paradigm assumes that speech comprehension is mediated largely in the dominant (usually left) hemisphere, in or near Wernicke's area. In direct contrast, Jackson's neurological model (Fig. 7.1) specified that different stages of comprehension take place on each side, starting preconsciously on the right, as seen in item (1) above. Therefore, in Jackson's model, a left-sided lesion will still leave part of the speech apparatus available to the patient—in the right hemisphere. The qualifier 'on matters simple to him' shows that Jackson recognized the clinical fact of altered comprehension in some patients with left-sided lesions.[199] Since he believed that it is words, not propositions, that are processed on both sides, it is important to understand how he thought about words as 'images'.

> Words are in themselves meaningless, they are only symbols of things or of "images" of things; they may be said to have meaning "behind" them. A proposition symbolises a particular relation of some images.[1] ...
>
> [1] The term "image" is used in a psychical sense, as the term "word" is. It does not mean "visual" images only, but covers all mental states which represent things. Thus we speak of auditory images ... What is here called "an image" is sometimes spoken of as "a perception."

---

[195] The last sentence ('no propositions') would not find wide agreement among modern aphasiologists. On Ogle's introduction of 'agraphia' see Henderson 2010, p.586.

[196] Presumably this means reading aloud, without considering comprehension.

[197] Jackson 1878g, pp.319–321; my square brackets.

[198] Jackson's use of 'also' is potentially confusing, because it could mean that comprehension takes place on both sides, or simply that the right side 'also' has a function. I agree with Sully's interpretation of Jackson's statement (Jackson 1880e, p.254, which is Sully's abstract of Jackson 1879t): 'it is the right half of the brain which acts when the first subconscious service of words begins, the left when there follows that verbal action which is speech'.

[199] He did not consider the issue of atypical dominance, but see Jackson 1879t, p.329.

> In this article the term perception is used for a *process*, for a "proposition of images," as speech is used for propositions, *i.e.* particular inter-relations of words.[200]

Despite Jackson's admonition to be cognizant of the boundary between the two parallel sides of the psychophysical divide, he often tended to slide back and forth without notice. In the above he acknowledged that he was doing his analysis on the psychological side, and then he continued: 'although we artificially separate speech and perception, words and images co-operate intimately in most mentation'.[201] From there he went on to a largely psychological discussion of the 'subconscious' processing of words. Written words, he said, are merely 'symbols of symbols of images'. Hence,

> For the perception (or recognition or thinking) of things, at least in simple relations, speech is not necessary, for such thought remains to the speechless man. Words are required for thinking, for most of our thinking at least, but the speechless man is not wordless; there is an automatic and unconscious[1] or subconscious service of words.[202]

In the footnote 1 Jackson tried to explain his difficulty with conceptualizing the comprehension of words. To do this he emphasized the physical side of his parallelism.

> [1] The expression "*un*conscious reproduction of words," involves the same contradiction as does the expression, "unconscious sensation." Such expressions may be taken to mean that energising of lower, more organised, nervous arrangements, although unattended by any sort of conscious state, is essential for ... energising of the highest and least organised – the now-organising – nervous arrangements, which last-mentioned energising is attended by consciousness ... (I use the term subconscious for slight consciousness).[203]

Note that 'energising' is clearly a physical process, but otherwise undefined. He assumed that expenditure of energy can occur only in a physical process, even if the 'reproduction of words' is '*un*conscious'. Conversely, of course, this implies that mental processes do not consume energy—at least not energy of a kind that physicists would recognize.[204] Going back to the mental side, Jackson said that speech is

> ... required for thinking on novel and complex subjects, for ordering images in new and complex relations (*i.e.*, to the person concerned), and thus the process of perception in the speechless, but not wordless, man may be defective in the sense of being inferior from lack of co-operation of speech ...[205]

Note also Jackson's emphasis on 'thinking on novel and complex subjects'. In contrast to the faculty psychology of Broca et al., classical associationism could account for learning in a mechanistic way at the psychological level, even before Spencer and Bain.

---

[200] Jackson 1878g, p.321. In the omitted part of this footnote Jackson mentioned 'Taine', i.e., Hippolyte Taine (1828–1893), French critic and historian, whose *De l'Intelligence* of 1870 was translated in 1871.
[201] Jackson 1878g, p.321.
[202] Jackson 1878g, p.323; Jackson's parentheses.
[203] Jackson 1878g, p.323; Jackson's italics and parentheses.
[204] On the issue of 'psychic energy' see Millett 2001.
[205] Jackson 1878g, pp.323–324.

The Ascendance of Physiological Associationism, October 1878

At the end of Chapter 8 we saw that in 1876 Jackson had pejoratively equated 'the most psychological of psychologists' with adherents to the faculty psychology.[206] In 1878, when he completed the first installment of his aphasia treatise, he invoked sensori-motor associationism to declare victory over earlier concepts of the 'Will' and similar entities, which were supposed to 'reside' in the cerebral hemispheres: 'There is no faculty of memory apart from things being remembered; apart from having ... now and again, these or those words, or images, or actions (faintly or vividly).'[207] And later, in a similar vein, he said: 'We seem to ourselves to Perceive, as also to Will and to Remember, without prior stages, because these prior stages are unconscious or subconscious.'[208]

> It is ... because speech and perception are preceded by an unconscious or subconscious reproduction of words and images, that we seem to have "faculties" of speech and of perception ... The evidence of disease shows ... that the highest mentation arises out of our whole organised states ... that Will, Memory &c., "come from below," and do not stand autocratically "above," governing the mind; they are simply the now highest, or latest, state of our whole selves.[209]

By the later 1870s, Jackson and his contemporaries had banished 'Will, Memory &c.' from discourse on the physical side of the psychophysical divide. In their place he had offered his neurological models of cognitive processing (Figs 7.1 and 8.1), involving a division of functions between the right and left hemispheres. He feared, however, that this anatomical division was 'too abrupt', pointing out that patients who have severe loss of speech from damage of the left hemisphere still have 'Occasional Utterances'. And equally to the point:

> ... from disease of the right half [of the brain], there is not loss of that most automatic service of words which enables us to understand speech. The thing which it is important to show is, that mentation is dual, and that physically the unit of function of the nervous system is double the unit of composition; not that one half of the brain is "automatic" and the other "voluntary."[210]

Here Jackson apparently recognized that right-sided lesions do not generally interfere with auditory comprehension. If he had pursued the implication of this clinical reality he would have been forced to question the validity of his neurological model of speech processing (Fig. 7.1), because his model predicted that right-sided damage should result in defects of comprehension. Perhaps he was so invested in his model that he did not want to go there. In any case, his immediate concern was to avoid the simplistic notion that each hemisphere is totally different from the other.[211] And there the first installment ended. He did not go on to draw the seemingly obvious conclusion that some auditory comprehension must be

---

[206] Jackson 1876v, pp.306–307.
[207] Jackson 1878g, p.322; Jackson's parentheses.
[208] Jackson 1878g, p.326.
[209] Jackson 1878g, p.325.
[210] Jackson 1878g, p.327; Jackson's quotation marks, my square brackets.
[211] Since the 'split brain' (callosotomy) work of the mid-twentieth century this simplistic view has been rife in our own popular press.

conducted in the left hemisphere, except when he said that the functional division between the hemispheres is not 'abrupt'.

Aphasic Utterances and Physiological Prescience, July–October 1879

The second installment of Jackson's treatise on aphasia was devoted to extensive treatments of 'Occasional Utterances'[212] and 'Recurring Utterances'.[213] This discussion was conducted almost entirely on the psychological side. He concluded that aphasic utterances with propositional value are possible but very uncommon.[214] At the more elementary end of the spectrum, he brought up the phenomena of 'oaths' (swearing) and other linguistic 'ejaculations'. Psychologically, they were understood as part of nonpropositional, 'emotional' language. At the neurological level, 'their utterance by healthy people is on the physical side a process during which the equilibrium of a *greatly* disturbed nervous system is restored ... All actions are in one sense results of restorations of nervous equilibrium by expenditures of energy'.[215] And on the last page of Jackson's second installment there is a speculation about the neurology of learning: 'the more automatic a process is, or becomes by repetition, the more equally and fully is it represented doubly in each half of the brain. But the utterances show ... that the speech possible by the right side of the brain is inferior speech.'[216]

In his third installment Jackson began with recurring utterances. Patients who use 'yes' and 'no' usually do so emotionally,[217] without propositional intent, but expressions such as 'come on to me' have potential meaning, because *'they were being said, or about to be said, when the patient was taken ill'.*[218] His psychological analysis of this phenomenon led him to some interesting insights, quoted here from Sully's *précis*.

> Speech is to be regarded as but the second half of a whole process which may be called *verbalising*.[219] We can say that it includes two propositions, a "subject proposition," followed by an "object proposition." It is supposed that the subject-proposition is the 'survival of the fittest' words in fittest relation during activity beginning in the right half of the brain," and that it "symbolises an internal relation of two images, internal in the sense that each of them is related to all other images already organised in us." On the other hand, the object-proposition symbolises relation of these two images as for things in the environment, each of which images is related to all other images then organising in the environment." Thus, "the two propositions together symbolise an internal relation of images in relation to an

---

[212] This second installment begins with a footnoted reference to Baillarger (Jackson 1879o, p.203), whom Jackson thinks he has neglected. Apparently no one else complained about it.

[213] Here (Jackson 1879o, p.205) Jackson said that one of the four kinds of recurring utterances is 'jargon', using the term as we would. I have not seen this usage by Jackson previously, and a very brief survey of writings about aphasia by his contemporaries yielded no other instances.

[214] In Jackson 1879o, p.213, Jackson remarked intriguingly, 'I find that I have led Kussmaul to misunderstand me on this matter', followed by a quotation from Kussmaul in English. However, he gave no citation to Adolf Kussmaul (1822–1902), whose *Die Störungen der Sprache* (*The Disturbances of Speech*) was published and translated in 1877.

[215] Jackson 1879o, p.216; Jackson's italics. In a footnote he added: 'It has been said that he who was the first to abuse his fellow-man [verbally] instead of knocking out his brains without a word, laid thereby the basis of civilization.'

[216] Jackson 1879o, p.222.

[217] Jackson 1879t, pp.323–324.

[218] Jackson 1879t, p.326; Jackson's italics.

[219] Jackson first used 'verbalising' in Jackson 1873a, p.85, with his own definition.

external relation of images." Dr. H. Jackson bases this distinction on Mr. Spencer's definition of a psychological proposition as compounded of two propositions . . .[220]

In the above, 'survival of the fittest' catches our eye immediately. In 1864 it was Spencer's
invention to designate the 'Darwinian' struggle for survival.[221] In describing his model for
processing auditory language in 1874 (Fig. 7.1), Jackson had implied that there is a competitive process of word order selection in the right hemisphere, but the implication was
not clearly acknowledged and the process was not defined.[222] Thus, it was in October–
November 1879 that Jackson first used 'survival of the fittest' in an explicit application to
the subject–object distinction on both sides of the mind-brain divide, albeit largely on
the mental side.[223] With regard to recurrent utterances as residuals of the patient's speech
output or his thoughts at the onset of the ictus, Jackson speculated about the neurological
basis of recurring utterances.

> . . . such utterances . . . correspond to the latest and newest nervous actions. We have to sup-
> pose that in the healthy man there remains after every last utterance for a short time a slight
> degree of independent organisation of nervous arrangements concerned; for without as-
> suming this we cannot understand how it is possible to recollect what has just been said . . .
> consecutively. In the case of the speechless man we must suppose that this normally tem-
> porary activity of nervous arrangements becomes permanent. There are strong reasons for
> saying that these recurring utterances are due to the activity of the right half of the brain.
> The left half is known to be extremely damaged.[224]

The prescience here is Jackson's *a priori* recognition that there must be some form of rolling
short-term memory prior to actual speech output, or propositional speech would be impossible. On the physical side, the short-term memory must have a neurological basis. On both
sides, the memory of what has just been thought or said constitutes a 'preconception' of the
next proposition. And there are similar preconceptions for all 'voluntary' actions. About this
Jackson pointed out

> . . . the bearing of Spencer's remark on the distinction betwixt voluntary and involuntary
> operations . . . In the voluntary operation there is <u>preconception</u>; the operation is nascently

---

[220] Jackson 1880e, p.254; my underlining, Jackson's quotation marks. This is Sully's summary of Jackson
1879t, pp.328–329. In the original Jackson cited Spencer's '*Psychology* I., p.162', which must refer to Spencer 1870,
but I find nothing similar at the cited page, nor is it found in Spencer's (1870) section §162, pp.354–357. In the
latter Spencer discussed the 'survival of the fittest' in regard to 'increasingly complicated impressions' and their
'increasingly complicated actions'.
　Also in the original (Jackson 1879t, p.329), Jackson made an important statement about cerebral dominance: 'in
one of the cases to be presently mentioned . . . there was left hemiplegia, and thus the inference is irresistible that
his speechlessness was caused by damage to the right half of his brain. But as he was a left-handed man, his case is
an exception proving the rule. It is admitted that there are cases of left-hemiplegia with aphasia in persons who are
not left-handed.'
[221] See Perrin 1993, pp.969–970, and Chapter 4. Jackson was using 'survival of the fittest' at the psychical
level in relation to survival of words in the process of comprehension. The phrase brings to mind a late twentieth-
century effort to apply Darwinian mechanisms to neurophysiological events; see Edelman (1987) on '*The Theory
of Neuronal Group Selection*'. Jackson (Jackson 1881s, p.400) again anticipated Edelman in 1881, when he said, 'The
survival of the fittest is the law both of healthy and of morbid mentation and of the concomitant cerebration'. For
further on Edelman see Raitiere 2012, p.234, footnote 58.
[222] Jackson used 'survival' of images with better definition in Jackson 1879u, pp.410–411.
[223] See Jackson 1879t, pp.328–329; and Jackson 1879v, p.410.
[224] Jackson 1880e, p.255; this is Sully's summary of Jackson 1879t, pp.330–332.

done before it is actually done . . . Before I put out my arm voluntarily I must have a "dream" of the hand as being already put out.[225]

This is a theoretical approximation to a phenomenon that is now called 'motor planning'. It is evidenced by preparatory signaling from cortical cells upstream from the primary motor cortices, before the actual movement begins.[226] Of course, Jackson could not foresee the details of twentieth-century neuroscience. He was still analyzing the implications of Ferrier's work for his own paradigm, especially with regard to seizures and epilepsy.

The Harveian Lectures 'On the Diagnosis of Epilepsy', January–February 1879

The above discussion of aphasia took us to October 1879. Now we must go back to January–February 1879, when Jackson delivered the annual tripartite Harveian Lectures, 'On the diagnosis of epilepsy', at the Harveian Society of London.[227] Like the Medical Society of London, the Harveian Society was founded to serve the needs of physicians in a particular geographic area of London. Its original name in 1831 was Western London Medical Society.[228] Among its founders was Marshall Hall, who was its second President.[229] 'In 1875 the Society was in a position to institute and endow the Harveian Society Lecture (or Harveian Lecture), to consist of two or three lectures, to be delivered annually . . .'[230]

Jackson used this occasion to tackle the long-festering issue of 'genuine' epilepsy, but first there were some preliminaries. In order to integrate generalized seizures into his paradigm he began by discussing some details of that framework, most of which we have already encountered. However, there were some new elements. After he reviewed his conception of the discharging lesion, he added: 'We must not forget the resistance offered to local discharges in our consideration of their effects. The "discharging lesion" may be likened to a fulminate which overcomes the resistance of less stable compounds.*'[231] 'Resistance' here is an analogy, 'likened' to a chemical process; Jackson was not proposing that the actual mechanism of neural resistance is strictly chemical. In April 1877, discussing the cerebellum, he had postulated resistances between neural centers as requisite parts of normal function.[232] Here, in January 1879, he inserted that concept into the pathophysiology of seizures when he said,

---

[225] Jackson 1879t, pp.348–349; my underlining. Jackson gave no direct citation of Spencer, and I have not found the corresponding section in Spencer's *Psychology*.

[226] See Krakauer and Ghez 2000.

[227] For my analysis I have used the version in the *BMJ* (Jackson 1879c, Jackson 1879f, Jackson 1879g). Other versions were in *The Lancet* (Jackson 1879b, Jackson 1879e, Jackson 1879i) and in the *Medical Times and Gazette* (Jackson 1879a, Jackson 1879d, Jackson 1879h, Jackson 1879j). These Harveian Lectures are not to be confused with the Harveian Oration of the Royal College of Physicians, which began in 1656.

[228] Bailey 1895, vol.2, p.100.

[229] 'The Harveian Society of London', *BMJ* 2:449, 1919.

[230] www.harveiansocietyoflondon.btck.co.uk/history, accessed October 25, 2013. Since 1903, only one lecture has been given annually. Since 1951 the Harveian Society's rooms have been in Lettsom House, with the Medical Society of London.

[231] Jackson 1879c, p.33. In Jackson 1884d, p.660, Jackson used 'physiological fulminate' as an analogy to a chemical reaction, but not as an actual explanation of a nerve cell's discharge. In the asterisked footnote he said (Jackson 1879c, p.33): 'The importance of considering resistances in our estimation of the consequences of nervous discharges in diseases of man . . . was . . . first stated in a methodical way by Sydney Ringer.' This is the Ringer (1836–1910) of 'Ringer's physiological solution'. Jackson gave no citation for Ringer's statement, and I have not found it (November 2013). For biographies of Ringer see Brown 1955, pp.186–187, and Orchard 2004.

[232] In Jackson 1877g, Jackson said: 'if some centres could not overcome the resistance of others – discharge them by their discharges – there would be no association of operations . . .'

'there are degrees of paroxysms of each kind, depending on the degree of the discharge of this or that part of the cortex, and on how much resistance it can overcome.'[233]

Classification and the Epilepsies, January 1879

Another relatively new feature in Jackson's first Harveian Lecture was a change of emphasis in his view of classification. He said that 'scientific or theoretical classification, whilst of value in extending and simplifying our knowledge, is worthless for practical purposes.'[234] In practice, 'we require quite a different classification from the scientific one, or rather we must have a mere arrangement; we must have types, not definitions, and consider cases presented as they approach this or that type.' He mentioned Moxon and [Charles] Handfield Jones (1819–1890), and then he continued: 'The clinical or empirical types are only the most frequently occurring cases; there is really no such thing as "genuine" or "real" epilepsy, or "epilepsy proper", except in this arbitrary sense.'[235] While thus denying the scientific reality of 'epilepsy proper', he went on to define its place in practical nosology.

The following is the first division in our empirical or clinical arrangement of cases of epilepsy. There are two types:

1. Epilepsy proper
2. Epileptiform seizures.

Partly in order to show that I do not advocate absolute separation of clinical from scientific investigation, but only the temporary separation, I will consider several broad differences and resemblances betwixt the two divisions of cases from a scientific as well as an empirical standpoint.[236]

'Epilepsy Proper' and the Anatomy of the 'Three Levels', January 1879

Following the above passage, Jackson compared 'epilepsy proper' with 'epileptiform seizures' in six clinical and pathophysiological categories. The first was *'As to Affection of consciousness'*, where he said: 'The distinction is ... that consciousness is lost at first, or very soon, in the paroxysm of epilepsy proper, and late or not at all in the epileptiform seizures.'[237]

His terms 'epilepsy proper' and 'epileptiform seizures' are largely synonymous with our current categories of 'generalized' and 'focal' seizures, albeit with some ambiguity about the boundary between them. Beyond his definition, we have already seen most of the phenomena that he described. In one category, however, we find advancing clarity of a concept that Walshe called Jackson's 'Hierarchy of Levels in the Nervous System'.[238] Among Jackson

---

[233] Jackson 1879c, p.33.

[234] Jackson 1879c, p.33. This passage continued: 'To arrange migraine along with ordinary epileptic seizures – with cases of loss of consciousness and convulsion – for practical purposes, would be ... absurd ...', but he still considered migraine to have the same cerebral pathophysiology as epileptic seizures.

[235] Jackson 1879c, p.33. On Moxon (1870) see Chapter 8. Jackson gave no citation for Handfield-Jones, but remarks of that kind are found in Jones 1870, pp.284–285.

[236] Jackson 1879c, p.34; Jackson's italics.

[237] Jackson 1879c, p.34; Jackson's italics.

[238] Walshe 1961, pp.127–128.

aficionados, this basic concept is commonly referred to as his 'three levels'. To understand its development in the 1870s, we need to go back a few years before 1879.

The idea of hierarchical levels within the cortices is inherent in Jackson's early evolutionary view of the nervous system, but Jackson began to give it anatomical specificity only after the advent of Ferrier's work of 1873–1874. In 1875, he speculated about a 'third centre' when he was working out his *xyz* theory.[239] In 1876 he defined the lowest and middle levels respectively as the 'corpus striatum, &c'. and 'Hitzig and Ferrier's [cortical] Region'. At that time he referred repeatedly to the 'highest centres', and he used the expression 're-re-representation'.[240] But he did not define the anatomy of the third level, so it is not surprising to find that in 1876 he complained that he had 'been misunderstood to believe that all epilepsies are owing to discharging lesions in Hitzig and Ferrier's region. I never believed the "genuine" epilepsy of authorities – that is, epilepsy beginning with loss of consciousness – to be owing to discharging lesions in this region'.[241]

In 1879, on the other hand, Jackson was straightforward about the anatomy. The lowest *cerebral* centers are subcortical, i.e., the striata and the thalami, and

> ... *As to Seat of Changes* ... [epileptiform seizure] depends on disease in some part of Hitzig and Ferrier's region ... [epilepsy proper] – this is <u>hypothetical</u> – on disease in some part in front of that region, or behind Ferrier's sensory region; that is, on disease in some part of what I suggest are the highest cerebral centres. The so-called motor and sensory regions are only ... middle motor and middle sensory cerebral centres; the parts in front of the middle motor centres being the highest motor centres; those behind the middle sensory [being] the highest sensory centres.[242]

Thus the primary cortical motor and sensory regions are in the middle level, while the highest motor regions are prefrontal, and the highest sensory region is parieto-occipital, posterior to the primary cortical sensory region. Hence, the 'movements of both sides of the body ... are re-re-represented in the highest cerebral motor centres ...'[243] In genuine epilepsy, then, the discharging lesion is in the highest centers, although he acknowledged that this idea was 'hypothetical'. That said, in the remainder of his lectures he proposed to 'consider only epilepsy proper—what most nosologists call genuine, or idiopathic, epilepsy. I exclude the epileptiform seizures ...'[244] Of course, Jackson's comparative method would not allow strict exclusion of all references to epileptiform seizures. He noted especially that

> Charcot and others have added very greatly to our knowledge of the anatomy and physiology of the brain, by their discoveries of the cortical origin of monoplegias corresponding to monospasms. Their researches merit the highest of all praise, that of introducing method, by a kind of work which can be rated highly as clinical, or physiological, or anatomical, or pathological.[245]

---

[239] Jackson 1875l, p.421; see also Chapter 8.
[240] Jackson 1876v, pp.292, 297–298; see also Chapter 8.
[241] Jackson 1876v, p.299.
[242] Jackson 1879c, p.34; Jackson's italics, my square brackets and underlining.
[243] Jackson 1876v, p.298.
[244] Jackson 1879c, p.34.
[245] Jackson 1879c, p.34. Charcot began his lectures on cerebral localization in 1875; see Goetz et al. 1995, pp.120–127. Guillain 1959, pp.123–124, summarizes the conclusions of Charcot and Pitres on monoplegia as of 1883.

Parsing 'Epilepsy Proper' and the Pathophysiology of '*le petit mal*', January 1879

When Jackson took up the problem of 'epilepsy proper' he immediately narrowed his focus:

> ... we now divide epilepsy proper ... because there are degrees of affection of conscious-
> ness and degrees of spasm, the division must be not only arbitrary but rough ... It is into
> slight and severe, or, using French names, into *le petit mal* and *le grand mal* – freely trans-
> latable as "little fit" and "big fit" ...
>   By the expression severe, we mean those cases in which there is very much spasm and
> often universal convulsion with tongue-biting. I exclude those cases.[246]

Jackson's use of *petit mal* was more inclusive than ours, but it was consistent with general
usage at the time. In 'little fit[s]' he saw an opportunity for fruitful analysis, which is reminiscent of his detailed attention to epileptiform seizures in the 1860s. Similarly, here he gave
petit mal a pathophysiology that could account for its clinical variability.

> ... discharge in the highest cerebral centres has ... to overcome the resistance of the middle
> cerebral centres before it can produce peripheral effects (spasm, etc.) If there be such a
> thing as epileptic loss of consciousness without any peripheral manifestations, I suppose
> the explanation is that the effects of the discharge are limited to the highest centres; the
> currents developed by the primary discharge of some part of the highest centres pass by lat-
> eral or integrating lines to other collateral parts of the highest centres and discharge them.
> This is equivalent to saying that the currents developed, whilst strong enough to overcome
> the resistance of collateral parts of the highest centres, are not strong enough to overcome
> the resistance of, that is to discharge, the middle cerebral centres.[247]

In fact, pure loss of consciousness in generalized epilepsy, without any 'peripheral manifestations', is uncommon. In using this phrase Jackson was referring to the frequency of
seemingly minor, focal symptoms, i.e., 'slight cases [of] sudden and transient loss of consciousness, closely followed or accompanied by but little spasm and that of small muscles,
such as is signified by pallor of the face (spasm of facial arteries), slight spasm of the eyes,
hands, etc.'.[248] Moreover, about 'epilepsy proper', in general

> ... we say that it is a paroxysmal loss of consciousness. That is only a statement from the
> psychical side ... We have, speaking of the physical side, to add that there is with the loss of
> consciousness more or less spasm of muscles (including in that expression spasm of mus-
> cular coats of arteries and the like), or equivalent effects of cortical discharges.[249]

Shades of Brown-Séquard! Jackson's remarks about 'arteries' are references to the vasomotor
nerves, which in 1852 were shown by Brown-Séquard to control arterial contraction.[250] That
basic idea played a prominent role in Jackson's *Suggestions* of 1863, where he also interpreted

---

[246] Jackson 1879c, p.35; Jackson's italics, my underlining.
[247] Jackson 1879c, p.35; my underlining.
[248] Jackson 1879c, p.35; Jackson's parentheses, my square brackets.
[249] Jackson 1879c, p.34; on p.35 he added: 'Instead of saying "small muscles", we should ... say "parts, the
movements of which require little force for the displacements they have to effect"'.
[250] See Chapter 3.

'pallor of the face' as an epileptic phenomenon.[251] In 1879, still following Brown-Séquard, he thought that epileptic discharges can spread to the vasomotor system, thus explaining the facial pallor and other autonomic phenomena. In the quotation immediately above, 'equivalent effects' means direct cortical discharge of the facial muscles, as compared to discharge through vasomotor innervation of their arterial supply.

The importance of Jackson's ideas about these ephemeral epileptic phenomena will be apparent when we get to his treatment of the 'dreamy state' in his third Harveian Lecture. In that same regard, his first Lecture also contained remarks about the facial appearance in *petit mal*.

> There is a kind of spasm which is not obvious … A loss of expression is essentially an unvarying expression … the so-called "vacant look" in a slight seizure may signify slight even-spread facial spasm, admitting that it may also signify relaxation of the facial muscles … It is important to notice these expressions; for possibly they will help us to account for the "form" of the actions which in some cases follow seizures.[252]

Thus, in 1879 Jackson considered the 'vacant look' to be an ictal phenomenon, and he proposed the same for the 'epigastric sensation' that is often reported by epileptics.

> It is well known that a common pre-cursor of affection of consciousness in a paroxysm of epilepsy proper (slight or severe fits) is a strange sensation at or near to the epigastrium … patients tell us that, for months before they had any affection of consciousness preceded by an epigastric sensation, they occasionally had that sensation alone … This … would be a … subtype of epilepsy; it would be for a time all [there is of] the paroxysm.[253]

Harveian Lecture II: Ephemeral 'Peripheral Effects of the Central Discharge', January 1879

Jackson's second Harveian Lecture was largely devoted to classifying the 'visible or inferable peripheral effects of the central discharge'. He did this at great length, and I will discuss only a few of his details, beginning with his definitions.

> Visible effects of the discharge are spasms. [In contrast,] Such an effect … as that the salivary glands secrete in excess is inferred from witnessing flow of saliva … We infer that the bladder contracts from finding that the patient has passed urine. There is a large and important class of inferable effects, from … the discharges; these are "crude sensations" … Of course, any sensation, healthy or morbid, is only to be called peripheral in the sense that it is referred to the periphery …[254]

Thus, 'visible effects' are motor actions or other observable phenomena, whereas, 'With regard to all "crude sensations", we can, since … they are psychical states, only translate what

---

[251] Jackson 1863a, pp.10, 44, 47.
[252] Jackson 1879c, p.35.
[253] Jackson 1879c, p.36; Jackson's parentheses, my square brackets.
[254] Jackson 1879f, p.109; my square brackets.

the patient tells us into physical conditions'.[255] Continuing his effort to provide hierarchical clinical categories he said:

> We divide the peripheral effects of epileptic discharges into three rough groups ... speaking ... only of slight fits ... (1) Affection of Animal parts; (2) affection of Organic parts. Then under each we consider (a) what we see, viz., spasms or equivalent effects of central discharge; (b) what we infer from the patient's statement about his crude sensations before he loses consciousness.[256]

Jackson's use of 'Animal' and 'Organic' was consistent with contemporary usage. A medical dictionary said, 'Most animals have the power of locomotion ...'[257] And 'organic' was defined as: 'Relating ... to beings possessed of organs. Hence Organic Functions are those possessed by both animals and vegetables.'[258] Finally, the third of Jackson's 'rough groups' was *Common to both Animal and Organic*. In a seeming paradox, his definition of '*Affections of Parts serving in Animal Functions*' involved 'those parts directly concerned in the most intellectual operations and most voluntary actions'. Exemplifying '*Affections of Parts serving in Organic Functions*' he listed autonomic phenomena, and in both 'Animal' and 'Organic' categories he gave examples of 'Crude Sensations'.[259] Ultimately, his supposedly practical distinctions of 'Animal' versus 'Organic' did not enter his neurological paradigm.[260] My purpose in discussing them is partly to show a 'blind alley' in his attempt at an empirical classification, and partly to provide background for a particular point in his reasoning.

> In these lectures, we deal with cases in which there is little more than loss of consciousness ... it is in these very cases that the slight symptoms ... are not only those referable to animal parts, but also symptoms referable to organic parts, as pallor of the face, flow of saliva, slowing and stoppage of the pulse. With either set of symptoms there may be stoppage of respiration, with little spasm of the limbs ... these facts show that <u>organic as well as animal parts of the body are represented in the cerebrum</u> ... in the very highest of the cerebral centres ... how would anyone set about explaining what occurs physically during the emotional manifestations of fear, joy, etc., unless he assumed that the organic parts are represented in the highest centres?[261]

Jackson's conclusion that animal parts and organic parts are both represented in the highest centres does not necessarily mean that he thought there are direct efferent connections from the cortices to the target structures in the periphery. Remember that he did not have the logic of the neuron theory, and he still thought that primary motor cortex connects to the periphery largely through relays in the striatum. Nor did he offer any speculation about the nature of these connections. He simply assumed that they exist. Indeed, he said, even organs such as the liver are represented in the cerebrum. It follows that sometimes symptoms that would ordinarily arise directly from those organs are actually cerebral in

---

[255] Jackson 1879f, p.109.
[256] Jackson 1879f, p.109.
[257] Dunglison 1874, p.57.
[258] Dunglison 1874, p.732.
[259] Jackson 1879f, p.109; Jackson's italics.
[260] Jackson did use 'Animal' and 'Organic' again in Jackson 1890e, p.765, where he equated 'animal' with 'voluntary'; see also Jackson 1895c, p.476, and Chapter 12.
[261] Jackson 1879f, p.110; my underlining.

origin, either epileptic or due to some other disturbances of brain tissue.[262] Finally, at the end of his Lecture II he reminded his audience that the 'morbid anatomy' of epilepsy was unknown.[263]

Harveian Lecture III: Further Analysis of the Dreamy State, February 1879

Jackson's third Harveian Lecture[264] was devoted to his advancing analysis of the 'dreamy state'—a subject that has attracted attention from numerous commentators.[265] When thinking about the dreamy state historically we must try to forget its modern association with the medial temporal lobe. He began to localize the dreamy state to the 'uncinate' (medial temporal) region only in the late 1880s. Here, in 1879, he was analyzing it within his category of generalized epilepsy 'proper'. In the previous lectures, he said, he had

> ... spoken of negative mental states in slight epileptic seizures. We said the patient had in, and also after, his attacks defect of consciousness, or loss of consciousness. But occasionally there is also an exactly opposite mental state, a positive one ... A patient seized with a slight fit suddenly becomes vague as to his present surroundings, and at the very same time, or in instant sequence, he has a "dreamy" feeling, often of some apparently former surroundings. This double mental state helps the diagnosis of slight seizures greatly.[266]

Continuing his effort to provide a clinical nosology, Jackson observed that:

> ... sometimes there is no "dreamy state," but there are actions; there is an "epileptic somnambulism" as well as an "epileptic dream" ...
> We have, then, two divisions of positive conditions in or after slight fits of epilepsy proper:
> 1. "Dreamy" states without actions;
> 2. Actions more or less elaborate ...
> There is a distinction betwixt the two classes* ... The rule is that the patient, in the cases under the first division ["without actions"], remembers his positive mental state – remembers his dream – or ... we should know nothing about it, there being nothing ... from which to infer it ... But when a patient does anything in or after his fits, he remembers no mental state during his actions, nor does he remember what he has done.[267]

So we can know about a patient's dreamy state from the patient's memory only if it occurs without any outward action on his part. If there are accompanying behaviors of any sophistication, we can see those actions, but the patient has no memory of them. In the asterisked footnote Jackson explained that this conclusion was derived from his conception

---

[262] Jackson 1879f, pp.110–111. He cited examples and similar etiologic statements from Trousseau and from Théodore Herpin (1799–1865). On Herpin see Eadie 2002; also Temkin 1971, pp.324–327, 391–392.

[263] Jackson 1879f, p.111.

[264] My arbitrary dating of this Lecture to February 1879 is based on its publication date of February 1 (Jackson 1879g); presumably the actual presentation was a few days or weeks earlier.

[265] See e.g. Hogan and Kaiboriboon 2003; Lardreau 2011; and indices in Temkin 1971, Dewhurst 1982, and Critchley and Critchley 1998.

[266] Jackson 1879g, p.141.

[267] Jackson 1879g, p.141; my square brackets.

of the pathophysiology of the observable actions in the dreamy state, which are release phenomena.

> * In no case do I believe it possible that elaborate states ("dreamy" states, "actions," or "movements,") can occur from an *epileptic* discharge; I believe all elaborate positive states ... arise during an increased energising of centres permitted by removal of control of higher centres ... In the case [of a patient with dreamy state] mentioned [above] in the text, we note that ... the patient had defect of <u>object-consciousness</u> (negative) and (positively) increase of <u>subject consciousness</u>; in another way of stating it, he had loss of function of the now-organising nervous arrangements and increased function of the earlier organised.[268]

In the last few sentences of his third Harveian Lecture, Jackson expanded the same conception.

> In no case can we suppose the "dreamy state" to be a symptom of the same order as the crude sensation which may go along with it; for the crude sensation attends the epileptic discharge; the dreamy state is infinitely too elaborate to have such causation. It is supposed to be owing to "loss of control," and possibly may depend on rise in activity of the <u>opposite hemisphere</u>.[269]

In these two quotations Jackson raised issues that were central topics in a series of papers that he published in the Fall of the same year. In that later series he discussed subject consciousness and object consciousness at length, remaining consistent with his theory that the neurological bases of those functions are in the right and left hemispheres respectively.

'Psychology and the Nervous System', September–November 1879

In September–November 1879 Jackson published a treatise on 'Psychology and the Nervous System' in five installments in the *Medical Press and Circular* (*MPC*).[270] Its title was exactly the same as that of his unsigned editorial of 1875,[271] and some of its contents were similar but much expanded. In truth, Jackson's title in 1879 was a misnomer. The treatise would be more accurately characterized as 'Psychophysical Parallelism and the Brain'.

Another problem with Jackson's title concerns the meaning of 'psychology'. He was using it as Spencer and we moderns would use it—to mean the *scientific* study of mental phenomena, which Spencer and Bain had begun in 1855.[272] However, in Dunglison's dictionary of 1874, 'Psychology' was defined as 'A treatise on the intellectual and moral faculties or sphere. Also the intellectual and moral faculties or sphere'.[273] Thus, Dunglison's primary definition was that of a piece of philosophical writing on those faculties. His secondary definition referred

---

[268] Jackson 1879g, p.141; Jackson's italics and parentheses, my square brackets and underlining.
[269] Jackson 1879g, p.143; my underlining.
[270] Jackson 1879q, Jackson 1879r, Jackson 1879s, Jackson 1879u, and Jackson 1879v. Recall that the publisher of the *MPC* was Albert Tindall's Baillière, Tindall & Cox, who had apparently been the intended publisher for Jackson's never-completed monograph on epilepsy in 1874–1876; see Chapter 8. Here again there may have been thoughts of another book, but nothing came of it; see Jackson 1879u, p.410, where Jackson used the phrase 'in this book'.
[271] [Jackson]1875b.
[272] See in Chapter 4 on Bain 1855 and Spencer 1855.
[273] Dunglison 1874, p.862.

to mental activities, but not specifically to the science that studies them. Dunglison's definition was representative of how 'psychology' was used by most of Jackson's contemporaries,
but he was trying to make a larger point about dualistic assumptions and parallelism.

First Three Installments: Issues Around Psycho-Physical Parallelism, September–October 1879

My initial impression on reading Jackson's first installment was that, for some reason, he
suddenly felt the need to defend himself against charges of materialism—and I was right.
There was widespread concern about scientific materialism throughout the 1870s, such that
even Huxley backed off from any hard position on it.[274] Since Jackson's work dealt with concepts of mental functions, which could involve immateriality, he apparently thought it best
to be careful. I noted above in this chapter that in 1878 he declared victory in the struggle to
repudiate the old faculty psychology, which had allowed such entities as 'Will' and 'Memory'
in physiological discourse.[275] Here, in his series on 'Psychology and the Nervous System', he
was trying to demonstrate the widespread acceptance of parallelism, which could be interpreted as a way to deal with materialism.

> In a scientific investigation of nervous diseases, it is essential to keep distinct psychology
> and the anatomy and physiology of the nerve [*sic*] systems. In epilepsy it is imperative.
> I have been misled by not having seen the distinctness of physical (nervous) states and
> psychical states in my earlier studies, and thus I feel bold to point out the evil results of the
> confusion of the two things.[276]

Before he explained the 'evil results', Jackson defined 'parallelism' twice in the same paragraph.

> The psychical and the physical states occur in parallelism, one does not change into the
> other. Two things are said: (1) psychical states are utterly different from physical states; (2)
> physical states always go along with psychical states. [And again,] There are two series of
> states: (1) an immaterial series, psychical [and] (2) a material series, physical; the latter are
> active states of nerve structures; that is, liberations of energy or discharges.[277]

Within his definition of parallelism, Jackson claimed that all 'properly educated' people are
materialists in a narrow sense, but not to the extent of denying mental experience.

> No properly educated person denies that along with every sort or degree of psychical state
> there is a corresponding physical state. We are all thoroughgoing materialists in that sense.
> "Within the limits of our experience no one supposes that thinking is done without a body.
> No philosopher of any school whatever, theological or scientific, maintains ... that there is
> such a thing as consciousness without brain. None will assert that ... we have any experi-
> ence of psychical manifestation apart from physical structure."[278]

---

[274] See Smith 2013, pp.5, 24–25.
[275] Jackson 1878g.
[276] Jackson 1879q, p.199; Jackson's parentheses, my square brackets.
[277] Jackson 1879q, p.199; Jackson's parentheses; my square brackets.
[278] Jackson 1879q, p.200. For the quotation in the quotation, Jackson cited '(Fiske, "Cosmic Philosophy"
vol.2, pp.436–437)'; it is found there in Fiske 1874.

The source of the quotation within this quotation was the American philosopher-historian John Fiske (1842–1901), whose *Outlines of Cosmic Philosophy* was *Based on the Doctrine of Evolution*. Fiske's enthusiastic version of evolution contained elements from both Darwin and Spencer, but he has been described primarily as a 'Harvard Spencerian – without-port-folio'.[279] He was the first of 14 authorities who Jackson quoted to support his position on the prevalence of parallelism. As usual with any controversial subject, Jackson himself claimed the middle ground between extreme materialism and rigid theology.

> From the names of the authorities cited, the reader will see that the matter has simply nothing to do with "orthodoxy" in any way … Some theologians seem to think the un-orthodox *must* be materialists, and on the other hand some materialists think that the in-sistence on the distinctness of the psychical and physical arises from a desire to uphold the theological systems of the day. Both fail to see that the question is a scientific one, or if the *nature* of the relation be a question, a problem in metaphysics; it has no necessary con-nection with theology … It is commonly supposed that those who hold the Doctrine of Evolution are materialists. This is a great mistake.[280]

Jackson's comments on theology and theologians are noteworthy, because he had not pre-viously said anything about those subjects in print. Clearly, however, he had been thinking about them. In 1879 the tenor of the times had changed from the mid-century. Science was ascendant but not really triumphant. When Jackson did broach theology he followed his usual practice of marshaling a thick pile of evidence, often from seemingly miscellaneous sources. Thus, his first two installments consisted largely of quotations from his authorities. All of them were supposedly in favour of parallelism, but there were no theologians. In order of appearance, and using Jackson's spellings, they were:[281]

Fiske	Ferrier
Spencer	Huxley
Sir William Hamilton	Du Bois Reymond
J.S. Mill	Tyndall
Clifford[282]	Herman[283]
Max Müller	Laycock
Bain	Lewes

The nationalities in this list are interesting. There were eleven subjects of Her Majesty, two Germans, and one American,[284] which leaves out the French. Since Jackson knew the French biomedical literature, this is a striking omission, but there is a likely explanation. Most of the French 'authorities' still adhered to the faculty psychology, so probably their opinions did

---

[279] Werth 2009, p.109. For further on Fiske see Werth 2009, pp.109–113.

[280] Jackson 1879q, p.200; Jackson's italics.

[281] For some of the quotations Jackson provided only the author's names, with no citations (e.g., Hamilton), and others were copied from publications by other authors (e.g., Max Müller from Spencer, Bain from Ferrier, Tyndall from Lewes).

[282] Presumably this is the mathematician and philosopher William Kingdom Clifford, who coined the term for his concept 'Mind-Stuff'; see Turner 1993, p.275.

[283] Martin N. Raitiere (2012, p.231, note 19) thinks that Herman is probably the physiologist Ludimar Hermann (1838–1914), and I agree, given Jackson's approach to German spelling.

[284] The American is Fiske; the Germans are Du Bois Reymond and Hermann. The originally German phil-ologist Max Müller was in the Queen's realm, at Oxford.

not support Jackson's argument. Suffice it to say that Jackson thought the listed names bolstered his opinion, and my reading of them is largely consistent with his purpose—as far as they go and given that they were only excerpts. Only Lewes might be questioned, because he could be characterized as a monist. Obviously Jackson thought that his friend was not disqualified on that account. Lewes had died in November 1878, after Jackson had published his accommodation with him a few years earlier, and Jackson did so again in this series.[285]

In the last part of his second installment, Jackson addressed four 'particular errors' committed, he said, by those who objected to his parallelism. In describing the first of those errors, he pointed to a common tendency.

> ... (1) We may very easily suppose ourselves to take a materialistic view of mind, and yet follow the psychological method to all intents and purposes ... To speak of mental states as being nervous states, to consider cerebral centres as being ideational, perceptive, and so forth ... is neither materialism nor psychology, but simply a mixture of both. To "solidify the mind," to talk of the brain as if it were a kind of mind made up of cells and fibres ... does not go far enough for medical purposes ...
>
> Ignoring the distinction betwixt physical and psychological states leads to ignoring anatomy and physiology of the higher parts of the nervous system ... [286]

To think in sensori-motor terms, he said, it is necessary to resist three further errors in the ordinary way of thinking.

> (2) It is very widely assumed that sensory nerves and centres are alone engaged during ideation or sensation, but it is very plain that a movement element also is represented in the substrata of tactual and visual images.
>
> (3) Active states of sensory (afferent) nerves and centres are often spoken of as if they were sensations ... the term Sensation (really the name of a psychical state) is of the same derivation as Sensory, [which] ... fosters the confusion that an active state of a sensory nerve or centre (a state of body) is a sensation (a state of mind) ...
>
> (4) Whilst nearly every body admits ideas (images) and sensations are psychical states, having correlative nervous states, it is taken for granted that movements ... have no psychical side. But ... there is a psychical side to movements ... a word is a psychical movement.[287]

While Hughlings Jackson was exhorting his readers to keep the above clearly in mind, I submit that he had powers of concentration which most of us don't enjoy. He could go back and forth across the psycho-physical boundary and keep track of where he was, but for most of us those tracks are very hard to follow. Indeed, he admitted that it took him years to learn to keep the boundary constantly clear in his own mind. Introducing his third installment, he said, 'I can illustrate the confusion very well from my own writings'.[288] Then he offered five self-incriminating examples, of which I will mention the first and the third. His first example came from his paper on 'Physiology of Language' at the British Association in 1868.[289] His mistake, he said, had been his use of 'the expression "psychical movements".'

---

[285] Jackson addressed the problem of monism and Lewes' relation to it in Jackson 1879s, p.284.
[286] Jackson 1879r, p.240. Jackson did not give a specific citation for 'solidify the mind'.
[287] Jackson 1879r, p.240; Jackson's parentheses, my square brackets.
[288] Jackson 1879s, p.283.
[289] Jackson 1868o, discussed extensively in Chapter 5.

For his third example he gave a long quotation from his 'Study' of 1870. Into it he now inserted additional words in square brackets to clarify the psychical–physical distinction: 'But of what "substance" can the [organ of] mind be composed ...'[290] Since there were many of these instances, Jackson asserted that his confessions gave him license to critique similar mistakes by others. 'These samples are enough to illustrate my blunders and leave me free to criticise such blunders more generally'.[291] 'More generally' is exactly how he did it—without mentioning names. The one exception was Lewes.

> ... for the sake of argument, let us grant ... that psychical states and nervous states *are* one and the same thing ... Lewes holds that view, but as a physician, I say nothing critical of his opinion, because he takes the other steps which medical inquiry demands; he studies not only psychology, but gives ... an account of what he considers to be the physical nature of the nervous states which he believes to be only another aspect of psychical states ...[292]

In effect, Jackson's definition of mind would require *ongoing* investigation of the neurological functions that accompany parallel mental states. Such a requirement was consistent with the positivist idea of progress, which was starting to be questioned among the Victorians,[293] but Jackson kept the faith.

> *To give a materialistic or morphological explanation of mental states is not to give an anatomical one.* Suppose that for clinical purposes it matters nothing whether we believe (1) that conscious states are parallel with active states of nerve fibres and cells, the nature of the association being unknown, or (2) that mental states and nervous states are the very same thing [Lewes], or (3) whether we believe that there is a soul acting through a mere mechanism. I wish to insist that to hold any one of these beliefs does not one whit justify us in omitting anatomy. Betwixt our morphology of the nervous system and our psychology there must be an anatomy and a physiology.[294]

Now we might ask, wouldn't such research on either side of the psycho-physical boundary be reductionistic? Jackson had already acknowledged this when he said at the outset, 'We are all thoroughgoing materialists' in day-to-day practice.[295] In his further elucidation of common errors involving the mind-body problem, he said the 'distinction betwixt the psychical and physical states is not a merely theoretical one ... its non-recognition, or if there be no such distinction its non-separation by artifice, leads to medical errors'.[296] In fact, errors in neurological diagnoses in the 1870s would have been largely theoretical, insofar as they would have involved incorrect science with little impact on therapeutics. This situation was illustrated by the contents of Jackson's fourth and fifth installments, which dealt mainly with his conceptions of 'Subjective' and 'Objective' as applied to ideation and perception. He had first discussed these ideas in 1876, when one of his purposes was to analyze loss of consciousness in seizures.

---

[290] Both examples are stated in Jackson 1879s, p.283; Jackson's square brackets.
[291] Jackson 1879s, p.284.
[292] Jackson 1879s, p.284.
[293] See Newsome 1997, pp.172–177.
[294] Jackson 1879s, p.284; Jackson's italics and parentheses, my square brackets.
[295] Jackson 1879q, p.200.
[296] Jackson 1879s, p.284.

Installments 4 and 5: Further Development of Subjective and Objective, November 1879

In Chapter 8, I quoted Harrington's statement about Jackson's idiosyncratic use of '*subject* and *object* consciousness'. In common usage at the time, she says, 'subject consciousness corresponded to introspection' and 'object consciousness' was 'directed outward'.[297] At the beginning of his fourth installment Jackson remarked that the terms were used 'variously'.

> Sometimes the term subjective is used for psychical states, and the term objective for the correlative physical states. Under this use of the terms colour is subjective, the correlative discharge in the visual centres is objective.
>
> Occasionally, however, the term subjective is used for a psychical state when the corresponding physical changes are centrally initiated, and the term objective for a psychical state when the corresponding changes in the centre are peripherally initiated. Under this use of the term when we think of colour (coloured thing) there is a subjective state; when we see a colour there is an objective state.[298]

These characterizations correspond to Harrington's assessment, but then Jackson went on to a further critique.

> ... it would almost seem to be held by some that when we think of a thing (ideation) there is a psychical change only, and that when we see it (perception) there is a physical change only. In each case there is both. The difference betwixt the two is only one of degree. The psychical state in the former [ideation] is faint, in the latter [perception] vivid. The physical state during the former is a slight nervous discharge, in the latter a strong nervous discharge.[299]

When Jackson then introduced his own definitions for subjective and objective, he was simultaneously apologetic and independent-minded.

> I hope no one will suppose that I imagine myself to be capable of declaring the right way in which these two venerable terms should be used. I am only about to state the way in which I shall use them ... Much of what follows is hypothetical. I should not venture on the inquiry were it not that I think we must study delirium, epilepsy, &c., on a deeper basis ...[300]

So his 'venture on the inquiry' was driven, as usual, by the pragmatism of the clinical. At this point in his exposition, when he defined subjective and objective, he was working explicitly on the psychical side of the mind-brain divide.

> I use them both as psychical terms. A subjective state is one which is the psychical side of what is physically the influence of the environment on the organism. The fuller definition

---

[297] Harrington 1987, p.228; her italics.

[298] Jackson 1879u, p.409. A similar statement is found in Jackson 1880j, pp.195–196, concluding with 'all mental action is a rhythm of subjective and objective states'.

[299] Jackson 1879u, p.409; Jackson's parentheses, my square brackets. This shows the continuing legacy of the associationist tradition in Jackson's thought, because 'faint' and 'vivid' are fundamental concepts in it; see Definition Section 7 in Chapter 5.

[300] Jackson 1879u, pp.409–410.

is to say that a subjective state is the psychical side, not only of the effect of the present environment on us, but of that in relation to the whole of what we are from past organisations of such effects, individually and racially. <u>Subjective states are in their totality subject consciousness</u>.

On the other hand, the term objective is used for the psychical side of the present reaction of the organism on the environment, and for that in relation to all possibilities of reaction, which we have organised individually and racially. <u>Objective states are in their totality objective consciousness</u>.[301]

Now here is a problem. Jackson has just said that he was using subjective and objective as psychical terms, but 3 years earlier, in 1876, he had given neurological bases to subject and object consciousness, as cartooned in Fig. 8.1. Was he now (in 1879) restricting subjective and objective to the psychical sphere? Trying to be helpful, he went on to say:

So, then, the two terms are not used as psychically corresponding to what are materially (1) organism and (2) environment, but as corresponding to (1) organism as affected by, and (2) organism as reacting on, the environment. As psychical states both are states of our minds; the two <u>corresponding physical states</u> are states of our bodies ... How it is that we got the notion of there being two separate things in relation, organism and environment, I do not inquire.[302]

Based on the underlined part of the above passage, I conclude that Jackson changed his usage of subjective and objective between 1876 and 1879. *By the later date he restricted those terms to the realm of the psychical.* This is confirmed in a footnote where he was writing about the neural basis of integration: 'The two kinds of [physical] organisation correspond to what on the psychical side are objective and subjective.'[303] So our analysis can proceed with this conclusion confirmed, but even then it's not straightforward.

Nothing justifies us in using the term subjective at one time as a name for psychical states, and thus in contrast to states of the nervous system and [the] rest of the organism, which latter states are then called objective; and at another time for mind, in contrast to the environment, which latter is then called objective.

The division just made is plainly too abrupt: there is no such absolute chopping in two. Let us approach the consideration of this admission by first trying to show what we do *not* mean by the two terms, subjective and objective.

The difference betwixt ideation and perception is not what we mean by the difference betwixt subjectivity and objectivity. Let us see how ideation and perception differ [from subjective and objective].[304]

301 Jackson 1879u, p.410; my underlining. Some help in understanding this difficult part of Jackson's thought is found in C.U.M. Smith 1982a, and in Harrington 1987, pp.226–234, 254–262. However, those analyses are without strict chronological discipline, so Jackson's definitions could have changed in the interval from one of his papers to another, and they did.
302 Jackson 1879u, p.410; my underlining.
303 Jackson 1879v, p.429.
304 Jackson 1879u, p.410; my square brackets.

Ideation and Perception: The Parallel Neurology of Subjective and Objective, November 1879

From this point on, *Jackson viewed ideation and perception as the physical sides of subjective and objective.* Physiologically, he said, there is resistance in the lower centers to the constant assaults from the higher, which is, in effect, a Darwinian mechanism.

> The resistance offered by the lower centres, to discharges beginning in the highest, is the physical side of effort, the basis of our knowledge of the difference betwixt ideation and perception. When it is not overcome there is ideation, when it is overcome ideation passes into perception.[305]

And those assaults on the lower centers are the products of prior, unconscious (preconscious) processes in the higher centers. In his further discussion, we get a sense of how he conceived the brain's normal operations.

> When ... we say that an image comes into our mind spontaneously, we mean that, being alive, something is always going on in our nervous system, and correspondingly in our minds. The so-called spontaneous image is a survival of the fittest image of the moment during conflicting energisings of all nervous arrangements which have been already organised in us. It is evidently the same when the conflict is aroused by a presented object.[306]

Here Jackson was going back and forth between the psychical and the physical, from one sentence to the next. In the final installment of 'Psychology and the nervous system', he did it habitually. There he elaborated on 'further differences betwixt ideation and perception'. Briefly, he said: 'the greater the ideation, the less the perception; the greater the perception, the less the ideation'.[307] Since ideation and perception were physical concepts, he could offer a 'speculation' about their neurological mechanisms.

> The highest centres being most differentiated will be those with most numerous "cross," or "lateral," lines of integration. When nervous discharges of parts of the highest centres are slight, as during ideation, they will only be able to overcome the resistances to discharge other parts of the highest centres, but not able to overcome the resistance of subordinate centres ... Wide[ly] spreading discharges throughout the highest centres are the physical side of association ... When discharges of the highest centres are strong, they will be able to overcome the resistance of ... the subordinate centres. When discharged the lower centres are *then* lines of least resistance; the currents will then "flow" more downwards, and less laterally; and thus the ideation ... will be less, and the perception ... greater.[308]

---

[305] Jackson 1879u, p.410.
[306] Jackson 1879u, p.411.
[307] Jackson 1879v, p.429. In the process he remarked parenthetically that, 'We think not only by the Association but by the Dissociation of ideas'.
[308] Jackson 1879v, p.429; Jackson's italics, my square brackets.

Invoking those speculations about spreading discharges was a way for Jackson to transition to the clinical data of epilepsy.

> I speak of the seizures that begin with loss of consciousness, or in which consciousness ceases very early, and mostly after a "warning" ... It is very common for the patient to have the slight attacks called *le petit mal* long before he has *le grand mal* ... he does not, the rule is, become subject to *le grand mal* by having seizures of intermittent degrees of severity. I believe that in the stage of *le petit mal* the discharges are nearly confined to the highest centres, and that when the big fit comes they have become strong enough to overcome the resistance of the subordinate centres.[309]

One of the epileptic phenomena that most interested Jackson, of course, was the 'dreamy state'. After the above he said:

> In some cases of slight epilepsy the patient has during the ceasing of object consciousness (or when he is simply forgetting what he is doing and where he is) an increase of subject consciousness (or simply ideas rise up in his mind ... of what has been [previously] organised in him). Now he remembers this "dream," or at any rate, [he] remembers that he did dream. In some cases of epilepsy, after the paroxysm, the patient acts; if so, the rule is, that he does not remember anything of the actions.[310]

On the psychical side Jackson was trying to understand the 'dreamy state' as a reversion from objective to subjective consciousness. On the physical side, he was saying that the patient in the dreamy state performs physical actions when the resistance of the lower centers is overcome.[311] Psychically, the dreamy state is a form of 'morbid mentation', which was a broader subject that he addressed briefly in terms of subjective and objective states.[312] He continued to pursue his analysis of the dreamy state throughout the 1880s, largely in relation to his evolving ideas about dissolution, but early in that decade most of his attention was on more tangible clinical problems.

---

[309] Jackson 1879v, pp.429–430; Jackson's italics.
[310] Jackson 1879v, p.430; Jackson's parentheses, my square brackets.
[311] Jackson 1879v, p.430.
[312] Jackson 1879v, p.430.

10

The Neurological Examination, the Epilepsies, an International Platform, and Dissolution, 1880–1884

In this chapter we move into the 1880s, when the earlier optimism of the mid-century Victorians was challenged by a more critical, darker view of life. Some of this was associated with the middle and upper classes' discomfort with their own prosperity, which was partly related to the 'progress' of the Industrial Revolution. On the other hand, as we've seen, the society's increasing secularism was important for Jackson and his colleagues,[1] because it freed them from the theological constraints of earlier decades. By and large, religion could no longer impose limits on scientific discourse—at least not overtly.[2] Jackson's outlook was upbeat. In 1884 he said, 'The doctrine of Evolution daily gains new adherents. It is not simply synonymous with Darwinism. Herbert Spencer applies it to all orders of phenomena.'[3]

On the physical side of the environment in the 1880s, the effects of the Industrial Revolution had been transformative for half a century.[4] Movement of people and goods was revolutionized by increasingly efficient steam engines in ships and railroads, although horses remained the primary source of power for intra-city transportation until the advent of the internal combustion engine in the early twentieth century. Without actually moving people or paper, communication was transformed by the increasing sophistication of the telegraph in the 1830s and 1840s. The first cross-channel cable to the continent was laid in 1850, and the first successful transatlantic cable was achieved in 1866.[5] Correspondence could then be transmitted over great distances in seconds or minutes rather than days or weeks.

Syphilis and Neurosyphilis in Victorian Medicine, *circa* 1880

By the 1880s, medicine was also perceived to be making rapid progress. The most spectacular evidence was the work of Louis Pasteur on bacteria in the 1860s and 1870s, which established the basic mechanism of contagious diseases. Those scourges had bedeviled people for millennia, and now they appeared to be coming within human control. Tuberculosis (TB) and syphilis were among the chronic conditions that were begging to be understood, so one of the most heralded achievements of modern medicine was Koch's demonstration of the

---

[1] On 'George Eliot and secularism' see During 2013.
[2] For a nuanced view of this relationship see Stanley 2014, especially pp.253–254.
[3] Jackson 1884b, p.591.
[4] See Bowler 1989, p.1: 'By the time Victoria came to the throne in 1837 the railways had begun to spread across the landscape'.
[5] www.submarinecablesystems.com/default.asp.pg-History, Accessed December 25, 2013.

tubercle bacillus in 1882.[6] Solid intracranial tubercles were among the foreign bodies that Jackson sometimes encountered during autopsies, but TB was a less prominent concern for neurology in his time.[7]

Syphilis, on the other hand, was a pervasive problem because of its devastating neurological symptoms.[8] It was separated from gonorrhea in 1837 by Philippe Ricord, who defined its three stages in 1838. However, its causative agent, the protozoan spirochete, *Treponema pallidum*, was not found until 1905. The first two stages of syphilis (primary and secondary) occur within a few months of exposure. They are manifested largely on the body's surface, but the tertiary stage usually occurs years or decades later. It can include the severe neurological symptoms of meningoencephalitis in general paresis (general paralysis of the insane) and/or tabes dorsalis, which latter was known clinically for many decades as 'locomotor ataxy'. A particularly distressing symptom associated with tabes is the phenomenon of 'lightning' pains—brief but terrible, lancinating pains in the legs, due to lesions in the spinal cord.[9]

The main pathological finding in tabes is degeneration of the dorsal (posterior) columns of the spinal cord—fiber tracts which carry afferent sensations of position and vibration to the brainstem. However, the same abnormality can be found in other, nonsyphilitic conditions, so dorsal column degeneration is a necessary but insufficient condition to make the diagnosis of tabes and tertiary syphilis. In 1875 Alfred Fournier (1832–1914) began to demonstrate the syphilitic etiology of tabes, and in 1879 he did the same for general paresis, but there was no universal agreement about the syphilitic etiology of either condition until the turn of the twentieth century.[10] Duchenne was also a leader in making the connection for tabes; he had distinguished it from Friedreich's ataxia in 1858.[11] On the other hand, Charcot and Vulpian did not connect tabes to syphilis; Charcot thought it was hereditary.[12] In the process of sorting out these issues, the participants added an important component to the modern neurological examination.

Toward the Modern Neurological Examination, 1880–1882

In the last decades of the nineteenth century neurology was one of the more exciting subspecialities of medicine—led by Charcot et al. at the Salpêtrière, and by the luminaries at the National Hospital. How much had changed is appreciated by contrasting Romberg's *Manual of the Nervous Diseases of Man* of 1853 with Gowers' *Manual of Diseases of the Nervous System* of 1886–1888. Both were popular in their days. To the modern neurologist, Romberg's strict separation of everything into 'Neuroses of Sensibility' and 'Neuroses of Motility' seems contrived, whereas the nosological arrangement in Gowers is familiar, even if its contents are old-fashioned. The growing technology that nourished this change was the development of the modern neurological examination ('neuro exam'), including ophthalmoscopy, because it enabled the search for focal lesions in living patients. Our standardized neuro exam began to

---

[6] The historical background in this and the next paragraph is based largely on Bynum et al. 2006, pp.123–132 ('Bacteriology') and pp.175–188 ('Three chronic conditions'). Porter 1997 is another useful source.

[7] Neurotuberculosis could be associated with aphasia and epilepsy; see Shafi 2015.

[8] For a description of 'Syphilis and the nervous system' in the work of Gowers see Scott et al. 2012, pp.123–129.

[9] But Jackson (1881v, p.140) cautioned, 'The pains called lightning may occur in cases which are not tabetic; they are only signs of disease of the posterior root zone ...'

[10] See Quétel 1990, pp.134–136, 162–164.

[11] See Adams in Haymaker, p.433; and Koehler et al. 2000, pp.316–320.

[12] See Goetz et al. 1995, pp.108–113.

take shape in the 1870s; by 1880 its form was clearly discernible.[13] In that light we can begin to understand a group of Jackson's papers whose titles would otherwise seem strange.

Jackson's Friend, Thomas Buzzard, and Deep Tendon Reflexes, 1880–1882

In *Brain* between July 1878 and October 1882, Jackson published a series of seven pieces that reviewed previous publications by his friend, Thomas Buzzard.[14] That kind of survey was common in medical publications, which often filled their pages with notices of interesting contributions from the literature. What is curious is the personal element in Jackson's titles. They all began with 'Buzzard on ...' I think the 'Buzzard papers' can be understood as the result of a combination of factors—personal, but also professional, technical, and scientific.

In Chapter 9 we saw that Jackson had an especially close relationship with Buzzard and his family. The two men first became acquainted at Queen Square in the 1860s, when Buzzard was working as a reporter for *The Lancet*. He was appointed to the staff in 1867.[15] According to Ferrier, 'Hughlings Jackson was the most intimate' of Buzzard's friends. Moreover, Buzzard had professional qualities that would have appealed to Jackson.

> Clinical work was Buzzard's forte, and nothing was more noteworthy than the laborious care with which he observed and recorded his patients' symptoms and the effects of treatment ... Not only in professional matters, but in affairs in general, Buzzard was a man of great caution and sound judgement, and was regarded by his colleagues of the National as the 'Nestor' of the staff.[16]

More to the present point, it was Buzzard who introduced Jackson to the patellar ('knee jerk') and Achilles ('ankle jerk') reflexes, and thus to the phenomena of deep tendon reflexes. The knee jerk was probably known to laymen as a curiosity for a long time,[17] but Wilhelm Heinrich Erb (1840–1921) and Carl Friedrich Otto Westphal (1833–1890), separately, brought it into medical practice in 1875.[18] Buzzard and Grainger Stewart (1837–1900) then introduced the knee jerk into British medicine in 1878.[19] In 1880 Jackson said:

> We owe a debt of gratitude to Westphal and Erb for their discovery of its significance, and for further researches on the matter to Grainger Stewart, Buzzard, Russell, Byrom

---

[13] This generalization is based on my survey of Louis 2002, and Fine and Darkhabani 2010; for Charcot it is supported by Goetz et al. 1995, pp.137–149.

[14] Jackson 1878c, Jackson 1880k, Jackson 1881c, Jackson 1881m, Jackson 1881n, Jackson 1881o, Jackson 1882h.

[15] See [T. Buzzard] 1919, Obituary; and Holmes 1954, p.96. Buzzard trained at King's College and graduated M.D. in 1860. He served on the Committee of Management of King's College Hospital, and he was elected a Fellow of King's College in 1880, but apparently he did not practice at the Hospital; see Lyle 1935, pp.68, 76–77.

[16] Ferrier in Buzzard Obituary 1919; Ferrier's 'symptoms' included the findings by examination. In Greek mythology, Nestor was the wise king of Pylos. Jackson was called 'the Nestor of English Neurology' when he received an L.L.D. at Edinburgh in 1905 (Critchley and Critchley 1998, p.185); see also Purves-Stewart 1939, p.41.

[17] In 1881 (Jackson 1881v, p.143) Jackson said, 'Every schoolboy knows, to use a favourite expression from Macaulay, that smart tapping just below the knee makes the leg jump up'.

[18] See Louis 2002. Their contributions were simultaneous but independent. For short translations from their original German publications see Clarke and O'Malley 1996, pp.355–359.

[19] McHenry (1969, p.349) says: 'The examination of the reflexes was introduced into British neurology in 1878 ...' The same statement is made in [Stewart] 1900, p.356. This chronology of the deep tendon reflexes puts the dates of their dissemination by Buzzard and Stewart earlier than those given by Louis 2002 or by Fine and Darkhabani 2010.

Bramwell, and Gowers; and here I gladly acknowledge that I have learned much about this symptom directly from my colleague, Dr. Buzzard...[20]

Buzzard's contribution was made in two nearly simultaneous publications in two different journals. In *The Lancet* of July 27 and August 10, 1878, he published 'Clinical lectures on some points in the diagnosis of [dorsal column] spinal sclerosis' where he described how he elicited both reflexes. The paper included drawings of an examiner doing the test without a reflex hammer.[21] Buzzard's other publication was in the first volume of *Brain*, dated July 1878, 'On a prolonged first stage of tabes dorsalis: amaurosis, lightning pains, recurrent herpes; not ataxia; absence of patellar tendon reflexes'.[22] There Buzzard referred to Westphal's hope that 'the test may prove useful in the early stage of tabes, before there is any ataxia'. Buzzard reported that, 'In all the cases of confirmed tabes in which I have used this test since I became acquainted with Dr. Westphal's suggestion, I have found ... that the knee-phenomenon was absent'.[23]

Jackson's second 'Buzzard paper' reviewed three of Buzzard's lectures that had been published in *The Lancet*, January–May 1880. His title was 'Buzzard on certain points in tabes dorsalis'.[24] The clinical problem was to differentiate tabes from other similar conditions, because they felt they had to treat syphilis suspects with potassium iodide and mercury.[25] What they really wanted, of course, was a reliably pathognomic sign of tabes.[26] Although deep tendon reflexes disappointed those hopes, they soon turned out to have wider utility.

In light of Buzzard's publications in 1878, it is reasonable to assume that Jackson started to use the knee jerk and the ankle jerk at that time. However, he published no report about it until 2 years later. In October 1880 he described a 22-year-old woman who was a remarkable 'Case of recovery from organic brain-disease'. Her only residuals were '*Anosmia and Absence of Patellar Tendon-Reflex*'.[27] Of course, the knee jerk is helpful toward localization only if its normal anatomy and physiology are understood. Concerning this patient, Jackson thought it was

... very likely that this woman's posterior columns are diseased ... at any rate, there must be some break in the loop betwixt her patellar tendon and her quadriceps; for as a certain kind

[20] Jackson 1880m, p.655; this paper contains the same case report as in Jackson 1881aa. Gowers' contribution is discussed in Fine and Darkhabani 2010, pp.222–223; and in Scott et al. 2012, pp.100–102,137–138,148–149. I have not investigated Russell or Bramwell.

[21] Buzzard 1878–1879; my square brackets. Buzzard's 'spinal sclerosis' referred to degeneration of the dorsal columns of the spinal cord seen in tertiary syphilis.

[22] Buzzard 1878a.

[23] Buzzard 1878a, pp.168–169. Jackson would have known Buzzard's modest monograph on *Clinical Aspects of Syphilitic Nervous Affections* (Buzzard 1874). Jackson's life-long interest in syphilis can be traced to Hutchinson, who had been studying congenital syphilis since 1853. Hutchinson's monograph of 1863 established his reputation on the subject; see Wales 1963, p.72.

[24] Jackson 1880k, dated July 1880, which reviewed Buzzard 1880. Jackson's first Buzzard paper was on blepharospasm; it contained nothing of compelling historical significance.

[25] See Jackson 1880i, and Jackson 1880m, p.656: 'I never run the risk of not using either the iodide of potassium or mercury, or both.'

[26] Jackson 1880k, p.268; Jackson recorded that Buzzard referred to a patient 'he had seen in private, in whom the absence of the reflex was the only symptom in addition to optic atrophy. There could be no doubt ... that these were cases of tabes dorsalis as yet in a restricted form.'

[27] Jackson 1880m, p.654; Jackson's italics. Gowers was using the knee jerk at least as early as 1879 (see Scott et al. 2012, pp.137–138).

of reflex action is absent, there must be a flaw in at least some one of the parts subserving it – tendon, afferent nerve, centre, efferent nerve, or muscle to be moved.[28]

In this statement about the reflex arc of the knee jerk, Jackson was agreeing with Erb's (correct) interpretation of the phenomenon's pathophysiology. Westphal, on the other hand, thought the knee jerk is simply due to sudden mechanical stretching of the quadriceps muscle.[29] Either interpretation could be generalized to reactions in other muscles or reflex arcs, but Erb's is more useful physiologically, because a local muscle reaction would not tell us much about the status of the attached nervous system. In his review of 'Buzzard on tendon reflex in the diagnosis of diseases of the spinal cord' in 1881, Jackson said that Buzzard's 'paper is a contribution to the arguments which the clinical facts afford in favour of the reflex mechanism of the phenomena.'[30]

Jackson was especially pleased when Buzzard defined a new deep tendon reflex in November 1880. He explained that Buzzard had a case which suggested 'the ingenious and original idea of comparing the tendon reflex in a muscle on each side of the face'. Buzzard realized that there could be a reflex arc through the brainstem, with the fifth cranial (trigeminal) nerve being the afferent part and the seventh (facial) cranial nerve being the efferent component. To test this arc he found that he could cause contraction of the zygomaticus major muscle by striking its tendinous origin on the malar bone.[31] The jaw jerk is now attributed to the masseter muscle, rather than the smaller zygomaticus major, and there are various techniques for eliciting it. Buzzard was the first to describe it, at least in Britain.[32] Doubtless it was this kind of thoughtful ingenuity that Jackson found so attractive in his friend.

Buzzard's influence is also seen in a report that Jackson published on February 12, 1881, 'On a case of temporary left hemiplegia, with foot-clonus and exaggerated knee-phenomenon, after an epileptic seizure beginning in the left foot'.[33] The patient was a 35-year-old man who 'came into one of my upstair rooms at ten o'clock, Sunday, January 16, 1881'.[34] He had previously experienced three focal seizures, beginning in November 1880. The first two had generalized to loss of consciousness. Within minutes of his arrival he had a fourth, which Jackson observed. The patient 'referred the sensation at the onset of each of his seizures to the outer side of the ball of the left big toe'. The motor march began with toe

[28] Jackson 1880m, p.655.

[29] In Jackson 1880o, p.968, Jackson said that the 'theory' of the 'patellar tendon-reflex' is 'much disputed and not accepted by the discoverer of the symptom'. He used 'Westphal's symptom' to mean 'absence of the knee phenomenon'. The reflex arc theory was accepted definitively by Gowers, when he introduced our current concepts of 'upper' and 'lower segments'; see Louis 2002, p.387; also York 2002, pp.371–373.

[30] Jackson 1881o, p.280.

[31] Jackson 1881o, pp.281–282; my square brackets. In the paper cited by Jackson, Buzzard (1880, dated 'Nov. 27, 1880', p.843) said of the jaw jerk, 'It occurred to me a few days ago …', so he was probably referring to late October or early November 1880.

[32] Fine and Darkhabani (2010, pp.223–224) discuss various reports of the jaw jerk in the mid-1880s.

[33] Jackson 1881a; it was actually published *after* Jackson 1881b, because Jackson referred to Jackson 1881a in Jackson 1881b, p.185. York and Steinberg 2006, p.97, give the date of '12 Jan 81' for Jackson 1881a, but the publication itself says 'Feb. 12, 1881'. The case was reported at the Harveian Society of London on February 3 or February 5; the former date is given in Jackson 1881a, p.183, footnote (a), and the latter in Jackson 1881d (published 'Feb. 26, 1881'). Jackson 1881d is a summary of Jackson's report, which says that after Jackson's paper, 'Dr. Ferrier and Dr. Buzzard spoke', and Jackson replied. I have used Jackson 1881a, which Jackson said (p.183, footnote (a)) was 'printed with additions'.

[34] Jackson 1881a, pp.183–184. After the seizure, the patient left at noon, but it required the help of Jackson and a servant to get him into a cab. Jackson then visited him at 'a quarter past four'. This was ordinary for managing a private patient. Cushing observed that, 'As is usual in English houses apparently … an M.D.'s waiting room is his dining room …' (Fulton 1946, p.164).

flexion and spread up the leg. Jackson was unsure about involvement of the left arm because, 'I had not only to make scientific observations, but to look after my patient'. Indeed, 'We talked together every now and then during it; there was no affection of consciousness'. The entire seizure 'lasted about eight or ten minutes'.[35]

The main point of Jackson's paper was to describe the reflex findings during postictal weakness. When the patient was in that state, Jackson said that he *'easily obtained foot clonus on the left side; the knee jerk on that side was very greatly exaggerated. There was no right-foot clonus … The clonus (left) was not at all like the spasm in the fit … the knee jerk on the right side was hard to get.'*[36] When Jackson saw the patient at 4:15 PM, 'His knee jerks were equal, easily obtained, and I believe normal. I refrained from trying for foot clonus, thinking it possible that another fit might be started.' Two days later, the patient's 'Patellar tendon reflex … was equal and normal … no foot clonus… I stupidly omitted to test deep reflexes of arms'.[37]

So how to account for the exaggerated reflexes in the postictally paralyzed leg—during but not after its paralysis? Using his comparative method, Jackson contrasted it to the pathophysiology of hemiplegia due to stroke. In the latter, when hemiplegia persists there is permanent rigidity and hyperreflexia, which is attributed to 'lateral sclerosis', i.e., to deterioration of the motor fibers from the cerebrum to the spinal cord. In that situation there is persisting hyperflexia because the controlling influence of the brain through the upper segmental fibers is eliminated. Analogously, while there is temporary exhaustion of the fibers in the postictal state, the deep tendon reflexes are exaggerated due to loss of inhibitory cerebral control. When the fibers recover, the reflexes return to normal.[38] With our neuron theory, we now attribute most of the mischief to exhausted neuronal cell bodies, but Jackson's basic idea is still valid.

Finally, when Buzzard published a book-length collection of *Clinical Lectures on Diseases of the Nervous System* in 1882, Jackson wrote an effusive review of the book and its author.

> The able work Dr. Buzzard has done in Neurology is so well known that it is not necessary to write an ordinary review of the contents of this volume. He has achieved a position such that a reviewer's praise or blame is to him of little import … we believe the book to be one of the most valuable contributions to the diagnosis and treatment of diseases of the nervous system we know of …[39]

A bit overwrought, eh! The book consists of 25 lectures, most published previously. Among the prominent subjects were tendon reflexes, tabes, other manifestations of neurosyphilis, and Charcot joints. As Buzzard said in his Preface, his book was not meant to be a full presentation of the entirety of neurological nosology.[40] Although Jackson's inflated view of Buzzard's contributions has not been perpetuated, in his own time 'Buzzard gradually obtained a very leading position as a consultant in neurology in London'.[41] I have emphasized

---

[35] Jackson 1881a, p.184.

[36] Jackson 1881a, p.184; Jackson's italics. Clonus is 'a rapid series of rhythmic contractions maintained for the duration of the stretch' (Nolte 2002, p.460), i.e., a form of hyperreflexia. Ankle clonus was known to Brown-Séquard in 1858, and Charcot understood that it has the same pathophysiological significance as hyperreflexia; see Mettler and Mettler 1947, p.590.

[37] Jackson 1881a, p.185. Jackson also mentioned this case in his Croonian Lecture II (Jackson 1884d, p.661); autopsy in 1882 (Jackson 1884l) revealed a 'gliomatous tumour' in the right frontal lobe.

[38] Jackson 1881a, p.186.

[39] Jackson 1882h, p.382.

[40] Buzzard 1882, pp.v–vi; see Gowers 1886–1888.

[41] [T. Buzzard] 1919. Obituary.

Jackson's relationship with Thomas Buzzard because it has not been explored in any depth,[42] and it was important to Jackson personally and professionally.

Ophthalmology, Ophthalmoscopy, and the Neuro Exam, 1880–1881

Another subject that was important to Jackson was ophthalmology. In Chapter 2 we saw that he was probably exposed to it as a medical student in York, and he was active in that field from his earliest years in London.[43] During 1881–1894, 20% of his papers had ophthalmological titles,[44] and he continued to publish on ophthalmology until 2 years before his death in 1911.[45] In 1885 Jackson gave the Ophthalmological Society's Bowman Lecture,[46] and he presented the Society's Presidential Address in 1889.[47] Here I will engage his ophthalmological work only where it served to shape his neurology. In fact, his contributions were essentially the same for both specialties: (1) routine use of the ophthalmoscope, including the problem of optic neuritis; and (2) the neurology of extra-ocular movements (EOMs).[48] He was especially concerned with EOMs in 1880 and with optic neuritis in 1881, so we'll start with EOMs.

Extra-Ocular Movements (EOMs), 1880–1881

Examination of EOMs has been an important part of the neuro exam since Jackson's time in the late nineteenth century.[49] Each EOM is innervated by a specific cranial nerve, which is therefore the efferent component of a reflex arc through the brainstem. So an isolated abnormality of the function of an EOM indicates the presence of a lesion somewhere along its reflex arc, but an abnormality of conjugate eye movements generally means that the responsible lesion is physiologically 'above' any individual arc. It was these complicated, suprasegmental abnormalities that Jackson and his colleagues were struggling to understand.

On the theme of diagnosing syphilitic tabes, Jackson read a paper on 'Eye symptoms in locomotor ataxy' at a meeting of the Ophthalmological Society on December 9, 1880.[50] The presentation contained nothing truly new, but it can be viewed as part of Jackson's continuing

---

[42] See Critchley and Critchley 1998, pp.48, 163.

[43] Jackson's first independent publication, outside of his medical reporting, was in the *Royal London Ophthalmic Hospital Reports* (*RLOHR*) of 1861 (Jackson 1861f). His first paper on 'The ophthalmoscope, as an aid to the study of diseases of the brain' followed in 1862 (Jackson 1862f).

[44] See York and Steinberg 2006, pp.97–126.

[45] Jackson 1909b is the last item in York and Steinberg's 2006 *Catalogue* (p.139). It was written with Leslie Paton (1872–1943), who was appointed Ophthalmic Surgeon to the National Hospital in 1907 (Holmes 1954, p.97).

[46] Jackson 1885e, Jackson 1885g, Jackson 1885h, Jackson 1885i, Jackson 1886h. On the history of the Society (founded 1880) and its Bowman Lecture see History in www.rcophth.ac.uk, accessed February 12, 2014. The professional circumstances of the Society's founding are explained in Casper 2014, pp.24, 30–37.

[47] Jackson 1889h, Jackson 1889i, Jackson 1889j, Jackson 1889l, Jackson 1890i.

[48] See Chance 1937, pp.282–283; Chance summarizes many details of the contributions in 89 of Jackson's publications with ophthalmological titles. See also Taylor 1915, pp.415–416.

[49] See Fine and Darkhabani 2010, pp.217–219.

[50] The texts in Jackson 1880o (*The Lancet*) and Jackson 1880p (*BMJ*) are essentially (not exactly) the same; Jackson 1881v is an expanded version, where Jackson said (p.140): 'for these cases "locomotor ataxy" is strictly a misnomer; tabes dorsalis is better, since it covers cases with and without abnormal gait. I, however, retain the term locomotor ataxy in the title, as the term tabes dorsalis is not yet commonly used in this country.' In 1883 (Jackson 1883b), commenting on a paper on tabes by Gowers, Jackson described the neuro-ophthalmological complexities in dizzying detail.

effort to flesh out the localization paradigm. In the process he utilized the data from 25 of his own cases to review and confirm information that was coming from many sources. For example, he referred to statements about lightning pains by Charcot, Pierret, and Buzzard,[51] and to the contribution of Argyll Robertson (in 1869) and a host of others regarding pupillary abnormalities,[52] which also involve reflex arcs through the brainstem.

Ophthalmoscopy and Optic Neuritis, March–April 1881

We've seen that Jackson began to advocate the routine use of the ophthalmoscope in the early 1860s.[53] Although he was soon joined in this effort by Clifford Allbutt,[54] they had not made much headway. By '1871 there was only a small number of physicians in the British Isles who did practice' ophthalmoscopy,[55] and the same was probably true for the rest of that decade. When the light source was a flame, the procedure required patience and skill, thus being a time-consuming nuisance. For Jackson and his small cadre of fellow devotees, that was simply in a day's work if the work were to be done properly. As they continued to promote the technique into the 1880s they were still trying to understand the pathogenesis and clinical connotations of optic neuritis. To all appearances—literally—it seemed to be a single entity, and yet some patients had normal vision, and others were severely impaired.

In March and April 1881, Jackson discussed optic neuritis in papers at the Ophthalmological Society. At the meeting of March 10, he delivered a paper 'On optic neuritis in intracranial disease'.[56] From his consulting physician's point of view, Jackson said, 'Optic neuritis interests me much as an important incident in many cases of intracranial disease, and comparatively little as an eye affection'.[57] Indeed, the most interesting part of his paper was subtitled 'Various Hypotheses as to the Mode of Production of Changes in the Optic Discs by Intra-cranial Adventitious Products'.[58] To explain optic neuritis as a single and/or double entity, there were many hypotheses, which Jackson summarized.

> Now comes the question, What is the secondary [pathogenetic] process? There is the hypothesis of Graefe that one variety of optic neuritis, or of swelling of the disc (*Stauungs-Papilla*) is produced by raised intracranial pressure – the "chocked disc" of Clifford Allbutt. It is … stated by Pagenstecher, who does not adopt it …[59]

---

[51] Jackson 1881v, p.140.

[52] Jackson 1881v, pp.146, 149; see also Fine and Darkhabani 2010, p.218. On third (oculo-motor) nerve lesions in tabetics see Jackson 1880o, p.969.

[53] See Chapter 6.

[54] The first edition of Allbutt 1871 was dedicated to Jackson; see Rolleston 1929, p.57.

[55] Chance 1937, p.269. Regarding Jackson's international influence, Chance (p.252) says, 'there are but few references to his writings in the accepted continental ophthalmological works'.

[56] Jackson 1881e and Jackson 1881f were the initial reports. Jackson 1881u was the delayed but definitive text, which I have used primarily. It included comments from the audience, which were summarized earlier in the *Medical Times and Gazette* of April 23 (Jackson 1881i).

[57] Jackson 1881u, p.60; in a footnote Jackson added: 'This paper is a brief *résumé* of what I have written on the subject during the last seventeen years. That sight may be good in cases of well-marked double optic neuritis I pointed out in 1865. This was first mentioned by Blessig.' There is no mention of R. Blessig in Jackson 1865g or Jackson 1865h. My only other information about him is his thesis at Dorpat (Tartu, Estonia) in 1855: *De retinae textura: disquisitionis microscopicae* (in Wellcome Library online catalogue, accessed May 7, 2014).

[58] Jackson 1881u, pp.85–92.

[59] Jackson 1881u, p.85; Jackson's parentheses, my square brackets. He also said (p.87): 'There is the hypothesis of Schmidt, which ascribes some cases of swollen disc to distension of the optic nerve sheaths.' Allbutt suggested 'choked disc' in place of 'stauungspapille' (Allbutt 1871); see Rolleston 1929, p.57. On the role of Albrecht von Graefe (1828–1870) see Lepore 1982, p.178, and Albert and Edwards 1996, pp.205–207. Assuming that 'Schmidt'

The theory that we now accept to explain papilledema, i.e., raised pressure in the optic nerve sheath secondary to raised intracranial pressure, was summarized and rejected by Jackson.[60] Instead, evincing Brown-Séquard's continuing influence, he thought that

> ... optic neuritis may be a doubly indirect result of local gross organic disease; that first there are changes of instability about the tumour; that next these lead on [to] discharges, by intermediation of vaso-motor nerves, to repeated contractions, with subsequent paralyses, of vessels of the optic nerves or centres, and thus, at length, to that trouble of nutrition that is optic neuritis ... in cases of epilepsy proper we see often ... effects produced by discharges on arteries and on viscera ...[61]

Although Jackson's paper was read on March 10, the Society's *Discussion on the relation between optic neuritis and intracranial disease* was scheduled for March 31.[62] At that later meeting, there were comments by Stephen Mackenzie (1844–1909) and many others. Buzzard agreed with Jackson,[63] and Hutchinson said, 'I am very glad that Dr. Jackson has spoken decisively as to the impossibility of drawing any definite line of distinction between the condition known as "choked disc" and other forms of neuritis, for I have myself regarded them as varying degrees of the same condition'.[64] On the other hand, Gowers said cogently, 'Is there ... any real ground for believing that inflammation at a distance from the source of irritation is ever produced by a reflex vaso-motor influence?'[65] From our standpoint, Gowers was on the right path, while Jackson was still searching for a single cause of the apparently similar funduscopic appearances. But Gowers said that sheath distension is probably the cause of *some cases* of optic neuritis.[66]

One of the major objectives that Jackson was pursuing through his interest in ophthalmology was a more accurate way to diagnose the existence and location of brain tumors. This concern can be seen in many parts of his Ophthalmological Society lecture of 1881,[67] and he was not alone. Ferrier and Gowers had similar motivations. The diagnosis of tumors was also part of Jackson's penchant to understand the localizing value of different kinds of seizures.

---

here is the same as 'Schmidt-Rimpler' in Jackson 1881u, p.106, Jackson was referring to Hermann Schmidt-Rimpler (1838–1915); see Morton 1961, p.521. (Ernst) Hermann Pagenstecher (1844–1832) of Wiesbaden, Germany, worked at Moorfields for a year and a half before he and Carl (Philipp) Genth (1844–1904) published their German–English *Atlas of the Pathological Anatomy of the Eyeball* in 1875, with the English translation by Gowers (Pagenstecher and Genth 1875). Albert and Edwards 1996, pp.82–83, state that cases were contributed to the *Atlas* by Bowman, Hutchinson, Jackson, and others.

[60] Jackson 1881u, p.87.
[61] Jackson 1881u, p.89; my square brackets.
[62] Jackson 1881u, pp.94–115. It was followed by two case presentations from Gowers.
[63] Jackson 1881u, pp.97–98.
[64] Jackson 1881u, pp.99–100.
[65] Jackson 1881u, p.105. In August 1881 (Jackson 1881y, p.610), regarding his 'acceptance of the vaso-motor hypothesis', Jackson said, 'I hold this hypothesis very loosely', since it was simply the 'most plausible' of the available theories.
[66] Jackson 1881u, p.106.
[67] See e.g. Jackson 1881u, pp.71–85.

Integrating the Pathophysiology of the Epilepsies and Dissolution, July 1880–November 1881

Integrating Genuine Epilepsy, Epileptiform Seizures, and the Dreamy State, July 1880

Our analysis of Jackson's ophthalmological interests has taken us into 1881, but now we must go back to July 1880, when he published an article 'On right or left-sided spasm at the onset of epileptic paroxysms, and on crude sensation warnings, and elaborate mental states'.[68] As the title implies, the paper contained a mixture of subjects, including: (1) genuine epilepsy, (2) unilateral hemispheric dominance (our term) for language and other functions, and (3) further analysis of the dreamy state, interpreted in accordance with his subjective/objective theory.

Jackson's article began with a clear distinction: 'In this paper I speak of the epilepsy of nosologists, sometimes called "genuine" epilepsy, or epilepsy proper. In this epilepsy consciousness is either lost first … or very early in the paroxysm.'[69] As far back as 1874 he had accepted the idea of genuine epilepsy as a nosological entity.[70] For both types he wanted to know the location of the unstable focus. Since he had already enjoyed considerable success in analyzing epileptiform seizures, he wanted to apply the same method of clinical analysis to genuine epilepsy.

> I think the time has come for recognising that many different epilepsies are grouped under one term epilepsy; we have come to recognise that at least several different epileptiform seizures are grouped under the term epileptiform … The seats of the "discharging lesion" must differ when there are … two different paroxysms. There are … as many different epilepsies as there are different warnings; the so-called warning … is the thing of most localising value … we should study – not the epilepsy of nosologists, but each different epilepsy as distinguished by its particular warning.[71]

As examples of his unifying approach, Jackson contrasted the auras of (1) vertigo with (2) epigastric sensations. Either could herald a generalized convulsion. Thus they could be part of genuine epilepsy, and their foci could be sought in the cortical localizations of those sensations. He also had a similar motivation in trying to understand dominance. In this regard, he promulgated a practical rule that is still clinically valid as a reasonable first assumption.

> Since most people are right-handed, the left cerebral hemisphere in most people represents the most objective movements, those movements for most specially operating on the environment. Moreover, speech is a process by which are symbolised relations of things in … the environment … or things considered objectively … the left cerebral hemisphere is in most people the one concerned during speech.[72]

---

[68] Jackson 1880j.
[69] Jackson 1880j, p.192.
[70] Jackson 1874jj, p.579.
[71] Jackson 1880j, p.193.
[72] Jackson 1880j, p.197.

Continuing on the same theme—differing localizations of dominance for different functions—Jackson considered auras to be subjective sensations. However, in examining some patients,

> It was a ... surprise to me to find evidence of left-sided spasm at the onset of convulsions with these "warnings." I used to think the more "subjective" of sensations were chiefly represented in the <u>posterior part of the left cerebral hemisphere</u>. The inference that they occur most often in cases when the first spasm is left-sided is from observations ... all of which cannot be certainly trusted, the reports of patients and their friends not being always to be relied on.[73]

The surprise was due to Jackson's earlier conceptualization of crude versus elaborate sensations in epilepsy.[74] He thought that crude auras are ictal phenomena, so they should have cortical foci. On the other hand, elaborate sensations like the dreamy state could not be localized, he said, because their behavioral complexity implies involvement of many brain areas at very high levels, so elaborate sensations are postictal release phenomena.[75] In the above quotation his statement about the 'posterior part of the left cerebral hemisphere' is a reference to his localization scheme for subject and object consciousness (Fig. 8.1). According to that scheme, crude sensations are forms of subject consciousness, localized in the left posterior brain region, but the occurrence of a crude aura with left-sided motor seizures implies a right-sided focus. Nonetheless, he was reluctant to alter or abandon his model unless the evidence was overwhelming, and it wasn't. This was partly because he had not personally observed a left-sided onset, and reports from families and friends are often incomplete.

When Jackson wrote about elaborate mental states in epilepsy in 1880 and beyond, he was usually referring to the dreamy state. He had addressed it in his papers on the diagnosis of epilepsy at the Harveian Society in February 1879[76] and in November 1879 he had applied his conception of subjective and objective to it.[77] Here, in July 1880, he was trying to figure out how the dreamy state—not localizable *per se*—might sometimes be triggered by events that could be localized.

> The elaborate mental state alluded to occurs sometimes without any crude sensation warning, but in some at least of these cases the first spasm or one-sided affection is [on the] left [body side]. In one case, with the dreamy state, the patient's head at the onset of every convulsion turned to the right. I was interested in finding that he was a left-handed man. This was the exception proving the rule.[78]

Despite the optimism in the end of this passage, Jackson was palpably frustrated by his inability to work out the principles of brain organization that ought to be revealed by localization of crude auras.

---

[73] Jackson 1880j, p.198, my underlining.
[74] Jackson 1880j, pp.198–200.
[75] This is my summary of Jackson 1880j, p.200.
[76] Jackson 1879g; see Chapter 9.
[77] Jackson 1879u.
[78] Jackson 1880j, p.200, my square brackets; see also Jackson 1880f. Head turning to the right can imply a left frontal focus, which would contradict his theoretical, subjective/objective localizations.

I doubt not that <u>there is some order throughout</u>, from the warning to the end of the post-paroxysmal stage. The above imperfect sketch, the best I can do, is the result of much labour, as a contribution towards discovering this order. I am far from asserting that I have done anything of value towards this end, and trust I have fairly acknowledged the difficulties and uncertainties necessary to investigations in which we have to trust so much to our patients [for critical information].[79]

Jackson felt thwarted because he was trying to use the initial auras of seizures with focal onsets to reason 'backwards' to an understanding of normal cortical organization for such sensations, and he could not make it work. Thus stymied, he turned to another aspect of epilepsy—its relation to dissolution.

Postictal (Todd's) Paralysis and Dissolution, January 1881

Jackson's growing attention to dissolution was signaled in January 1881 with a paper in *Brain*, 'On temporary paralysis after epileptiform and epileptic seizures: a contribution to the study of dissolution of the nervous system'.[80] At the outset he offered a defense of the word: 'The term Dissolution has long been used by Herbert Spencer as the opposite of Evolution ... Great objections are made to this application of the term, but I submit that it is inexpedient to coin a new word ... when Dissolution has been used for at least fifteen years ...' Actually, it had been 19 years since Spencer introduced 'dissolution' via a discussion in his *First Principles* of 1862.[81] In the second edition of 1867 he added a penultimate chapter on Dissolution, where he applied the concept to everything in the universe, including biological organisms.[82] Jackson's interest in the idea was engendered, or at least heightened, by his reading of Spencer's second edition,[83] which was published 14 years before Jackson's remark about 'fifteen years'.

Jackson's first published use of dissolution had occurred in an article of January 1873,[84] and he had expanded it in a paper of May 1873.[85] Up to 1881 he used it several times, generally in relation to specific clinical problems, such as drunkenness, mania, and insanity. And we have epistolary evidence that Spencer knew about Jackson's efforts with dissolution and agreed with them. On January 9, 1883, Spencer addressed a letter to his American admirer and factotum Edward Livingston Youmans (1821–1887).[86]

> I enclose some pages from the *Medical Times and Gazette* [6 Jan.], sent to me the other day by Dr. Hughlings Jackson. The initiative he made years ago by applying the doctrine of dissolution to interpretation of nervous diseases ... seems likely to lead to other results. The

[79] Jackson 1880j, p.206; my square brackets and underlining.
[80] Jackson 1881b; for its dating see above in this chapter (ftn 33).
[81] Spencer 1862/1864, pp.351–352.
[82] Spencer 1867a, pp.518–537. Despite Jackson's remark about 'Great objections', Spencer's friends and critics alike gave little attention to dissolution at the time, and it has attracted only limited discussion since; see Walshe 1961, pp.129–130. Perrin (1993, p.117) mentions dissolution in his summary of Spencer's sixth edition of *First Principles* (1904), but Francis' (2007) study of Spencer does not list dissolution in its index. Dissolution was mentioned briefly by Spencer in his *Autobiography* (1904, vol.1, pp.553, 554; and vol.2, p.168) and once in his *Life and Letters* (Duncan 1908/1911, p.227).
[83] See Jackson 1881h, p.330, where Jackson cited Spencer 1867a.
[84] Jackson 1873a, p.85; see also Chapter 7.
[85] Jackson 1873k, p.532.
[86] Youmans founded *Popular Science Monthly* in 1872, and Spencer wrote dozens of articles for it (Wikipedia, accessed July 25, 2019).

paper is very clearly and conclusively argued; and is to me just as much a revelation as that which Hughlings Jackson made of the doctrine.[87]

Clearly Spencer appreciated Jackson's use of dissolution. It is hard to know whether he had known about it before 1882, but such prior knowledge does seem likely. Now getting back to 1881, Jackson began his analysis of dissolution in relation to postictal motor paralysis with a summary of contemporary theories about the etiology of the paralysis. Then he explained his theory of a discharging lesion, using the example of a foreign body causing instability of adjacent brain cells.[88] One reason to expand his conception of dissolution, as applied to postictal paralysis, was to generalize the applicability of the idea as widely as possible. Another was a further effort to bring genuine epilepsy into the same etiologic framework as epileptiform seizures, by showing that they share a common pathophysiology.

> We have so far ... spoken only of epileptiform seizures. Logically, if Todd and Robertson's hypothesis is to be sustained, there ought to be paralysis after seizures of epilepsy proper. It would usually be said that there is none. So that whilst after the comparatively slight seizures called epileptiform, there is often decided paralysis, there is, according to current opinions, none after the much severer paroxysms of epilepsy proper ... But ... there is such a thing as paralysis spread all over the body. The patient, after a severe paroxysm of epilepsy proper ... is not hemiplegic. He is ... biplegic ... I mean that there is some ... paralysis of both sides of the body ...[89]

This passage is a good example of Jackson's ability to think about clinical phenomena in unconventional ways, and the same applies to his explanation of why others had missed the seemingly obvious.

> How does it happen that such paralysis is ignored? One reason ... is, that being slight, evenly spread, and transient ... it is not easily recognisable as paralysis. Another reason is, that ... abnormal physical conditions are erroneously "explained" as being owing to abnormal psychical states. After a very severe fit of epilepsy proper, the patient does not move his limbs ... As he is then comatose, it would generally be said that he does not move because he is unconscious ... this is an explanation which verbally explains everything, and yet in reality explains nothing.[90]

Such explanations, Jackson said, involve common 'psychologico-materialistic confusions'. Furthermore, 'It is ... inexpedient in a scientific exposition to attempt to explain physical conditions by invoking crude popular psychological doctrines'.[91] Using insanity as an

---

[87] Duncan 1908/1911, p.227. Concerning 'Medical Times and Gazette [6 Jan.]'. The bracketed date appears to be an erroneous insertion by the editor (Duncan), but the journal title may be Spencer's error, because the papers that Jackson sent to Spencer most likely were those published in the Medical Press and Circular on November 15 and 22, 1882 (Jackson 1882i, Jackson 1882j).

[88] None of this was new, but in the process Jackson theorized the existence of an epileptic phenomenon that we now call 'synchrony' or 'hypersynchrony' (Jackson 1881b, p.436; see Engel and Pedley 2008, vol.1, p.5). He said: 'the cells rendered unstable occasionally "explode" or liberate much energy, or ... discharge excessively, and all of them much more nearly simultaneously than the comparatively stable cells do in health'. Here, in a footnote (Jackson 1881b, p.436), Jackson also expanded his ideas about the role of 'small cells' in focal motor seizures; see Chapter 8.

[89] Jackson 1881b, pp.438–439.

[90] Jackson 1881b, p.439.

[91] Jackson 1881b, pp.439–440.

example, he asserted 'that in every case of insanity, however slight it may be, there is, so long as it lasts, defect[1] of consciousness.'[92] This statement required a definition of consciousness: 'A person has not got a consciousness in addition to will, memory, and emotion; these are only names applied to artificially distinguished aspects of consciousness; defective judgment, &c., is defect of consciousness.'[93] Neurologically,

> The highest centres are not consciousness, they are only the anatomical substrata of consciousness. Since the anatomical substrata of consciousness are … made up of sensorimotor arrangements, there should be wide-spread, however slight, paralysis in every case of insanity. I believe there is … Some of those who might deny there to be any in a case of insanity might nevertheless admit it by saying that there was loss of expression, shambling gait, and slowness of movement.[94]

So, according to Jackson the problem was related to the degree of the paralysis. In his 1874 editorial on 'reduction' due to intoxication, he defined 'three arbitrary degrees' of reduction (dissolution) in the postictal state, and he applied them to intoxication.[95] Here, in 1881, he repeated that grading system, with further definitions that are applicable to all forms of epilepsy.

> … there are many degrees of Dissolution consequent on exhaustion of different amounts effected by epileptic discharges of different degrees of severity … there is (1) post-epileptic "ideation;" (2) post-epileptic action (mania for example); and (3) post-epileptic coma … There is a negative and a positive element in each degree. Along with post-epileptic ideation there is – (*a*) defect of consciousness; with the post-epileptic actions, there is (*b*) loss of consciousness, and in the third degree there is (*c*) coma … the central condition being "shallow," "deep," and "deepest" exhaustion of nervous elements of the highest and perhaps also of lower centres.[96]

From these clinical considerations, he went on to a larger issue.

> … the psychological "explanation" is really no explanation of the comatose patient's immobility; [because] the explanation of a materialistic condition should be in materialistic terms … the <u>absolute distinction betwixt mind and body is insisted on</u> … *The distinction is made in order that we may be thoroughly materialistic in our dealings with disease*, and that we may methodically consider the nervous system from top to bottom as a mere sensori-motor mechanism.[1][97]

And Jackson's footnote 1 at the end took his argument again into the cultural debates about materialism.

> [1] Scientific materialism is quite a different thing from crude popular materialism. Scientific materialism distinguishes betwixt mind and nervous system in order to study each

---

[92] Jackson 1881b, p.441; Jackson's footnote 1 is explained below.
[93] Jackson 1881b, p.442.
[94] Jackson 1881b, p.442.
[95] Jackson 1874p, p.653; and see Chapter 8.
[96] Jackson 1881b, p.443, footnote 1. With regard to genuine seizures, Jackson (Jackson 1881b, p.444) said: 'Even after slight epileptic attacks (le petit mal) there is veritable paralysis; the patient is weak ("unfit for anything," "thoroughly done up" are the kind of expressions patients use).'
[97] Jackson 1881b, pp.444–445; Jackson's italics, my square brackets and underlining.

thoroughly ... Scientific materialism is only materialistic as to what is material, the nervous system. Popular crude materialism, making no distinctions, confuses two utterly different things, psychical states and physical states.[98]

Jackson first used the word 'materialistic' in print in 1875 in a privately printed pamphlet.[99] In 1879 he proffered his psychophysical parallelism as a defense against intimations of materialism—the material and the immaterial are parallel but never interacting phenomena.[100] Here, in 1881, he was relatively comfortable with the issue of materialism, but he was still struggling to understand the pathophysiology of seizure discharges. He knew that there are different seizure thresholds (our term, not Jackson's) among individuals and in different areas of brain. Beyond that, he said, the rate and range of discharge are also determinants of the clinical phenomena, because the same amount of energy may be distributed slowly or quickly and over larger or smaller amounts of tissue. Large amounts of energy distributed quickly over a large amount of tissue will result in generalized seizures and hence postictal generalized prostration.[101] True to his own advice about the utility of materialism, Jackson went on to a discussion of epileptic pathophysiology at the molecular level. But even as he tried to use the idea of 'force' he was unsure about its meaning.

> The more rapid short liberation ... of greater force ... will overcome greater resistances than currents of less force over a larger time from slow, lengthy liberation ... I do not use the term force as synonymous either with momentum or energy; it is, however, difficult for me to use the term force without misgivings, since ... it is a term used differently by different people ...
>
> The movements of external parts which any centre *most* specially represents are, physiologically speaking, those united to it by lines of *least* resistance.[102]

Jackson's thoughts about normal and abnormal physiology in January 1881 are background to his further analysis of the pathophysiology of dissolution, which he explored to great depths in a series of papers that began in April 1881.

Dissolution and Epilepsy in Another Unfinished Book: First Three Installments, April–July 1881

Jackson expanded his analysis of dissolution in serialized 'Remarks on dissolution of the nervous system as exemplified by certain post-epileptic conditions'.[103] They were published in the *Medical Press and Circular* (*MPC*), for which they appear to have been specially prepared. The series had not previously been presented as lectures or in any other form. It is reminiscent of Jackson's earlier attempt in 1876 to produce a book on epilepsy for the publisher of the *MPC*, Albert Alfred Tindall.[104] Here it appears that Tindall was again trying to cajole a book out of Jackson. In the second installment, Jackson said, 'In this book ...'[105] Be that as it may, the first

---

[98] Jackson 1881b, p.445.
[99] [Jackson, J.H.] 1875a, pp.xxviii and xxix.
[100] Jackson 1879q; see also Chapter 9.
[101] This paragraph summarizes Jackson 1881b, pp.448–449.
[102] Jackson 1881b, pp.449–450; Jackson's italics.
[103] Jackson 1881h, Jackson 1881k, Jackson 1881l, Jackson 1881r, Jackson 1881s, Jackson 1881t.
[104] See Chapter 8.
[105] Jackson 1881k, p.399; the very next paragraph starts: 'In this paper ...'

three installments were published in April–July 1881 and the last three in November. The entire series was presented with labeled sections, as one might do in a textbook or a monograph. Table 10.1 is an outline of the existing sections, using Jackson's headings.

Table 10.1 Outline of Jackson's extensive 'Remarks on dissolution of the nervous system as exemplified by certain post-epileptic conditions', 1881.[a]

Jackson's titles for each section	Citations in Jackson's Bibliography
(April–July 1881)	
'Introduction.' (many acknowledgments)	Jackson 1881h
'I. – The Definition of Epilepsy.'	Jackson 1881k
'II. – The Importance of the Study of Post-Epileptic Conditions.'	↓
'1. Clinically.'	
'(2) Socially or Medico-Legally.'	
'III. – Three degrees of the post-epileptic condition.'	Jackson 1881l
'IV. – The symptomatic condition in each degree is double.'	↓
'V. – On Nomenclature of the Negative Elements.'	
'VI. – Justification of the Study of the Three Degrees in Relation.'	
'VII. – No Dreamy State in Some Cases.'	
'VIII. – On Range of Concomitance of Psychical and Nervous States.'	
'IX. – The Nature of the Negative Elements.'	
'(a.) Physically.'	
'(b.) Psychically.'	
'X. – The Nature of the Positive Element.'	
'XI. – The Nature of the Positive Element (continued) Illustrated by a case of partial aphasia.'	
(November 1881)	
'XII. – The Nature of the Positive Elements (continued) Anatomically Considered.'	Jackson 1881r
'XIII. – The Nature of the Positive Elements (continued). – The Positive Element cannot be said to be always Abnormal from Over-activity.'	↓
'XIV. – The Nature of the Positive Element (continued). – Its Psychical Side.'	
'XV. – Difference betwixt the Negative and Positive Elements.'	Jackson 1881s
'XVI. – Two Aspects of the Negative Element.'	↓
'XVII. – Two Aspects of the Positive Element.'	
'XVIII. – Two Aspects of the Positive Condition (continued). – Illusions.'	
'XIX. – Re-statements and qualifications.'	Jackson 1881t
'XX. – Re-statement of the Differences betwixt the Negative and Positive Elements in the First and Second Degree.'	↓
'XXI. – Various Uses of the Terms Subjective and Objective.'	
'(to be continued.)'	
(But it wasn't.)	

[a] Jackson 1881h, Jackson 1881k, Jackson 1881l, Jackson 1881r, Jackson 1881s, Jackson 1881t.

A survey of Jackson's bibliography shows that dissolution was a major theme from 1881 to 1884. The culmination of that work was his presentation of the prestigious Croonian Lectures at the Royal College of Physicians in 1884,[106] which I will examine below. Beyond dissolution, Jackson's 'book' of 1881 can be interpreted as a further effort to unify neurological nosology by bringing everything into a single pathophysiological framework. We have seen that during the four and a half years after his wife's death he continued his clinical and theoretical work quite vigorously, and the intellectual effort in his 'Remarks' went to an even deeper level. As he explained: 'We have to find some fundamental principle under which things so superficially different as the diseases empirically named hemiplegia, aphasia, acute mania, chorea, melancholia, permanent dementia, coma, &c., can be methodically classified.'[107] For this he proposed the principle of dissolution as the basis for the quest.

> I have long thought that Herbert Spencer's hypothesis of dissolution will enable us to develope [sic] a science of disease of the nervous system ... At any rate, there is no harm in trying to see how far the hypothesis of Dissolution will apply to some diseases of the nervous system. I have long ago applied it to the elucidation of cases of aphasia ... to cases of the ordinary form of hemiplegia and to cases of epileptiform seizures ... I suppose these to be examples of Dissolution beginning in different lower cerebral centres, as insanity is ... Dissolution beginning in the highest of all centres.[108]

Part of Jackson's 'Introduction' served to acknowledge his many predecessors. With regard to his leading muse, he said: 'Readers will not ... judge Spencer's doctrines from my application of them. I should take it as a great calamity were any crudities of mine to be attributed to this distinguished thinker.'[109] This sentence is sometimes cited to show Jackson's excessive deference to Spencer.[110] Although it is obvious that Jackson owed special thanks to Spencer, I think too much has been made of it. After he cited many other authors on epileptic insanity, including Spencer, Jackson said:

> ... it is not inconsistent to acknowledge that much of what I have to put forward has been said in principle before, and yet to take full responsibility, because I am saying it in a different way ... no one has advanced any claim to priority on the points I mention.
>
> The foregoing must not be taken as an admission that I have not worked quite independently at most parts of the subject.[111]

---

[106] See York and Steinberg 2006, pp.97–107.

[107] Jackson 1881h, p.330.

[108] Jackson 1881h, p.329. He also said: 'I have been misunderstood to have put forward the Hypothesis of Dissolution as a basis for classification of cases of Insanity for clinical purposes, and have been asked to go to some lunatic asylum and show how the cases of patients there could be classified under it.' Needless to say, he refused the request. On the other hand, Jackson took the psychiatrist George Savage (1842–1921) on rounds at the London, and he went to Bethlem hospital with Savage on occasion (Savage 1917). According to Savage, Jackson tried to avoid seeing purely insane cases, because he could not help them.

[109] Jackson 1881h, p.330.

[110] See Raitiere 2012, pp.129–133, for a discussion of this issue; I agree with his general conclusion—Jackson's dependence on Spencer has often been over-stated.

[111] Jackson 1881h, p.332.

In the last sentence Jackson was again defending his intellectual independence. Beyond that, in the penultimate sentence he raised the issue of priority without disclaiming it, which he probably would have done when he was younger. Although he was only 46 in April 1881, I think he was beginning to think about his legacy.[112] A major part of that legacy, of course, was his reconceptualization of seizures and epilepsy, and for that he needed the clarity of a definition.

> *The Definition of Epilepsy.* – I have defined epilepsy as a condition in which there is a sudden excessive transitory discharge of some part of the cortex. Under this definition epileptiform convulsions are included … By epilepsy here shall be meant solely what are called cases of epilepsy proper or genuine epilepsy, the epilepsy of nosologists.[113]

Since genuine seizures were defined nosologically as manifesting early loss of consciousness, he said: 'Anatomically, they are cases in which the discharge begins in some part of the highest centres, these centres being the anatomical substrata of consciousness.'

> … it follows … that strictly we ought to speak of several kinds of epilepsy which are grouped under the term epilepsy proper. Doubtless there are as many kinds as … there are kinds of epileptiform seizures … the "discharging lesion" may be of different parts of any of the several divisions of the highest centres … anatomically, the discharging lesion may be in the highest motor or highest sensory centres of either side … [in the terms of] psychology [it may be] in the motor or sensory substrata of either object or subject consciousness. There will be at least as many epileptic seizures, differently seated discharging lesions, as there are 'warnings' of the paroxysm.[114]

Three aspects of this passage invite comment. First is Jackson's brain science, i.e., his clinical conception of the functional anatomy of the hemispheres. The main point here is that he did have such a conception, which he had worked out over the preceding decade. Second, he was trying to bring most cases of genuine epilepsy into the same pathophysiological category as epileptiform seizures, because he was looking for focal onsets of all seizures. And third, his integrative goal had clinical implications.

> We may occasionally be consulted because a person suddenly acts strangely, violently, or passes into a state which resembles somnambulism, and nothing will be volunteered as to epileptic attacks. Unless we have very carefully studied the phenomena of very slight seizures of epilepsy we shall … dwell … on the striking and neglect the essential; the thing is to ferret out the <u>quasi-trifling signs of a transitory fit.</u> It is of more importance for diagnosis and treatment to inquire about such symptoms as transient pallor, movements of

---

[112] Jackson also mentioned priority in Jackson 1881k, p.399: 'On some parts I have worked for years in ignorance of what prior workers had done.' He listed Todd and Robertson (postictal paralysis), Thompson Dickson ('loss of control'), and Anstie. Then he said, '… I do not know of any previous attempts to study Insanities on the principle of Dissolutions'.

[113] Jackson 1881k, p.399.

[114] Jackson 1881k, p.399, my square brackets.

mastication, turning up of the eyes, than to note with care the "interesting" symptoms of elaborate quasi-somnambulism.[115]

At the conjunction of practical clinical nosology and pathophysiology, Jackson's interpretation of these transitory subtleties was an essential part of his effort to integrate the two approaches. One part of his strategy was to define a spectrum of three 'degrees' of postictal dissolution, which could be characterized both clinically and scientifically. Unfortunately, his Section III—'*Three degrees of the post-epileptic condition*'—is quite confusing, because it does not start with definitions. On the other hand, he had been using a version of the same tripartite scheme since 1874,[116] and he had provided definitions of his three levels of postictal dissolution in a footnote to his paper in *Brain*, January 1881. There his '*Three degrees*' of dissolution were, hierarchically from the highest: '(1) post-epileptic "ideation"; (2) post-epileptic action (e.g., mania); and (3) post-epileptic coma ...'[117] By (1) 'ideation' Jackson meant dreamy states or other complex mental operations; by (2) 'action' he meant cruder actions, usually motor in nature; and in (3) 'coma' the postictal patient's physical status is reduced to 'vital' actions, such as breathing. Hence, he said, 'We may name these three duplex conditions respectively Highest, Middle and Lowest post-epileptic conditions ... They are ... significant of three "depths" of Dissolution, each beginning in the highest nervous arrangements ...'[118]

Jackson was usually at pains to point out the positive and negative aspects of any neurological condition. In the above definitions of postictal states it is the positive aspects that are commonly emphasized, but he said, '*The symptomatic condition in each degree is double*'. His text on this point is difficult to understand,[119] partly because his view of seizure propagation and postictal states is so dynamic, but dynamism in analyzing the pathophysiology of epileptic seizures is surely a virtue. The following is a paraphrase of how I believe he was thinking.

In Jackson's conception as of 1881, a seizure can start from a focus anywhere in the cortex. Its initial symptom is determined by the normal function of the tissue in which it starts. However, its propagation can be extremely variable, depending on its amount of force, and especially on the relative levels of resistance of the efferent paths to which it is connected.[120] During the seizure there are positive actions and negative features, the latter generally amounting to depressed levels of consciousness. During the postictal state, the same is true: mania is a positive feature, and again the negative features are depressed levels of consciousness. The dynamic feature of this conception is Jackson's observation that seizing patients can be in different states at different times, often with rapid and repeated changes. Regarding the degrees of dissolution, he said, 'We may see all three in the same patient in connection with one full paroxysm'.[121] However, it is not necessarily the case that all postictal patients go through all stages. In particular, there is

---

[115] Jackson 1881k, p.399; my underlining. A discussion of criminal responsibility followed.
[116] Jackson 1874r, p.653; see also in Chapter 8 on De Quincey.
[117] Jackson 1881b, p.443, footnote 1; this is repeated from above in this chapter.
[118] Jackson 1881l, p.69.
[119] Jackson 1881l, Sections IV, V, VI, pp.68–69.
[120] See Jackson 1881r, p.381: 'a more rapid liberation of energy gives rise to nerve currents of greater force – that is, to currents capable of overcoming lines of greater resistance – than does a slower liberation of an equal quantity of energy'.
[121] Jackson 1881l, p.69.

… *No Dreamy State in Some Cases* … it is not asserted that there is ideation ("a dreamy state") at or about the onset of all epileptic attacks; on the contrary, it is asserted that in some cases there is none … some patients remember no dream. Is there nevertheless, an "unremembered dream" in these cases? Some would doubtless consider an unremembered dream to be equivalent to nothing … there is total lack of evidence of the existence of any sort of mental state when the patient … remembers nothing.[122]

Now remember that all of this is primarily concerned with genuine epilepsy, so the above shows that Jackson and/or others had entertained the idea that the dreamy state might be present at the onset of all epileptic seizures that originate from the highest levels. That would be the likely reason for his statement above, in which he felt compelled to reject that idea. But the idea is not unreasonable, as he pointed out in the next section.

… *On Range of* Concomitance *of Psychical and Nervous States.* – The question mooted in the last section is not one to be carelessly dismissed as being nonsensical. Whilst accepting the ordinary doctrine that psychical states are different from, and yet concomitant with, nervous states, nothing was said for or against the doctrine of Lewes, that active states of all nervous centres have a psychical side. The question is, how far down in the nervous system there are psychical states during nervous activity. Is the brain the organ of mind, or only the chief part of that organ? I give no opinion on this difficult question.[123]

This was Jackson's first published use of 'concomitance', although he had been developing the concept for many years. In thus applying psycho-physical parallelism to neurology he made one of his major contributions.[124] After the above passage he gave the example of a man in a postictal state who apparently behaved as an automaton, laying a fire in a bread-pan and lighting it. Then he continued:

Mental states have always concomitant physical states – that is … discharges of, or liberations of energy by, nervous elements; but can we say the reverse – that nervous states always have concomitant psychical states? Observe, psychical states are not functions of any nervous elements, but attend the functioning of at least some nervous arrangements of those, at least, by which the *most special* … adjustments of the organism as a whole to the environment is effected. That consciousness arises during the activity of the highest arrangements … is not disputable. But now comes the question – Is there any sort of subconsciousness or sensibility or any sort of psychical state, however rudimentary, attending functioning of any lower nervous arrangements? And, if this be answered in the affirmative, comes the further question – How low down in the nervous system is the concomitance?[125]

In his next paragraph Jackson said again, 'I express no opinion on this difficult question', and then he went on to give one: 'But were I to make an abrupt limit to the concomitance of

---

122 Jackson 1881l, p.69; Jackson's italics, parentheses, and quotation marks.
123 Jackson 1881l, p.69; Jackson's italics, my underlining.
124 See e.g. Walshe 1961, p.121; and York and Steinberg 2011, pp.3110–3111.
125 Jackson 1881l, p.69; Jackson's italics.

psychical with nervous states I should place the lower limit at the lower Motor (Hitzig and Ferrier) and lower Sensory (Ferrier's) centres.'[126] So he appeared to be declaring that mind emerges from the activity of the hemispheric cortices and not from lower levels. This formulation is somewhat helpful in trying to understand a fundamental difficulty of psycho-physical parallelism in neurological terms.

> ... consciousness *attends* activity of certain nervous arrangements, and ceases when those nervous arrangements are *hors de combat*. That consciousness attends activity of some nervous elements is disputed by nobody. What the nature of the relation is nobody knows ... we speak of concomitance only. To say that those elements are of sensori-motor nervous arrangements adds nothing to the difficulty of the question, and yet clears up much of the difficulty in studying disease.[127]

In Jackson's series of 'Remarks on dissolution of the nervous system' there was a 3-month gap between the publication dates of his first three and his last three installments,[128] but his stream of thought continued.

Dissolution and Epilepsy: Final Three Installments, November 1881

In the above passage, Jackson's remark about clearing up the 'difficulty in studying disease' presumably refers to the role of 'sensori-motor nervous arrangements' on the physical side of concomitance. In a footnote on November 2 he repeated his anatomical conjecture.

> ... we speak of three motor centres of different grades of evolution. 1. Highest (the motor substrata of consciousness, or of most vivid consciousness). 2. Lower (Hitzig and Ferrier's centres). 3. Lowest (Spinal and higher homologous motor nuclei) ... I wish now to mention explicitly that this double order of centres is not supposed to correspond to our three degrees of post-epileptic conditions.[129]

On the psychological side, according to Jackson, the dreamy state is a negative (release) phenomenon. Its corresponding positive element on the physical side is release of activity in some part of the highest brain level 'which the epileptic discharge had not reached', i.e., that is not exhausted.[130] To illustrate 'Two Aspects of the Negative Element', i.e., loss of function in the releasing level and released activity in the next lower level, Jackson used a political analogy.

> Were the highest governing people in this country suddenly destroyed, we should have to lament the loss of their offices; the loss of them is the analogue of our post-epileptic patient's negative condition. But we should also have to lament the now permitted anarchy

---

[126] Jackson 1881l, p.69. This would limit concomitance to *neocortex*, but I don't think he thought about it phylogenetically in that way.

[127] Jackson 1881l, p.70; Jackson's italics.

[128] From July 27 (Jackson 1881l) to November 2, 1881 (Jackson 1881r).

[129] Jackson 1881r, p.382, footnote (*a*) in column 1.

[130] Jackson 1881s, p.399.

of the now ungoverned people consequent on that loss; the anarchy is the analogue of our patient's positive condition.[131]

As a political statement Jackson's analogy depends on his assumption that the 'ungoverned people' will be anarchical. However, having impugned the social stability of the lower classes, he then showed some limited faith in his countrymen.

> ... when control is slowly removed, the positive condition may be normal in degree ... if, in this country, the highest governing people were slowly removed, the "positive condition" of the rest of the country would not be ... anarchical. The lower governing bodies would ... gradually become efficient substitutes for general purposes.[132]

Having thus illustrated 'Two Aspects of the Negative Element', Jackson went on to '*Two Aspects of the Positive Element*'.

> We have also to look at the positive element from two points of view. There is the result of what ... we may call the "permitted" over-energising of the now uncontrolled and thus over-active nervous arrangements. The outcome of this is the <u>survival of the fittest</u> states in what is left of the nervous system. (The survival of the fittest is the law of both healthy and of morbid mentation and of the concomitant cerebration) ...
>
> What we called the "survival of the fittest" is here the resultant of two factors; (1), of permitted activity of what is already organised in what is left of the patient, and of (2) the influence of external things, or peripheral conditions interfering with, modifying, that activity of that already organised ... [so that] a *more elaborate* state is produced ...[133]

In Chapter 9 we saw that Jackson's first use of 'survival of the fittest' occurred 2 years earlier, in October–November 1879.[134] At that time he clearly understood that the principle applies to competing processes within the organism, as well as to the organism's relation to its external environment. In the last published installment of his 'Remarks' of 1881[135] Jackson attempted to bring together his underlying themes of survival of the fittest, dissolution, and subjective–objective. About dissolution, he said, '... we have now spoken of three factors in Dissolution (1) 'Depth' of the dissolution; (2) Rapidity with which it is effected; (3) Influence of local bodily states, &c.'[136] In his final section, 'Re-statement of the Differences betwixt the Negative and Positive Elements in the First and Second Degree', he wove in the subject–object distinction for a patient in a postictal state.

> There often is after a slight epileptic seizure (our first degree) a defect of object consciousness – so far negative – and [there are] positively remains of object consciousness with

---

[131] Jackson 1881s, p.399. This analogy was repeated in Jackson 1884d, p.662.
[132] Jackson 1881s, p.400; my square brackets. In 1884 (Jackson 1884d, p.660) Jackson made another analogy, using the 'Navy Board', whose 'highest navy centres – consists of twenty-four members, each one of which governs the whole of the Navy, through the intermediation of middle and lower officials'.
[133] Jackson 1881s, p.400; Jackson's italics, my square brackets and underlining.
[134] In Jackson 1879t, pp.328–329.
[135] Jackson 1881t.
[136] Jackson 1881t, p.421. The text continues: 'We shall later on consider ... "the person in whom dissolution occurs ... "' 'Later on' implies that more discussion of this point would be forthcoming, but it never appeared.

sometimes increase of subject consciousness, that is, "a dreamy state" – so far positive. In other words, "the positive condition" is itself duplex; it is an abnormal mental state; one imperfect by deficit and [also] imperfect by excess.[137]

If the reader—then and now—feels inundated by a multitude of confusing theoretical constructs, Jackson was aware of the difficulty, although his meliorative efforts were limited.

> As the last paragraph may be thought a little obscure, especially since further terms (subjective and objective) are introduced, I must illustrate what is said. But before that can be properly done, some important terms have to be defined …
> … *Various Uses of the Terms Subjective and Objective.*
> The words subjective and objective are used in different senses by different medical men. Hence I must say how they are to be used in this work. First, let me state several contrasted ways in which they are used, in which ways I shall *not* use them.[138]

Surely Jackson's clarification of how he used objective and subjective would have been most welcome, but it never happened. Immediately after the above he gave six examples of ways in which his medical contemporaries used the terms, affirming that he would not assume 'that my definition is superior to some of those …'[139] His last installment ended abruptly there, with the usual '(*to be continued*)', but alas, his promised definition was *hors de combat*.[140] At this point we have reached the full extent of Jackson's incomplete treatise of 1881, on dissolution and postictal states. Now I will go back to look at events that occurred during the interregnum, from August through October 1881.

Epilepsy and Localization at the Seventh International Medical Congress, London, August 1881

On the Continent a biennial series of physicians' conferences began with the first International Medical Congress in Paris in 1867. Although British participation in the meetings had been spotty, a decision to cross the Channel was taken at the sixth Congress in Amsterdam in 1879.[141] Accordingly, the Seventh International Medical Congress was held in London, August 2–9, 1881.[142] In July 1880, a year before the event, the Executive Committee voted to 'expressly indicate in the letters of invitation that only male members of

---

[137] Jackson 1881t, p.421; my square brackets.
[138] Jackson 1881t, pp.421–422; Jackson's italics.
[139] Jackson 1881t, p.422.
[140] In November 1882, Jackson began another series of installments on the same subject ('On some implications of dissolution of the nervous system') in the *MPC* (Jackson 1882i). Although he referred to his 'recent paper in this journal (1881)', the new series did not start with definitions of objective and subjective.
[141] See Bartrip 1990, pp.141–145.
[142] The four volumes of *Transactions* of the Congress (Mac Cormac 1881) were a monumental accomplishment. According to the editor's Preface (vol.1, pp.ix–x), they were published in December 1881, much sooner than Osler would have expected (Osler 1881, p.125), but they do not include the precise dates for each section's activities. There is no comprehensive historical analysis of this landmark event; but see Bynum 1994, pp.142–146.

the medical profession would be eligible for attendance ...', although that had not been the previous practice.[143]

A month later it was announced proudly (and apparently without any sense of gendered paradox!) that 'Her Majesty the Queen has most graciously given a fresh proof of her sympathy with the cause of medical science, and our efforts in its furtherance, by authorising us to place the Congress under her Royal Patronage'.[144] Pride swelled in British chests.

A Brief Overview of the Congress, August 1881

According to the official count, there were 3,182 (male) 'members' of the Congress, two-thirds from the United Kingdom and the 'English Colonies', plus 220 from the United States, 203 from Germany, 201 from France, and most of the rest from Western Europe.[145] The entire affair was presided over by its President, Sir James Paget, Jackson's friend and former mentor at Barts.[146] The presence of such public luminaries as Charcot, Huxley, Lister, Pasteur, and Virchow brought extensive coverage by the medical and lay press.[147] In addition to the numerous official receptions and dinners, there were many private parties.[148] In a letter to his wife during the Congress, Huxley complained about too much socializing.[149] He had a point. Sir James and Lady Paget kept continuous open house for the week—breakfast, lunch, and dinner.[150] Before the Congress Hutchinson had written to his wife that part of the purpose of 'these Congresses' as 'great religious gatherings' was 'to promote the general sentiment of good brotherly feeling'.[151] Nonetheless, when Lord and Lady Lister entertained they had to invite the French members and the Germans on different days.[152]

Despite Jackson's aversion to large throngs he could not avoid being drawn into the swirl, because he was one of the lesser luminaries. Indeed, there is some evidence that he attended one of the most lavish of the private parties. In February 1881 Baroness Angela Burdett-Coutts, aged 67, had caused a delicious Victorian scandal by marrying a 30-year-old American.[153] On the seventh day of the Congress, Monday, August 8, their guests included Charcot and Jackson, as well as Jackson's friends Allbutt, Hutchinson, and Wilks.[154]

---

[143] News item about 'International Medical Congress, 1881' in *BMJ* 2:182 (July 31). After an unexpected 'smart discussion', the vote was 27 for the prohibition and 19 against it, with 'many members of the Committee present abstaining from voting'. Nonetheless, 'At previous Congresses ... lady physicians have been eligible to attend and have attended'.

[144] Paget et al. 1880.

[145] Mac Cormac 1881, p.xxxi.

[146] See Chapter 2.

[147] *The Times* of London gave extensive coverage from August 3 to August 10, but largely for the plenary sessions and social events (see *The Times Digital Archive*. Website accessed July 11, 2015). There was nothing in those reports for 'Jackson' or 'Hughlings Jackson'.

[148] For a short summary of the whole event see Spillane 1981, pp.393–396.

[149] Huxley L. 1900, vol.2, p.33.

[150] S. Paget 1902, pp.317–318.

[151] Sakula 1982, p.184.

[152] Godlee 1918, p.441; see also Fisher 1977, p.272.

[153] Sakula 1982, pp.185–186; Queen Victoria is reported to have said, 'The woman must be crazy!' Other reactions, in the Queen's diary, are given by Healey 1978, p.207.

[154] See Sakula 1982; Sakula's figures 2 and 3 purport to identify Jackson among the many attendees in a large composite painting. The figure does look like Jackson, but it is hard to be sure. Sakula (p.188) says that, 'No official or original key to the group-portrait exists'. Burdett-Coutts' biography reproduces the painting without mention of the Congress (Healey 1978, p.208). The original painting is in the Wellcome Collection, London. Another reproduction in color is in Hunting 2002, plate 21.

Among the members of the Congress, one of the attendees was the 'Baby Professor' of medicine from McGill University, William Osler (1849–1919), aged 32.[155] His report of the Congress to the *Canada Medical and Surgical Journal* was dated August 10, 1881.[156] It can serve as a guide to some of the most important activities. Osler spent his time 'chiefly in the pathological, physiological and medical sections'.[157] In the Pathological section he heard 'very interesting discussions' on 'Tubercle' and on 'Germs', but 'It is apparent that Osler, like many other physicians, did not appear at this time fully to grasp as Lister did the significance of Pasteur's work, or to show great interest in Koch's remarkable contributions ...'[158]

About the Physiological section, Osler observed that: 'The time of the ... section was occupied chiefly in discussing certain set topics; very few papers were read. An animated discussion on Cerebral Localization took place, in which Goltz of Strasburg, Brown-Séquard, Ferrier and others participated.'[159] This was the famous episode in the history of localization when Friedrich Goltz (1834–1902), an anti-localizationist, exhibited a clinically intact dog whose motor cortex had been removed. Ferrier then showed a hemiplegic monkey who had been treated similarly. When Charcot saw the monkey, he exclaimed, 'It is a patient!'[160] Expeditious autopsies were performed on the animals, and it turned out that Ferrier's description of his monkey's lesion was accurate, whereas Goltz' dog had spared cortex that accounted for its better clinical status.[161] This episode can be seen as a turning point toward general acceptance of cerebral/cortical localization. There is no direct evidence that Jackson attended any of the Physiological sessions, though it would seem likely. In any case, Osler heard Jackson's major contribution in the section on Medicine.

Jackson's Presentations at the International Medical Congress, August 1881

In the medical section Charcot and Jackson were among the 51 members of the international Council, which included many others who had strong neurological interests.[162] The Inaugural Address for the section was given by its President, Sir William Withey Gull (1816–1890), who had been Jackson's friend since his days as a medical reporter.[163] Gull showed that he had been absorbing Jackson's ideas when he said, 'epilepsy ... is traceable to apparently trifling changes

---

[155] On 'Baby Professor' see Bliss 1999, p.80.

[156] Osler 1881.

[157] Osler 1881, p.123.

[158] Cushing 1926, vol.1, p.190.

[159] Osler 1881, p.123. For the official record of the 'Discussion on the Localization of Function in the Cortex Cerebri' see Mac Cormac 1881, vol.1, pp.218–242d.

[160] Mac Cormac 1881, vol.1, p.237, recorded this remark in English, in which Charcot was fluent (see Hierons 1993, p.1590). If Charcot had made the remark in French, it would have been: '*C'est un malade!*' and that French is often quoted (e.g., in Finger 2000, p.157, citing Spillane 1981, p.395, but Spillane gives the English). Since French was one of the official languages, I conclude that Charcot made the remark in English, because Mac Cormac would have recorded Charcot's exclamation in French if it had been said that way.

[161] See Mac Cormac 1881, vol.1, pp.218–242d; summarized in Spillane 1981, pp.394–396, in Finger 2000, pp.155–158, and in Morabito 2017, pp.152–156.

[162] Mac Cormac 1881, vol.2, p.xvi. Four members of the Council had appointments at Queen Square: T. Buzzard, Jackson, Radcliffe, and Reynolds; see Holmes 1954, p.96.

[163] See Chapter 2.

in a few grey nerve-cells'.[164] Next after Gull's Address was Jackson's invited contribution on 'Epileptiform convulsions from cerebral disease'.[165] Apparently Jackson esteemed the honour, because this paper is much better organized than usual. As a succinct summary of his views on 'Epileptiform convulsions' his paper is highly recommended, but to repeat its contents here would be tedious. Although he had proposed to integrate the pathophysiologies of epileptiform and genuine seizures, I suspect he chose this narrower topic to avoid the controversy that might have arisen if he had brought up his views about 'epilepsy proper'.

The paper immediately after Jackson's was given in German by Franz Müller, of Graz, Austria. It was titled 'Zur Jackson'chen Epilepsie und Localisation des Armcentrums ...'[166] Müller described a case with Jacksonian seizures beginning in the left arm. At autopsy the patient had a circumscribed glioma in the right convexity, exactly where it should have been according to Ferrier's localization figures, i.e., in the pre- and post-rolandic cortex of the 'arm area'. In his introduction Müller described Jackson as 'England's greatest neuropathologist' ('den grossen Neuropathologen Englands').[167] Since Charcot had introduced the term 'Jacksonian epilepsy', circa 1877,[168] Müller's use of 'Jackson'chen' shows that Charcot's usage had penetrated the German-speaking world quite quickly. In the published discussion that followed Jackson's and Müller's papers, the adjective 'Jacksonian' appeared frequently.[169]

One of the discussants was Brown-Séquard, whose views on cerebral localization were sceptical. In the discussion Jackson replied: 'I have never acceded to the doctrine that the third left frontal convolution (or any convolution or limited region) is "the centre for speech;" my belief is that Broca's convolution is chiefly concerned during speech. I have never believed in abrupt localization of any kind.'[170] Jackson also commented on the use of 'positive' and 'negative' by Allen Sturge (1850–1919),[171] and he used some of Gull's remarks as an entrée to bring up his ideas about the sensori-motor nature of the nervous system, about hierarchical release, and about concomitance. After Jackson's remarks, the next series of six papers in the Medical section were concerned with tabes, led off by Thomas Buzzard.[172] Regarding Jackson's other participation in the Congress, we know only that he attended the section of Ophthalmology, where he commented in a discussion on optic neuritis.[173]

Three months after Ferrier's triumph at the Congress he had to face prosecution by the anti-vivisectionists under the Cruelty to Animals Act of 1876. The summons was issued on November 3, returnable at the Bow Street Police Court on November 17, 1881.[174] On the appointed day there was much commotion outside the courthouse.

---

[164] Mac Cormac 1881, vol.2, p.4. Later in his Address (p.5) Gull anticipated other neurological contributions to the section: 'In the matter of diagnosis, we have invited contributions on the pathognomonic and diagnostic value of the localization of disease in the brain and spinal cord, which will be an occasion for a review of our knowledge of cerebral and spinal mechanism ...'

[165] Jackson 1881w.

[166] Müller 1881.

[167] In German the term 'Neuropathologen' could refer to a clinician who uses the clinico-pathological method.

[168] See Critchley and Critchley 1998, p.65; see also Chapter 9.

[169] Mac Cormac 1881, vol.2, pp.19–21.

[170] Jackson 1881x, p.21.

[171] Mac Cormac 1881, vol.2, pp.19–21. This is the Sturge of Sturge–Weber syndrome, which can involve severe seizures. He had been Registrar at the National Hospital in 1874 and studied with Charcot in 1876 (Barlow 1919; Holmes 1954, p.98)).

[172] Mac Cormac 1881, vol.2, pp.22–55.

[173] Jackson 1881y.

[174] See [Ferrier 1881a], p.552, which states that the summons was made a 'fortnight' before November 17. This episode is reviewed in French 1975, pp.198–205; Finger 2000, pp.169–172; Stiles 2012, pp.67–70; and Morabito 2017, pp.160–163.

The interior of the court presented a no less unusual aspect than its exterior. Seven chairs on either side of the magistrate gave accommodation to a favored few, among whom there were five ladies, besides Dr. Hughlings Jackson, Professor Lister, Curnow ... the Baroness Burnett-Coutts was in the court, and this I regret to say is only too probable, for in this matter her kindliness of heart has conspicuously eclipsed that calm judgement which should have led her to accept the unanimous verdict of her late guests, who, during the recent International Medical Congress, so unhesitatingly declared themselves opposed to the whole principle of the anti-vivisection legislation in this country. The audience ... included ... Michael Foster, Gerald Yeo, Burden-Sanderson ... and others, especially the defendant's colleagues at King's College.[175]

In the course of the brief proceedings it turned out that the potentially painful operations were actually performed by Ferrier's colleague at King's, Professor Gerald Yeo (1845–1909). He had followed the Act properly in registering himself and in caring for the animals, so Ferrier was acquitted. In fact, the Congress itself had been a turning point in the profession's finally getting organized to resist the anti-vivisectionists.[176]

A Lecture on Pathology, and Further on Dissolution and Compensation, August 1882–August 1883

From January through July 1882 Jackson produced just two short pieces, which were presentations at local societies.[177] For that period, then, we know only that he was following his usual habit of attending such meetings, while he was also managing a busy consulting practice. Apparently that was enough. In the year from August 1882 to August 1883 his major productivity consisted of (1) a single lecture on pathology, which was largely a recapitulation of previous themes, and (2) a series of four articles 'On some implications of dissolution of the nervous system'. The main topic in the latter was a new and more extensive analysis of his theory of compensation.

A Lecture on Pathology, August 1882

In August 1882, 'At the annual meeting of the British Medical Association, in Worcester', Jackson gave 'An address delivered at the opening of the section of pathology'.[178] He emphasized the importance of autopsies, partly as essential to the clinico-pathological method, but also to control the hubris of diagnosticians. Another theme was his assertion that a knowledge of general pathology is essential to all medical specialties, because their diseases are all

---

[175] [Ferrier 1881a], p.552. The magistrate deciding the case was Sir James Taylor Ingham (1805–1890), who was a Yorkshireman. He had practiced at West Riding before removing to London. In 1876 he became chief magistrate of London and was knighted (http://www.oxforddnb.com, accessed October 30, 2015). 'Curnow' was John Curnow, M.D., F.R.C.P., dean of King's College Hospital Medical School; see Brown 1955, pp.255–256.

[176] Rupke 1987, pp.189–194.

[177] Jackson 1882b was a brief case report at the Medical Society of London, and Jackson 1882c was 'Observations on migraine', given to the 'Epidemiological Society. South-eastern branch: East and West Surrey districts'. Jackson's presence at the latter was likely due to the location of Hutchinson's residence in Haslemere, Surrey, where Jackson was a frequent guest; see Hutchinson 1911, p.1552. In effect, Jackson retracted Jackson 1882b later, when he learned more about the patient's multifocal seizures; see Jackson 1882g, p.370.

[178] Jackson 1882d and Jackson 1882e are the same title in different journals.

affected by systemic processes. Using his tripartite method and the example of epilepsy, he issued a challenge.

> ... the man who finds out by what pathological process it comes to pass that certain parts of the nervous system become so physiologically abnormal that they occasionally discharge excessively, will have done ... the best medical work on epilepsy ... the question is: "In what tissue of nervous organs does the abnormal nutritive change begin?" It is often assumed, without evidence, that it begins in nervous tissue.[179]

In the last sentence Jackson struck another old theme. Since most neurological diseases begin in their 'subordinate elements, blood-vessels and connective tissue ... Most of them are not in a strict sense nervous diseases at all.'[180] He had emphasized this point in 1875, when he said that he had understood it in 1864.[181] At the end of his Address he touched on some larger issues, concluding with a digression on metaphysics. Provocatively, he asserted that medical students should be taught metaphysics—so they could recognize it and reject it when they see it. To explain, he offered an allegory.

> A good deal under the guise of practicality is pure metaphysics. There was once a man who could conceive an abstract Lord Mayor. The conception he had, so he averred, had neither head, arms, legs, nor corpulence; it was not an image of any particular Lord Mayor, nor a fusion of several, but an abstract Lord Mayor. Well, we think this metaphysician was too confident in his powers of conception. But do we not imagine ourselves capable of the same kind of marvellous feats? Let us look at a case of aphasia. A man does not speak, and yet can understand what we say to him, and can think – on ordinary things, at any rate. These are the facts; no one disputes them. Now comes the metaphysician, who proffers the explanation that the patient has lost words, but retains the memories or ideas of words. There are, it seems, words, and also memories or ideas of words, which latter, somehow, are not words. Now, what is an idea of a word which is not a word? It is, like the abstract Lord Mayor, simply nothing at all.[182]

As befits a true Yorkshireman, John Hughlings Jackson would have no truck with idealism. He was a solid British empiricist. After all, what is—or should be—more empirical than an autopsy? On September 9, 1882, an editorial in the *BMJ* praised Jackson's address on pathology, including its emphasis on '*post mortems, post mortems, and more post mortems*'.[183] The author described Jackson as 'One of the most distinguished of living specialists ...' and he referred to neurology as 'that obscure nervous department, which Dr. Jackson himself cultivates so successfully ...'[184] The editorial ended with a plea for a more rational nomenclature

---

[179] Jackson 1882d, p.307.

[180] Jackson 1882d, p.307, where he also said: 'a study of pathology corrects specialism', which latter was then a pejorative term. Although he was recognized as a specialist, Jackson denied that he was guilty of specialism because of his broad pathological outlook. This statement exemplifies Casper's (2014, p.23) claim that British 'physicians and scientists in the nineteenth century did not regard neurology as a medical specialty or scientific discipline ... they emphasized the broadness ... of inquiries into the nervous system. In some sense, they modeled themselves upon the great naturalists and philosophers of their age'.

[181] Jackson 1875kk, p.488, and Jackson 1864h; the latter is discussed in Chapter 3.

[182] Jackson 1882d, p.308; my square brackets.

[183] Jackson 1882f; italics in original. York and Steinberg 2006, p.102, include this item as if it were written by Jackson, but that is unlikely because the piece lauds him so effusively.

[184] Jackson 1882f, p.494. Probably the author was Ernest Hart, the *BMJ*'s editor. Note the contrast in Hart's description of Jackson as a specialist to Casper's (2014, p.23; see above footnote 181) statement that neurology was not considered a speciality.

in neurology, which Jackson had not stressed. What Jackson's writings emphasized next was his 'Principle of Compensation'.

Dissolution and Compensation, November 1882 and July–August 1883

In November 1882, Jackson published the first two installments of a four-part treatise, 'On some implications of dissolution of the nervous system'.[185] The first installment had three parts: (1) a series of 15 'principles' of cerebral organization and its dissolution.[186] They were stated as physiological propositions, based on clinical observations, but without explanations of how they were derived. In his writings they had been long established, so they will not be repeated here; (2) conversion of the principles into the nomenclature of his *xyz* theory;[187] and (3) some interesting remarks about his position in the holist–localizationist debate,[188] where, as usual, he claimed a studied neutrality.

When Jackson first introduced his *xyz* theory in his 'Study' of 1870, he used lowercases *x*, *y*, and *z* to stand for *both* the movements of some region of the body *and* for that region's representation in the brain.[189] Here, in 1882, he used uppercases *X*, *Y*, and *Z* to stand for the movements (not individual muscles) and lowercases *x*, *y*, and *z* to represent brain areas directing those movements. This is easier to follow. To illustrate how his theory worked, he posited an 'artificial scheme'.

> We speak of but one [cerebral] centre ... and of a [muscular] region represented by it. The region has ... only three muscles, each of which is different in size, shape, and has different attachments from the others. We suppose the centre to represent seven different movements, in every one of which all the three muscles serve, but that in each of the seven movements the three muscles serve differently. We symbolise this in the subjoined expression of seven terms from $x^{21}y^2z$ to z^7yx. (b)[190]

Footnote (b) listed the details of all seven hypothetical 'terms', which was the word that he used (instead of *xyz* 'units') to stand for individual cerebral centers devoted to specific movements. He conceived that such 'terms' were always located among others with similar but not exactly the same functions. Thus, when the first term, $x^{21}\,y^2\,z$, is destroyed, the muscle X appears weakest because it is most represented in $x^{21}y^2z$, so

> ... there *appears* to be decided paralysis of the *muscle* X, but really there is only loss of a movement in which that muscle serves more largely than it does in any other of the

---

[185] Jackson 1882i and Jackson 1882j; Jackson 1883h and Jackson 1883i appeared in July–August 1883. Circumstantial evidence suggests that Jackson had an agreement with Albert Tindall to publish his papers on dissolution in the *MPC*, at least in some years (see Rowlette 1939, pp.84–87, and Chapter 8). In 1881–1883 there were 10 items in Jackson's bibliography with 'dissolution' in their titles, but none with that word in their titles in other journals (York and Steinberg 2006, pp.97–105).

[186] Jackson 1882i, pp.411–412.

[187] Jackson 1882i is the subject of Greenblatt 1988, where the discussion and analysis are largely still valid, including my critique of Jackson's *xyz* theory.

[188] Jackson 1882i, p.414.

[189] Jackson 1870g, pp.190–191; see also Chapters 6 and 8.

[190] Jackson 1882i, p.412; my square brackets.

seven movements – of one in which, however, Y serves but yet slightly, and Z also but very slightly, so that the *muscles* Y and Z do not *appear to be* appreciably paralysed.[191]

As each of the seven terms is successively destroyed, the muscles/movements appear to be progressively weaker—and they are—but some representation still remains in terms not fully destroyed. Here again Jackson used the graded and overlapping (weighted and ordinal) features of his theory to explain the paradox that violent seizures can occur in muscles/movements which otherwise appear to be paralyzed.[192] Indeed, he asserted, 'Such cases are in complete harmony with the Principle of Compensation', because seizures can arise from intact terms that have some representation of the otherwise paralyzed movements. Referring to this resolution of the paradox, and using the word 'universaliser' where we would use 'holist', he went on to a related subject.

> The foregoing statements imply that I am not what has been called a Universaliser ... I have never believed that in any centre ... external parts are represented uniformly through it. The universaliser's representation would be symbolised by terms representing X Y and Z, such as $x^{21} y^{11} z^9 + x^{21} y^{11} z^9 + x^{21} y^{11} z^9$, &c. – that in some centres ... external parts are represented ... uniformly. Such can scarcely be called localisation at all.[193]

In this example, the terms $x^{21}y^{11}z^9$ are simply repeated seven times, which is physiologically absurd. Having thus shown that the holistic position is untenable, Jackson then applied his *xyz* theory to the strict localizationists.

> Nor am I a Localiser. The Localiser's symbolisation would be $x^{54} + y^{34} + z^{26}$.[194] On this view there is a centre for, let us instance, the movements of the face only, one for those of the arm only, and one for those of the leg only. This seems to me to ignore that there is in healthy operations co-operations of movements of different regions.[195]

Saying that he was 'neither a universaliser nor a localiser', he maintained his independence while exhibiting a bit of pique in a footnote.

> (*a*) In consequence I have been attacked as a Universaliser and also as a Localiser. But I do not remember that the view I really hold as to localisation has ever been referred to. If it is, it will very likely be supposed to be a fusion of, or compromise betwixt, recent doctrines. I stated it plainly many years ago, so that it is independent of any recent doctrines on localisation ... I derived it from Herbert Spencer. If any one [s]hould by chance take the trouble to refer to that article[196] he is asked to remember that it was written fifteen years ago, and to note that the word "movement" is there used less precisely than I now use it, and further that I did not then so carefully distinguish betwixt the psychical and the physical as I now try to do.[197]

---

[191] Jackson 1882i, p.413.

[192] Jackson 1882i, p.414; see also Jackson 1883h, p.65. This point was discussed in Jackson's 'Study' (Jackson 1870g, pp.189–191).

[193] Jackson 1882i, p.414.

[194] These superscript numbers are the totals of the *x*'s, *y*'s, and *z*'s in the seven 'terms' that Jackson listed in a footnote (*b*) in Jackson 1882i, p.412.

[195] Jackson 1882i, p.414.

[196] I.e., to Jackson 1867i.

[197] Jackson 1882i, p.414; my square brackets.

Given Jackson's usual level of civility, this was a bit nasty, but probably with justification. He was accusing some commentators of not having read his papers, at least not thoroughly, and doubtless he was right. As we saw in the section on Physiology at the International Congress, cerebral localization was hotly debated, and probably some of Jackson's statements were selectively invoked by some of the disputants. When he went on to discuss Compensation in his next installment, he felt compelled to defend himself against similar accusations.

> I have been said not to take note of the "Suppleance" (I use the word Compensation) of one part of the cortex for another. As a matter of fact I have, so far as I know, long ago carried the doctrine of compensation ... further than any other physician; for example, *Edinburgh Medical Journal*, Oct., 1868 ... [and also in] ... the *Medical Mirror*, Oct., 1869 ... [I then implied] absolute compensation, whereas I believe now that there is no such thing. There are many degrees of compensation, from slightest to seemingly complete.[198]

Considering Jackson's earlier disdain for priority, it is worth noting that the underlined phrase is such a claim. After two decades of surviving professionally in the rough and tumble of medicine in Victorian London, it is no surprise that he had lost some of his youthful idealism about the purity of science.[199] In any case, to illustrate Compensation he postulated the destruction of one term in his theoretical seven.

> The loss of the movement x^{21} y^2 z^1 is largely compensated in time by greater activity of the six remaining terms. Compensation does not ... mean that nervous arrangements take on duties they never had before, but that ... they serve ... next as well as those destroyed. Plainly, the compensation is in no case ... absolute ... In many cases we may say that compensation is "practically["] perfect ... Prompt recovery in some cases leads to the hypothesis that there is a 'functional lesion'. I contend that recovery follows when some nervous arrangements are gone, never to be restored.[200]

Jackson's Compensation thus implied a mechanism for plasticity, but his 'terms' themselves were not plastic. In the last part of this second installment he again explained the clinical phenomena of seizures within the conceptual framework of his *xyz* theory, including discharge of 'collateral *healthy* terms'.[201]

The third installment of Jackson's treatise on dissolution was published 7 months later, in July 1883. Much of it recapitulated the first two installments. However, a relatively new element was Jackson's explication of the 'Compound Order' of paralysis due to a negative lesion—just as he had earlier pointed out the '*compound sequence*' of Jacksonian seizures.[202]

> ... the progress of paralysis from increasing extent of a negative lesion is a ... compound order of a different kind according to the particular part of the centre in which that lesion begins. There appears more paralysis in the part of the region suffering first, and also greater range of paralysis the more the lesion extends. From increasing extent of a positive

---

[198] Jackson 1882j, p.433; Jackson's parentheses, my square brackets and underlining. His self-citations are respectively to Jackson 1868r and to Jackson 1869l. The French *suppléance* means 'substitute', which would be consistent with Jackson's meaning of Compensation, albeit less precisely.

[199] See Jackson 1864j, p.389, which is quoted in Chapter 3

[200] Jackson 1882j, pp.433–434; my square brackets.

[201] Jackson 1882j, p.434; Jackson's italics.

[202] See Jackson 1870g, p.166; in Jackson 1868v he had described the 'sequence' of the march without using the word 'compound'.

lesion there is compound order of spreading of convulsion, and a different order according to the particular part of the centre first affected.[203]

From this more extensive analysis of Compensation, Jackson maintained that it reinforced his previous position with regard to the effect of tissue loss in the highest centers. For example,

> ... a part of the highest motor centres (*a*) may be destroyed without obvious permanent paralysis resulting – many would say without any. I submit that there is universal slight paralysis from such lesions. On the other hand, an excessive discharge (*b*) beginning in a part of these centres, as in cases of epilepsy proper, convulses the whole body ...[204]

In his footnote (*a*) Jackson addressed an assumption that still seems counterintuitive.

> (*a*) It has long been admitted that large parts of the brain may be destroyed without there resulting any <u>striking</u> symptoms. It has been said that there may be no symptoms in such cases. This is untenable unless on the supposition that some parts of the brain are without function, a supposition that no one is likely to entertain.[205]

In the above, 'striking' might better be rendered as 'detectable'. Although Jackson did not say it in so many words, the 'large parts of the brain' that are without known function were likely to be in his highest evolutionary levels.

Further Definition of Three Hierarchical Levels, July–August 1883

Toward the end of his third installment Jackson again brought up his theory of levels in the nervous system. He started by saying that there are 'three orders of centres – highest, middle and lowest', which constitute 'what I suppose to be the hierarchy of nervous centres according to the doctrine of Evolution. (*a*)'.[206] Using 'morphological' as a static term, without functional implication, he said: 'This scheme is, not ... as I have in some former papers erroneously said, after the morphological divisions, into spinal cord, medulla oblongata, pons varolii, cerebral hemispheres, and cerebellum.' Rather, 'It is an anatomical division. By anatomical I mean that it is after the different degree of complexity ... of representation *of parts of the body* by different centres. The nervous system is a representing system, and even the centres "for mind" represent parts of the body.' Moreover,

> The doctrine of Evolution repudiates all schemes which make piebald divisions into Ideational, &c., centres ... Nor does it divide motor centres into centres for representation

---

203 Jackson 1883i, p.65; my square brackets.
204 Jackson 1883i, p.65; Jackson's italics. Footnote (*b*) said that his use of 'discharging lesion' had led to 'misunderstandings', because 'It has been taken to imply that a pathological product discharges', whereas 'The correct statement of my opinions would be that "the theory of discharges" is *not* the <u>pathology</u> of epilepsies. The "discharging lesion" is an <u>hyper-physiological</u> condition of cells' (Jackson's italics, my underlining).
205 Jackson 1883h, p.65; my underlining.
206 Footnote: '(*a*) I should say that a very great part of this paper is nothing more than an application of certain Herbert Spencer's principles, stated in his Psychology, were it not that I dare not risk misleading readers by imputing crudities of my own to this distinguished man.' This and similar statements are often quoted to demonstrate Jackson's excessive deference to Spencer, but I submit that it served to express appreciation *and* to maintain his intellectual independence.

of movements, and centres for co-ordination of movements; the two things – representation and co-ordination – are really one. The whole nervous system is … a co-ordinating system from top to bottom.[207]

This was in the last paragraph of Jackson's third installment, which was in effect an introduction to the fourth installment. For heuristic reasons, he said: 'I shall state the scheme … *only as regards the motor centres*, assuming for simplicity, which I do not believe, the middle and highest centres to be purely motor … Another simplification is that … we speak of the cerebral system only; we almost ignore the divisions of the cerebellar system …' Then he defined his three levels.

Lowest Centres. – A lowest centre is one which represents some limited part of the body most nearly directly; it is a centre of simplest, and yet is one of compound, co-ordination … Not only are the spinal anterior horns lowest centres, but so also are the higher homologous [brainstem] nuclei. Thus the nuclei representing … the ocular muscles, [and] the nuclei representing … parts concerned during circulation [vagus], are some lowest centres, as certainly as the lumbar nuclei are some others. The sum of these representations … is the first, most nearly direct representation of the whole body.

Middle Centres. – A middle centre represents over again in still more complex … combinations what … the lowest have represented in comparatively simple combinations; thus it represents a less limited part of the body. The middle centres … are centres of doubly compound co-ordination. They are supposed to be made up of the parts in the so-called psycho-motor region, and also of the ganglia of the corpus striatum. The sum of these representations of wider districts … is a doubly indirect representation of the whole organism. (*a*)

Highest Centres. – The highest [motor] centres … are supposed to be parts in front of the middle. They represent over again in more complex … combinations, the parts which all the middle centres have re-represented, and thus they represent the whole organism; they are re-re-representative … This statement implying that the highest motor centres of each half of the nervous system represent both sides of the body is an anticipation of what will be said when considering Broadbent's hypothesis.[208]

The most important part of this is Jackson's effort to define his '*Middle Centres*'. From the text of that section, and that of the highest centers, we can conclude that the middle level extends from the 'so-called psycho-motor region' (Ferrier's motor region) downstream to the basal ganglia. The thalami were not mentioned, presumably because they do not have motor functions. Despite the improving knowledge of neuroanatomy, he was frustrated about uncertain details of the middle level.

(*a*) I do not pretend to be able to speak with accuracy of the exact parts which make up the middle centres. Artificial excitation of only certain convolutions produces movements; in these convolutions most large cells are found; it is from destructive lesions of fibres

---

[207] Jackson 1883i, p.66; Jackson's italics. His next lines continued: 'The Evolutionist can take a brutally materialistic view of disease of any part of the nervous system, for the reason that he does not take a materialistic view of mind … The doctrine of Evolution has nothing whatever to do with the nature of the relation of psychical to the physical states of these centres …'

[208] Jackson 1883ij, p.85; Jackson's italics, my square brackets and underlining.

connected with these convolutions that descending wasting occurs, and this stops at the lowest [spinal] centres. <u>Lesions in front</u> do not produce descending wasting into the cord; whether or not they produce wasting 'descending' to the middle centres I do not know. These facts, however, are read by most physicians, not only as proving that the convolutions in question are motor, but that those in front of them are not motor … I believe the latter to be also motor.[209]

On the motor side, Jackson had begun to define his middle and highest levels in 1876,[210] when he had extended them into the sensory side,[211] and he repeated those definitions in 1879.[212] But in 1883, he had something new and fundamental—neuroanatomical evidence of direct connections of fibers from Ferrier's motor cortex to the spinal cord, i.e., the nearly complete corticospinal (pyramidal) tract. This was 7 years after Flechsig's (1876) initial demonstration of the tract, but Flechsig's method was myelogenetic, and Jackson was citing evidence from Wallerian degeneration.[213] Since he gave no citation for the Wallerian findings he must have assumed that all of this was common knowledge at the time. Indeed, we will see in the next section that such an assumption was probably correct. We must also remember that this was at the least 8 years before widespread acceptance of the neuron theory. Although Jackson was clearly referring to the Betz cells ('large cells') in the motor cortex, he said nothing about degeneration of those cells. Since 'Lesions in front' refers to (our) prefrontal cortices, he was saying that he had no information about fibers from prefrontal motor cortices to the basal ganglia. In general, his preference was to establish principles, regardless of the details, and that is what he did for hierarchical levels in the brain.

We have also seen that Jackson had a habit of abruptly discontinuing serialized papers without announcing their terminations. In the paragraphs that defined his levels he twice promised later consideration of Broadbent. And in the last sentence of his fourth installment he said, 'Resistances will be considered later', followed by '(To be continued.)'. In fact, the series was not continued in the *Medical Press and Circular*, but the subject was carried into a major address in the following year.

The Croonian Lectures on Evolution and Dissolution, March–April 1884

The full title of Jackson's major publication in 1884 was 'The Croonian lectures on the evolution and dissolution of the nervous system. Delivered at the Royal College of Physicians'.[214] To this day there are still two different Croonian Lectures in London. They occur in

209 Jackson 1883ij, p.85, footnote (*a*) in column 1; my square brackets and underlining.
210 Jackson 1876v, pp.297–298; see Chapter 8.
211 Jackson 1876v, p.296
212 Jackson 1879c, p.34; see Chapter 9.
213 See McHenry 1969, pp.174–176. Flechsig's myelogenetic technique involved developmental studies of axonal myelination in the nervous systems of humans, from fetuses to adults, rather than following Wallerian degeneration of already-myelinated axonal tracts.
214 The three lectures were published simultaneously and identically in the *BMJ* (Jackson 1884b, Jackson 1884d, Jackson 1884g) and *The Lancet* (Jackson 1884a, Jackson 1884f, Jackson 1884j). In the *Medical Times and Gazette* (Jackson 1884c, Jackson 1884e, Jackson 1884h) they were abstracted, and there was a laudatory editorial (Jackson 1884i). I have used the *BMJ*'s version. In November 1884 the American *Popular Science Monthly* reprinted Jackson's Croonian I (Jackson 1884k); the editor was Edward L. Youmans, who was a Spencer devotee (see Werth 2009, p.xv, etc.).

alternating years because that's the way they were endowed at two separate institutions by the widow of William Croone in the early eighteenth century. At the Royal Society the Croonian is considered to be 'the premier lecture in the biological sciences'.[215] At the Royal College of Physicians (RCP) they are also highly prestigious and, unlike the Royal Society, they must be given by a fellow.[216] Thus the audience for Jackson's three lectures would have been largely from the fellowship of the College.

In Jackson's publication record there is nothing from the end of the *MPC* series about dissolution on August 1, 1883, until the publication of his first Croonian Lecture on March 29, 1884. From this 8-month gap we can infer that he received the invitation sometime in the middle of 1883. By the time of the lectures' actual delivery, in March–April 1884, Jackson was 49 years of age and considered by his colleagues to be quite senior—his hair was gray and his luxuriant beard was nearly white.[217] It was 21 years after his first effort to reform neural pathophysiology in his *Suggestions* of 1863. He had been writing and lecturing about dissolution since 1873, but few physicians had really absorbed what he was trying to say. The officers at the RCP obviously thought that his ideas were appropriate for a general medical audience, so this was an opportunity to introduce them more widely.[218] From the broader cultural perspective we might perceive some consonance between Jackson's 'dissolution' and the late Victorians' concern with decadence and degeneration, although I doubt that Jackson thought he was addressing those societal issues.[219] Evolution, of course, was a hot topic, but his emphasis was on dissolution.

Given the interconnected nature of Jackson's theories, presumably the RCP expected that he would use the lectures to review many of his main ideas, not just dissolution.[220] By and large, that is what he did, although he said relatively little about aphasia and nothing about the cerebellum or the subjective–objective distinction. Most of what he had to say had been published in his major treatises of 1881–1883, but frequent repetitions were required. Fortunately, his many months of preparation conferred a benefit. Jackson's Croonians were relatively well organized. In my analysis I will deal with the lectures sequentially, more or less.

Croonian Lecture I: Five New Elements in the Paradigm, Published March 29, 1884

After the usual pleasantries and acknowledgments, Jackson began with a review of his theory of dissolution. Within that review there were at least five new or modified elements:

(1) distinction of 'Uniform' versus 'Local' dissolution;
(2) expansion of the concept of the 'compound' (temporally over-lapping) order of focal seizures to compound patterns in dissolution and in other clinical conditions;

---

[215] Website accessed August 16, 2015.

[216] Website accessed August 16, 2015.

[217] See the1886 group photograph in Gowers 1960 (Illustration 32 on p.63); the same photograph is labelled 1887 in Holmes 1954 (Plate III) and 1888 in Shorvon 2014, p.229.

[218] The President of the RCP at the time was Sir William Jenner, who had attended Mrs. Jackson in her fatal illness (see Cooke 1972, p.1130, and Chapter 9). Jackson's friend Sir Andrew Clark became President in 1888, so he would have been deeply involved in the RCP in 1883, when Jackson was appointed to the Croonian.

[219] On 'decadence' see immediately above in this section; 'degeneration' was a biological concept applied to the deterioration. See Chamberlain and Gilman 1985; also Newsome 1997, pp.248–250, and Burrow 2000, pp.62, 181–190.

[220] I suspect that another attraction of Jackson as a lecturer was his willingness to politely but firmly disagree with the other 'authorities', which is seen especially in his second Croonian (J84-04, pp.660–661).

(3) a new pathophysiology of hemiplegia!

(4) citation of recent experimental evidence for representation of unilateral movements in both hemispheres; and

(5) changed nosological *and* pathophysiological usages of 'epilepsy' and 'epileptiform'.

Although the first two of these new elements can be identified separately, they are best discussed together.

Regarding elements (1) and (2), in the first part of his first lecture Jackson proposed 'two broad divisions of cases of dissolution, Uniform and Local'. Starting with the former, he said:

> In Uniform Dissolution the whole nervous system is under the same conditions ... the evolution of the whole nervous system is comparatively evenly reversed ... but the different centres are not equally affected. An injurious agent, such as alcohol ... flows to all parts ... but the highest centres, being least organized, "give out" first and most; the middle centres ... resist longer; and the lowest centres ... resist longest.[221]

In trying to explain how 'Uniform' dissolution actually works, Jackson offered a theoretical example which was an expansion of another, older concept, though one might wonder if it really helped his cause.

> ... increasing uniform dissolution follows a "compound order;" these stages may be rudely symbolised ... using the initial letters of, highest [*h*], middle [*m*], and lowest [*l*] centres. First stage ... of dissolution, *h*; second stage, $h^2 + m$; third stage, $h^3 + m^2 + l$; etc.... in cases of uniform dissolution, it is important, especially with regard to clear notions on localisation, to recognize that the order of dissolution is a compound order.[222]

Let me hasten to explain that the formulaic system (*hml*) in the above is not another theory of localization, different from Jackson's *xyz* theory. Rather, it is his way of emphasizing the compound nature of Uniform Dissolution with a summary version of *xyz*. His use of 'compound' was an expansion of its application in his 'Study' of 1870, but it was not a change of meaning. It still referred to temporally overlapping, not strictly sequential phenomena. We will encounter this expanded use of 'compound' often in his Croonians, but not just then, when he went on to define 'Local Dissolution'.

> Obviously, disease of a part of the nervous system could not be a reversal of the evolution of the whole; all that we can expect is local reversal of evolution, [i.e.] that there should be loss in the order from voluntary towards automatic in what the part diseased represents ... dissolution may be local in several senses. Disease may occur on any evolutionary level, on one side or on both sides; it may affect the sensory elements chiefly, or the motor elements chiefly ... there are local dissolutions of the highest centres, [because] in every case of insanity, the highest centres are morbidly affected. Since there are different kinds, as well as

---

221 Jackson 1884b, pp.591; Jackson's quotation marks.

222 Jackson 1884b, p.591; Jackson's italics and quotation marks, my square brackets. Later in Croonian I (Jackson 1884b, p.593) he used a similar notation system to summarize the compound spreading of epileptiform seizures, where *a* is for arm, *f* for face, and *l* for leg. About this he said, 'Degrees of epileptiform seizures illustrate different depths of dissolution ... This compound order of spreading, which any adequate doctrine of localization has to account for, may be symbolised thus: *a*, then $a^2 + f$, then $a^3 + f^2 + l$, etc.'

degrees, of insanity ... it follows ... that different divisions of the highest centres are morbidly affected ... Different kinds of insanity are different local dissolutions of the highest centres.[223]

After his definitions of uniform and local dissolution, Jackson gave several examples, including 'delirium in acute non-cerebral disease. This, scientifically regarded, is a case of insanity.'[224] However, his penchant for orderly, hierarchical dissolution led him to a questionable generalization in his first example.

Starting at the bottom [caudal end] of the [central] nervous system, the first example is the commonest variety of <u>progressive muscular atrophy</u>. We see here that atrophy begins in the most voluntary limb, the arm; it affects, first, the most voluntary part of that limb, the hand, and first of all, the most voluntary part of the hand; it then spreads to the trunk, in general to the more automatic parts.[225]

Before the classical work of Charcot in 1874, the term 'progressive muscular atrophy' was something of a wastebasket. From a confusing group of similar presentations, Charcot defined *amyotrophic lateral sclerosis* (ALS) by correlating specific clinical findings with histologically definable lesions of the spinal cord (motor tract and ventral horn cells) and ventral roots.[226] Presumably ALS was what Jackson meant by the 'commonest variety of progressive muscular atrophy', because he referred to the 'anterior horns' of the spinal cord,[227] which are affected in most of the disorders that are now grouped together as *motor neuron disease*, including ALS. However, the clinical presentation of ALS is much more variable than Jackson described in the above quotation.

Even at the time, Charcot's delineation of ALS was recognized as a transformative event in the developing science of medical neurology—on the same order as the experimental achievements of Fritsch and Hitzig and Ferrier. Those events were part of the general excitement in the biomedical sciences of the late nineteenth century. Notwithstanding the work of Ferrier and a few of his countrymen, most of the basic neuroscience was happening in France and in the German-speaking countries. Since Jackson could read French, that part of the rapidly growing science was available to him, and he used it.

Regarding element (3), returning to the hemispheric end of the neuraxis, Jackson offered hemiplegia as an example of dissolution. Almost in passing, he mentioned that hemiplegia was 'owing to a lesion of the internal capsule ...'.[228] *Voila!* His first Croonian of 1884 is where Hughlings Jackson inconspicuously dethroned the gray matter of the corpus striatum as the site of the lesion that is commonly responsible for hemiplegia. He gave no citation for this new information, but its source is not far to seek. It was the team of two French neurophysiologists, Charles Emile François-Franck (1849–1921) and Jean Albert Pitres (1848–1928).

---

[223] Jackson 1884b, pp.591–592; my square brackets.

[224] Jackson 1884b, p.592.

[225] Jackson 1884b, p.592; my square brackets and underlining.

[226] See Goetz et al., pp.100–108.

[227] Jackson 1884b, p.592.

[228] Jackson 1884b, p.593. The internal capsules on each side are the places where the densely packed fibers of the corticospinal (pyramidal) tracts pass through the gray matter of each striatum. However, in the absence of the neuron theory, accepting the internal capsule in this way does not automatically implicate cortical cells as the origins of the fibers in the internal capsule.

The former was a pupil of Brown-Séquard, and both were pupils of Charcot.[229] Lawrence McHenry states that François-Franck 'was the first to map the motor fibres in the motor [internal] capsule',[230] and Meyer lists François-Franck and Pitres together in 1878 as first among those who 'incriminated the internal capsule rather than the corpus striatum for any resulting movements' during (unsuccessful) experimental attempts to stimulate the striatum.[231] In January 1879 Jackson had devoted a long footnote to experiments by the two French investigators, so he knew their work.[232]

Regarding element (4), since François-Franck and Pitres used both electrical stimulation and Wallerian degeneration in their studies, their work had a bearing on Jackson's concerns about hemiplegia *and* cortical representation of unilateral movements. With regard to the 'compound order of spreading' in focal seizures, which 'illustrate different depths of dissolution', Jackson said, 'these cases … supply further evidence that both sides of the body are represented in each half of the brain. Certain experiments of Franck and Pitres (*Arch. de Phys.*, August 15th, 1883, No.6) bear in a most important way on the question as to double representation.'[233] Then he summarized the French paper, emphasizing the different patterns of degeneration that the authors had found in the two hemispheres after unilateral lesions. About this he said, 'Here seems to be evidence that both sides of the body are represented in each half of the brain, and also that the two sides are differently represented in each half'. He stressed this result because it was 'a matter of extreme importance for the doctrines of evolution and dissolution'.[234]

Regarding element (5), the significance of the different hemispheric patterns of motor representation for the same movement was also related to Jackson's changing conceptions of 'epileptic' and 'epileptiform' seizures. In his first Croonian he redefined his use of those terms. In essence, he localized focal epileptiform seizures to his middle cerebral level and genuine/proper epileptic seizures to his highest level. One indication of this change occurred in his fourth example of dissolution, when he said: 'Next we speak of epileptiform seizures, which are unquestionably owing to disease in the mid region of the brain (middle motor centres).'[235] In 1881 he had nominated the 'highest centres' as the site of the focal lesions responsible for 'epilepsy proper',[236] but here in 1884 his use of 'unquestionably' indicates that he had also settled on the middle level as the site of the lesions responsible for epileptiform seizures. In a footnote to a discussion of 'Degrees of epileptiform seizures' in Croonian I he said:

I am not speaking of epileptic attacks, which depend, I think, on discharges beginning in parts of … the highest level of evolution. A man long subject to very limited epileptiform seizures may at length have seizures beginning in the same way and becoming universal, but these are not epileptic seizures, they are only more severe epileptiform seizures.[237]

---

[229] On François-Franck see McHenry 1969, p.223, and Aminoff 2011, p.221; on Pitres see McHenry 1969, p.296, and Goetz et al. 1995, pp.123–125. Morton 1961, p.126, says, 'Three papers by Charcot and Pitres in 1877, 1878, and 1883 left no doubt as to the existence of cortical motor centres in man'.

[230] McHenry 1969, p.223.

[231] Meyer 1971, p.40; my square brackets.

[232] See Jackson 1879c, p.34. In Croonian II (Jackson 1884d, p.661) Jackson referred to 'Franck and Pitres for whose highly scientific work I have a most respectful admiration …'

[233] Jackson 1884b, p.593. I have not analyzed the paper of François-Franck and Pitres.

[234] Jackson 1884b, p.593.

[235] Jackson 1884b, p.592; Jackson's parentheses.

[236] Jackson 1881k, p.399; see also above in this chapter.

[237] Jackson 1884b, p.593.

And near the end of the lecture he elaborated.

> ... the middle motor centres (a discharge beginning in parts which cause ... epileptiform seizures) of each half of the brain represent movements of both sides of the body... the highest motor centres (frontal lobes) re-represent, in more intricate combinations, all that the middle centres have represented in simpler combinations; a discharge beginning in part of these more evolved centres produces an epileptic seizure, which is, so to speak, a "more evolved convulsion" than an epileptiform seizure.[238]

Nowadays we might be uncomfortable with the proposition that *grand mal* seizures are somehow 'more evolved'—i.e., of a higher order—than others. In the end Jackson did not push this idea, but it does highlight his inclination to follow out the logical consequences of his theorizing. Since he was constantly re-evaluating his theories, they were always under construction, and there were bumps in the road.

Croonian Lecture II: Depths of Dissolution and Postictal States, Published April 5, 1884

Jackson's constant reworking explains the miscellaneous feeling of the five new elements that I identified in his first Croonian. It seems like a list for tying up loose ends, but remember that I was looking mainly for new elements among the old. Overall, in his first Croonian he was laying the groundwork for the central theme of his second Croonian,[239] which might have been subtitled 'Three Depths of Dissolution, illustrated by epilepsy, epileptiform seizures, and insanity'. He was trying to further the integration of dissolution into his paradigm for all epileptic disorders. Of course, there were some new elements, which will be discussed within a more comprehensive analysis.

The Main Themes in Jackson's Croonian II

(1) review of his hierarchical/evolutionary *levels* in the brain;
(2) review of his *pathophysiology of epileptic seizures* in relation to (1);
(3) review of *epileptic mania* in relation to (2);
(4) definition and discussion of *three depths of dissolution*, using epilepsy and epileptiform seizures as illustrations; and an
(5) inconclusive discussion of the *limits of consciousness* in the second and third depths.

Regarding elements (1) and (2), in reviewing his concept of hierarchical levels, Jackson slipped in a statement about the 'physical basis of consciousness', which clarified his ideas about the distinction of epileptic versus epileptiform seizures:

---

[238] Jackson 1884b, p.593; Jackson's parentheses and quotation marks. In Lecture II (Jackson 1884d, p.660) Jackson repeated: 'An epileptic paroxysm depends on a sudden and excessive discharge, or liberation of energy, beginning in some *part* of the highest centres.²' And in footnote 2 he said: 'It must be clearly understood that I am not speaking of epileptiform seizures; they depend on discharge beginning in some part of the middle centres – so-called motor region – centres of a lower degree of evolution.'

[239] Jackson 1884b.

That the middle motor centres represent over again what all the lowest motor centres have represented, will be disputed by few. I go further, and say that the highest motor centres (frontal lobes) represent over again … what the middle centres represent … The main conclusions are (1) that the highest (chiefly) sensory centres – parts behind Ferrier's sensory region – and also the highest (chiefly) motor centres – parts in front of the so-called motor region – make up – the physical basis of consciousness; and (2) that just as consciousness represents, or is, the whole person psychical, so its anatomical basis (highest centres) represents the whole person physical … States of consciousness attend survivals of the fittest states of centres representing the whole organism.[240]

Here we see Jackson's reasoning for assigning epileptic (but not epileptiform) seizures to foci in the highest centers—because the highest centers are the 'physical basis of consciousness', and epileptic seizures begin with alterations of consciousness.

Regarding element (2), in reviewing his conception of the epileptic discharge at the physiological level, Jackson said again that 'certain cells … gradually attain very high tension … and suddenly liberate a large quantity of energy, and then gradually re-attain high instability'.[241] The sudden discharge, he said, is the result of a 'physiological fulminate',[242] which seems closer to a chemical analogy than he had conjectured in his 'Study' of 1870.[243] The energy in this fulminate spreads laterally to healthy cells and downwards, where resistance is greater in lower levels. Although the clinically derived idea of postictal physiological exhaustion goes back at least to Todd and to Robertson,[244] in 1884 Jackson could also cite experimental evidence from François-Franck and Pitres, who had 'found that after epileptiform convulsions induced in dogs, the part of the cortex which had been artificially discharged, remained for a time unexcitable'.[245]

Regarding element (3), for Jackson the idea of a *refractory period* after a motor seizure was central to his reasoning about postictal mania—and it is in keeping with our current conceptions.

It is well known that some epileptics, after their fits, are maniacal. The condition is called "epileptic mania," but it should be called "epileptic unconsciousness with mania" … Since the fit is over, and as the patient remains unconscious, there is … on the physical side, loss of function of some of the highest arrangements of his highest centres – let us say, of the highest two [hypothetical] layers. The co-existing mania is, I contend, the outcome of greatly raised activity of the next lower level of evolution remaining, the [hypothetical] third layer, which is normal, except for hyperphysiological activity. But now comes the question, Why is an unconscious man furiously active? Why, on the loss of function of the highest two layers, is the next, the third, layer in the state of hyperphysiological activity …[246]

---

[240] Jackson 1884d, p.660; Jackson's parentheses, my underlining.
[241] Jackson 1884d, p.660.
[242] Jackson 1884d, p.660.
[243] See Chapter 6.
[244] On Todd see Chapters 4 and 6. On Robertson see Chapter 8, where Jackson 1876u and Jackson 1876v are cited. This Robertson is (Charles) Alexander (Lockhard) Robertson (1825–1897; see Brown 1955, p.165), not his brother Argyll, of pupillary reflex fame.
[245] Jackson 1884d, p.661. About François-Franck and Pitres, McHenry (1969, p.223) says they were 'Working at a time when new physiological tools had become available, [so] they were able to show by careful timing that there was a delay in response after stimulating the gray matter which disappeared when the white matter alone was stimulated'.
[246] Jackson 1884d, p.660; my square brackets and underlining.

To understand Jackson's thinking in this passage it is crucial to recognize that his 'highest two layers' and his 'third' layer are *hypothetical* layers *within* the 'highest centres'. If he had meant 'third' to refer to his lowest *level*, he would have said 'lowest level', rather than 'layer'. Purely for the sake of argument he is postulating the existence of three layers within the highest level. This heuristic device goes back at least to 1881, when he said that 'there may be different parts of any of the several <u>divisions of the highest centres</u> …'.[247] And in 1883 he said, 'there are many lowest, many middle, and many highest centres'.[248] However, late in 1881, discussing 'three motor centres of different grades of evolution' (i.e. levels), he had cautioned 'that this … order of centres is not supposed to correspond to our three degrees of post-epileptic conditions'.[249] That is, the successive three *depths* of exhaustion—to be defined shortly—are not necessarily assigned to the three *levels* of the brain; there will be only one depth in relation to any individual *layer*, because the latter is hypothetical.

As an example of local dissolution, in his first Croonian Jackson had discussed 'delirium in acute non-cerebral disease', whose

> … negative mental state signifies, on the physical side, exhaustion, or loss of function … of some highest nervous arrangements of his [the patient's] highest centres. We may conveniently say that it shows loss of function of the topmost "layer" of his highest centres. No one, of course, believes that the highest centres, or any other centres, are in layers; but the supposition will simplify exposition.[250]

This is the first place where Jackson used the idea of a high cortical 'layer' as a hypothetical, heuristic device. Assuming that his audience understood his use of the word, in his second Croonian he went on to an assertion about the postictal state.

> It is commonly said … of epileptic mania … that it replaces … an ordinary epileptic paroxysm. Further, what I shall shortly speak of as the first depth of dissolution … remaining after … an epileptic discharge would … be considered by most medical men to be, or to be part of, a paroxysm. I do not accept these hypotheses … I shall state a counter-hypothesis …[251]

Jackson's 'counter-hypothesis' was his statement that 'the sudden and excessive discharge in an epileptic paroxysm produces exhaustion of nerve-tracts which have been travelled by excessive currents in that paroxysm'.[252] This was his counter-poise to a 'doctrine of replacement', which would have been inconsistent with his theory of release.

> I have been said to accept the doctrine of replacement – to believe that "psychoses" occur instead of ordinary epileptic paroxysms. In reality, I entirely disbelieve that doctrine; I gave

[247] Jackson 1881k, p.399; my underlining.
[248] Jackson 1883i, p.85.
[249] Jackson 1881r, p.382.
[250] Jackson 1884b, p.592; Jackson's quotation marks; my square brackets. Jackson's hypothetical, hierarchical layers within the highest level were not meant to imply somatotopy.
[251] Jackson 1884d, p.660.
[252] Jackson 1884d, p.660. Here he again cited clinical examples and the experimental work of François-Franck and Pitres. A clinical example was a case of postictal paralysis after focal left leg seizures due to a tumor in the 'right middle region of the brain'. This seems like the autopsied tumor case that Jackson reported in Jackson 1884l, but that patient's tumor was on the left.

it up many years ago. I believe that <u>all elaborate, suddenly-occurring states in epileptics</u> ... <u>follow a paroxysm</u>.[253]

Regarding element (4), beyond the 'primary' seizure focus, he said: 'there is a far wider negative state from running down of the parts secondarily discharged, and from exhaustion of central nerve-fibres effected by these primary and secondary discharges'.[254] Continuing with his hypothetical example of three layers in the highest level, Jackson returned to epileptic mania, for which,

> ... exhaustion of the highest two layers of the highest centres being a purely negative state [it] cannot account for the superpositive state, mania. Nothing cannot be the cause of something ... the maniacal actions are ... the outcome of the activity, on the lower level of evolution remaining – third layer – of nervous arrangements which ... are healthy ... they are manifestations of the survival of the fittest states on the lower ... level of evolution... we must speak of <u>three degrees of exhaustion</u>, [i.e.,] <u>three increasing depths of dissolution</u>, which are effected by epileptic discharges of different degrees of severity, taking count of the corresponding three degrees of decreasing shallows of evolution.[255]

Jackson then gave succinct definitions of his three depths of postictal dissolution, which were consistent with his definitions of 3 years earlier.[256]

> First Depth. – There is <u>defect of consciousness</u> significant of dissolution of the topmost layer along with the rise of a certain kind of ideation significant of increased activity of the second layer ... <u>roughly analogous to ordinary sleep with dreaming</u> ...
>   Second Depth. – There is so-called <u>loss of consciousness</u>, significant of dissolution of the topmost and second layers, along with <u>actions of more or less elaborateness</u> (one example of which is postepileptic unconsciousness with mania) significant of increased activity of the third layer ...
>   Third [Depth]. – There is <u>coma</u>, significant of dissolution of the first, second, and third layers, with which ... there is <u>persistence only of "vital" operations</u>, such as respiration and circulation, significant of retention of activity of the <u>fourth layer</u> ... analogous to deep slumber, to so-called dreamless sleep.[257]

In recording Jackson's further discussions of these three depths, the reporter gave only a condensed summary of the first.

> [The first depth was then remarked on. The ideation or "dreamy state" was usually called an intellectual aura, and was by most physicians considered to be part of the paroxysm. Particular attention was drawn to the frequent occurrence of the "dreamy state," with or

---

[253] Jackson 1884d, p.661, footnote 3; Jackson's quotation marks, my underlining. To support his statement about giving it up 'many years ago', Jackson cited the title of Jackson 1875ll, 'On Temporary Disorders *after* Epileptic Paroxysms'.

[254] Jackson 1884d, p.661; he said nothing about exhaustion of muscle.

[255] Jackson 1884d, p.661; my square brackets and underlining.

[256] In Jackson 1881l, pp.68–69. The following three definitions were originally printed in one continuous paragraph; I have separated them for clarity.

[257] Jackson 1884d, p.661; Jackson's parentheses, my square brackets and underlining. Note that in discussing the third depth Jackson slipped a hypothetical 'fourth layer' into the highest centers.

after movements of chewing, or tasting, and sometimes of spitting – movements believed to imply an excitation of central gustatory elements.][258]

Since the above included a reference to the dreamy state, we would conclude that it can occur in the first depth. Indeed, following the above definitions, Jackson said that the dreamy state occurs when there is 'dissolution of the topmost layer'—not simply 'highest'—and 'increased activity of the second layer'. In his discussion of the second depth he included another example of the dreamy state.

> *Second Depth.* – There has been a stronger discharge, which has effected deeper exhaustion. Now, there is no ideation, at least none is remembered on recovery; but there are actions. There are really subdegrees or subdepths of the second depth, and no doubt of the first and third depths, of dissolution ... As to the second depth, there are ... actions of different degrees of elaborateness, from such highly special and complex actions as that of a fisherman, unconscious after an epileptic fit, occurring at dinner, pulling out a line from a reel, untying a knot, taking out a hook from his pocket, affixing it and baiting it (doing all this pantomimically), down to such actions ... as sprawling on the floor.[259]

Here the dreamy state has occurred in the second depth, so we can infer that it can be seen whenever there is preservation of some layer of the highest level. However, the dreamy state cannot be due to release of the middle or lowest levels, because the actions in it are too complex to be represented in those levels. Jackson supported this conclusion when he said he would

> ...remark on some differences in the two [highest] depths ... in the first, the ideation is remembered, or of course we should know nothing about it. From the second, as in somnambulism, nothing is remembered. But it comes to be a question of importance ... whether or not ... in the second depth there is some ideation, in spite of the expression, "*loss of consciousness*." That there is activity of some nervous arrangements of the highest centres, we are supposing of the third layer, is, I submit, quite certain.[260]

Regarding element (5), so far Jackson's conclusion about release of the third layer in the second depth was relatively straightforward, but the clinical 'elaborateness of the operation' in the second depth raised a much more difficult problem.

> The question is this: "Do states of consciousness attend ... [the dreamy state] ... or not?["] There will be two views on this matter. Let me return to the case of the fisherman ... Had that man ... any states of consciousness attending the nervous activities which were producing his elaborate actions? One view would be that the fact that the patient remembered nothing was proof that there were no mental states. Another view would be that the very elaborateness of the operation implied some co-existing states of consciousness. We must carry each view to its logical conclusion.[261]

---

[258] Jackson 1884d, p.661; square brackets inserted by the reporter.
[259] Jackson 1884d, p.661; Jackson's italics and parentheses.
[260] Jackson 1884d, p.662; Jackson's italics and quotation marks, my square brackets.
[261] Jackson 1884d, p.662; my square brackets and underlining. The open quotation mark in the first line was never closed.

At this point Jackson's discussion turned from the clinical characteristics of the second depth to the implications of consciousness or its absence.

> Those who take the first view – most medical men, I believe – must say that the patient was a mere machine; that, having no consciousness, he was a mere automaton … this view is that elaborate and universal movements may occur without a trace of consciousness. On the second view, it would be admitted that the man was … an imperfect automaton … having lost the highest parts of his nervous machinery; but it would be asserted that some degree of consciousness attended activities of the nervous arrangements on the lower level of evolution remaining. Each of these two views has consequences …[262]

Jackson started to explore those consequences in his next section, on the 'Third Depth', which he supposed to be due to 'a severest discharge; when it is over, the patient is comatose … [he] has seemingly no movements excepting "vital" movements, such as the respiratory and the circulatory'.[263] About this conundrum he repeated his earlier opinion: 'The current explanation of the post-epileptic comatose patient's immobility is, that he does not move, because he is unconscious … My belief is that the postepileptic immobility is … universally spread paralysis.'[264] But how can a patient be widely paralyzed and yet thrashing about? Jackson's explanation had long depended on his *xyz* theory, which was assumed but not stated.

> … in post-epileptic mania there is some degree of paralysis all over the body, or, more precisely, loss of some movements of all parts, and … at the very same time there is persistence and over development of some other movements of all parts … [a] severe convulsion … is nothing other than a sudden excessive development of the movements remaining.[265]

Jackson had made essentially the same statement in 1881,[266] albeit with less emphasis on 'movements remaining', which means remaining in the *xyz* theory. I have reiterated his repetition here because it was relevant to the unanswered question about 'automaton' versus 'imperfect automaton'. He never said explicitly that he preferred the latter, but his subsequent discussion leaned heavily in that direction. This is seen in his discussion of: (1) a hypothetical resolution of the problem of consciousness in the second depth, and (2) a statement about 'defect of consciousness in every case of insanity'. About (1), in a discussion of the third depth he said:

> The following difficulty, taking the case of the fisherman, has to be met. There was so-called loss of consciousness, implying a deep dissolution, and yet his very elaborate doings implied a very high level of evolution remaining. I hold that in post-epileptic states there are local dissolutions, meaning that the post-epileptic exhaustion is in … one cerebral hemisphere. Thus, whilst there is a low level of [remaining] evolution in the highest centres of one half of the brain, there is a perfect or very high level in those of the opposite half. If so, the discrepancy disappears.[267]

---

262 Jackson 1884d, p.662; my underlining. Here Jackson was willing to use 'automaton' a decade after Huxley (1874) loaded it with materialistic implications; see Chapter 8.
263 Jackson 1884d, p.662; Jackson's italics, my square brackets.
264 Jackson 1884d, p.662.
265 Jackson 1884d, pp.662–663; my square brackets and underlining.
266 In Jackson 1881b, pp.438–439, quoted and discussed above in this chapter.
267 Jackson 1884d, p.663; my square brackets and underlining.

The 'discrepancy' here was a clinical observation—convulsions in otherwise paralyzed limbs—but the proposed solution was entirely hypothetical. He did not offer any clinical or experimental data beyond the clinical phenomenon itself, nor did he say anything about an imperfect automaton, which might be inferred from this passage. Rather, he went on to a discussion of (2) insanity, where the implication seemed to be that while insane persons are in depths 1 or 2, they retain some consciousness.

> Since I say ... that there is some defect of consciousness in every case of insanity, I ought to hold the opinion that, in every case of insanity, there is some degree ... of universal or widely distributed paralysis ... So I do. That I could not demonstrate its existence in many cases, I admit ... In cases of dementia [insanity] the patient's "lethargy" might be put down to his negative mental state ... I should call dementia the chronic analogue of what acutely is post-epileptic coma, and attribute the lethargy to the negative condition ... of the patient's highest centres ... [268]

If the reader has the feeling of drowning in a sea of hypotheticals, that is because your author feels likewise, and the same was probably true for Jackson's audience. I have tried to follow his theorizing faithfully, but it seemed to be extending beyond the warrant of his available data, which, involving consciousness, would be entirely clinical. The virtue of Jackson's model was its dynamism—its ability to account for many different abnormalities in a single framework, but the price of dynamism is the risk of bewilderment. I think he recognized this problem in his final Croonian, because he multiplied his examples of each distinction that he proposed.

Croonian Lecture III: A Series of Broader Issues, Published April 12, 1884

Jackson started his third Croonian by invoking Spencer as a defense against charges of materialism.

> Spencer says, "the doctrine of evolution ... does not involve materialism, though its opponents persistently represent it as doing so" ... he writes ... "Of course, I do not mean that material actions thus become mental actions ... I am merely showing a *parallelism*" [italics in original] "between a certain physical evolution and the correlative psychical evolution" ... as to mind ... [it] is not material at all. [269]

Immediately after this passage Jackson inadvertently showed how difficult it is to keep to strict parallelism.

> A man, physically regarded, is a sensori-motor mechanism. I particularly wish to insist that the highest centres – <u>physical basis of mind or consciousness</u> – have this kind of

---

[268] Jackson 1884d, p.663; my square brackets. Dunglison (1873, p.302) defined dementia: 'In common parlance, and even in legal language, the word is synonymous with insanity. Physicians, however, have applied it to ... cases of unsound mind ...' In 1884 there was a proposal to admit cases of insanity to the National Hospital (Rawlings 1884). It was apparently rejected, and the name of the proposer was not given.

[269] Jackson 1884g, p.703; Jackson's parentheses, my square brackets. For his source of the Spencerian passages Jackson cited 'Psychology, vol.i, p.403', which actually refers to the *Psychology*'s third edition of 1880, where these passages are found.

constitution, that they represent innumerable different impressions and movements of all parts of the body, although very indirectly … It may be rejoined that the highest centres are "for mind." Admitting this, in the sense that they form the physical basis of mind, I assert that they are "for body," too.[270]

The expression 'physical basis of mind or consciousness' belies the distinction between mind and body by saying, in effect, that the mind has a physical basis—he said 'basis', not 'correlate'. Therein lies the fundamental difficulty of Cartesian dualism in relation to modern physical science.[271] This is the ultimate challenge to modern neuroscience. By the 1880s the reductionist program of experimental neuroscience was claiming superior authority over clinical data. This phenomenon is seen at a point where Jackson and Ferrier had a disagreement about the motor functions of the frontal lobes, and Ferrier would not go beyond his primate evidence.

Recently … Ferrier and Yeo … have concluded, from experiments on monkeys, that the frontal lobes represent … lateral movements of the eyes and head … many epileptic paroxysms … begin by turning of the eyes and head to one side … Whilst … Ferrier agrees with me in thinking that the whole anterior part of the brain is motor, and that … "mental operations … must be merely the subjective side of sensory and motor substrata" (*Functions of the Brain*) … he does not agree with me in thinking there to be a division into middle and highest cerebral motor centres … he thinks that what I call the highest motor centres represent only movements of the eyes and head, and not movements of all parts of the body …[272]

Immediately after the above passage Jackson quoted Ferrier again: 'This view has been repeatedly and clearly enunciated by Hughlings-Jackson, with whose physiological and psychological deductions from clinical and pathological data I frequently find myself in complete accordance.'[273] Eight years later some of the 'accordance' was less complete, though not severely. Of course, some discordance would be expected within the self-correcting paradigm of modern science, but here we see evidence of an early separation between the experimental and the clinical parts of neuroscience. This tendency was further evidenced when Jackson pleaded: 'If the highest centres do not represent movements, it seems to me that the phenomena of an ordinary epileptic fit are unintelligible.'[274] Among many 'very different kinds of [clinical] evidence' that Jackson invoked to support his position, he cited some of the autonomic phenomena that may be seen in many 'minor' seizures, including ' "crude sensations" of smell, sight, hearing, and taste. Besides these we find palpitation, a peculiar sensation referred to the epigastrium.' Moreover,

The existence, in some cases of *le petit mal*, of the voluminous mental states, so-called intellectual aura … guarantees … that the cruder effects … are owing to abnormal activity of the highest centres. The elaborate mental states … which … no one will hesitate to ascribe

---

[270] Jackson 1884g, p.703; my underlining.
[271] Currently known as the 'hard problem'; see Smith and Whitaker 2014.
[272] Jackson 1884g, p.703, citing Ferrier and Yeo 1884. The quotation followed by '(*Functions of the Brain*)' is found in Ferrier 1876, p.256.
[273] Ferrier 1876, pp.256–257.
[274] Jackson 1884g, p.703.

to activity of the 'organ of mind' (highest centres), never ... occur in or after epileptiform seizures (discharges of middle motor centres).[275]

Jackson intended this passage to reinforce his view that any kind of 'elaborate mental states' related to seizures must be due to released cortical activity in the highest levels. But his use of 'aura' raises a related issue: What is the relationship between an intellectual aura and the dreamy state? Are they one and the same? He first used dreamy state in print in 1876, when he had also used the term 'so-called intellectual aura'. The latter was preceded by the statement that:

> It is not very uncommon for epileptics to have vague and yet exceedingly elaborate mental states at the onset of epileptic seizures, or, rather ... just after the very earliest part of the discharge ... all elaborate, although morbid, mental states arise during activity of centres which are healthy, except for loss of "control."[276]

So, according to Jackson in 1876, intellectual auras are ictal in the sense that they arise during a seizure, but they are not strictly epileptic. They come from normal tissue whose functions are released by the epileptic activity in the level just above them. A fine distinction, really, and yet an important one. Three years later, in 1879, he again equated intellectual auras and the dreamy state. When he discussed '*Dreamy States without Actions*' he said: 'There is ... some defect of consciousness, and, at the very same time, some mental activity of a sort – what is commonly called an Intellectual Aura, but which is here called "a dream" ...'[277]

Getting back to 1884 and Jackson's third Croonian, there is nothing to indicate that he had changed his mind about the equivalency of intellectual auras and the dreamy state. Throughout his lecture he was primarily concerned to prove his point about the origin of elaborate mental states in the highest centers. To that end he adduced 'several kinds of evidence [which] point to the conclusion that the highest centres – the physical basis of consciousness – represent the whole organism'.[278] Since it is sensori-motor information that is represented in the highest centers, some of his theoretical arguments were based on explicitly associationist principles.

> It may be objected that, during most mentation, there are no movements ... [but] I said that ... together the highest centres represent, parts of the body triply indirectly [re-re-representation] ... to take the case of visual ideation, and neglecting the sensory element ... there are slight excitations of nervous arrangements triply indirectly representing movements of the ocular muscles, but excitations not strong enough to overcome the resistance of the middle centres. When ideation rises to perception, there is, physically, a stronger discharge of the same nervous arrangements of the higher centres, so that the middle and then the lowest centres are overcome.[279]

---

[275] Jackson 1884g, p.703; Jackson's parentheses. '*Petit mal*' then encompassed a wider clinical spectrum than we now give it.

[276] Jackson 1876u, p.702. This passage is part of a larger quotation which is in Chapter 8.

[277] Jackson 1879g, p.141; Jackson's italics.

[278] Jackson 1884g, p.703; my square brackets.

[279] Jackson 1884g, p.704; my square brackets and underlining.

By implication this passage says that ideation occurs in the middle or lowest level, whereas conscious perception happens in the highest levels.[280] As signals go up or down, they have to overcome resistance, and 'as to the highest centres … there is no difficulty in supposing that these centres may be the most complex, and, at the same time, the least organized'.[281] Jackson's conception of complexity was also closely related to his view of the difference between voluntary and automatic, which led him back to his earlier view of emergent consciousness and thence to some resolution of the automaton issue. About conscious volition he cited Spencer.

> … the "cessation of automatic action and the dawn of volition are one and the same thing" (*Psych.*, vol.i, p.497). Volition arises during activity of the least automatic nervous arrangements; or, rather, "a kind of mental action arises which is one of memory, reason, feeling, or will, according to the side of it we look at" (Spencer, vol.i, p.495). So now we say that the progress in evolution is from the most to the least automatic, and thus that the highest centres are the least automatic … [This] … does not imply an abrupt division into the voluntary and the automatic, but implies degrees from most to least automatic, and that a man, physically regarded, is an automaton, the highest parts of his nervous system … being least automatic …[282]

One might interpret this passage to mean that humans are just automatons, at least to some extent, but that would go very much against Jackson's centrist grain. In the next paragraph his view was stated a little more clearly.

> A perfect automaton is a thing that goes on by itself. There are degrees from those nervous arrangements, which almost go on by themselves to those which come into activity by the aid of other, lower, more organized, nervous arrangements. To say that nervous arrangements go on by themselves, means that they are well organized; and to say that nervous arrangements go on with difficulty, if at all, by themselves, is to say that they are little organized.[283]

Jackson's discussion of disorganization in the highest centers included an original insight: 'If the highest centres were already organized, there could be no new organizations, no new acquirements.'[284] That is, there would be no neurological mechanism for learning, which is the essence of evolution—but he could postulate a biological mechanism for it.

> … there is what I will call <u>Internal Evolution</u>, a process which goes on most actively in the highest centres … there is, on the physical side, an organization of many different nervous arrangements of our highest centres, during actual converse with the environment. When, as in sleep and in "reflection," this actual converse ceases, the quasi-spontaneous slight activity of the highest sensory centres is uninterfered with by the environment … and, consequently, there are no reactions on the environment … in such case (sleep, reverie, reflection, etc.),

---

[280] In 1876 (Jackson 1876g, pp.174–175) Jackson said that an idea arises when we think of something, but 'To perceive a thing is *to refer it to the environment* or to some part of the body'. In 1881 he said (Jackson 1881l, p.12, footnote (d)): 'Ideation … is of course a psychical state. Perception is … simply a further development of Ideation, or part of it.'

[281] Jackson 1884g, p.704.

[282] Jackson 1884g, pp.704–705; my square brackets. Jackson's citation of Spencer's *Psychology* is to the third edition (1880). He had adopted Spencer's emergent theory in 1866 (see Jackson 1866o, p.605; and Chapter 4). In 1868 he made a similar statement (Jackson 1868u, p.527, footnote (c); see also Chapter 5).

[283] Jackson 1884g, p.705.

[284] Jackson 1884g, p.704.

the very highest nervous arrangements of the highest centres, those in which entirely new organizations can be made, will be in least activity, and the next lower of those centres in greater activity [of resistance]. The nervous arrangements of the highest centres … are "left to fight it out among themselves;" new combinations arise, the survival of the fittest … new, although evanescent combinations, are made during dreaming; but I contend that permanent rearrangements (internal evolutions) are made during so-called dreamless sleep.[285]

This was Jackson's first published use of 'Internal Evolution', but he had applied 'survival of the fittest' to cerebral events in 1879,[286] and he used 'survival' again in the same context in 1881.[287] Here in 1884 he drew a prescient inference. That is, there has to be a consolidation process for retention of memories. He proposed that the evolutionary struggle for survival among competing memories takes place in a layer of the highest brain level just below the highest layer. Of course, at that time there was no way to see this kind of activity in the brain. Needless to say, that did not stop his speculating further—in this case about the histological basis of memory consolidation.[288] Then he went on to a different subject, claiming broad support for his 'doctrine of concomitance'.

It seems to me that the doctrine of concomitance is … convenient in the study of nervous diseases. It, or an essentially similar doctrine, is held by [William] Hamilton, J.S. Mill, Clifford, Spencer, Max Müller, Bain, Huxley, Du Bois Raymond, Haycock [sic], Tyndall, Herman, and David Ferrier.[289]

Two names that are notably absent from this list are Darwin and Lewes. Darwin's views were not much different than Huxley's or Spencer's,[290] but Lewes was another matter.

The next question is as to range of concomitance. How "far down" in the nervous system does [concomitant] consciousness extend? Lewes thought that some degree of consciousness or "sensibility" attended activities of even the lowest centres. The current view is, that it only attends activities of the highest parts of the nervous system, although no lower limit is agreed upon. Some … speak of "unconscious states of mind," as if, below consciousness, there were some faint mental states. I am not sure that I state this view with verbal correctness, as I do not understand it … whether the activities of the lower nervous arrangements have attendant states of mind, however faint or not, is disputable.[291]

Most of the rest of Jackson's third Croonian was concerned with his theory of localization, which he explained with a direct quotation about his *xyz* theory from his 'Study' of 1870.[292] In summarizing the 'current hypothesis' about localization among his colleagues, he again said there were two opposing views: the 'Universaliser' (holist) and the strict 'Localizer'. Rejecting both extremes, he issued a methodological challenge to anyone who would dispute his view,

---

[285] Jackson 1884g, p.705–706; Jackson's parentheses, my underlining. Jackson's next sentence said, 'I believe that the late Dr. Symonds, of Bristol, stated this in effect'. John Addington Symonds (senior; 1807–1871) wrote *Sleep and Dreams* (1851).

[286] See Jackson 1879t, pp.328–329, which is discussed in Chapter 9.

[287] See Jackson 1881s, p.400, and Jackson 1881t, which are discussed above in this chapter.

[288] He invoked Lewis' small cells (Lewis 1878); see Chapter 8.

[289] Jackson 1884g, p.706. He corrected 'Haycock' to 'Laycock' in Jackson 1887e, p.38.

[290] See C.U.M. Smith 1999 and C.U.M. Smith 2010. Jackson never used 'Darwin' in print; see Chapter 1.

[291] Jackson 1884g, p.706; Jackson's quotation marks, my square brackets.

[292] Jackson 1884g, p.707, quoting Jackson 1870g, pp.190–191.

saying: 'the current hypothesis did not account for all the facts. Any adequate hypothesis had to account for the following', and he gave a list of eight clinical observations that he had used over the years to formulate his conception of cerebral organization and its disorders:

(1) that from a <u>destructive lesion</u> of motor centres the paralysis was especially of the more <u>voluntary</u>, etc.;
(2) that from a <u>discharging lesion</u>, the development of <u>movements</u> (convulsion) was the same: an epileptiform seizure starting in the arm began, first of all, in the hand; one starting in the leg began in the foot; one starting in the face, in the side of the mouth;
(3) that the progress in each (1 and 2) was in <u>compound</u> order;
(4) that a part might be permanently imperfectly paralyzed, and yet the whole of it might be occasionally convulsed;
(5) that recovery, or some recovery, follows on permanent destructive lesions producing paralysis; there is often at least some <u>compensation</u>;
(6) that a small destructive lesion of a motor centre may entail little or no obvious paralysis, whilst a sudden and excessive discharge beginning in such part produces (indirectly) very great convulsion;
(7) that from discharges beginning in different parts of the <u>mid-cortex</u>, we have fits affecting the same regions, but their parts in different order ('isomeric seizures');
(8) that a patient, who has no paralysis before a convulsion, has much (temporary) paralysis after it.[293]

Within Jackson's description of each of the eight clinical observations the underlined words are his names for the conceptions that he drew from them. For example, 'destructive' in (1) means his distinction of 'positive' versus 'negative' lesions. In Table 10.2 the names

Table 10.2 Correlations of terms in Jackson's final paragraph of his Croonian III with parts of his comprehensive paradigm of cerebral organization.

'Destructive lesion'—functional distinction of 'positive' versus 'negative' (destructive) lesions

'Voluntary'—conscious actions, contrasted to automatic movements that involve 'less' consciousness, or none

'Discharging lesion'—Jackson's foundational idea about a 'unit' of histological elements that becomes unstable and causes an abnormal manifestation of that tissue's normal function

'Movements'—which are what is represented in gray matter, not individual muscles

'Compound'—the situation of separate movements that are occurring simultaneously with other separate movements

'Compensation'—his theory of how recovery occurs, based on xyz theory, which latter postulated multiple (but still limited) representations of movements

'Mid-cortex'—the middle level in Jackson's theory of three levels in the cerebrum

---

[293] Jackson 1884g, p.707; Jackson's parentheses and quotation marks, my underlining. In the original these eight items were written in narrative form in a single paragraph. I have broken out each part separately, keeping Jackson's wording. On 'isomeric seizures' see Jackson 1870g, p.184.

have been pulled out and given their meanings in Jackson's conceptual framework of normal and abnormal neurological functions.

All of these conceptions together constituted a major part of Jackson's mature neurological paradigm. For cerebral localization and seizures the utility of the paradigm was dramatically demonstrated in 1884. Those exciting events will mark the beginning of the next chapter.

11

Brain Surgery, Ophthalmology, Evolution, and an Active Professional Life, 1884–1888

On November 25, 1884, the most famous operation in the history of neurosurgery was performed in London, at the Maida Vale Hospital for Epilepsy and Paralysis in Regent's Park.[1] At a minimum, Jackson was involved indirectly, because localization of the patient's brain tumor depended on interpretation of Jacksonian seizures. It is often said that he was present at the operation, but there is no reliable documentation about that possibility. Thus his activities in regard to that patient must be reconstructed from lesser sources. Using what is available, I will try to tell the story of early modern brain surgery as Jackson would have experienced it.[2]

When modern brain surgery began in 1879, and for some decades thereafter, there were two main indications for its use: (1) treatment of severe posttraumatic epilepsy, and (2) localization and treatment of intracranial tumors, especially when there were no external stigmata. For both purposes the logic of surgery followed directly from Jackson's conception of the discharging lesion and from his *xyz* theory of cerebral localization. The crucial background to all of this was Ferrier's primate work.

Jackson, Ferrier, Horsley, and the Beginnings of Modern Brain Surgery, 1879–1886

Localization and Brain Surgery in the later 1870s

Historians of neurosurgery are generally agreed that three technologies were required to establish the *feasibility* of operating on the brain—that is, for safely entering and exiting the intradural space. They were, in order of historical appearance: (1) anesthesia; (2) Listerian antisepsis/asepsis; and (3) cerebral localization.[3] Chloroform, ether, and nitrous oxide were used for general anesthesia in the 1840s, and Lister's initial contribution can be dated to 1867. 'Listerism' was highly controversial at first, but by the late 1870s it was gaining adherents rapidly throughout Europe and North America.[4] Before Lister, surgeons dared not open any body cavity (cranial, thoracic, or abdominal) for fear of nearly 100% mortality.[5] So the remaining requirement in the 1870s was cerebral localization, which also gained acceptance as the decade went along. In 1871, before Ferrier, Broca used his knowledge of aphasia to

---

[1] Bennett and Godlee 1884 and 1885b. Maida Vale was not Queen Square; see Feiling 1958, Shorvon et al. 2019, pp.262–268, and Chapter 2.

[2] The history of early modern neurosurgery (1871–1886) is summarized by Finger and Stone 2010; a similar, older version is in Greenblatt et al. 1997, pp.137–166.

[3] Neurosurgery became *successful* in the early twentieth century, when Harvey Cushing lowered its mortality rate with a fourth technology: control of intracranial pressure (Greenblatt 1997, 2003).

[4] Bynum et al. 2006, pp.158–159.

[5] We know that prehistoric trephiners avoided opening the dura, because many of their patients survived to grow new bone; see Saul and Saul 1997, p.31.

locate an intracranial abscess in a patient who had been kicked in the head by a horse, but that was pre-Listerian.[6]

Owsei Temkin long ago pointed out that surgery *per se* has always been localizing.[7] A surgeon has to operate *somewhere* in the patient's body—in a defined place. In the 1870s Broca's localization of aphasia was still controversial, so by itself it was not sufficiently dependable to justify the daunting risks of intradural surgery. Ferrier's motor localizations were also controversial, but his experimental data were potentially more useful. In cases of posttraumatic seizures, there are often healed external signs of the injury, so deciding whether and where to operate depended mainly on establishing correlation of the patient's seizure pattern with the known functions of the brain at the injury site. In the middle and late 1870s surgeons were beginning to operate for debridement of intracranial injuries in patients who were having posttraumatic seizures. Ferrier was consulted about such a case in 1879, and 'He advised that trephining should be practiced...'[8]

The ultimate goal of the localizationists was to be able to locate intracranial lesions in patients who had no external signs—where the localization was decided by means of applied physiology. Lazar has shown that Ferrier's publications were widely cited in the Anglo-American literature as early as 1874,[9] but, given the risks, operating on theory alone was controversial. It was Ferrier who convinced some young surgeons to try it. He himself was 33 when he published *The Functions of the Brain* in 1876. Its last chapter ended with a section on '*Relations of the Convolutions to the Skull*', where he tried to homologize cerebral anatomy from his primates to the human brain, and thence to human crania.[10] About this he said: 'The determination of the exact relations of the primary fissures and convolutions of the brain to the surface of the cranium is of importance to the physician and surgeon, as a guide to the localization and estimation of the effects of diseases and injuries of the brain and its coverings...'[11]

Now why would the information be important to surgeons unless they were planning to use it? In 1878 Ferrier gave the Gulstonian Lectures at the Royal College of Physicians, with the title 'The localization of cerebral disease'.[12] In those lectures he was especially concerned with making localizations in the face of clinical and experimental results that were not always consistent from one case to the next. Despite such uncertainties he asked:

> But what would be the practical effects of this [uncertainty], say as regards surgical treatment? Supposing it were a question of trephining (a question which may arise more frequently at no distant date) ... would it be a very hazardous thing to operate, granting the advisability of the operation? ... In medical practice, as in life generally, we have to act on probabilities more than on certainties...[13]

As Ferrier predicted ('no distant date'), in the following year just such an opportunity arose for a self-confident young surgeon in Glasgow. William Macewen (1848–1924) was 31 at the

---

[6] Broca published the case in 1876; see Stone 1991; Finger and Stone 2010, pp.190–191.

[7] Temkin 1951.

[8] Lees and Bellamy 1880.

[9] Lazar 2009a.

[10] Ferrier 1876, pp.308–314; capitals and italics in original.

[11] Ferrier 1876, p.308. There is an important technical point about opening the skull in those days. The circular trephines removed buttons of skull that were only an inch or two in diameter, so multiple trephinings were needed to gain wider exposures. The larger, 'osteoplastic flap' of the skull was invented by Wilhelm Wagner in 1889 (Lyons 1997, p.158).

[12] They were published in the *British Medical Journal* (*BMJ*) (Ferrier 1878a) and as a monograph (Ferrier 1878b).

[13] Ferrier 1878b, p.9; my square brackets. In 1883 Ferrier (p.805) included Jackson among those who believed 'that the apparent discrepancies between human pathology and experimental physiology would one day be cleared up and dispelled'. Despite the inadequacies of cerebral localization, Ferrier (1883, p.807) asked, 'is there any reason why a surgeon should shrink from opening the cranial cavity, who fearlessly exposes abdominal viscera?'

time. For the first combined use of the three technologies the dates usually proposed are between 1879 and 1884. The earlier year (1879) is for reports by Macewen, and the later date is for the famous case in London by Bennett and Godlee. I will now outline some of the events in that 5-year span, trying to understand what Jackson would have known and when.[14]

William Macewen, Glasgow, 1879

In March 1879 Macewen found and removed a right fronto-parietal subdural hematoma in a 9-year-old boy whose focal seizures began in the left face. There was mild right facial swelling extending into the scalp, but deciding whether and where to operate was also based on localization of the seizures. The boy recovered completely.[15] In July 1879 Macewen exposed and removed a left prefrontal *en plaque* meningioma in a 14-year-old girl. In this case there was recurrence of a tumor of the left orbit, sticking out above the eyeball, and a separate, 'pea-like node' causing 'a slight prominence on the brow'.[16] However, Macewen did not trust the external signs as guides to localization. Therefore the patient was 'placed under the observation of an educated skilled nurse'.[17] Some weeks later the nurse observed focal seizures of the right face and arm, with Jacksonian marches. At 11 PM on July 27, 1879, the patient was in status epilepticus.[18] Macewen trephined 'midway between the centre of the ascending convolutions and the anterior aspect of the cranium', also using the small lesion in the brow as one of his guides.[19] The tumor was removed and the patient's seizures remitted.[20] With apologies for self-quotation, my previous interpretation of these two cases claimed that:

> Macewen … used every piece of … information he could find to make the best possible decision. This tactic is seen clearly in his placement of the patient under a nurse's observation until the appropriate pathophysiological data … were obtained … he also used another ageless device of clinical judgement. He fudged a little. According to his later drawings of the lesions, the [boy's] subdural hematoma of March 1879 was directly over the motor strip, but the entire mass of the *en plaque* meningioma of July 1879 was anterior to it … He obviously made the judgmental decision that it was not necessary to expect absolute geographical correspondence between an epileptogenic region and the experimentally known site of the normal functions that it is aberrantly eliciting. Such a position would have been entirely consistent with Jackson's … [*xyz* theory].[21]

Macewen reported these two cases at a meeting of the Glasgow Pathological and Clinical Society on November 11, 1879, with 'Alexander Robertson, M.D., President, in the Chair'.[22]

---

[14] Macmillan (2004) has made a thorough analysis of Macewen's cases and his claims about them, which are largely confirmed.

[15] Macewen 1881, pp.542–543. For detailed analysis of this case see Macmillan 2005, pp.32–35.

[16] Macewen 1879a, p.211.

[17] Macewen 1888, p.304. See also Greenblatt 1997a, p.150, and Macmillan 2005, pp.36–39. Analogizing the nurse to our seizure monitoring is irresistible.

[18] Status epilepticus is a life-threatening condition of unremitting seizures.

[19] Macewen 1888, p.304. Macmillan (2005, p.39) concludes that Macewen used *all* of the patient's symptoms to localize the lesion; and 'when he selected the frontal nodule as the starting point for the operation he anticipated it might lead to an internal dural tumor'.

[20] General anesthesia is still a last-ditch treatment for status epilepticus, and it's not clear if Macewen understood that probably that's what stopped the girl's status epilepticus.

[21] Greenblatt et al. 1997, p.151; my square brackets.

[22] Macewen 1879b. In 1876–1877 Jackson (Jackson 1876v, p.266) referred to postictal paralysis as 'Todd and Robertson's hypothesis'. See details in Chapter 8.

An extensive description of the successful tumor case was published in the *Glasgow Medical Journal*,[23] apparently before a report of the two cases in the *BMJ* of December 27, 1879.[24] Given Jackson's interest in Robertson's ideas about postictal paralysis, it is possible that Jackson found Macewen's report in the *Glasgow Medical Journal*. In any case, he would not have missed it in the *BMJ*. Further to the point about Jackson's knowledge of Macewen's cases, on September 24 and October 1, 1881, Macewen published two serialized articles in *The Lancet*, titled 'Intra-cranial lesions, illustrating some points in connexion with the localization of cerebral affections and the advantages of antiseptic trephining'.[25] Since this series was apparently written specifically for *The Lancet*, the question arises why Macewen did that. Beyond establishing priority, the answer, I think, is in the timing.

Recall that the International Medical Congress had recently been held in London in late August, 1881, and Macewen was there. He contributed papers and discussion in the section on Diseases of Children, concerning genu valgum (knock knee) and tracheal intubation.[26] We don't know if he attended any of the sessions where cerebral localization was discussed, but, given his interest in it, we can presume that he either attended those sessions or he heard about them second-hand. Their surgical implications would have been quite apparent. With regard to timing, note that Macewen's series in *The Lancet* was published after the Congress but before Ferrier's prosecution by the anti-vivisectionists. The trial where Ferrier was exonerated was held on November 17. On November 19, 1881, the *BMJ*'s lead editorial was titled 'Dr. Ferrier's localization: for whose advantage?'[27] The author referred to Macewen's report in the *Glasgow Medical Journal* of September 1879 without mentioning Macewen's name! Be that as it may, all of this was in the professional air that Jackson was breathing.

Hughes Bennett and Rickman Godlee, London, November 1884

We come now to the famous tumor operation of November 25, 1884, generally known as the 'Bennett and Godlee case'. Alexander Hughes Bennett (1848–1901), age 36, was an Edinburgh medical graduate who settled in London in the 1870s. In addition to appointments at the Westminster Hospital, 'He was also physician to the [Maida Vale] Hospital for Epilepsy and Paralysis, Regent's Park, and made neurology his chief interest'.[28] Some weeks before the operation, Bennett was consulted by a 25-year-old farmer, for paralysis of his left hand and arm. Subsequently he developed paroxysmal paresthesias in the left face and tongue, with head turning to the left and at times a motor march, sometimes eventuating in loss of consciousness. Six months before admission he had developed 'spasmodic twitching of the left hand and arm'.[29] After an extended period of hospitalization, with no relief of severe pain and vomiting, surgical exploration was recommended and accepted.

The surgeon, Rickman John Godlee (1849–1925), age 35, was a nephew of Joseph Lister and a medical graduate of the University of London. The main centers of his professional activities were at University College Hospital and Brampton Hospital for Consumption and

---

[23] Macewen 1879a; by internal evidence this was published after August 15, 1879.

[24] Macewen 1879b.

[25] Macewen (1881) described seven cases; the first was actually an autopsied cerebral abscess in 1876; cases 2 and 3 were the 14-year-old girl and the 9-year-old boy.

[26] Mac Cormac 1881, vol.4, pp.190–191, 205–207, 212–213.

[27] Ferrier 1881b.

[28] Brown 1955, p.299; my square brackets. On Bennett see [Bennett, A.H.] 1901.

[29] Bennett and Godlee 1885a, p.244. There was an old history of blunt trauma to the left side of the head, but Bennett correctly ignored it.

Diseases of the Chest, but in 1881–1884 he was also Surgeon to Maida Vale.[30] In contrast to Macewen, who did his own localization, Godlee followed Bennett's instructions when he

> … trephined the [right] skull [thrice], and removed a triangular piece of bone over the region corresponding with the upper part of the fissure of Rolando … the cortex of the brain [was] exposed, [but] no tumor was visible. The ascending convolution … seemed to be somewhat distended. An incision about an inch long was made into the grey matter … and a quarter of an inch below the surface a morbid growth was found. This was carefully removed, and proved to be a hard glioma, about the size of a walnut. The superficial part of this was distinct from the brain matter and was easily enucleated.[31]

Unfortunately, the patient died 4 weeks later, on December 23, due to brain fungus (extrusion of brain tissue through the wound) and meningitis, but surely he did not die in obscurity. His case was followed avidly in the medical and lay press, and it was discussed extensively in medical meetings after his death. The first published notices in the medical journals were identical, one-paragraph reports in the BMJ and The Lancet, both on November 29, 1884, 4 days after the operation. The news items explained the basic facts of the diagnosis and procedure, ending on a hopeful note: 'Up to the present time the patient has progressed favourably in every respect. We shall be glad to learn the future progress of the case.'[32]

On December 6, both journals sounded the same worrisome notes: 'The latest information about this case is that the surgical condition of the wound is causing some anxiety; otherwise the man is in a satisfactory state …' And the BMJ continued: 'The future progress of this important and unique case is being watched with the greatest interest and anxiety by the whole profession.'[33] On December 20, a medical reporter for The Lancet gave the first full-length report of the case in some detail, as of December 15, when the preoperative paresis of the left leg had worsened. Regarding 'the state of the wound', he said, 'a hernia [fungus] has formed … which was shaved off. This caused the flaps in the scalp to gape open, and these have not yet healed.'[34] On January 3, 1885, both journals reported the patient's death on December 23, 1884, due to meningitis, which was a complication of the brain fungus.[35] In the midst of the reports in the medical journals, and before the outcome was known, the case was prominently deployed against the anti-vivisectionists in the lay press. On December 16, 1884, The Times of London carried the following letter, dated December 11.

BRAIN SURGERY.

TO THE EDITOR OF THE TIMES

Sir, – While the Bishop of Oxford and Professor Ruskin were, on somewhat intangible grounds, denouncing vivisection at Oxford last Tuesday afternoon there sat at one of the

---

[30] Feiling 1958, p.42; [Godlee] 2013.

[31] Bennett and Godlee 1884, p.1091; my square brackets. Probably the lesion was an oligodendroglioma (E. Stopa, personal communication), based on its microscopic appearance in Bennett and Godlee 1885a, p.251.

[32] BMJ 2:1084; Lancet 2:971.

[33] BMJ 2:1150 (1884; misprinted in original as p.1050); Lancet 2:1017 (1884).

[34] Bennett and Godlee 1884; my square brackets. A brain fungus (hernia cerebri) occurs when brain tissue pushes outward through a wound. If the hernia breaks through the scalp, infection and meningitis follow almost invariably.

[35] Bennett and Godlee 1885b and 1885c (both January 3). When the autopsy was fully reported in May 1885 (Bennett and Godlee 1885a, pp.258–264) there was no mention of any organs other than the scalp, skull, and brain.

windows of the Hospital for Epilepsy and Paralysis, in Regent's-park, in an invalid chair, propped up with pillows, pale and careworn, but with a hopeful smile on his face, a man who could have spoken a really pertinent word upon the subject, and told the right rev. prelate and great art critic that he owed his life, and his wife and children their rescue from bereavement and penury, to some of these experiments on living animals which they so roundly condemned.[36]

The letter went on at great maudlin length, describing the importance of Ferrier's experiments for the feasibility of the operation and then the scene at the surgery.

Mr. Godlee, surgeon to University College Hospital, in the midst of an earnest and anxious band of medical men, made an opening of the scalp, skull, and brain membranes of this man at the point where Dr. Hughes Bennett had placed his divining finger, the point corresponding to the convolution where he declared the peccant body to be and where sure enough it was discovered.[37]

The author of this Victorian missive was identified only as 'F.R.S.' until 1934, when Sir James Crichton-Browne revealed himself. Half a century after the fact, he said he had

... perceived that the operation opened up new vistas of hopefulness to those hitherto doomed to misery and darkness. He determined that it should not be hidden in the pages of the medical journals. He therefore wrote a letter to *The Times*. That letter ignited a controversy which raged in the columns of *The Times* for three months and evoked 64 letters and two brilliant leading articles in support of the scientific position. He scarcely remembered a non-political discussion in *The Times* that attracted more attention.[38]

Crichton-Browne certainly achieved his intended effect. One result of the controversy in the lay press was his condemnation in the medical press for drawing the attention of the laity to the medical arguments.[39]

Jackson's Limited Role in the Bennett and Godlee Case, 1884–1885

So where was Jackson in the midst of this hubbub? That is, (1) how much, if at all, did he participate in the preoperative evaluation of the patient; (2) was he present at the surgery; and (3) beyond the ultimate misfortune of the patient, what did he think about the 'success' of the entire undertaking? Given the hubbub, we can presume that he talked about it with his colleagues, but we have no records of those informal conversations. Aside from whether Jackson was there—to be discussed further below—what we do have is documentation of

---

[36] F.R.S. 1885. The Bishop of Oxford in 1870–1889 was John Mackarness (1820–1889; see *Dictionary of National Biography* 1906/1965, p.817), whose immediate predecessor was Samuel Wilberforce. John Ruskin (1819–1900; see *Dictionary of National Biography* 1906/1965, p.113) was Slade professor of art at Oxford 1870–1879 and 1883–1884.

[37] F.R.S. 1885; my underlining. 'Peccant' means 'morbid, not healthy'. It was sometimes used in reference to the ancients' humors (Dunglison 1874, p.767).

[38] [Crichton-Browne] 1934.

[39] *BMJ*, January 3, 1885, p.48; *Lancet*, January 3, 1885, p.23.

the first medical forum where the case was discussed in detail. It was half a year later, at a meeting of the Royal Medical and Chirurgical Society (RMCS) on May 12, 1885. In addition to presentations by Bennett and by Godlee, there were extended comments by Jackson, Ferrier, Macewen, and Victor Horsley (1857–1916).[40]

We have seen that Jackson took a special interest in brain tumors as early as 1872.[41] That experience served him well, because it enabled him to suggest criteria for deciding on the diagnosis of tumors and thus on indications for their surgical removal. At the RMCS:

> Dr. Hughlings Jackson congratulated Dr. Hughes Bennett on the accuracy of his diagnosis. The operation Mr. Godlee performed showed that Dr. Bennett was right in saying that a cerebral tumour might, so far as the operation itself goes, be safely removed … Dr. Hughlings Jackson also warmly congratulated Dr. Ferrier, from whose valuable researches the tumour was localized. Speaking more generally of localization of cerebral tumours with regard to trephining, Dr. Hughlings Jackson said that there was a kind of monoplegia, often passing into hemiplegia, which was almost certain evidence of cerebral tumour; a paralysis beginning very locally, for example, in the thumb and index finger and spreading very slowly week by week. In such a case he should not advise trephining, since there would be great probability of a large tumour in the centrum ovale, not certainty, for he had seen such hemiplegia in a case of tumour of the dura mater pressing down on the cortex.[42]

Jackson then explained why his distinction of epileptiform seizures versus epilepsy proper was so important. In fact, observation of Jacksonian seizures was one of the most important factors in clinical localization for neurosurgical explorations until the 1920s and beyond.[43] Here in 1885 Jackson said:

> The convulsive seizures of localizing value were not cases of epilepsy proper, but epileptiform seizures, – convulsions beginning one-sidedly and very locally … Whilst these seizures pointed with certainty to disease of the opposite cerebral hemisphere they did not always occur from such gross disease as tumour. In some there was local softening [stroke]. When, however, there was also double optic neuritis such gross disease as tumour might be confidently predicted. Even yet there is not evidence of exact position. Dr. Hughlings Jackson had not seen a case of epileptiform seizure caused by disease outside Ferrier's motor region. But such cases were reported by great authorities … repeating … what Charcot and Pitres had urged, we required also some local persisting paralysis of the part convulsed – persisting, since temporary paralysis after a seizure was not further help towards localization. So far, then, three things were required: local persisting paralysis, epileptiform convulsion, and double optic neuritis.[44]

---

[40] Bennett and Godlee 1885a and 1885d. On Horsley see below in this chapter. The question arises, why at the RMCS, since Jackson had not previously been active in that group? In fact, he had received the Society's first Marshall Hall Prize in 1878; see Baily 1895, p.26, and Hunting 2002, p.117 (the latter cited in Chapter 9). Hunting says there were efforts to revive the Society in the 1870s and especially in the 1880s.

[41] See Jackson 1872o, Jackson 1872p, Jackson 1872q, Jackson 1872s, and Jackson 1872t.

[42] Jackson 1885, which is in Bennett and Godlee 1885d, p.439.

[43] Plain X-rays (discovered in 1895) were sometimes helpful but seldom definitive. Walter Dandy's (1886–1946) invention of ventriculography and pneumoencephalography in 1918–1919 enabled visualization of many intracranial masses. See Walker 1951, pp.26–30; Gobo 1997, pp.223–228; and Kevles 1997, pp.100–103.

[44] Jackson 1885; my square brackets.

Referring to the discussion at the RMCS on May 12, an editorial in the *BMJ* on May 16 invoked Jackson's reputation for sagacity—and his carefully worded endorsement of the surgery—as antidotes to the reckless polemic by 'F.R.S.' in *The Times*.

> The discussion ... of a case in which Dr. Hughes Bennett diagnosed ...[and] ... correctly localized a small cerebral glioma ... and advised its excision by Mr. Godlee, which was accomplished successfully so far as the operation was concerned, showed the rapid advance of cerebral surgery, and gave some glimpses into the benefits that may be derived from it. The operation was commented on ... in many public papers, as recklessly hazardous and almost criminally unjustifiable; and in that connection it was very important to notice the carefully considered but emphatic approval given to the operation by Dr. Hughlings Jackson, the most prudent and learned master of the functions and capabilities of the brain, trained by the bedside, and not in the experimental laboratory. He contributed what is perhaps the most important element to the discussion of a new operation, namely, a sketch of the cases where it should not be attempted.[45]

At the least, it is reasonable to surmise that Jackson knew about the surgery soon after it was done, or maybe before, and his opinion about it is quite clear—he approved, albeit with caveats. But the question of his actual presence at the surgery remains unresolved. In his letter to *The Times* Crichton-Browne described an 'anxious band of medical men'[46] looking on, and Jackson's attendance is frequently asserted.[47] However, such statements were made only by people of later generations, and that is the stuff of which myths are easily made. The earliest statement of Jackson's presence that I have found is by the neurosurgeon Wilfred Trotter (1872–1939) in 1934.[48] Trotter had worked with Horsley, who probably would have known if Jackson were present at the Bennett and Godlee surgery, so Trotter's statement must be taken seriously. But frankly I don't trust it, partly because Maida Vale was entirely separate from Queen Square—corporately, physically, and in staffing. Perhaps more to the point, in the discussion at the RMCS Ferrier said plainly that he was present at the surgery, but Jackson made no such statement. I conclude that we don't know if Jackson was among the 'anxious band of medical men' at the Bennett and Godlee operation, but the lack of positive evidence speaks against it.[49]

Another perpetually unresolved issue concerns the competing claims of priority for Macewen versus Bennett and Godlee. Taking a step back, it seems fair to say that Macewen started the process of relying on physiological localization, and Bennett and Godlee brought it to fruition.[50] In any case, it is clear that Bennett and Godlee get credit for bringing 'successful' brain surgery to the attention of the entire medical profession. Nonetheless, 'Godlee

[45] [Bennett and Godlee] 1885e, p.1006; my square brackets.

[46] F.R.S. 1885, and see above in this chapter.

[47] See e.g. Pearce 1982, p.241; Finger and Stone 2010, p.197.

[48] Trotter 1934, p.1208.

[49] Macmillan (2000, p.227) also doubts that Jackson was there, saying: 'only Ferrier says he was there whereas Jackson's remarks read as if he were not'. However, Macmillan confuses the issue by incorrectly connecting Jackson's comment about putting a joke in a Scotsman's head to this (Bennett and Godlee) case rather than to Horsley's case in 1886 (see below), where it actually happened. I suspect that some who assert Jackson's presence at Maida Vale have been confused by his role in the discussion at the RMCS in May 1885 (Jackson 1885).

[50] Successful removal of an olfactory groove meningioma on June 1, 1884, was reported in Italy by Francesco Durante (1844–1934) 3 months later. Durante's case was also presented to the 'Surgical Section of the International Medical Congress held at Washington, U.S.A., September 1887' and thence published in *The Lancet*; see Durante 1887, and Tomasello and Germanò 2006.

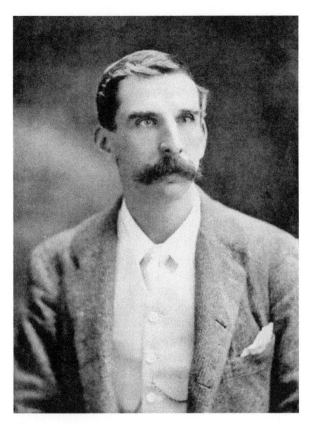

Fig. 11.1 Portrait of young Victor Horsley.
(Reproduced courtesy of J. B. Lyons.)

never did another brain operation, although it is not clear why'.[51] Rather, the neurosurgical torch was picked up quickly and carried swiftly by an even younger surgeon, aged 29, who operated on patients who were directly under the care of Ferrier, Jackson, and others at Queen Square.

Victor Horsley's First Three Cases, May–July 1886

Victor Alexander Haden Horsley (1857–1916; Fig. 11.1)[52] was an important actor in Jackson's story, so it will be interesting to know something about him before we describe his first cases, which were done in 1886. The social circumstances of his parents are evinced by an explanation of how he got his name. When he, their 'third child was born, on the same day as [Queen Victoria's] Princess Beatrice, their friend Miss Skerret, who had an important position at Court, mentioned the coincidence to Queen Victoria. Her Majesty graciously requested that the boy be given her own names' (Alexandrina Victoria), and she became his godmother.[53]

---

[51] Powell 2016, p.632.
[52] For biographies see [Horsley] 1916, S. Paget 1919, F.W.M. 1920, Sachs 1958, Lyons 1966, and Lyons 1967.
[53] Lyons 1967, p.362; see also Powell 2016, p.632.

Horsley became a brilliant student at University College Medical School (M.B., B.S., 1881) while qualifying M.R.C.S. in 1880 (F.R.C.S., 1883). At University College Hospital he was surgical registrar 1882–1884 and Assistant Surgeon 1885–1893, then Surgeon to 1900. From 1884 to 1890 he was also Professor-Superintendent of the Brown Institution, a biomedical research entity within the University of London. In addition to all of this, 'In February 1886, the Board of Governors of the National Hospital ... appointed a new surgeon to take forward the then newly topical cranial surgery, as their two surgeons in the staff were never going to do so'.[54] Apparently the powers-that-be at Queen Square were feeling the hot breath of competition from Maida Vale.[55] Horsley was certainly the right man for their job. In March 1886, in conjunction with Edward Albert Schäfer (1850–1935),[56] he presented his initial work on localization in the motor cortex to the Royal Society of London.[57] Their experiments included exploration of the hemisphere's mesial surface. In the same year, Horsley was elected to Fellowship of the Royal Society (F.R.S.) for the totality of his work on the thyroid, rabies, and cerebral localization.[58]

Between May 25 and July 13, 1886, Horsley performed three successful brain operations at Queen Square—two for posttraumatic epilepsy (Cases I and III) and one (Case II) for a tumor (tuberculoma) that was associated with seizures. According to the published records, Jackson had major roles in the diagnostic efforts and surgical recommendations of Cases I and II, but less involvement in Case III. I will now look at those three cases more closely, trying to learn as much as possible about Jackson's contributions.

Horsley's Case I: Focal Posttraumatic Seizures

This case was admitted 'under the care of Dr. H Jackson and Dr. Ferrier'.[59] At age 7, this 22-year-old man was 'run over by a cab, in Edinburgh ...' At the Royal Infirmary he was found to have

> ... a [left paramedian] depressed comminuted fracture, with loss of brain-substance ... [after debridement the wound] ... ultimately healed ... The patient was hemiplegic for some time, but gradually (seven weeks) the paralysis disappeared. At about 15 years, the patient began having fits ... He was admitted into the [National] hospital in 1885 ... and for some days was in [focal] *status epilepticus* ... and for three days before [re-]admission [May 1886] he was again in *status epilepticus.*[60]

The patient's seizures usually began in the right leg and spread in complex patterns into the right arm and face, which corresponded with Horsley's localization and with the location

---

[54] Powell 2016, p.631. Regarding the appointments of staff Surgeons at Queen Square, there are discrepancies of dates and spellings among: (1) Holmes' narrative (Holmes 1954, p.40), (2) his listing of the honorary staff (p.96), and (3) Powell's statement of 'two surgeons in the staff'. According to Holmes' staff listing, the only staff Surgeon in the 1880s before Horsley was William Adams (appointed 1872), who had a strong reputation in orthopedic deformities. His obituary in the *BMJ* ([Adams 1900]) said nothing about Queen Square, but see S. Paget 1919, p.117. Holmes (p.40) explains that the duties of the Surgeons had been 'limited to dealing with accidents and with deformities resulting from, or associated with, paralysis and to treating any surgical emergencies ...' See also Holmes 1954, pp.69–73.

[55] The Board of Management of the National Hospital paid for the transportation of Horsley's three patients to be presented at the annual meeting of the British Medical Association in Brighton in October 1886, in 'an effort to aid the progress of medicine'. See Horsley 1886, p.670, footnote 2.

[56] For biography see Sparrow and Finger 2001. 'Schäfer' was later 'Sharpey-Schafer' (Sparrow and Finger, p.46).

[57] Horsley and Schäfer 1884.

[58] F.W.M. 1920, p.xlvi.

[59] Horsley 1886, p.672. Horsley's (1887, p.864) later summary lists only Ferrier.

[60] Horsley 1886, pp.672–673; Jackson's parentheses, my square brackets.

of the patient's left scalp scar. Horsley concluded, 'that the focus of discharge was situated around the posterior end of the superior frontal sulcus ...'[61] At operation on May 25, 1886,

The scar in the brain was found to be ... about 3 centimètres long and 2 broad ... The scar, and about half a centimètre of surrounding brain substance was excised to the depth of 2 centimètres. It was then found that the scar tissue penetrated a few millimètres further into the corona radiata fibres of the marginal convolution. This portion was then removed and the wound closed.[62]

Through all of this,

The physicians watched the operation with keen interest: and when it was over, Hughlings Jackson let himself enjoy the relaxation of the strained mind. He beckoned to Ferrier: 'Awful, perfectly awful,' he said. Ferrier was shocked: the operation had seemed to him faultless. Again Hughlings Jackson murmured that an awful mistake had been made. 'Here's the first operation of this kind that we have ever had at the Hospital: the patient is a Scotsman. We had the chance of getting a joke into his head, and we failed to take advantage of it.'[63]

In contrast to the uncertainties about Jackson's presence at the Bennett and Godlee operation in 1884, this is clear evidence for Jackson's presence at Horsley's first case in 1886. The passage was written by Stephen Paget (1855–1926), whose father, James, had been a mentor to Jackson.[64] And Jackson himself 'drew particular attention to the fact that he had advised operation in this case ...'[65] The patient had had no postoperative seizures when reported by Horsley in April 1887.[66]

Horsley's Case II: Lateral Right Fronto-Parietal Tumor (Tuberculoma)

The case was admitted to Jackson. In January 1884 this 20-year-old man began to have '"cramps" in the left thumb and forefinger', which became severe in March 1884. His seizures

... began by clonic spasmodic opposition of the thumb and forefinger (left), the wrist next, and then the elbow and shoulder were flexed clonically, then the face twitched, and the patient lost consciousness. The hand [sic] and eyes then turned to the left, and the left lower limb was drawn up. The right lower limb was next attacked, and, finally, the right upper limb ...[67]

The patient was admitted to the care of Jackson on December 4, 1885. He apparently stayed in the hospital until his surgery on June 22, 1886—and beyond! During that long interval his focal seizures were observed and recorded. He was thoroughly examined, and 'The *Optic Discs*, examined by Mr. Marcus Gunn, appeared to be normal, though very pink

---

[61] Horsley 1886, p.673. In more detail: 'the parts affected [by seizures] were so in the order of [right] lower limb, upper limb, face, and neck; the character of the movements was, first, extension, then confusion, finally flexion ...'

[62] Horsley 1886, p.673.

[63] S. Paget 1919, p.120. Later Jackson said (Jackson 1888j, p.1): 'Everybody has heard of Sydney Smith's remark— that it requires a surgical operation to get a joke into the head of a Scotchman.' Smith's daughter said of him (Austin 1855, vol.1, pp.31–32): 'It requires ... a surgical operation to get a joke well into a Scotch understanding.' The Reverend Sydney Smith (1771–1845) was known for his 'manliness, honesty, and exuberant drollery and wit' (Lee 1965, p.1216).

[64] See Chapter 2.

[65] Jackson 1886d, p.674.

[66] Horsley 1887, p.864.

[67] Horsley 1886, p.673. My square brackets; probably 'hand' is a 'typo' for 'head'.

(physiological hyperæmia)'.[68] From Horsley we get a sense of the preoperative discussions about this case.

> Dr. Beevor and myself have shown [in monkeys] that the movement of opposition of the thumb and finger can be elicited by minimal stimulation of the ascending frontal and parietal convolutions at the line of junction of their lower and middle thirds. Dr. Hughlings Jackson witnessed one of our experiments ... and expressed his belief that this patient (Case II) was suffering from an irritative lesion ... in the part of the brain thus indicated.[69]

At surgery:

> The border of the tumour stood out about one-eighth of an inch from the surface of the brain ... as the brain-substance all round it for more than half an inch appeared dusky and rather livid, I removed freely all the part apparently diseased ... This procedure was fully justified, since the growth spread very widely under the cortex ... Before closing the wound, the centre of the thumb area was removed ... This detail Dr. Jackson and myself had resolved to carry out in the possible event of there being no obvious gross organic disease, in order to prevent, as far as possible, recurrence of the epilepsy.[8][70]

In his footnote 8 Horsley said: 'I wish to point out that, as strongly urged by Dr. Jackson, the removal of an epileptogenous focus is not only justifiable, but called for'. Postoperatively, the patient had left arm paralysis and facial weakness, as well as 'left hemianæsthesia to light touch'. However, at 7 weeks after surgery 'the patient had regained everything, except that the grasp of the left hand was not quite so good as before, and the fine movements of the fingers remained hampered'. There had been 'no fits since operation'.[71] Jackson gave a 16-month followup in October 1887: 'whereas before the operation, the lad had had as many as fifteen attacks in thirteen days, he had only had eleven attacks since the operation, only one of which was severe enough to lead to loss of consciousness'.[72]

Horsley's Case III: Paramedian and Mesial Localization of Posttraumatic Seizures

Since this patient was admitted to Thomas Buzzard it is inconceivable that he did not discuss it with Jackson, but there is nothing about Jackson's participation in the published record. This 24-year-old man had multiple scalp scars, especially in the 'upper anterior angle of the left parietal bone, close to the middle line'. On examination, 'There was almost complete right hemianæsthesia, the patient feeling neither a touch, nor a prick with a pin'. This was not physiological, as shown when 'Dr. Buzzard ordered the application of a strong faradic current to the affected side, which completely dispersed the hemianæsthesia, but left the fits unaltered'.[73]

---

[68] Horsley 1886, p.673; Horsley's italics and parentheses. Robert Marcus Gunn (1850–1909) was appointed Ophthalmic Surgeon to the National Hospital in 1886 (Holmes 1954, p.96). Jackson (J74-11, p.235) had earlier quipped that: 'Many very good ophthalmoscopists of my acquaintance are unwilling to admit that any optic disc is normal.'

[69] Horsley 1886, p.673; Horsley's parentheses, my square brackets. He was referring to Beevor and Horsley 1887, which was 'Read June 10, 1886' at the Royal Society. At Queen Square, Charles Edward Beevor (1854–1908) was appointed Registrar in 1880 and successively Assistant Physician and Physician.

[70] Horsley 1886, p.673.

[71] Horsley 1886, p.674.

[72] Jackson 1887i, in the *BMJ*. Jackson 1888k is the same in the *Proceedings of the Medical Society of London*, where Jackson gave his brief report from his presidential chair.

[73] Horsley 1886, p.674.

On the other hand, the patient's seizures exhibited many clinical features that Jackson had described in 'epileptiform' fits, including an abdominal aura. 'The head (and frequently the eyes) then turned to the right; the right arm was jerkily protruded, and the patient lost consciousness ... After the fit, the patient stated that the right arm felt weak for some time.'[74]

For localization in this case Horsley referred to his paper with Schäfer in 1884, which showed that, 'situated in the marginal convolution on the mesial surface of the hemisphere are motor areas for the muscles of the trunk, and that the abdominal centres are just opposite the hinder end of the superior frontal sulcus'.[75] Together with data in Ferrier's *Functions of the Brain*,[76] 'These facts led Dr. Buzzard to diagnose an irritative lesion situated in the posterior third of the superior convolution, that is, just under the slight depression in the skull'. At the '*Operation*, July 13th, 1886' there was 'splintering of the inner table [of the skull], with dural tears and a "cavity in the brain"', which 'was ... situated exactly where diagnosed ... the cavity was then removed'. Postoperatively, as of April 1887, the patient had only 'three slight attacks of *petit mal*'.[77] However,

> One week after the operation, the patient complained of weakness in the whole right upper limb. All movements were affected, especially those of the hand. This paresis is ... without the slightest doubt, an example of male hysterical paralysis, and its connection with the functional anesthesia before the operation is obvious. The interval of six or seven days before its appearance exactly coincides with that given recently by Professor Charcot. This paresis had, at the date of the meeting [August 13, 1886], completely disappeared.[78]

This problem of clinical presentations that are admixtures of physiological and hysterical phenomena can still present challenges for modern neurology. We will see shortly that Horsley's description of it probably was not coincidental, because Charcot was in the audience when Horsley presented his first three cases.

Horsley, Jackson, et al., at the British Medical Association, Brighton, August 1886

Horsley lost little time in announcing his success. All three patients were brought in person to the Surgery section of the BMA's annual meeting in Brighton on August 13, 1886,[79] where his presentation caused quite a stir. *The Lancet* observed: 'What may truly be called *the* surgical paper of the meeting was read by Mr. Victor Horsley, entitled "Advances in the surgery of the central nervous system".'[80] When Horsley finished, the President of the Section, John Eric Erichsen (1818–1896), said, 'it would be difficult to overrate the interest of Mr. Horsley's paper, which he might characterize as pure science applied to the advancement of practical surgery'.[81] Erichsen is little remembered now,

---

[74] Horsley 1886, p.674; Horsley's parentheses.
[75] Horsley 1886, p.674.
[76] This could have been a reference only to the first edition (Ferrier 1876), because the Preface to the second (Ferrier 1886) is dated '*October* 1886'. There is no page citation.
[77] Horsley 1886, p.674.
[78] Horsley 1886, p.674; my square brackets.
[79] Horsley 1886, p.670, footnote 2.
[80] In Horsley 1886a; italics in original.
[81] Horsley 1886, p.674.

but he was then senior Surgeon Extraordinary to the Queen, and a major figure in British surgery.[82] After Erichsen's brief remarks,

> Professor Charcot (Paris) said it had given him very great pleasure to ... listen to the interesting demonstration given by Mr. Horsley. He thought that British surgery was to be highly congratulated on the recent advances made in the surgery of the nervous system. Not only had English surgeons cut out tumors of the brain, but here was a case in which it was probable that epilepsy had been cured by operative measures. The cure was very creditable not only to the surgeon who operated, but also to the surgeon and the physicians who had so accurately diagnosed the case.[83]

Charcot's congratulations were obviously a great compliment to British national pride. One major source of that pride, Hughlings Jackson, spoke next, when he discussed Horsley's Case II, the tuberculoma.

> Dr. Hughlings Jackson warmly congratulated Mr. Victor Horsley on the success of his operations on the brain. He (Dr. Jackson) had long felt confident that there was in every case of epileptiform seizures a very local change of some kind. Very often there was tumour (frequently syphilitic), but occasionally no such coarse product [is present] ... that [a] "discharging lesion" was produced by tumour might be confidently diagnosed in cases where there was double optic neuritis and severe headache. When there are epileptiform seizures without these complications, we cannot tell whether there is tumour or not. In the case of his patient operated on by Mr. Horsley, there were no signs of tumour ... Dr. Hughlings Jackson drew particular attention to the fact that he had advised operation in this case, bearing well in mind the possibility of there being no tumour.[84]

Because the surgical success in Case II had verified Jackson's reasoning, he was confident of his ability to prognosticate other, nontumoral cases.

> ... in any future case of epileptiform seizures of the same kind, could he be certain ... that there was no tumour, he would still advise operation. Believing that the starting point of the fit was a sign to us of the seat of the "discharging lesion," he would advise cutting out that lesion ... He had formerly said that operation should not be attempted in cases of epileptiform seizures ... unless there was also double optic neuritis ... Here was a change of opinion. In this patient's case, cells of the "thumb centre" having become highly over-unstable ... Dr. Hughlings Jackson advised that the centre should be cut out. The tumour was found and removed ... [and] the "thumb centre," or part of it, was cut out too.[85]

In an earlier report of Jackson's comments about this case in a different journal, Jackson explained why 'He thought in removing the tumour that the adjoining portions of the brain ought to be removed ... He would cut out too much rather than too little'.[86] I think he put 'thumb centre' in quotation marks to signal his ambivalence about the idea of any delimited center, but

[82] [Erichsen] 1896 (Obituary), p.886.
[83] In Horsley 1886, p.674; parentheses in original.
[84] Jackson 1886d, p.674; parentheses in original, my underlining.
[85] Jackson 1886d, p.674; my square brackets and underlining.
[86] Jackson 1886c, which is a more succinct summary of his remarks than Jackson 1886d.

Table 11.1 Admitting Physicians for Victor Horsley's ten brain surgeries at Queen Square in 1886.[a]

Admitting Physician
    Ferrier[b]—4
    Jackson—2
    Bastian—2
    Buzzard—1
    [T.S.] Savill—1

Postoperative Diagnosis
    Trauma—4
    Tumor—4
    Cystic lesion in motor cortex (? old hemorrhage)—2

Followup Status (4 months to 11 months)[c]
    'Improved' or 'Much improved'—6
    Unchanged ('as before')—3
    Dead—1

[a] Derived from tabular summary in Horsley 1887, where the cases are numbered with Arabic rather than Roman numerals, so Cases I, II, and III in Horsley 1886 are the same as Cases 1, 2, and 3 in Horsley 1887. For a thorough analysis of 'Sir Victor Horsley's 19th century operations at the National Hospital', Queen Square, see Uff et al. 2011.

[b] In Horsley 1886, p.672, he said that Case I was admitted 'under the care of Dr. H. Jackson and Dr. Ferrier', but in Horsley 1887 it says only Ferrier.

[c] Calculated from surgical date to publication on April 23, 1887, so most follow-up intervals were actually shorter.

he did not indicate the source of his confidence. In fact, his *xyz* theory implied: (1) that cortical representation of individual limb movements is widespread, so limited excision would not be likely to remove all of the normal tissue, and (2) the graded and overlapping nature of the *xyz* theory also predicts that some function will return—compensation.[87] In Horsley's published remarks at the BMA he did not say anything about Jacksonian localization theory, but he demonstrated his confidence in it by performing seven more surgeries in the same year.

Horsley's Ten Cases at Queen Square, May–December 1886

In September–December 1886 Horsley did another seven brain cases with only one death (Case 10), and that patient was *in extremis* from tuberculosis. Table 11.1 shows some relevant data for all ten patients.

There must have been palpable excitement in the air at Queen Square in the Summer and Fall of 1886. It would have been literally a heady time! The news of Horsley's successes also induced a flood of attempts by other surgeons to do 'brain cases' in the decade 1886–1896. That was followed by 'discouragement and a beginning return to sanity' in 1896–1906.[88]

[87] See Chapter 10, and Greenblatt 1988.
[88] Scarff 1955, p.421.

The discouraging outbreak of sanity was due to the realization that operating on the brain could be associated with terrible morbidity and mortality.[89] Although Horsley had given explicit instructions for carefully handling scalp, bone, and brain tissue,[90] many of his imitators did not grasp their importance, nor did they or their medical consultants understand the intricacies of preoperative cerebral localization. Of course, the people at Queen Square could enjoy the sanctuary of 'safe' surgery afforded by Horsley.[91] Jackson hoped for even greater surgical success, because the outlook for any other therapy was not good, and the surgical efforts had severe limitations.

> It is notorious that our treatment of epilepsy is deplorably unsatisfactory, and if my hypothesis be correct – there is a persisting local lesion in the highest centres of one side of the brain – there are good reasons for it. The radical cure of [genuine] epilepsy, as of epileptiform seizures, is for the surgeon to cut out the "discharging lesion;" but in no case of epilepsy proper do we as yet know its exact position . . .[92]

There are two important points about Jackson's endorsement of a 'radical cure of epilepsy' by surgery. First, surgery for cases of 'genuine' epilepsy was not available because its localization was unknown;[93] and second, Jackson's *xyz* theory predicted some compensation for lost functions if some motor cortex is removed, whereas strictly mosaic localization would contraindicate such ablations.

Jackson's Bowman Lecture, November 1885

For the sake of historical continuity I have followed Horsley's early neurosurgical efforts to the end of 1886. In the process, however, I skipped over another important event. During the interval between the Bennett and Godlee case (November 1884) and Horsley's first case (May 1886), Jackson delivered the Bowman Lecture at the Ophthalmological Society.

The Founding of the Ophthalmological Society and its Bowman Lecture, 1880–1883

Ophthalmological Society of the United Kingdom
The Ophthalmological Society of the United Kingdom was formed at a meeting of the Medical Society of London on June 23, 1880, which was chaired by William Bowman (1816–1892). Jackson seconded the motion, which was unanimously agreed. 'Bowman was elected

---

[89] Greenblatt 2003, p.792.
[90] Horsley 1886, pp.670–672.
[91] Horsley's adherence to Listerism put him in the minority; see Scott et al. 2012, p.65.
[92] Jackson 1888d, p.116; my square brackets. In Jackson 1888d, p.112, Jackson gave surgeons advice that we still follow: '. . . on account of the "speech centre," operations on the left cerebral hemisphere are more serious than operations on the right'.
[93] Also in 1888, Jackson (Jackson 1888e, p.189, footnote 2) said: 'I have suggested that the radical cure of fits in such cases is for the surgeon to cut out the "discharging lesion," as well as the tumour, if there be one . . .' Daras et al. 2008, p.34, refer to this as 'Jackson's famous footnote'. It was, they say, the 'first suggestion of a potential surgical cure' of epilepsy by surgery. In view of everything above in this chapter, this priority statement of Daras et al. is not correct. Note: Daras' citation of Jackson 1888e is to p.179, but the footnote is on p.189.

the first President'.[94] In September 1883 a resolution of the Society's Council proclaimed the establishment of the annual ' "Bowman Lecture," which shall consist of a critical résumé of recent advances in ophthalmology or in such subject ... as the Council shall select ...'.[95]

Specialization, Spencer, and Epileptic Mental States in the Bowman Lecture, November 1885

On November 13, 1885, Jackson delivered the Bowman Lecture on 'Ophthalmology and diseases of the nervous system'[96] before 'a very large audience'.[97] Although most of his presentation was directed at the ophthalmological aspects of epilepsy, broadly interpreted, he began with a justification of specialization. About this he had first offered a spirited defense in 1877.[98] In his Bowman Lecture his argument was forthrightly Spencerian.

> It was long ago said that division of labour, or, more generally, differentiation, is an [*sic*] universal law ... Differentiation is well seen ... in the social organism. It would be very remarkable if there were an exception in the case of one part of the social organism, the body medical ... [It] is now very complex; there are alienist physicians, obstetric physicians, neurologists, ophthalmic surgeons, aural surgeons, dentists, physiologists, chemists, etc.; the speciality of each ... is a differentiated part of, a wide general knowledge.
>
> Specialists have ... to justify their differentiation ... The factors in progressing evolution, according to Spencer, are increasing (1) differentiation, increasing (2) definiteness, increasing (3) integration, and increasing (4) co-operation.[1][99]

The first sentence of Jackson's footnote 1 is intriguing: 'I am using terms more familiar to medical men than those Spencer uses; for this change, of course, Spencer is not answerable...'[100] So what Spencerian terms did Jackson convert to words 'more familiar to medical men'? I think he substituted 'differentiation' and 'definiteness' for Spencer's slightly different usages of 'homogeneity' and 'heterogeneity'. That is, differentiation is the evolutionary process and definiteness is its result. In any case, Jackson followed Spencer in thinking that the four principles are equally applicable in the realms of the biological *and* the social. Given the many different specialties already in existence, he addressed the second factor.

> Increasing differentiation without increasing definiteness would be only confusion. That the ophthalmic surgeon has justified himself in the second factor of evolution [definiteness]

---

[94] Bailey 1895, p.102; parentheses in original, my square brackets and underlining. For biography of Bowman see [Bowman] Obituary 1892.

[95] [Ophthalmological Society] 1975.

[96] I have largely used the version in the *BMJ* (Jackson 1885f); other, nearly identical reports were in *The Lancet* (Jackson 1885e), *Medical Times and Gazette* (*MTG*) (Jackson 1885h), and *Transactions of the Ophthalmological Society* (Jackson 1886h). The *MTG* folded in 1885; see Bynum et al. 1992, p.181.

[97] The large audience was noted in [Ophthalmological Society] 1885.

[98] Jackson 1877j, p.575; he also mentioned 'Division of labour' in Jackson 1882d, p.306, and a defence of 'specialism' on p.307; on the latter see Chapter 10.

[99] Jackson 1885f, p.945; my square brackets. Jackson gave no citation to Spencer for these factors, presumably because they are found throughout Spencer's writings.

[100] Jackson 1885h, p.695, and Jackson 1886h, p.2; with very slight alterations, this same footnote is found in Jackson 1887e, p.31 (also in the text of Jackson 1887j, p.461). The last sentence is missing in Jackson 1885e and Jackson 1885f.

needs no proof. I will instance, however, his highly definite work on paralyses of ocular muscles and on abnormalities of refraction … And here I must say … that by definiteness I mean definiteness which connotes exactness.[101]

The essence of Jackson's application of evolutionary principles (3) and (4) to ophthalmology, and to medicine in general, is summed up in his two sentences with Spencerian undertones: 'Division of labour necessitates the co-operation of labourers. The whole of one disease is better understood by bringing to bear on its direct investigation and treatment different workers in different fields.'[102]

Most of the rest of Jackson's lecture was an extensive review of the current status of epilepsy, considered from his evolutionary and pathophysiological points of view.[103] Although there was nothing fundamentally new here, it would be a rare public lecture where Hughlings Jackson had absolutely nothing new to say. In his Bowman we find a new twist on the pathophysiology of the dreamy state and similar phenomena.

> Now for the mental symptoms of … the discharge beginning in part of the "organ of mind." During the epileptic discharge there is defect or cessation of consciousness. Some think that also during it … there arise the exactly opposite mental states of "overconsciousness," "dreamy state," alterations in size and stance of external objects, "seeing faces" and "hearing voices." I believe these superpositive mental states … at the onset of different epileptic attacks, to arise during slightly raised discharges of healthy nervous arrangements untouched by the epileptic discharge.[104]

But a question arises from the last sentence. If the 'slightly raised discharges of healthy nervous arrangements' are 'untouched by the epileptic discharge', then why are they 'slightly raised'? I think he was referring to normal tissue that is recruited during propagation of the seizure: 'Admitting that crude sensations arise *during*, and that convulsions occur *from*, the epileptic discharge, I urge that elaborate mental states arise *during*, and that movements, properly so called, occur *from*, but slightly raised discharges of ['healthy'] nervous arrangements.'[105]

Immediately after the lecture Sir William Gull said that Jackson was 'the greatest living worker, as he was also the most honest and most disinterested, in the field of neuropathology … he has given us … as he never fails to do in all his public utterances, much food for thought, and many suggestions to guide future observation and research.'[106] A week later an editorial writer in the *MTG* lamented the absence of a comprehensive book to present the totality of Jackson's ideas. However, in a word of caution he said: 'It cannot be denied that … almost any lecture by Dr. Jackson, is intimately dependent on his previous utterances … [so] every reader who is to profit by anything fresh that Dr. Jackson has to say must first have

---

101 Jackson 1885f, p.945; my square brackets.
102 Jackson 1885f, p.945.
103 Expressing some frustration 5 months later, Jackson (Jackson 1886b, p.11, footnote 1) said, 'I have been said to have put forward the "theory of discharges" as the *pathology* of epilepsies. I have really tried very hard to show that certain pathological processes only *induce* "discharging lesions" which are *hyperphysiological* states.'
104 Jackson 1885f, p.946; Jackson's quotation marks.
105 Jackson 1885f, p.946; Jackson's italics, my square brackets.
106 Jackson 1885g.

possessed himself of a neurological "Grammar of Assent" as an introduction to the higher teaching set before him from time to time.'[107]

Acknowledging this difficulty, the editorial writer was concerned about the challenging intellectual depth of Jackson's conceptions. The book would need 'a greater attention to consecutive arrangement, and possibly a little more <u>sympathy with what is called average intellect</u>, [which] would not only make Dr. Jackson's finished work one of the most valuable treatises on scientific neurology … but would also gain for him the sincere recognition of many practical physicians and earnest students'.[108] Indeed, Jackson already had an abundance of 'sincere recognition'.

Professional Life in the Middle 1880s

In Table 11.2 I have cobbled together a chronological list of most of the honors and offices that Jackson accumulated over his lifetime, *not* including first qualifying (licensing) titles by examination, hospital staff positions, or teaching appointments at the London. From this it can be seen that in the middle 1880s, when he was around age 50, Jackson's professional situation began to change. His career as an invited lecturer continued, but positions as office-holder and honoree increased. Also around this time there were some potentially explosive tensions between the medical staff and the hospital management at Queen Square—including a staff threat to resign *en masse*—but we know little about Jackson's role in those troubles.[109] His attention was focused on a more productive professional event.

The Founding of the Neurological Society of London, November 1885–March 1886

This Society originated at a meeting held on November 14th, 1885, when, on the proposition of Dr. Broadbent, <u>seconded by Dr. Hughlings Jackson</u>, the desirability of forming such a Society was agreed … A Committee was appointed to draw up rules and to nominate a Council and officers. The report of this Committee was agreed to … on January 14th, 1886. The first ordinary meeting was held at the National Hospital, Queen Square, on March 24th, when <u>Dr. Hughlings Jackson, the first President</u>, delivered an [i]naugural address on the Scope and Aims of Neurology, and the manner in which a Society like the Neurological might be utilised for the advancement of science.[110]

The original membership of the Society numbered 95,[111] which is an indication of neurology's appeal at the time. It is most unfortunate that Jackson's address was never

---

[107] Jackson 1885i; my square brackets. *An Essay in Aid of a Grammar of Assent* (1870) by John Henry Newman was a widely circulated introduction to the logic of Catholic belief (assent).

[108] Jackson 1885f; my square brackets and underlining.

[109] Holmes 1954, pp.41–45.

[110] Bailey 1895, pp.102–103; my underlining. Schurr 1985, p.146, dates the first meeting of the Society to '14 June 1888', but this is likely a misunderstanding. Bailey was Librarian of the Royal College of Surgeons, so he was writing only a decade after the event.

[111] Hunting 2006, p.263.

Table 11.2 Chronology of Jackson's professional offices and honors, 1869–1906. From numerous sources.

Year(s)	Organization	Activity
1869	Royal College of Physicians	Fellow (F.R.C.P.)
1869	Royal College of Physicians	Gulstonian Lecturer
1871	Royal Medical and Chirurgical Society	Fellow
1877	Medical Society of London	Orator
1878	Royal Society [of London]	Fellow
1878	Royal Medical and Chirurgical Society	Marshall Hall Prize[a]
1881	American Neurological Association	Honorary member
1882	British Medical Association, Worcester	President of Section on Pathology and Bacteriology
1884	Royal College of Physicians	Croonian Lecturer
1885	Opthalmological Society of the United Kingdom	Bowman Lecturer
1885–1887	Royal College of Physicians	Councilor[b]
1886	Neurological Society of London	(First) President
1886	Harveian Society	President
1887	Medical Society of London	President
1887	University of Glasgow	L.L.D., h.c.
1888–1889	Royal College of Physicians	Censor
1889	British Medical Association, Leeds	Address in Medicine
1889	Opthalmological Society of the United Kingdom	President
1890	Royal College of Physicians	Lumleian Lecturer
1892	Hunterian Society	Lecture (annual)
1894	London Hospital	Retirement Testimonial
1897	Neurological Society of London	Hughlings Jackson Lectureship established
1897	Neurological Society of London	(First) Hughlings Jackson Lecturer
1903	Royal College of Physicians	Moxon Medal
1904	University of Leeds	Sc.D., h.c.
1904	Neurological Section, Royal Society of Medicine	Honorary Member[c]
1905	University of Edinburgh	L.L.D., h.c.
1906	*Brain*	Vol.29, Part IV, dedicated to Jackson
?	Royal College of Physicians, Ireland	Honorary Fellowship
?	University of Bologna	Honorary doctorate
?	Yorkshire University	Honorary D.Sc.[d]

[a] Bailey 1895, p.26.

[b] Presumably the duties of the Councillors and the Censors were similar to those of the period 1858–1861 when 'The Censors and College Officers attended probably at intervals of days, the Council at intervals of weeks …' (Cooke 1972, p.803). The Censors dealt with disciplinary matters.

[c] Critchley and Critchley 1998, p.158.

[d] Taylor 1925, p.21. Apparently this was Yorkshire College, which became part of the University of Leeds; see Wikipedia ('University of Leeds', p.1), accessed January 18, 2017.

published—it might have explained some of neurology's attraction.[112] Regarding 'the advancement of science', the surgeon John Bland-Sutton (1855–1936) remembered:

> In 1886 the Neurological Society was founded, and I was an original member. In the early days of this Society the meetings were not merely conferences where papers were read and discussed; they were laboratory meetings, and some of the most successful were held in the Physiological Laboratory of University College. I remember well the demonstrations of Professor Sharpey-Schafer who, at that time was localizing experimentally the centre for hearing in the cerebral cortex of monkeys.[113]

In many respects the Ophthalmological Society was the model for the Neurological Society. There was significant overlap in membership, and it was Jackson who seconded the motions for both of their respective foundings. However, there was one major difference in their cultures.

> The members of the Ophthalmological Society ... advocated a wholly specialist profile; [whereas] the members of the Neurological Society ... never aligned themselves with a specialist identity ... and scrupulously cultivated a generalist appearance in order to mitigate any pejorative charge that neurology was a narrow field of enquiry.[114]

In ordinary conversation the neurologists were recognized as specialists by themselves and by others, so the contrast to the ophthalmologists may be overdrawn.[115] Still, the differences were real. When Jackson defended specialization at the Ophthalmological Society he was preaching to the choir. Casper observes that the early specialist societies 'emerged in a culture hostile to specialisation. Such societies sought to maintain the values and practices of their generalist peers while simultaneously instigating a quiet but radical change into the unified structure of medicine.'[116] Those considerations contributed to the prominence that Jackson gave to specialization in his Bowman Lecture. But the question is, why did he feel compelled to offer his defense in November 1885, when the issue had been roiling around for decades? I think he was trying to head off charges of specialism in the Neurological Society.[117] And beyond that, there were larger cultural concerns.

---

[112] I searched vols. 7–10 of *Brain* and all items listed in York and Steinberg 2006. George York (personal communication) has seen no such item in the Library and archives at the National Hospital. During the 3 weeks following the meeting on March 24, there is no report of the Society's meeting in the *BMJ* or *The Lancet*. A general idea of Jackson's outlook for neurology is found in Jackson 1888c (published July 14, 1888), which is discussed below.

[113] Bland-Sutton 1930, p.147. He was at the meeting of the Royal Medical and Chirurgical Society on May 12, 1885, when the Bennett and Godlee case was discussed. About that event he said (p.148), 'I feel sure that the foundation of the Neurological Society was the outcome of that meeting'. On Bland-Sutton see Power and Le Fanu 1953, pp.88–91.

[114] Casper 2014, p.31; my square brackets.

[115] See e.g. an editorial in the *BMJ* in 1882 (Jackson 1882f, p.494), where the writer praised Jackson as 'One of the most distinguished of living specialists ...'

[116] Casper 2014, p.31.

[117] In 1907 the RMCS was transformed into the present-day Royal Society of Medicine (RSM) by amalgamating 13 medical societies of various kinds. One of its purposes was to combat perceptions of specialism in the profession at large. The Neurological Society was one of the first specialty groups to join and thus

Jackson's Relationship to Late Victorian Culture

In late Victorian culture—roughly, from the late 1870s to Victoria's death in 1901—there were many intellectual currents and cross-currents.[118] Here I will try to explain briefly how four of them were, or were not, relevant to Jackson: (1) the 'supernatural', i.e., all extra-scientific belief; (2) materialism; (3) progressivism; and (4) decadence and degeneration. Among them Jackson tried to steer middle courses as usual. His main concern was to protect the integrity of his entire approach—his paradigm—which was guarded, he thought, by his theory of concomitance.

The Supernatural

Within the term 'supernatural' Jackson included all forms of belief that invoked the miraculous. In Chapter 2 we saw that Hutchinson described Jackson's life-long, 'simple' agnosticism,[119] but he was surrounded by swirling theological controversies. Given his aversion to open discord, he tried to keep away from those conflicts as much as possible. In such circumstances his use of 'supernatural' accommodated the religious feelings of others without giving any ground if the only choice were theology *or* science.

Materialism

In Chapter 8 we saw that Jackson began to show some concern about potential charges of materialism in 1874,[120] although I have no information about who might have attacked him personally, or if any one actually did. Thereafter he made many comments about his perception of materialism, because he lived in a culture that was increasingly vexed about it. An understanding of his perception can be facilitated by comparing his view to a standard dictionary definition, in which 'materialism' is 'The theory or belief that nothing exists except matter and its movements and modifications; (more narrowly) the theory or belief that mental phenomena are nothing more than, or are wholly caused by, the operation of material or physical agencies'.[121]

Now comes the middle course. Given Jackson's theory of concomitance, it is clear that he would not have accepted full-blown materialism as thus defined, because he did not believe that 'nothing exists except matter'. However, that was for him the only scientific/neurological reality, i.e., 'scientific materialism'. He discounted 'crude popular materialism'.[122] The idea of material progress, on the other hand, was important and subject to change over time.

Progressivism

The term 'progressivism' is not exactly synonymous with the idea of progress, but they were related. In the middle Victorian period, when Jackson was young, there was a general sense of

---

became the Neurological Section of the RSM (Schurr 1985; Hunting 2002, pp.172–173, 263–269). The Medical Society of London and the Ophthalmological Society have retained their independence into the twenty-first century.

[118] In the large literature on this subject see e.g. Chamberlin and Gilman 1985, Young 1985, and Conlin 2014, p.125.
[119] Hutchinson 1911, p.1553.
[120] Jackson 1874aa, pp.348–349.
[121] *Oxford English Dictionary (OED)* online, accessed April 4, 2018.
[122] See Jackson 1881b, p.445, which is quoted in Chapter 10.

optimism.[123] Progress was thought to be inevitable, so evolution became entangled with the idea of progress. When Darwin's *Origin* was published in 1859, many people—perhaps most—initially ignored its darker implications. By the 1880s those implications were becoming more obvious. In a paper of December 1887 Jackson showed that he was well aware of his culture's evolving view of evolution. It was moving away from the teleological idea that evolution is always progressive: 'Evolution generally is a passage from the most to the least organised, the ever organising. But Evolution is not a necessary or inevitable or "even" process ... it depends on conditions. (*a*).'[124] In footnote (*a*) there was a quotation from Spencer to the effect that evolution is not always progressive, despite that 'erroneous assumption' by many people.[125] That is, dissolution is part of the evolutionary process, but others could interpret it as degeneration.

Decadence and Degeneration

'Decadence' and 'degeneration' are two words often used to characterize parts of the cultural milieu in the late Victorian period. They are English renditions of French expressions, which are labels for societal concerns about the materialistic and pleasurable aspects of degeneration. This was a feature of French high society at the *fin de siècle*, around 1900. Decadence was then a popular theme in French literature and art, and some Victorians had similar feelings.[126] According to Harrington, the French, 'like their English counterparts, were acutely aware of the "beast in man" specter raised by evolutionary theory ... This awareness probably was articulated most clearly in the French concept of degeneration, the perceived sinister flip-side of the evolutionary process.'[127] Degeneration was not in the vocabulary of Spencer's Synthetic Philosophy, and he used 'dissolution' only sparingly.[128] It was Jackson who picked up dissolution and ran with it, but he did not use 'degeneration' in any cultural context.[129] Nonetheless, the relative absence of the word 'degeneration' on the English side of the Channel does not mean that the British had no worries about it. As Harrington testifies, they did, though perhaps with less angst than the French.

Jackson's efforts to fend off charges of materialism could be interpreted as his way to avoid the issue of societal degeneration. Beyond that, however, it would be silly to suggest that his ideas about neurological dissolution had any *direct* effect on the surrounding culture. They were too technical. Still, technical influences can course through cultures in circuitous ways. Jackson's most direct connection to Victorian culture was through Spencer, Eliot, Lewes, and their circle, when both Spencer and Eliot were near the zeniths of their reputations, and we know that Jackson was in private contact with Spencer in the 1880s.[130] Additionally, Spencer

---

[123] See Newsome 1997, p.50, which is discussed in Chapter 2.

[124] Jackson 1887n, p.618.

[125] Jackson 1887n, p.618. As his source for this passage in Spencer, Jackson cited '"First Principles," p.574'. It is indeed found in Spencer 1880a, p.574.

[126] See Bowler 1989, especially pp.192–202; also Burrow 2000, pp.96–102 (on degeneration) and pp.182–187 (on decadence).

[127] Harrington 1987, p.101.

[128] See Collins' 1889 Index, pp.550–551, which I have relied on for these statements about Spencer's use (or not) of 'disintegration' and 'degeneration'. The current *OED* online (accessed April 4, 2018) cites Spencer 1862 for its first definition of 'dissolution'.

[129] Jackson used 'degeneration' in relation to Wallerian degeneration in neural tissue, which does not imply anything about evolutionary dissolution. For its second definition of 'dissolution' the *OED* online (accessed April 4, 2018) lists three citations, all from Jackson.

[130] For example, he served as an intermediary between Weir Mitchell and Spencer when Mitchell wished to meet Spencer in London in 1888; see Burr 1929, pp.209–210.

would have known about the activities at Queen Square because his 'friend Henry Charlton Bastian, M.D', was one of the trustees in his will.[131] In any case, Jackson's productivity continued unabated.

Lowest Level Fits and the 'Epileptic' Guinea Pigs Again, 1886

A Change in the Physiological Conception of Seizures: To Include the Lowest Level, April 1886

In the issue of *Brain*, dated April 1886, Jackson published 'A contribution to the comparative study of convulsions',[132] which contained a major change in his thinking about the classification of seizures. In the 1860s, he said, he had started with acceptance of the medulla as the 'seat of epilepsy'. Then, in his 'Study' of 1870, and after the work of Hitzig and Ferrier, he believed that

> ... no variety of convulsion in man arose from any sort of change below the cerebrum proper. But very lately I have come back to the belief, that *some* convulsions (I do not call them epileptic) in children (and, I suspect in some adults which are *called* epileptic) depend on lesions of the pons or medulla oblongata. The fits in children ... are "inward fits," otherwise called laryngismus stridulus; they are "respiratory convulsions."[133]

Laryngismus stridulus is now called 'pseudocroup'. It involves brief spasmodic closure of the glottis, with crowing inspiration, and it is not now considered to be epileptic. However, given Jackson's conception of any discharging focus as the pathogenesis of fits of any kind, his declaration about the 'pons or medulla oblongata' would have to imply that the focus for these 'inward fits' is in the respiratory center in the brainstem. Furthermore, there is a '*Scale of Fits*'.

> I believe (1) epileptic fits (epilepsy proper) to depend on "discharging lesions" of parts of the highest level of evolution, and (2) epileptiform seizures to depend on "discharging lesions" of parts of the middle level of evolution. Both ... are "cortical." (3) Inward fits (respiratory convulsions) and some other fits depend ... on discharges beginning in parts of the lowest level of evolution.[134]

---

[131] Spencer 1903, pp.3–4; see Duncan 1911, p.ix, and Compston 2015, p.3449. Raitiere 2012, pp.293–294, has some interesting information about Bastian and Spencer, although I do not accept his interpretation of it.

[132] Jackson 1886b; there is no evidence that this paper was presented orally before its publication or that its actual publication was not in or near April.

[133] Jackson 1886b, pp.1–2; Jackson's italics, my underlining. According to the laryngologist R. Scott Stevenson (1951, p.212), in the 1870s 'the teaching hospitals regarded laryngology with complete indifference, and diseases of the throat were in the charge of the most junior physician or surgeon on the staff. Thus Hughlings Jackson, "the Socrates of neurology," was in charge of the throat department at the London Hospital ...' A similar situation obtained at University College Hospital; see Merrington 1976, pp.157–158.

[134] Jackson 1886b, pp.2–3; Jackson's parentheses. This leaves open the possibility of cerebellar foci, but Jackson said only (p.5): 'the lowest level of evolution is at once lowest cerebral and lowest cerebellar'. Also, citing Moxon he said (Jackson 1886b, p.10): 'There is, in severe epileptic fits, a sequence of discharges of four levels of motor evolution—highest, middle and lowest nervous centres and of "muscle centres" – muscles being in one aspect ... nervous centres ... I continue, however, to speak of three levels of evolution.'

In discussing the experimental evidence for his changing conception, Jackson began by saying: 'I knew long ago that Brown-Séquard had demonstrated that in guinea-pigs a *liability* to convulsions could be experimentally produced ... and that the fits could be artificially brought on when the <u>brain proper had been taken away</u>.'[135] Actually, in most of Brown-Séquard's experiments he transected the spinal cords only partially, so Jackson's statement was an exaggeration. But his main point was evolutionary: '... we should have to consider the vast differences in the degree of evolution of the nervous centres in man and in the guinea-pig.'[136] In his footnote 1 Jackson advanced his argument with a single case and a bit of sarcasm.

> [1] <u>Since writing this sentence</u>, I have seen fits in a boy whose case is ... very like ... Brown-Séquard's guinea-pigs. A boy of seven, falls suddenly to the ground <u>when his head or face, either side, is touched</u>: his face flushes, his eyes turn up and to the right, his respiration stops, and there is a sudden jerk of his limbs. Since his fits began a few months before the age of two and a half years ... [and] as he has [partial] left hemiplegia ... the supposition of ... [pretending] is about as reasonable as that Brown-Séquard's guinea-pigs should pretend to have fits when the epileptogenous zone is touched.[137]

All of this raises an obvious question: What impelled Jackson to reconsider his previous rejection of lowest level fits? The answer appears to have been a confluence of at least two circumstances, amounting to the importance of a prepared mind. First was the issue of laryngeal representation. Among Bland-Sutton's memories of the early years of the Neurological Society, he said: 'Horsley and Felix Semon gave demonstrations at such meetings on the centres in the cerebrum for movements of the vocal cords.'[138] We don't know exactly what year Bland-Sutton was recalling, but Semon and Horsley began their work in 1886. They gave a 'preliminary' report of their results in 1889 and an extensive report in 1890,[139] so it is likely that Jackson knew about it well before 1890.

Second, in the indented quotation above, the initial phrase 'Since writing this sentence' can be taken to mean that Jackson was that far along in writing his 'Contribution' of April 1886, when he first saw the 7-year-old boy. That consultation happened on January 19, 1886.[140] I think he had started to review his conception of seizures in relation to his theory of three levels when he realized that there was an asymmetry. There were three levels of the brain, but only two correlated with any type of seizures. Although he never said it in print, this was incomplete. It violated his sense of symmetry. Just before his footnote about the boy, in a section titled '*Varieties of Lowest Level Fits*', he said: 'Speaking roughly, there are supposed to be lowest, middle and highest "level" fits.'[141] Since he knew the work of Brown-Séquard and

---

[135] Jackson 1886b, p.2; my underlining. Brown-Séquard's experiments are described in Aminoff 2011, pp.189–193. In our conception the guinea pigs were not epileptic; see Chapter 8.

[136] Jackson 1886b, p.6

[137] Jackson 1886b, p.6; my square brackets and underlining.

[138] Bland-Sutton 1930, pp.147–148. Felix Semon (1849–1921) was appointed Laryngologist to the National Hospital in 1887; see Holmes 1954, p.96; also Brown 1955, pp.307–308.

[139] Semon and Horsley 1890, pp.187–192.

[140] Jackson 1886f, p.962, and Jackson 1887o, p.79. The case is reported briefly in Jackson 1886e, somewhat more in Jackson 1886f, and extensively in Jackson 1887o. The latter contains a thorough record of the discussion after Jackson's presentation.

[141] Jackson 1886b, p.5.

others, he could have been thinking about them as he considered the problem of correlating seizures with the lowest level.

> … what we call respiratory convulsion should in many cases … be called <u>respiratory be-ginning</u> convulsion … Ordinary spasmodic asthma … is a respiratory convulsion, and it is also a lowest level fit. Both it and inward fits are … owing to sudden … <u>discharges begin-ning in some part of the respiratory centres</u> [in the medulla] … the fits induced by Brown-Séquard and Westphal in guinea-pigs, and by Kussmaul and Tenner in rabbits, are lowest level fits in those animals.[142]

According to Aminoff's summary of Brown-Séquard's experiments, 3 or 4 weeks after the cord lesions were made there were 'convulsive movements resembling seizures that occurred spontaneously or following stimulation of certain regions of the skin … At the onset of such attacks, animals often uttered hoarse cries, as if the vocal cords were partially closed'.[143] Although Jackson did not mention the 'hoarse cries', the epileptic focus for them would have to be in the lower brainstem. Most of the remainder of his 'comparative study' is concerned with lowest level fits in children, in view of their developing nervous systems, all of which was meant to support his conclusion that some seizures originate in the lowest level.

Another form of support came from some fast work by Horsley. At the boy's second visit, on January 25, 1886, Jackson 'had the help of Dr. James Anderson and Mr. Victor Horsley in investigating the case more fully'.[144] In the interval between that visit and Jackson's report of the case at the Medical Society of London on November 15, 1886, Horsley repeated the guinea pig experiments. He reported his results to the Society immediately after Jackson's report on November 15.[145] In the end, 'Mr. Horsley fully endorsed Dr. Jackson's opinion … So far, he had found that the cortex as well as the medulla was concerned.'[146] All of this was consistent with a noticeable trend in Jackson's thinking around that time—some of his attention was shifting to the lowest level.

'Remarks on Evolution and Dissolution of the Nervous System', April and November–December 1887

In April 1887, and separately in November–December 1887, Jackson published two major papers with the same title, 'Remarks on Evolution and Dissolution of the Nervous System'.[147] However, they were in different journals and their contents were quite different. Given the interval between them, and given Jackson's tendency to be constantly rethinking his ideas, it is reasonable to analyze them sequentially.

---

[142] Jackson 1886b, p.5; my square brackets and underlining. On Kussmaul and Tenner see Chapters 7 and 8. I have not been able to find any references to Westphal's experiments.

[143] Aminoff 2011, p.189.

[144] Jackson 1886f, p.963; also Jackson 1887o, p.81. James Anderson (1853–1893) had appointments at Queen Square and at the London; see Holmes 1954, p.96, and Brown 1955, pp.319–320.

[145] Horsley 1887a. A similar report by Horsley is also contained within Jackson 1886e, p.975.

[146] Jackson 1887o, p.85.

[147] Jackson 1887e, and (in installments) Jackson 1887j to Jackson 1887n.

'Remarks on Evolution and Dissolution of the Nervous System', April 1887

The subjects of this paper were mainly of long standing in Jackson's thinking, involving epilepsy/seizures, the highest centers, their evolution and dissolution, and concomitance. With regard to focal pathophysiology for all kinds of seizures, he restated this idea with a clarification: 'In all cases of epileptiform and epileptic seizures the "discharging lesion" is supposed to be of some small part of <u>one half of the brain</u> ...'[148] Thus, there must be focal lesions in all cases of genuine epilepsy. Furthermore, he said, 'although I shall continue to speak for the most part of [genuine] epilepsy as if there were one such clinical entity, there are really many different epilepsies ... each dependent on a "discharging lesion" of some part of the highest centres'.[149] Hence the pathophysiological implication.

> ... in <u>post-epileptic insanities</u> the dissolution is local in the sense that it preponderates in the highest centres of <u>one half of the brain</u>. If so, it follows that the level of evolution remaining is a lower one in one half of the brain, and a very high collateral one in the other ... I submit that the seeming exceptions to the law of dissolution which some of these cases present (the coexistence of great negative affection of consciousness with highly special actions) is accounted for by the hypothesis of there being <u>deep dissolution in one hemisphere, and a high level of evolution in the other</u>.[150]

Beyond that theoretical insight, Jackson was also continuing his effort to understand normal neurological function, the better to grasp its dysfunctions. This is seen when he was trying to justify his use of the generic term 'fits'.

> I use here the most general term I can find, "fits," advisedly, because I do not, as I should when working clinically, care, as an <u>evolutionist</u>, to know whether any paroxysm is or is not "a case of epilepsy," nor how near it approaches the clinical type of "genuine" epilepsy. As an evolutionist, I wish to learn how cases shew [*sic*] *departures from normal states*, and how the three classes of fits resemble and differ as results of discharges beginning on three different evolutionary levels.[151]

Here 'evolutionist' means a scientist who studies normal evolutionary processes, including dissolution. From that perspective Jackson thought that the available experimental evidence about cerebral localization was incomplete, and some of its interpretations were simplistic. In a footnote about '*The Process of Evolution*' he proclaimed: 'The formula of evolution states a doctrine of localization, and one very different from the current one. <u>Integration</u> ... is ignored by the current doctrine.'[152] In explaining this point he said, 'The highest level consists of highest motor centres (præ-frontal lobes), and of highest sensory centres (occipital lobes) ...'[153] His remark about 'Integration' was a complaint about the

---

[148] Jackson 1887e, p.27; my underlining.

[149] Jackson 1887e, p.26; my square brackets.

[150] Jackson 1887e, p.28; Jackson's parentheses, my underlining.

[151] Jackson 1887e, pp.26–27; Jackson's italics, my square brackets and underlining.

[152] Jackson 1887e, p.31; my underlining.

[153] Jackson 1887e, p.29; on p.30 Jackson said that Ferrier had found only eye/head movements in the pre-frontal lobes (in Ferrier 2 ed.) Also, in Jackson 1887e, pp.30–31, Jackson said that Ferrier was not sure that the occipital lobes are 'the highest sensory centres'. In Jackson 1887l, p.511, footnote (*b*), he discussed his agreements and disagreements with Ferrier.

tendency of Ferrier and others to present their experimental findings in motor cortices with fixed boundaries. Strict parcellation is reminiscent of phrenology—it suffers the same inability to explain integration between pieces in the mosaic, except by proximity of the individual centers to each other.[154] In contrast, Jackson's sensory-motor associationism obviates that problem—at least in theory. His perception of the problem is apparent when he used an interesting term.

> ... the *physical basis* of the Ego represents – that is, that the highest centres represent – or co-ordinates the whole organism in complex, &c., ways. Just as the consciousness of the moment is, or stands for, the whole person psychical, so the correlative activities are of nervous arrangements, representing the whole person physical.[155]

This was written before Sigmund Freud (1856–1939) made the Ego so famous. Jackson's Ego was a stand-in for the totality of unified consciousness. That was consistent with the contemporary meaning of the term, as explained by William James (1842–1910) in 1890, when he said that there were three 'theories of the Ego': '1) The Spiritualist theory' ['*The Theory of the Soul*'], '2) The Associationist theory', and '3) The Transcendentalist theory'.[156] So Jackson's use of Ego as a unifying psychical entity was consistent with the Associationist tradition. Further on he launched into a discussion of concomitance, offering summaries of three doctrines about the 'metaphysical question of the *nature* of the relation of mind to nervous activities'. Among them: 'It seems to me that the third doctrine, that of concomitance, is at any rate convenient in the study of nervous diseases'.[157] In defense of concomitance he said:

> A critic of my Croonian Lectures, who in all other respects dealt with my opinions very good-naturedly, says that I state this doctrine in order to evade the charge of materialism. It, or an essentially similar doctrine is held, so far as I can make out, by Hamilton, J.S. Mill, Clifford, Spencer, Max Müller, Bain, Huxley, Du Bois Raymond, Laycock, Tyndall and Herman. The critic referred to says that the doctrine of concomitance is Leibniz's "two clock theory." It may be; it matters nothing for medical purposes ... The evolutionist does not, however, invoke supernatural agency.[158]

Staying on the physical side of concomitance, Jackson shifted his attention from scientific to practical medicine with a puzzling disclaimer: 'Our concern as medical men is with the body. If there be such a thing as disease of the mind, we can do nothing for it. Negative and positive mental symptoms are for us only signs of what is not going on, or of what is going on wrong, in the highest sensori-motor centres'.[159] At first sight this apparent renunciation of psychiatry seems anomalous—surely Hughlings Jackson valued psychiatry and contributed

---

[154] I am indebted to Stanley Finger (personal communication) for this information about the only available mechanism for integration in phrenology.

[155] Jackson 1887e, p.35.

[156] James 1890, vol.1, p.342; my square brackets. In his discussion of the associationist theory (pp.350–360) James was largely concerned with Hume and J.S. Mill.

[157] Jackson 1887e, pp.37–38. The first two were interactionism and monism *à la* Lewes).

[158] Jackson 1887e, p.38. I have not pursued identification of the 'critic'. This list of names is the same as in Jackson 1884g, p.706. It implies that Jackson had read some writings of those authors, but not Leibniz. The latter's 'monads' have been interpreted as a form of psychophysical parallelism. Chirimuuta 2017, p.26, resolves the differences among this lot by saying they are all '*deniers of distinctly mental causation*'. See also York and Steinberg 2002.

[159] Jackson 1887e, p.39.

much to it. By this statement, however, I think he was trying to be consistent in his application of concomitance.

> ... *The Range of Concomitance.* – What is the range of concomitance? For my part I think the whole body is 'the organ of mind' ... when speaking of the dynamics of the chain of centres. I shall, however, continue to speak of the highest centres as being the 'organ of mind'. Here the question recurs: "How far down" in the highest centres is there consciousness attending nervous activities?[160]

In 1881 Jackson had asked the same question, when he introduced the term 'concomitance'. First he had said, 'I give no opinion on this difficult question', and then he went on, 'But were I to make an abrupt limit to the concomitance of psychical with nervous states I should place the lower limit at the lower Motor (Hitzig and Ferrier) and lower Sensory (Ferrier's) centres'.[161] So in 1881 he had declared that mind correlates with the activity of the highest *and* intermediate levels, but not with the lowest cerebral level. Here, in 1887, when he addressed the range of concomitance, he appeared to exclude conscious mind from the intermediate level by not mentioning it. His single paragraph on the subject started with the observation that: 'A distinction is made by many between mind and consciousness.*' And the footnote continued, '* I admit the distinction in Subject and Object consciousness, and also that into faint and vivid states of consciousness'.[162] Referring to the 'many' other authors, he said, 'I suppose they would say that consciousness shows activities of the highest and mind [*sic*] activities of the lower nervous arrangements of the highest centres. I take consciousness and mind to be synonymous terms ... if all consciousness is lost all mind is lost ...'.[163] In all of this he was implying that subjective ideas *might* be concomitant with activities of the intermediate level, but objective ideas can be concomitant with activities no further down than the lower layers of the highest centers. On the other hand,

> Unconscious states of mind are sometimes spoken of, which seems to me to involve a contradiction. That there may be activities of lower nervous arrangements of the highest centres, which have no attendant psychical states, and which yet lead to [the] next activities of the very highest arrangements of those centres whose activities have attendant psychical states, I can easily understand. But these prior activities are states of the nervous system, not any sort of states of mind.[164]

Now John Hughlings Jackson might 'easily understand' those complexities, but most of the rest of us mortals are likely to be bewildered. In an apparent attempt to help us—and to further explore the normal—he offered a discussion of 'subjective'.

> The term subjective is used in different senses in medical writings. It is sometimes used for psychical states in contrast to the correlative nervous states, which latter are then called objective; sometimes [it is used] for faint states of consciousness, as in ideation, in contrast to vivid states of consciousness, as in perception, which [latter] are then called objective;

---

160 Jackson 1887e, p.39; Jackson's italics, my underlining.
161 Jackson 1881l, p.69; see also Chapter 10.
162 Jackson 1887e, p.39.
163 Jackson 1887e, p.39; my underlining.
164 Jackson 1887e, pp.39–40; my square brackets and underlining. For a succinct statement of Jackson's position on 'Unconscious states of mind' see York and Steinberg 2006, pp.22–23; also York and Steinberg 1993.

sometimes [it is used] very crudely, for mind and brain together in contrast to "real things," that is, objects in themselves coloured, shaped, &c., which are then called objective.[165]

Jackson did not say which of the three meanings he favored—no surprise there—but we can speculate that it was the second, because 'faint states of consciousness' would be best consistent with associationism. In any case, in this paper he devoted only the one paragraph to a consideration of 'subjective', and that definition was essentially the same as he had given in 1876 and 1879.[166] He repeated it here because it was requisite background to his discussion of clinical problems, including postictal 'negative states of consciousness'.

> There is very often a stage of ... defect of consciousness before what we call ... loss of consciousness. These negative affections of consciousness occur during the sudden ... discharge; for whilst consciousness arises during slight sequent [sic] discharges, it ceases during sudden ... discharges of many nervous arrangements at once.*
>
> * When there is the "dreamy state" there is double consciousness ... there being remains of consciousness as to present surroundings (remains of object consciousness), and increase of consciousness as to some former surroundings (increase of subject consciousness).[167]

Thus, on the psychical side of the dreamy state normal object consciousness is partially suppressed, while normal subject consciousness is enhanced enough to reach some level of awareness—that is, the individual has at least a faint ideation of the subject. Toward the end of Jackson's paper of April 1887 he also used the psychical distinction of subjective and objective to address another old problem—people's tendency to continue to use the terms of the faculty psychology. First he said: 'During activities of the least automatic centres (highest centres), Will and other elements or states of (object) consciousness arise ...'[168] And later he named four basic faculties: 'Will, Memory, Reason, and Emotion', which are 'really four different aspects of object-consciousness ...'[169] When Jackson was young and trying to establish his intellectual independence he would not have dignified any terms from the faculty psychology by using them for anything. Here, at age 52, he had mellowed, as seen in his use of terms like 'genuine' epilepsy and in his naming of the four faculties. But intellectual mellowing does not exclude new ideas.

'Remarks on Evolution and Dissolution of the Nervous System', November–December 1887

In Table 11.3 I have extracted Jackson's section headings from his paper of November–December 1887.[170] Here we are dealing with consciousness, subjective–objective, 'constants', and neuro-cardiology (my neologism), where the latter two are new but only theoretical. They are of interest because they show the way in which he used a series of speculations

---

[165] Jackson 1887e, p.41; my square brackets and underlining.

[166] Jackson 1876g, p.174; see also Chapter 8; and Jackson 1879u, pp.409–410; see also Chapter 9.

[167] Jackson 1887e, pp.43–44.

[168] Jackson 1887e, p.41; Jackson's parentheses.

[169] Jackson 1887e, p.48; see also Jackson 1887j, p.461.

[170] For the first time the author's byline in Jackson 1887j, p.461, was 'J. Hughlings Jackson, M.D., LL.D., F.R.S.', which shows his pride in his recently acquired L.L.D. from Glasgow.

Table 11.3 Section headings extracted from 'Remarks on evolution and dissolution of the nervous system', November–December 1887.[a] They are grouped by published installments.

Jackson 1887j

Preliminary

I. Abrupt Beginning – Perception and Ideation

II. 'Breaking up' and 'Making up' of States of Object Consciousness

III. Restriction and Extension of the term Memory

IV. The Duality of Consciousness

V. Various ways in which the terms Subjective and Objective are used in Medical Writings

Jackson 1887k

VI. Subject Consciousness – The Introspection of Consciousness

VII. The Anatomical Substrata of Subject consciousness

VIII. On 'Sensations' and on Association of Ideas

IX. On Constants

X. On Estimation of Time

Jackson 1887l

XI. General Remarks on Parts of the Body, and on their Representation by Nervous Centres – Peripheral or Statical Co-ordination – Fixation of Limits; Things given by Inheritance to start with

XII. Peculiarities of the Heart[b]

XIII. Representation; Re-representation and Re-re-representation of the Heart, in Lowest, Middle, and Highest Centres Respectively

Jackson 1887m

XIII (Continued)

XIV. On Three Different Kinds of Representation of the Heart in the Highest Centres

Jackson 1887n

XV. The Fourth Kind of Representation of the Heart in the Highest Centres. Representation of the Cardiac Systole in the Physical Basis of the Time Constant

XVI. General Remarks on Constants[c]

XVII. Subject-Consciousness and its Anatomical Substrata – Pseudo Explanations of Psychical States

XVIII. On 'Prolongation of Time'

A70, pp.38–40[d]

XIX. On Detachment and Independence of the Highest Cerebral Centres and on Internal Evolution

---

[a] Jackson 1887j to Jackson 1887n; italics in original. Once again Jackson published extended discussions of theoretical issues in the *MPC*.

[b] This Section XII (J87-12, p.512) is expanded in the pamphlet reprint (A70, pp.16–19), largely with references to McWilliams 1888 on cardiac rhythm. That extra text is included in Jackson's *Selected Writings*, vol.2 (1932), pp.102–104, as if it were in the original.

[c] In Jackson 1887n, p.618, there is a footnote (*b*) that is not reproduced in Jackson 1932, p.112, nor is it found in the pamphlet of this article (A70, p.32).

[d] This last section is listed in York and Steinberg (2006, p.143) only as pamphlet A70, pp.38–40. It is not in the original article in the *MPC*. In Jackson's *Selected Writings* (1932), vol.2, pp.116–118, it was taken from the pamphlet. Taylor's footnote 1, p.92, in *Selected Writings* vol.2, says: 'Section XIX is not in the *Journal*', where 'the *Journal*' apparently means the *MPC*.

to advance a conception about the brain's integrative function, even when those particular ideas were stillborn.

On the physical side of concomitance, Jackson's basic insight was to recognize that *all* of the behavioral manifestations of any physical/affective state *must* be represented somewhere in the cerebrum at some level, because that is how their integration takes place. Without integration each component of a behavior would simply occur in splendid isolation. This may seem obvious, but that's because we are now Sherringtonians. It was not so obvious then.

This paper of late 1887 introduced or expanded a number of Jackson's new or recent theoretical conceptions. It also shows his attention to the changing views of evolution. Since it was one of his last major expositions of this part of his paradigm, it was one of the sources for his thought that was read by succeeding generations. From that point of view, his '*Preliminary*' section restated some of his fundamentals. Those included the comparative method applied to evolution and dissolution, concomitance, and the sensori-motor nature of the entire nervous system.[171] At the outset he emphasized the reality of the categories of 'Will, Memory, Reason, and Emotion', which he had started to resurrect in April.[172] At the end of that earlier paper it is not clear whether he had intended the four faculties to encompass *all* of object consciousness. Here this question was resolved in the affirmative, because the division into the four faculties is artificial. Actually,

> It is more correct to say that Ideation or Perception is an element in a state of object consciousness … A state of object consciousness is a thing to the different aspects of which we give the names Will, Memory, Reason, and Emotion. In other words, there are not two things – (1) Object consciousness and also (2) Will, Memory, Reason, and Emotion. The Will, Memory, Reason, and Emotion of the moment make up the object consciousness of the moment … it is often convenient to speak as if states of object consciousness were made up of the four "faculties," and to deal with them separately. But … it is to be tacitly taken that there is really a state of object consciousness in which Will only preponderates. And so, *mutatis mutandis*, for Memory, Reason, and Emotion.[173]

This dynamic conception is typical of Jackson's thinking—we find the same pattern in his statement that perception and ideation are forms of memory. Perception, he said, is 'mainly memory. There is nothing paradoxical in this statement … when it is said that recognition (a synonym of perception) is having relations of likeness and unlikeness'.[174] Going further, he expanded on the dynamics of subject–object.

> Two different states of object consciousness often enough co-exist for one Subject. This mode of having two distinct objective states is a quite different kind of "double consciousness" from that which is meant when subject and object consciousness are spoken of. I shall abandon the term "double consciousness" … because … it is equivocal.[175]

After that disclaimer, Jackson's discussion of subject–object continued with the title '*Subject Consciousness – The Introspection of Consciousness*'.[176] This might seem to evoke Harrington's

---

171 Jackson 1887j, p.461.
172 Jackson 1887e, p.48.
173 Jackson 1887j, p.461; Jackson's italics.
174 Jackson 1887j, p.461; Jackson's parentheses.
175 Jackson 1887j, p.462.
176 Jackson 1887k, p.491; Jackson's italics.

characterization of the standard use of 'subjective' at the time, which meant introspection.[177] But, with a nod to the Irish penchant for clever paradox, he actually said something rather different.

> What is called the Introspection of Consciousness is of states of Object consciousness already "come out of" Subject consciousness. Subject consciousness, that which has these states, is not to be known in any such way. To put the matter Hibernically; we only know … Subject consciousness, on its ceasing to be … Subject consciousness – on its becoming Object consciousness.[178]

So there is such a thing as 'Subject consciousness', but we can't know it *per se*. On the physical side, and acknowledging that 'What follows must be taken as speculative', he continued:

> I submit that the units making up that division of the highest centres which I call the anatomical substratum of Subject consciousness … re-re-represent … all parts of the body … *in relation to one another*. Each unit is the whole division in miniature, but each is … the whole of it in different miniature …
>
> The anatomical substrata of Subject consciousness … are made up of nervous arrangements in comparatively fixed relation to one another, they are comparatively … unmodifiable in new ways.[179]

'Constants' and Cerebral Representation of the Heart, November–December 1887

After the above passage about subject consciousness Jackson returned to his epistemological argument for it—and he quietly introduced a new theoretical concept.

> Subject consciousness is something deeper than knowledge; it is that by which knowledge is possible … it is an awareness of our existence as individuals, as persons having the objective states making up for each, the (his) universe. Subject consciousness is the comparatively unchanging, the most unchanging. It is thus a <u>Constant</u> to Object consciousness which is the continually changing.[180]

Jackson's Constants are innate 'Forms of Thought'. Apparently with the issue of materialism in mind, he said: 'if forms of thought are <u>supernaturally</u> given, it is reasonable to infer that their physical bases were given with them …'[181] And with or without the supernatural, he added: 'I accept Herbert Spencer's doctrine of the inheritance of Organized Experiences (*a*) …'. And the substance of footnote (*a*) was a direct quotation from Spencer.

> "If there exist certain external relations which are experienced by all organisms at all instants of their waking lives – relations which are absolutely constant, absolutely universal

---

[177] Harrington 1987, p.228; see also Chapter 8.
[178] Jackson 1887k, p.491.
[179] Jackson 1887k, p.491; Jackson's italics.
[180] Jackson 1887k, p.491; Jackson's parentheses, my underlining.
[181] Jackson 1887k, p.492; my underlining.

– there will be established answering internal relations that are absolutely constant ... Such relations we have in those of Space and Time."[182]

Again declaring himself to be an 'Evolutionist', Jackson pursued his investigation of innate Constants. This led to another new element—a role for the heart—which aligned well with Spencer's view, although Spencer had not mentioned the heart specifically.

> I adopt Herbert Spencer's opinions on the origin of the physical bases of the Constants – that they have been slowly evolved, organismally and racially; they are inherited imperfect and are perfected after birth ... what is said on Constants may be ... correct ... even on the hypothesis that a man was created with them fully developed. The term Constant is one of my own devising as a synonym for Forms of Thought ... the Time Constant ... is ... a ... representation of the cardiac systole in the highest cerebral centres.[183]

So the inborn cardiac rhythm is a Constant by which to evaluate the 'objective standards' of the external world: 'We inherit rhythms, the bases of the Constant Time (Subject), and choose objective standards to measure "external sequences" by.'[184] As Jackson said later, his entire analysis was 'hypothetical'.[185] Moreover, in his discussion there was a source of potential confusion about 'the Lowest Level of Evolution of the whole organism'.[186] Previously, when he said 'lowest level' he was referring only to the central nervous system, but of course the rest of the body is itself a level of evolution. Here he made an important distinction: 'it is not the heart, but a certain kind of representation of its systole in the highest centres, which is supposed to be the physical basis of that Constant ...'[187] What this meant was representation of the *heart's actions*, not the organ itself.

To make his theory work Jackson needed to nominate some organ whose function could serve as the inborn fiducial for the Constant, and the heart was the obvious choice.[188] Physiologically, he said of the heart: 'It is the most nearly perfectly rhythmical organ; having in normal states nearly a succession of similar movements at equal intervals.' And a little later: 'The heart is the most autonomous of all organs. A frog's heart, cut out of its body, beats for two and a half days ... an excised dog's heart beats ninety-six hours ...' Clinically, 'The heart holds out longest in general injurious influences such as the coma of acute alcoholism'.[189] Thus it was an appropriate vehicle for exploration of cerebral representation.

Starting with the lowest level, Jackson said, 'That the heart is represented in the Lowest Level of [Cerebral] Evolution is accepted doctrine. There are supposed to be a cardio-inhibitory

---

[182] Jackson 1887k, p.492, footnote *a*; Jackson's quotation marks. For this passage from Spencer, Jackson cited 'Spencer, Princ. Psych. Vol.1, p.467'; it is indeed found there in Spencer 1870, vol.1, and in Spencer 1880, vol.1.

[183] Jackson 1887k, p.492; my underlining. Presumably 'a man' referred to the biblical Adam. Although Spencer had used 'constant' in the passage that Jackson quoted above in (*a*), Jackson was claiming independent invention for his use of 'Constant'.

[184] Jackson 1887k, p.492

[185] Jackson 1887o, p.618.

[186] Jackson 1887l, p.511.

[187] Jackson 1887l, p.512; my underlining.

[188] Probably the obviousness of the choice was enhanced by the fact that the heart was the subject of some outstanding British research. Jackson (Jackson 1887m, p.586, footnote *b*) acknowledged his debt to the work of Walter H. Gaskell (1847–1914), who was at Michael Foster's Cambridge School of Physiology; see Geison 1978, especially pp.280–296, 314–319. Jackson said Gaskell's (1886) research helped him 'in the analysis of epileptic fits, and in many other ways'.

[189] Jackson 1887l, p.512; see Geison 1978, pp.280–289.

and an accelerating centre in the medulla oblongata. This is Representation (first representa-tion).'[190] Then he moved on to the heart's representation at the second level.

> ... in the Middle Level of Evolution, the so-called "motor region" ... the arterial system as well as the heart is represented ... I long ago arrived at the conclusion ... that the circu-latory organs and all other parts of the body are represented in units of the cerebrum ... Keeping ... to the "motor region" ... experiments on some lower animals supply the most definite evidence of representation of the circulatory apparatus in those centres.[191]

For validation of the heart's representation in the highest level of the cerebrum Jackson had to rely on clinical observations and deduction, because he admitted that he could not cite any experimental evidence.

> We now consider the third Representation of the heart ... in the highest centres ... it is certain that it is represented in those centres. The facts of emotional manifestations (phys-ical effects *during* emotions) seem to me to demonstrate it ... An emotion is an element in a state of (object) consciousness ... and of necessity the highest centres are concerned during it ... I submit that the *physical basis* of ... an emotion is of nervous arrangements of the highest centres especially *representing those parts of the body concerned in the manifest-ations of that emotion.*[192]

To illustrate, he used the example of anger. He argued that its physical components must be represented in the highest centers, although 'There is, as yet, no experimental evidence', because the experiments of Francois-Franck and Pitres applied only to the middle cerebral level.[193] Then he laid out his plan for the remainder of his paper, which would deal with four kinds of representation in the highest centers.

> So far we have spoken of representation of the heart in the three Levels of Evolution, re-gardless of _kind_ of representation. In the next Section we shall speak of three different kinds of representation ... in the highest centres. In a later Section we shall speak of a fourth kind of representation of it, that which is supposed to be, in the highest centres, the physical basis of the Time Constant.[194]

Jackson's phrase '*kind* of representation' signified qualitative differences among representa-tions. The four kinds are each different in the sense of exactly what is represented. In the 'First Kind of Representation' the nervous centers are 'represented in their most general character as tissues ... Muscle ... is most represented in that physical basis, the heart among other muscles, but only as so much muscular tissue'.[195] In the 'Second Kind of Representation' he presented the heart as a mere machine. Using Spencer's sociological terminology, he viewed

---

[190] Jackson 1887l, p.512. At the place of my square brackets the published text says 'Central', but that makes no sense. Jackson never used that term physiologically, so it is a misprint. There are indeed cardio-inhibitory and accelerating centers in the brainstem.

[191] Jackson 1887m, p.586. He quoted extensively from the work of Charles Émile Francois-Franck (1849–1921) and Pitres, whose experiments showed 'autonomic visceral changes in pulse rate, blood pressure and respir-ation following cortical stimulation' (McHenry 1969, p.223).

[192] Jackson 1887m, p.586; Jackson's italics and parentheses.

[193] Jackson 1887m, p.587.

[194] Jackson 1887m, p.587; Jackson's italics, my underlining.

[195] Jackson 1887m, p.587.

it 'as an organ doing menial work'. That is, 'The heart is represented on this level as a pump ... It is one of the Industrial Organs of Spencer, being one of the analogues of the Industrial parts of the Social Organism'. But, he added, 'here we cannot limit attention to the heart; we must take into account the whole circulatory apparatus'.[196]Jackson's 'Third Kind of Representation' involved the heart's role in emotion.

> The highest centres during emotional states have an effect on the heart, sometimes an enormous effect. The kind of representation of the heart in the physical bases of emotion ... is obviously vastly different from the second kind of representation ... For in so far as the heart is engaged during emotions, in so far does it for the time being cease to be of service as an industrial organ, that is as an organ doing menial work.[197]

The last sentence in the above is ambiguous. Obviously the heart continues to pump during emotional states, and its rate varies in the process. That problem had been lurking in the background of Jackson's discussion of the heart as a fiducial Constant. He acknowledged this confounding element in his theory and attempted to deal with it in his next section, *The Fourth Kind of Representation of the Heart in the Highest Centres. Representation of the Cardiac Systole in the Physical Basis of the Time Constant*.[198]

> ... the heart, as an organ doing menial work, varies in rate according to the needs of the system ... An organ, or centres for it made thus to vary, by agencies external to it, could not be a Standard for ... sequences which vary according to very different conditions ... any nervous arrangements ... of the Highest Level ... which can make the heart alter in rate ... could be no Standard ... I do not ... say that there is absolutely no such representation; I am in doubt on the matter.[199]

However, there was no doubt in Jackson's mind about the need for neural representation of the Time Constant. He acknowledged that his idea 'on the kind of Representation of the heart as the physical basis of the Time Constant is purely hypothetical. But I submit that Forms of Thought, even if supernaturally given, must have *some* physical basis. That basis cannot be anything else than *some* nervous arrangements representing *some* part or parts of the body in *some* way'.[200] Logically, then, 'Nervous elements which are independent, and which do not vary, and cannot be made to vary in their rate of activity, can alone be the physical basis of the Time Constant'.[201] Arguing for the independence of systole's representation in the highest level, he said:

> ... we may say that the physical basis of the Time Constant ... is of nervous elements in the highest centers which are the most Simple, and the most strongly Organised. They are the most Independent and most autonomous of all nervous elements, having become "detached" from the lowest centres out of which they have been evolved.[202]

---

[196] Jackson 1887m, p.587. On Spencer's idea of a society as an organism see Collins 1889, pp.389–391; on Spencer's theory of the 'Industrial Type of Society' as an evolutionary stage of social development see Collins 1889, pp.485–489.

[197] Jackson 1887m, p.587; on p.588 Jackson made another statement to the same effect.

[198] Jackson 1887n, p.617; Jackson's italics.

[199] Jackson 1887n, p.617; my underlining.

[200] Jackson 1887n, p.618; Jackson's italics.

[201] Jackson 1887n, pp.618–619.

[202] Jackson 1887n, p.618; Jackson's quotation marks, my underlining.

So Jackson's basic idea is that the highest centers, containing representations of cardiac systole, are somehow 'independent' from the lower centers. From there he went on to claim similar representation for other Constants: 'The physical bases of the other Constants (Space, Mass (force) and Weight) are *mutatis mutandis*, similarly explicable...'[203] In theory,

> As evolution ... progresses, the highest centres ... become more and more detached from ... the lower centres out of which they have been evolved. The detachment ... is never complete, except hypothetically, in cases of Constants ... By the double process of increasing complexity and increasing detachment of the highest centres, we gradually 'get above' our lower, mere animal selves.[204]

This passage was taken from Jackson's final section '*On Detachment and Independence of the Highest Cerebral Centres and on Internal Evolution*'. In 1888 it was added to the pamphlet reprint of Jackson's 1887 paper, extending his discussion with quotations from Spencer and Fiske.[205] In truth, his argument for the independent existence of the Constants is tortuous at best. After 1888 he did not mention them in any substantive way in his publications,[206] and I have not seen them discussed by any of his commentators. Presumably he knew that his conception was stretched beyond viability. On the other hand, in 1888 his production of more lasting contributions was immense—so much so that I have struggled with the problem of how to present them coherently. Part of the solution is to keep to chronological order, which is done in Table 11.4. But keeping to strict chronology for discussion could produce artificial results, so some of Jackson's prodigious output in 1888 and beyond will be analyzed later, in Chapter 12.

Other Significant Papers, *circa* 1887–1888

In Table 11.2 we saw that Jackson held leadership positions in several professional organizations in the years 1885–1890. At the same time, here in Table 11.4 we see that he was working intensely on preparation of several different papers in 1888–1890. In addition, he had a busy practice, as well as obligations at Queen Square and the London. From the beginning he had always worked simultaneously on multiple neurological problems. For that reason my chronological approach to Jackson's development can sometimes seem miscellaneous, but there is a way to tie these themes together. They are all part of the process of creating a paradigm and then extending it by application to other problems.[207] Of note, the extension can be happening at different times for different problems.

---

[203] Jackson 1887n, p.619; Jackson's italics and parentheses. He also postulated a role for the cerebellum in the Constants, because it is part of the whole integrated system. Half-way through this section, in footnote (*b*), concerning 'different degrees of objectivisation', Jackson (Jackson 1887n, p.619) said: 'I adopt Spencer's doctrine of Transfigured Realism'. His source for the latter is Spencer 1872 and 1880, pp.489–503; they are summarized in Collins 1889, pp.312–314.

[204] A70 (York and Steinberg 2006, p.143), p.38. The extension of Jackson 1887n into the pamphlet of 1888 (A70) is included in the reprinting of Jackson 1887n in Jackson 1932, vol.2, pp.116–118. See footnote at the end of Table 11.3.

[205] He cited Spencer 1870/1880, vol.1, p.546; and Fiske 1884, pp.46–47.

[206] There is a mention of the Constants' 'detachment and independence' in Jackson 1888g, p.362.

[207] Kuhn 1996, pp.10–22, called the latter 'normal science'.

Table 11.4　Chronology of the first presentations and/or publication dates of Hughlings Jackson's major papers, 1888–1890.

Month/year	Venue	Short title/subject	Citations in Jackson's Bibliography
Feb. 1888/Oct. 1888–Jan. 1889	Medico-Psychological Association	Post-epileptic states: comparative study of insanities	1888b, 1888g, 1889a
July 1888/July 1888	British Medical Association branches	Diagnosis and treatment of diseases of the brain	1888c, 1888d
July 1888	Publication only (*Brain*)	('Intellectual aura '), one case, no autopsy	1888e
(?) May 1888/ Oct. 1888	Neurological Society	Comments on Mercier on Inhibition	1888f
Feb. 1889	Medical Society of London	Epilepsy with olfactory aura – tumor	1889c, 1889k
Aug. 1889	British Medical Association, Leeds	Comparative study of diseases of the nervous system	1889d, 1889e, 1889g
Oct. 1889	Ophthalmological Society	Ophthalmology and general medicine	1889h, 1889i, 1889j, 1890i
Mar.–Apr. 1890	Royal College of Physicians	Lumleian Lectures on convulsive seizures	1890b, 1890c, 1890d, 1890e, 1890f, 1890g

Discussion of Bastian on the 'Muscular Sense', Published April 1887

Part of the fun of presenting a paper at a meeting is the opportunity for discussion afterwards. Jackson cherished that kind of give-and-take, whether he was making a presentation or commenting on someone else's. He did this throughout his career, but we know the details only when his comments were recorded and published, and that began to happen with some frequency in the 1880s. In *Brain*, 1887–1888, there were three such commentaries by Jackson. I will review them here because they have acquired some importance as expressions of his thought, and they illustrate some points in the progression of his paradigm.

'Bastian on the "Muscular Sense"' was 'read before the Neurological Society of London, on December 16, 1886' and published in April 1887.[208] In the analysis of E.G. Jones, 'Bastian seems to have been alone among his colleagues in anticipating modern knowledge that a considerable amount of sensory information arising at the periphery, and particularly in the muscles, need not be registered in consciousness yet may still be used by the central nervous system to coordinate motor acts'.[209] From that realization Bastian developed a theory that flew in the face of his contemporary neuroscience. He

> . . . felt that the only true motor centers in the brain were the lower motor neurons, or as we might now say, following Sherrington, 'the final common path.' He was, therefore, inclined

---

[208]　Bastian 1887; Jackson's comments (Jackson 1887f) are on pp.107–109 of Bastian 1887. Jones (1972) and Compston (2015) have analyzed Jackson's (Jackson 1887f) response to Bastian.

[209]　Jones 1972, p.301. I would argue that Jackson understood this to a considerable extent, because of his hierarchical conceptions.

to believe that the regions around the Rolandic fissure ... were not so much 'motor centers' as the arrival zones for unfelt muscle sense impressions and centers for the ideal revival of 'kinaesthetic images.' A lesion in these kinaesthetic regions would thus cause paralysis only because of the inability of ideal recall.[210]

Compston's summary of Bastian's position is perhaps overly succinct: 'In short, there are no motor centres.'[211] Needless to say, Jackson did not agree. He thought that the entire central nervous system is sensori-*motor*, so motor elements do reach consciousness, and 'There is no a priori reason why states of consciousness should not attend activities of motor as well as activities of sensory cells.'[212] Jackson implied, only a little obliquely, that Bastian was perpetuating the same mistake as the 'popular psychologist', who 'makes a confusion betwixt active states of sensory elements (physical states) and sensations'. Hence, 'The common expression "ideas of movement" is very objectionable.'[213] With regard to neural activity attending consciousness, Jackson assumed 'the activity of sensory elements ... [but] there is activity of motor elements as well ... the expressions "motor ideas," "ideas of movement," and "muscular sense" (if "muscular sensations" be intended) are illegitimate compounds of physiological and psychological terms'.[214] Never one to shrink from a fight, Bastian hit back with even stronger language.

> Dr. Hughlings-Jackson ... reiterates his well-known views, but unfortunately ... having given them the fullest consideration, I have felt compelled to come to the very opposite conclusions. He does not in any way endeavour to show me where I am wrong, or attempt to explain away the difficulties which, as I have pointed out [,] now make his favourite doctrine untenable.[215]

Jackson was indeed reiterating his 'well-known views', but it was another matter to summarily dismiss his 'favourite doctrine' as 'untenable'. It is easy to see why Bastian was not a favorite among his colleagues—he was prickly, whereas Jackson had a well-tuned sense of humor.

An Address on the Psychology of Joking, October 1887

While Jackson was preparing his 'Remarks on evolution and dissolution' in November–December 1887, he was also having some fun with a lighter application of evolution. As President of the Medical Society of London, he gave the Opening Address on October 17, 1887. His title was 'Remarks on the Psychology of Joking'.[216] He set the tone in his opening paragraph, where he offered a parody of his own evolutionary theories, while poking mild

---

[210] Jones 1972, p.304. Jones' use of 'neuron' for events before 1891 is anachronistic; see Definition Section 1 in Chapter 3. On Sherrington's 'final common path' see Clarke and O'Malley 1996, pp.370–371, 375–377.

[211] Compston 2015, p.3453. See also Finger's (1994, pp.203–204) summary of Bastian.

[212] Jackson 1887f, p.107.

[213] Jackson 1887f, p.108.

[214] Jackson 1887f, p.108; my square brackets.

[215] Jackson 1887f, pp.130–131.

[216] Jackson 1887g (*Lancet*), Jackson 1887h (*BMJ*), Jackson 1888i (*Proceedings* of the Society). I have used Jackson 1888j simply because its font is larger. York (2015) has analyzed Jackson's address extensively.

fun at one of his closest colleagues. From this paper we can surmise that Jackson's tripartite view of cerebral levels was sufficiently well known to be used as a theme for humor in addressing the general medical audience at the Medical Society—and it is important to remember that humor is culturally loaded.

> I think punning does not receive enough attention. In spite of Dr. Johnson's well-known dictum, we should not despise punning. Sydney Smith says that it is the foundation of all wit. Supposing three degrees of evolution, I submit that punning is the least evolved system of joking, that wit is evolved out of punning, and that humour is evolved out of wit. Everybody has heard of Sydney Smith's remark – that it requires a surgical operation to get a joke into the head of [a] Scotchman. But ... The Scotch have a great appreciation of those highly-evolved jocosities displaying the humorous, although, no doubt, a scorn of simple, lowly-evolved jocosities, such as plays on words. It is difficult to form a conception of a Scotch punster. Yet I have heard an Aberdonian, a physician of world-wide reputation, make a pun.[217]

Jackson claimed to be serious when he said, 'Punning is very worthy of the psychologist's attention. I seriously mean that the analysis of puns is a simple way of beginning the methodical analysis of normal and abnormal mentation.'[218] And so he continued, half tongue-in-cheek, but only half. Beneath the whimsical evolutionary hypothesis about punning, wit, and humor—lowest to highest—there was an element of seriousness, and yet even his seriousness was playful.

> Jocosities of all degrees of evolution ... are the "play of mind;" play in the sense in which the word has been used in the remark that the "æsthetic sentiments originate from the play impulse." A further definition of play ... is given in the following quotation from Spencer: – "The activities we call play are united with æsthetic activities by the trait that neither subserve, in any direct way, the processes conducive to life [survival]." There ... [was] ... a great intellectual advance ... when man began to value things for their beauty apart from their use ... For it showed that ... he had some surplus mind for greater ends of life. So I contend that our race owes some respect to the first punster.[219]

Toward the end of his Address, Jackson acknowledged that he had been playing 'one big poor joke' on his audience, and yet, 'If I had time I could ... show that ... what has been said applies closely to the study of "mental symptoms" in serious diseases'.[220] In the next few years he did go on to further discussions of mental disease, but not from the perspective of humor.

---

[217] Jackson 1888j, p.1; my underlining. The 'Aberdonian', of course, was David Ferrier, who was probably in the audience. Samuel Johnson supposedly called puns the lowest form of humor. On Sydney Smith see York 2015, p.2, and above in this chapter.

[218] Jackson 1888j, p.1.

[219] Jackson 1888j, p.2; Jackson's quotation marks, my square brackets. The quotation from Spencer is found in Spencer 1880, vol.2, p.627, and also in Spencer 1872, p.627.

[220] Jackson 1888j, p.6.

Discussion of Bennett on 'Muscular Hypertonicity in Paralysis',
Published January 1888

This paper was 'read before the Neurological Society of London, on July 7, 1887'. Bennett said that he had selected the 'general subject' of the 'apparently paradoxical condition of increased muscular tonicity as associated with motor weakness'.[221] The published version (*Brain*, January 1888) included comments by Jackson, Buzzard, Ferrier, and others.[222] Jackson's themes included hyperreflexia, of course, but he also ranged much further afield. Within that broad range I have identified four topics for analysis: (1) 'hypertonicity' (hyperreflexia), (2) the role of the cerebellum, (3) the meaning of 'functional', and (4) Jackson's recognition of the pathophysiology of the internal capsule.[223]

By 'muscular hypertonicity' Bennett meant both exaggerated deep tendon reflexes, especially at the knees, *and* muscle contraction ('irritability') after direct cutaneous percussion. The latter would not now be a major clinical concern, because the finding can be quite variable. Often there is simply no response, but Bennett was trying to figure that out. The knee reflex, on the other hand, is usually consistent with the patient's pathophysiology. As we saw in Chapter 10, the deep tendon reflexes were being integrated into the developing neurological examination in the early 1880s, so Bennett's paper of 1888 was a continuation of that process. Among the various theories that had been proposed to explain the clinical phenomenon, Bennett preferred 'The theory of the French school', which maintained 'that the symptoms of hypertonicity present in spastic paralysis are due to an irritative process, produced in the ganglion cells by the degenerated contiguous fibres of the lateral columns'.[224] This idea of proximity to irritation is long since rejected. Bennett also described another explanation— the one that we now accept.

> Another theory, and perhaps <u>the most popular</u> one, assumes that the increased excitability of the cord centres which leads to hypertonicity of muscle is the result of simple severance of the cerebral from the spinal centres, by which the controlling influence of the former is removed from the latter.[225]

Broadly interpreted, this theory could include much of the others, because it does not specify the source(s) of the 'controlling influence'. Hence Gowers' idea of lesions in lower or upper motor neuron lesions is at home in 'the most popular' theory.[226] Bennett also summarized a

> theory, which ... receives the support of Hughlings-Jackson, Bastian, and others... [It] assumes that when cerebral influence is suppressed, the uncontrolled action of the cerebellum (which is believed to be the excitor of tonic muscular action) becomes predominant, and so produces the exaggeration of muscular tonicity.[227]

---

221 Bennett 1888, pp.289–290.
222 Bennett 1888. Jackson's comments (Jackson 1888a) are on pp.312–318.
223 See Definition Section 2 in Chapter 3.
224 Bennett 1888, pp.303–304.
225 Bennett 1888, p.304; my underlining.
226 See Scott et al. 2012, pp.100–101. Chronologically, Gower's original formulation was made before full acceptance of the neuron theory; see also Chapter 12.
227 Bennett 1888, pp.305–306; Bennett's parentheses, my square brackets.

In addition to the 'hyper-physiological condition' of 'the knee-jerks in cases of hemiplegia', Jackson said: 'I have suggested, too … that by the taking off of cerebral influence from the anterior horns, the cerebellar influence on them is no longer antagonized'.[228] Except for the role of the cerebellum as the direct 'exciter' (it isn't) this idea is compatible with our current conception. Jackson also made further remarks on the cerebellum, and those ideas led to a digression, where he discussed the roles of the cerebrum and the cerebellum in normal movements and in Parkinson's disease.

> … we note that those parts suffer tremor before rigidity which are most under cerebral and least under cerebellar influence (fingers, hand, arm); and that those parts (neck and back), which are least under cerebral and most under cerebellar influence, pass into rigidity without a prior stage of tremor. That both the cerebrum and the cerebellum are engaged in any operation will … not be doubted. In manipulating [an object], the cerebrum will be only *chiefly* engaged; in walking the cerebellum will be only *chiefly* engaged. There is co-operation of only <u>amicable antagonism</u> between two large divisions of the nervous system…[229]

Jackson's speculations on the pathophysiology of Parkinson's have not been borne out. It's much more complicated, especially regarding the role of the cerebellum. Still, his ability to turn a phrase is delightfully exhibited in his description of normal physiological antagonism as 'amicable', and that is part of the next subject.

At the end of his paper Bennett outlined a long list of unanswered questions about the pathophysiology of hypertonicity, including the possibility of 'so-called <u>functional</u> disorder, consisting of definite symptoms without appreciable tissue change in the nervous system',[230] and that is where Jackson began his discussion. He said: 'I wish first to remark on a common use of the term functional … by most physicians. It is sometimes used as if there could be nervous symptoms … without abnormal changes in the nervous system… [but] this … misuse … of the term is to be deprecated.'[231] After giving several examples, he said:

> … the term functional should be used as the adjective of the word function … Function is a physiological term; it deals with the 'storing up' of nutritive materials having potential energy, with … liberations of energy by <u>nerve-cells</u> … with the rates of those liberations, with the resistances encountered, and with the different degrees of those resistances. Abnormalities of function are of two kinds, minus and plus.[232]

Note that Jackson said 'nerve-cells', not 'neurons'. Nonetheless, here in 1887–1888 his conceptual framework and its terminology were much closer to our own than they had been in the 1860s. Using two of his favorite examples from that earlier time, he said:

> After an epileptiform seizure … there may be … loss or defect of function of some fibres of the <u>pyramidal tract</u> – exhaustion of them consequent on the prior excessive discharge

---

[228] Jackson 1888a, p.315.

[229] Jackson 1888a, p.317; Jackson's italics and parentheses, my square brackets and underlining.

[230] Bennett 1888, p.312; my underlining. In common medical parlance now, 'functional' is sometimes used to imply unphysiological or even hysterical etiology.

[231] Jackson 1888a, p.312; my square brackets.

[232] Jackson 1888a, pp.312–313; my underlining. I don't know why he substituted 'minus and plus' for negative and positive—and he did the same in Jackson 1888d, p.116. In discussing the 'plus kind of functional change' in seizure discharges, Jackson referred to 'Horsley's term, an "epileptogenic focus."' So Horsley apparently gets credit for introducing our use of 'focus', but I've not yet found it in his writings. In Jackson 1888e, p.189, footnote 2, Jackson referred to Horsley's term as 'A most excellent name for what I call "discharging lesion" …'

beginning in some part of the mid-cortex [middle level]. In cases of hemiplegia from breaking up of the <u>internal capsule</u> by clot or softening, there is destruction of fibres and also, of course, loss of function.[233]

To the modern neurologist this feels familiar in both conception and terminology. Jackson has acknowledged that a lesion in the striatum causes hemiplegia because it interrupts the fibers of the pyramidal (motor) tract as they pass downward through the internal capsule, where they are surrounded by the gray matter of the striatum.[234] Hence the hemiplegia is due either to damage in the motor (rolandic) cortex or to interruption of its efferent fibers somewhere along their path to the anterior horn cell in the spinal cord. Either way, the inhibitory influence of the upper motor segment on the lower motor neurons is removed. Note that the paper and its discussion were delivered in highly technical terms. License to do this was inherent in the specialized nature of the Neurological Society, whose members shared similar levels of sophistication. Such was not the case for the next paper that we will consider.

'Remarks on the Diagnosis and Treatment of Diseases of the Brain', July 1888

In July 1888 Jackson read this paper to a general medical audience. It was '*Delivered at a Meeting of the Worcestershire and Herefordshire, Bath and Bristol, and Glouctershire [sic] Branches*' of the British Medical Association.[235] In the first of the paper's two installments he dealt with the old nosological issue of empirical versus scientific classifications. The second installment was largely an exercise in applying his tripartite method to his old favorites, hemiplegia and epilepsy, not including aphasia. Withal, there were several themes on which he offered new thoughts. Among them were: (1) 'scientific' nosology based on his three evolutionary levels in the brain; (2) migraine and his non-Baconian deductive method using hypotheses; and (3) application of evolutionary nosology and related hypotheses to epilepsy proper. As usual, he mustered clinical observations and theories from many different subject areas, so these three themes were commingled among themselves and with others. Hence it is not possible to deal with each of them separately. I can only follow them in the order in which he presented them, more or less.

At the outset Jackson equated studying disease 'on the principle of Evolution' with scientific classification. And then he said:

> But I have urged equally strongly that we should not follow this plan for direct practical purposes, but we should for those purposes have empirical arrangements ... of cases by Type. (In no part of this address do I use the term scientific as implying superiority, nor do I ever use the term empirical with its conventional evil connotations.)[236]

---

[233] Jackson 1888a, p.313; my square brackets and underlining.

[234] In 1884 (Jackson 1884d, p.661; my underlining), regarding a case of 'convulsion of the left leg' due to a focus in the right 'middle motor centres', he said, 'the nerve-currents developed must travel ... down the <u>internal capsule</u> into the opposite lateral column of the cord ...'

[235] Jackson 1888c and Jackson 1888d. The meeting's date and venue were not given. The first installment was published on July 14, so probably it would have been delivered approximately 2 weeks earlier.

[236] Jackson 1888c, p.59; Jackson's parentheses. At that time, 'empirical' often connoted quackery.

Jackson's protestation of parity between empirical and scientific classifications seems disingenuous—clearly he was trying to convert the former into the latter. Using 'Type' to refer to empirically classified disease entities, he worried about their profusion: 'Our knowledge of ... diseases by "cases" is becoming so minute ... that ... our empirical arrangements by type almost break down ... these types become so complicated that they almost cease to be typical.'[237] Now, more than a century later, this sounds familiar. For neurology in his time Jackson proposed a classification based on his theory of three evolutionary levels in the brain, and he introduced that idea with some interesting remarks: 'Fully believing that we must continue to study diseases by type, I wish <u>some one with great authority</u> would endeavor to define our types of the "progressive" diseases involving the spinal system more narrowly. I submit a plan which will, I hope, help us to a less empirical arrangement ...'[238]

Now who might be that 'great authority'? There was at least one potential candidate on each side of the Channel. However, by 1888 Charcot was more interested in hysteria, and he was beginning to suffer declining health. The English candidate was William Gowers, whose first volume of *A Manual of Diseases of the Nervous System* was devoted to 'Diseases of the spinal cord and nerves'. It was published in 1886.[239] Jackson's request for a 'great authority' could be an indirect criticism of Gowers, but actually I think it was a broader criticism. Like most other comprehensive texts on neurology, Gowers' classic was arranged by standard anatomical regions, with many types within each region. Systemic entities that didn't fit in any one region had their own sections.[240] But Jackson's idea—'evolutionary nosology'—meant organizing texts according to his three evolutionary levels of the nervous system.

> Were I writing a book on diseases of the nervous system, I should not have in it distinct sections on diseases of the spinal cord, medulla oblongata, and pons Varolii, but one section including diseases of all these parts, the three morphological divisions being considered together as making up one anatomico-physiological unity. This unity I have called the lowest level of evolution of the central nervous system ...[241]

Further along Jackson again suggested that he was thinking about a book.

> I have just been urging that we should take up for particular study cases in their order of simplicity. Were I to write a book I should follow this plan; for the ambitious aim of the work would be to help people in practice to examine for themselves in scientific ways for practical ends. We cannot learn for ourselves if we begin with complex problems; if we do, we shall run the risk of making vague, and often verbal, explanations.[242]

The totality of Jackson's 'Remarks' of 1888 constitutes his assessment of the state of neurology *and* his vision for where it could go, but there was a frustrating limitation.

> The plan suggested – that of studying diseases of the cord and of the other morphological divisions as diseases of the level – cannot be carried out fully, because our

---

[237] Jackson 1888c, p.59.
[238] Jackson 1888c, pp.59; my underlining.
[239] Gowers 1886–1888. Volume II on diseases of the brain was published in 1888.
[240] See e.g. Osler 1892.
[241] Jackson 1888c, pp.59–60. Jackson said that his idea was 'pretty much what Marshall Hall called the true spinal system', but Hall's spinal system was not in the same continuity with the cerebrum, whose localized functions were not known to Hall; see Clarke and Jacyna 1987, p.120.
[242] Jackson 1888c, p.62.

anatomic-physiological knowledge of its elements is not as yet complete. But I hope that ... we shall soon ... have a rational formula ... of the class of diseases to which tabes belongs and a nomenclature corresponding ... analogous to that in chemistry ...[243]

Another threat to Jackson's plan was his perception of widespread ignorance about his classification of the epilepsies. Here, before an audience of general 'medical men', he vented persisting frustration about his two types of 'epilepsy proper'.

We should have two types of this morbid affection. I find, however, that many medical men have but one type – loss of consciousness with severe universal convulsion. But the great thing in the diagnosis of epilepsy is not the 'quantity' of the symptomatology, but paroxysmalness. A sudden transitory loss of consciousness with very little physical manifestation, often enough suffices for the diagnosis of epilepsy. It may be said that there are 'all degrees'[4] of epileptic seizures from slightest to severest.[244]

In footnote 4 Jackson argued against the *necessity* for intermediate evolutionary stages ('all degrees'), i.e., against the idea that evolution must always proceed by 'insensible gradations'. In effect, he was saying that genuine epilepsy was an instance of saltatory change.

[4] The law of continuity – that things increase and decrease by insensible gradations – is ... in many medical matters applied without due thought ... Slight fits of epilepsy ... do not pass into severe fits ... by there occurring fits of ... intermediate degrees between the slightest and most severe ... Increasing evolution is not a process of increase by insensible gradations; there are ... occasional "stoppages," which are "re-beginnings." The division into *le petit mal* and *le grand mal* ... is ... a natural division ... answering to the evolutionary constitution of the nervous system. *Le petit mal* passes suddenly into *le grand mal* when the discharge beginning in some part of the highest centres has become strong enough to overcome the resistance of lower (middle) centres.[245]

Evolutionists have long argued about the pace of the changes that it entails. Are they sudden, or gradual, or both? Here Jackson seems to have preferred the former, but I think it was only in this particular case—about epilepsy proper. In general, he preferred spectra. Discussing migraine and evolution, he said, 'I have seen cases intermediate in type between migraine[,] epileptiform seizures and epilepsy proper ("missing links")'.[246] And more broadly, he said,

Using for the moment the term epilepsy generically, I should class migraine, epilepsy proper, and epileptiform seizures as epilepsies, on the basis that in each there is a "discharging" of some part of the cerebral cortex. Their differences are sufficiently accounted for by the different "seats" of those lesions ...[247]

---

[243] Jackson 1888c, p.60.
[244] Jackson 1888c, pp.60–61.
[245] Jackson 1888c, pp.60–61; Jackson's italics and parentheses.
[246] Jackson 1888c, p.61; Jackson's parentheses, my square brackets.
[247] Jackson 1888c, p.61. Jackson had suggested that migraine is epileptic in Jackson 1874jj, p.519 (see Chapter 8), and in Jackson 1879c, p.33 (see Chapter 9). For a review of the historical relationship between migraine and epilepsy, including Jackson's role, see Eadie 2012a, pp.150–153.

Since the 'seat' of migraine is cortical but otherwise different from genuine or epileptiform seizures, there are three types of epilepsy: 'It may be said that classification of the three different diseases on the basis mentioned is purely hypothetical. It is not so far as epileptiform seizures are concerned, and is … not for the two cases [types] of the variety of epilepsy proper.'[248] Then he interjected a methodological issue, saying that he would be

> … sorry to have it implied … that I repudiate hypotheses in scientific research … The use of hypotheses is the method of science. To suppose that we can make discoveries by the Baconian method is a delusion. No discovery, we are told by good authority, has been made on that method … Huxley [the "good authority"] writes … "Bacon's 'via' has proved hopelessly impracticable, while the 'anticipation of nature' by the invention of hypotheses based on incomplete deductions, which he [Bacon] specially condemns, has proved itself to be … an indispensable, instrument of research."[249]

The second installment of Jackson's 'Remarks' was largely a disquisition on the current state of knowledge about hemiplegia and 'epileptiform' seizures. He invoked his tripartite method, but in the nosological context that he had been discussing, i.e., where the method defines disease entities: 'what we call *a* disease is threefold – anatomical, seat of lesion; physiological, functional nature of lesion; pathological, disorder of the nutritive process …'[250] On that note we move on to Jackson's discussion of a more technical paper by a younger member of his circle.

Discussion of Mercier on 'Inhibition', Published October 1888

Charles Mercier (1852–1919) studied medicine at the London Hospital, 'where he had a brilliant student career', culminating in qualification in 1874.[251] Thus, 'he assimilated very early the doctrines of Herbert Spencer and the personal teaching of Hughlings Jackson'.[252] Osler recalled of Mercier that: 'When last with me [before they both died in 1919] … he … entertained us with stories of his student days and anecdotes of Hughlings Jackson and Jonathan Hutchinson'.[253] In January 1887 Mercier published a paper on 'Coma',[254] which Jackson praised for its dealing with insanity 'realistically and in a very masterly manner'. Further, said Jackson: 'It is a great satisfaction to me to find that Dr. Mercier agrees with me in many of the opinions that I have formed on insanity, considered as dissolution beginning in the highest centres of the cerebral system.'[255] Given Jackson's early influence on Mercier, such praise might seem like giving thanks for the achievement of a self-fulfilling prophecy. However, by 1887 Mercier was on his way to a substantial reputation on his own, so Jackson could well have been proud that his former student still agreed with his views. In Mercier's paper he

---

[248] Jackson 1888c, p.61; my square brackets and underlining.

[249] Jackson 1888c, p.61; my square brackets. The quotation was taken from Huxley 1887, p.325.

[250] Jackson 1888d, p.111; Jackson's italics. See Chapter 3.

[251] Within Mercier 1888, Jackson's comments are on pp.386–393 (which is Jackson 1888f). From the 'Discussion' it is clear that Mercier's paper was presented to a meeting of the Neurological Society, but there is no indication of the date. Much of Mercier's practice and writing involved asylum and legal work.

[252] [Mercier, C.A.] 1919, p.364.

[253] [Mercier, C.A.] 1919, p.365; my square brackets.

[254] Mercier 1887.

[255] Jackson 1887e, pp.34–35; my square brackets. Mercier (1887, p.469) said that his paper on coma was 'inspired by the teachings of Dr. Hughlings-Jackson, who must be credited with whatever of value the article contains'.

... developed a "dynamic" view of function into a general theory that all parts of the nervous system were continuously excitatory and inhibitory. He claimed that "Every nervous centre is at all times subject to continuous control or inhibition; so that while its intrinsic tendency is ever to discharge, this tendency is continuously counteracted by an extrinsic [tendency] which curbs it into quietude."[256]

Mercier's idea of a tendency for nerve cells to discharge spontaneously is generally correct. In recapitulation at the end of his long paper, he submitted eight 'propositions', the ultimate one being that, 'The nerve-centres are arranged in a hierarchy'.[257] Needless to say, Jackson found this to be quite agreeable, but he also used his discussion of Mercier's paper to advance his own ideas about nerve cell discharges in seizures.

... it would be best to use the term "force" as a name for the rate of liberation of energy by ... nervous discharges ... It ... is ... of great importance for our ... interpretation of some of the phenomena of epileptiform and epileptic seizures, and of their after-conditions ... particularly on ranges of convulsion, on sequence of convulsion, and ultimately on the interpretation of certain ... symptoms found when the fits are over (after conditions). It is with regard to the nature of these after-conditions that we are mainly concerned with inhibition ...[258]

This was new. It is the first instance when Jackson emphasized the *rate* of nerve cell discharges as a factor in the sequence and speed of seizure manifestations. To ground his physiological speculations in clinical data, he offered the example of a focal seizure beginning in the thumb. It might spread very little to adjacent body parts, or it could spread widely and even generalize. This was his *entrée* to an analysis of cellular firing rates in the 'primary' focus.

We shall speak of rapid and slow discharges in epileptiform seizures. All discharges producing paroxysms of convulsions are very rapid ... But the abnormally rapid discharges producing convulsion differ in rate ... I do not mean that "nerve impulses," after discharges which produce convulsion, "'travel" faster than those after discharges in health; but that in the former [unhealthy] case more numerous "nerve impulses" are emitted in a given time, or else that [more] cells are simultaneously discharging upon the same part ... in a given time.[259]

So by 'rapid' and 'slow' discharges Jackson was referring to the *frequency* of cellular discharges, not to what we now call axonal conduction velocity, which he asserted to be the same in health and in seizure propagation.[260]

If the primary discharge in a fit be slow [slower rate of firing] ... the "currents["] developed will "flow" more exclusively to that part which is most specially represented

---

[256] R. Smith 1992, p.170; my square brackets. The quoted passage is from Mercier's *The Nervous System and the Mind* (Mercier 1888a, p.76), which was dedicated to Jackson.

[257] Mercier 1888, pp.385–386.

[258] Jackson 1888f, pp.386–387; Jackson's parentheses, my underlining. Here he spoke only of 'nerve cells', without attributing any independent firing to 'fibres'. On Jackson's early conception of 'force' see Chapter 2.

[259] Jackson 1888f, pp.387–388; Jackson's quotation marks, my square brackets and underlining.

[260] Regarding how nerve impulses 'travel', Shepherd (1991, p.196) says: '... during the 1880s and 1890s, it was accepted that in peripheral nerves the nerve impulse is a brief propagating electrical event, and there was a consensus that this must be the main type of activity within and between nerve cells in the central nervous system.'

by the cells of the nervous arrangements of the "discharging lesion" … say, to the thumb only. If the primary discharge be rapid (the same quantity of energy being liberated as in the former case, that of slow discharge), the currents will "flow" also to parts less specially represented by cells of those nervous arrangements, not only to the thumb, but to other digits also; the convulsion will be of greater range [of body parts].[261]

However, 'when a convulsion starting in the thumbs spreads greatly in range … the supposition is that the primary discharge upsets the equilibrium of … *normal* cells … and compels them to "co-operate in its excess" …'[262] This idea about propagation to normal cells was not new, but it was now placed in his conception of 'slow' and 'rapid' conduction, which was also used to explain

… post-paroxysmal states. After epileptiform seizures there is paralysis. I submit that after slow discharges (slight fits long continued and limited in range), the paralysis is very local and decided, and therefore obvious; after rapid discharges (severer shorter fits) it is wide-spread, "diffuse," and therefore easily ignored.[263]

Here again an older idea of Jackson's—diffuse paralysis after generalization of epileptiform seizures—was extended by applying the newer idea (slow and rapid discharges) to it. And it was only logical to make the same extension for epilepsy proper: 'I now apply this generalisation to after-conditions of paroxysms of epilepsy proper … We have to do here with the highest cerebral centres … epileptic paroxysms being owing to "discharging lesions" of small parts of these centres. These after-conditions are, scientifically regarded, cases of insanity …'[264]

My analysis of Jackson's work on insanity will continue into the next chapter, but here I will refer back to the intensity of his professional activities in the later 1880s, as shown in Tables 11.2 and 11.4. There is poignant evidence that they were taking a toll on him. In 1887, or soon after, he enjoyed a bittersweet surprise, recounted many years later by Crichton-Browne.

A Respite in Yorkshire, *circa* 1887

My friend Sir Wemyss Reid told me of a singular experience … after he had … come to London. He went to spend the weekend at Clapham in Yorkshire … There was only one other guest in the hotel … Reid said to his new acquaintance, "Dr. Hughlings Jackson … I should like you to know why I have come to this out-of-the-way place in wintry weather … I spent my honeymoon here many years ago … I married my cousin; it was a very happy marriage. She passed away and I have come here … to revive some old associations." "Incredible!" exclaimed Dr. Hughlings Jackson. "Your case is mine! I spent my honeymoon

---

[261] Jackson 1888f, p.388; Jackson's parentheses, my square brackets.
[262] Jackson 1888f, p.389.
[263] Jackson 1888f, p.389; Jackson's parentheses, my underlining.
[264] Jackson 1888f, p.390; my underlining.

here many years ago … I married my cousin; it was a very happy marriage. She is dead and gone … I have come here out of the stress and anxiety of professional life in London to stir up some dormant emotions."[265]

The respite apparently helped. Jackson was able to continue his professional activities at a strenuous pace into the 1890s.

---

[265] Crichton-Browne 1926, pp.84–85. The journalist and biographer Thomas Wemyss Reid (1842–1905) moved to London from Leeds in 1887; he was knighted in 1894.

12

Last Years

The Dreamy State, the Insanities, Major Lectures, 'Fragments', and Honors, 1888–1911

In his last years Jackson continued to publish almost to the end. Beyond those who he taught personally, his ideas were transmitted to later generations largely through his lectures and publications of the 1880s and 1890s. In this penultimate chapter I will analyze the new elements in the later development of his paradigm. One could say that it was largely mature by 1884, when he delivered his Croonian Lectures on evolution and dissolution of the nervous system. However, at that time the data for localization of the dreamy state were indirect at best. Autopsy evidence began to accumulate in 1886, but at first it was inconclusive. In fact, as early as 1874, when he described the 'cocoa-mixing affair', he was thinking about the 'limited parts of the brain' in which the clinical phenomena originated.[1] His resolution of this problem came about in 1898–1899. It was a contribution that has resonated long after his death in 1911.

Localizing the Dreamy State, Part 1, 1874–1889

In 1888 Jackson defined his criteria and terminology for the semiology of seizures involving the dreamy state.

> There are cases of very slight epileptic fits in which occurs what is commonly called an "intellectual aura;" I call it "dreamy state." One variety of it is the feeling of "reminiscence" … Now if with the "dreamy state" occurring suddenly, there be a "warning" of smell or of taste or a sensation referred to the epigastric region, there is certainly epilepsy; there is always defect of consciousness, but loss of consciousness does not always follow. These seizures are often so slight, so odd, so short, so little incapacitating, and are sometimes, strange to say, positively agreeable, that the patient may disregard them until a severe fit comes to tell him what they mean. Medical men … may not recognise the epileptic nature of these quasi-trifling seizures …[2]

Where Jackson said 'reminiscence' we have long used *déjà vu*,[3] and sometimes he used 'aura' for 'warning', as we do now. Needless to say, he did not achieve this heuristic clarity without

---

[1] Jackson 1874ff, p.410.
[2] Jackson 1888c, p.61.
[3] Critchley and Critchley 1998, p.70, state that Jackson used neither *déjà vu* nor *présque vu* (never seen). In Jackson 1879h, p.142, footnote *b*, about 'Reminiscence', Jackson remarked, 'I use it "without prejudice", as the lawyers say'.

a struggle, which was partly due to the unpredictable availability of autopsy data. To understand his efforts to localize the dreamy state, it is first necessary to review his experiences from 1874 to 1888, beginning with a short contribution by an anonymous author.

The Chronology of Jackson's Encounters with the Dreamy State, 1874–1889

The monthly journal called *The Practitioner* was—and still is—a popular source of reviews for general practitioners. Its issue of May 1874 contained a short piece about 'A prognostic and therapeutic indication in epilepsy. By Quærens [The Seeker]'.[4] It began with quotations from Coleridge, Tennyson, and Dickens, the last of whom described the experience of *déjà vu*.[5] The author said he had recently realized that he had been having episodes of *déjà vu* (not his words) since childhood, but 'Last year I had the misfortune to become … subject to occasional epilepsy'. In 1874, of course, 'epilepsy' meant generalized convulsions. Nonetheless, Quærens said, the lesser phenomenon 'probably ought to be regarded as showing disturbance of brain-function'. He called it 'a minimized form of *petit mal*', thus implying that his *déjà vu* was epileptic, but he was not explicit about it. He simply wanted his readers to understand that *déjà vu* is a warning to rest before it could lead to a generalized seizure.

Given Jackson's predilection to devour the medical press, it would make no sense that he missed this little bombshell in *The Practitioner*. More to the point, when Quærens' piece was published the editor of *The Practitioner* was Francis Anstie, who was brother-in-law to Jackson's close friend Thomas Buzzard.[6] Nonetheless, Jackson has left us nothing about it in print until 1880, when he mentioned 'a medical man, who reports his own case – epileptic attacks beginning by "reminiscence"'.[7] Jackson's restraint may be related to the fact that Quærens became his patient in 1877.[8]

The story of how Jackson ultimately integrated the dreamy state into his localization paradigm is one of fits and starts, with many chronological gaps. Table 12.1 is intended to mitigate those difficulties for 1874–1889. In essence, he was trying to figure out the pathophysiological relationships among: (1) 'crude sensations', such as abnormal odors, tastes, and epigastric sensations; (2) brief 'sensations' like *déjà vu*, with few if any external signs; and (3) elaborate behavioral actions like those in the cocoa affair.

Looking at the events of 1874, we see that Jackson published the cocoa affair 6 months after Quærens' piece in *The Practitioner*. At the time Jackson paid little attention to the cocoa mixer's transient aura of *déjà vu*. He considered it to be separate from the overt behaviors of

---

[4] [Myers] 1874; my square brackets. On *The Practitioner* see Rolleston 1943 and Bynum et al. 1992, p.244. In Jackson 1888e, pp.185–186, Jackson reprinted Quærens' entire narrative of 1874, and on pp.201–207 Jackson published Quærens' notes on his own case up to late 1887.

[5] Lennox and Lennox 1960 (p.275, footnote) were not able to find the passage cited by Quærens, supposedly from *David Copperfield*.

[6] Rolleston 1943, p.323. Anstie died on September 12, 1874, but Quærens' piece had been published in May.

[7] Jackson 1880j, p.199, footnote, where Jackson gives the date of Quærens' piece incorrectly as 1870. Raitiere 2012, p.371, makes the same mistake, perhaps based on Jackson.

[8] In 1898, referring to this patient, Jackson (1898c, p.580) said plainly that he 'first saw the patient, a medical man … in December, 1877'. Taylor and Marsh (1980, p.758) cite the same passage from Jackson and come to the same conclusion about 1877. Dewhurst (1982, pp.91–92) interprets Jackson's (Jackson 1888e, p.185) remark about Quærens 'when he consulted me, Feb.1880' to mean '[first] consulted me', so he concludes that Quærens became Jackson's patient in 1880, but Jackson's latter statement simply meant 'visited me [again]'.

Table 12.1 Chronology of Jackson's encounters with the dreamy state, 1874–1889.

Month/year	Event	Citation
May 1874	Quærens' self-description of *déjà vu*	Quærens 1874
November 1874	'cocoa-mixing affair' (see Chapter 8)	Jackson 1874ff, p.410
November 1876	Coats' case of dreamy state	Coats 1876
December 1876	Jackson's first published use of 'dreamy state'	Jackson 1876u, p.702
December 1876	Jackson cited Coats' case	Jackson 1876u, p.702
December 1877	Quærens became Jackson's patient	Jackson 1898c, p.580
July 1880	Jackson's citation of Ferrier 1876 on mesial temporal localization of taste and smell	Jackson 1880j, p.195
July 1880	Jackson's first citation of Quærens	Jackson 1880j, p.199, footnote
August 1885	Jackson admitted Anderson's case to the London Hospital	Anderson 1886, p.388
March 1886	Autopsy of Anderson's case: giant pituitary tumor impinging left temporal lobe	Anderson 1886, pp.390–392
October 1886	Publication of Anderson's case	Anderson 1886
July 1888	Short discussion of 'dreamy' in 'Remarks'	Jackson 1888c, p.61
July 1888	Jackson cited Anderson 1886 and mentioned case with Beevor	Jackson 1888c, p.61; Jackson 1888e, p.182
July 1888	Review of dreamy state and Jackson's publication of Quærens' notes on himself	Jackson 1888e
October 1888	Comments on Mercier on Inhibition	Jackson 1888f
February 1889	Autopsy of right temporal tumor case presented briefly to Medical Society	Jackson 1889c (with Beevor)
October 1889	Published full autopsy of right temporal tumor case	Jackson 1889k (with Beevor)

the dreamy state. Clinically they are obviously different. The cocoa affair was a case of 'elaborate mental automatism after very slight epileptic discharges',[9] whereas Quærens' aura was sometimes followed by generalized convulsions. In hindsight from 1888, Jackson admitted that in 1874 he had recorded the cocoa patient's *déjà vu* or something like it. But he had 'omitted to state what I found in my notes of this case, that at the onset of his fits the patient had 'a sort of dreamy state coming on suddenly'. I fear I then thought this symptom too indefinite to be worth enquiring into and recording . . .[10]

By contrast, in 1876 Jackson recognized Joseph Coats' 'Case II' as a clear example of the dreamy state. The patient had a peculiar 'thought'—apparently *déjà vu*—before his episodes of elaborate behavior. A month after Coats' publication, which was without autopsy, Jackson cited it when he first used the term 'dreamy state' in print in December 1876.[11] This was also

---

[9] Jackson 1874ff, p.410.

[10] Jackson 1888e, p.188. Regarding the quotation within this quotation (in my single quotation marks; double marks in original) from Jackson's notes of 1874, it is not clear if he was transcribing the patient's words or his own. Either way, it would mark the first time we know that he used 'dreamy state', albeit unpublished at the time.

[11] Jackson 1876u, p.702, citing Coats 1876; see Chapter 8. The Glaswegian Joseph Coats (1846–1899) was a general pathologist with wide interests; he had read Jackson 1875ll and others of Jackson's papers. See [Coats, J.] 1899 (Obituary).

the paper in which Jackson postulated a hierarchy of levels *within* the highest level, thus explaining the dreamy state as release of one of the lower levels among the highest. Coats did not mention this point. He did restate Jackson's theory of three cerebral levels, but without any speculation about localization of the dreamy state.

In the same paper of 1880 where he first mentioned Quærens, Jackson also quoted a passage from Ferrier's *The Functions of the Brain*. As quoted by Jackson, Ferrier had said: As regards taste ... the phenomena occasionally observed in monkeys on irritation of the lower part of the middle temporo-sphenoidal [temporal] convolution, viz. movements of the lips, tongue, and cheek-pouches, may be taken as reflex movements consequent on the excitation of gustatory sensations.'[12]

The next sentence in Ferrier's text, not quoted by Jackson, says: 'The abolition of taste coincided with destruction of regions situated in close relation to the subiculum.' The subiculum is part of the cortex of the hippocampus which is in the deep medial temporal lobe. Ferrier said the 'centres both of smell and taste' are located there.[13] His findings ultimately gave Jackson the clue he needed to localize the dreamy state together with complex behaviors like the cocoa affair. In 1880 he tried to establish left hemisphere dominance for both crude sensations and the dreamy state, but without success.[14] Recognizing the likelihood of failure, he was patently frustrated.

> I doubt not that there is some order [of seizure propagation] throughout, from the warning to the end of the post-paroxysmal stage. The above imperfect sketch, the best I can do, is the result of much labor, as a contribution towards discovering this order. I am far from asserting that I have done anything of value towards this end ...[15]

The First, Inconclusive Autopsies of the Dreamy State, 1886–1889

Jackson's frustration was probably still simmering in 1885, when he encountered the patient reported later *with autopsy* by his younger colleague at the London Hospital, James Anderson (1853–1893).[16] There in the outpatients Anderson met 'G.B., aged 23 years ... [who] was sent to me ... [in] August, 1885, by Mr. Waren Tay, whom he had consulted for loss of vision in his left eye.'[17] The patient was admitted to Jackson's service at the London Hospital on August 27.[18] In Anderson's report there is nothing about Jackson's actual relationship with the patient, but Jackson knew what Anderson was finding.[19]

---

[12] Ferrier 1876, p.189, quoted in Jackson 1880j, p.195; my square brackets.

[13] Ferrier 1876, pp.183–184. There is olfactory representation in the cortical structures that Ferrier was stimulating, and cortical representation of taste is in nearby areas.

[14] Jackson 1880j; summary on p.206.

[15] Jackson 1880j, p.206; my square brackets.

[16] [Anderson 1893] (Obituaries). He became Assistant Physician to Queen Square in 1888.

[17] Anderson 1886, p.385; my square brackets. This is the Waren Tay (1843–1927) of Tay–Sachs disease. He was Surgeon to Moorfields (1877–1904); see Collins 1929, p.218.

[18] Anderson 1886, p.386. As Assistant Physician Anderson had no admitting privileges.

[19] Anderson 1886, p.390, said: 'in writing Dr. Jackson I ventured to say that I believed the tumour would be found in the same position as Mr. Nettleship's ...' The ophthalmological pathologist Edward Nettleship (1845–1913) was a close associate of Hutchinson; see Parsons 1913. His patient with a similar but smaller tumor had sudden 'fits' of 'suffocation in the nose and mouth', but nothing else to suggest the dreamy state.

The full title of Anderson's paper encapsulated its interest for both Anderson and Jackson: 'On sensory epilepsy. A case of basal cerebral tumour, affecting the left temporo-sphenoidal lobe, and giving rise to a paroxysmal taste-sensation and dreamy state'. In this context, 'sensory' included (1) auras of abnormal smells and/or tastes, (2) *déjà vu* ('childish' scenes), and (3) sensory marches involving the right arm, right shoulder, and back of the head.[20] Before the autopsy Anderson summarized his clinical conclusions.

> The ocular symptoms in this case pointed definitely to a basal tumour pressing on the left optic nerve in the first place ... I believed also, from my acquaintance with Dr. Hughlings-Jackson's observations, that the paroxysmal taste-sensation and dreamy state, &c., justified the diagnosis that this tumour in some way ... involved the left temporo-sphenoidal [temporal] lobe ... in the region of Ferrier's centre for taste (possibly also his centre for smell), and in neighbouring highest centres.[21]

The patient died on March 6, 1886. At autopsy by Anderson his clinical conclusions were confirmed. In the basal view an enormous mass extended from beneath the posterior frontal areas to impinge the left medial temporal lobe, and to a lesser extent the right. When the tumor was removed its origin in the pituitary gland was obvious, but 'the most important bearing of the case is on the doctrines as to the localization of cerebral function'.

> From the position and relations of the pituitary body, it is clear that the first part of the cortex involved by the tumour would be the anterior part of the inner border of the temporo-sphenoidal lobe – in other words, the area in which Ferrier has had grounds for locating the centres of taste and smell, at the tip of the gyrus uncinatus. Producing by pressure an instability in the grey matter of this area, I believe that the tumour was the cause of the paroxysmal taste-sensations which commenced the attack, and that from this point the discharge spread to neighbouring centres.
>
> Dr. Hughlings-Jackson has observed and noted, although not published, numerous cases of paroxysmal sensation, combined with dreamy state ...[22]

So, in Jackson's total experience, Anderson's case of 1886 was the first to be autopsied. Unfortunately, its localizing value was limited by the tumor's massive size. In July 1888 Jackson again cited Anderson's case, and he gave preliminary notice about a second one with autopsy.

> As yet there have been but two necropsies ... of patients who have been subject to such fits ... The only one published ... is recorded by Dr. James Anderson (taste warning and "dreamy state") ... another observed by myself and Dr. Beevor (warning of smell and "dreamy state"), has not yet been published; in each, tumour in the temporo-sphenoidal lobe was found. It is by ... cases of gross local organic disease, and by the investigations of Ferrier, that we shall ultimately be able to consider all "varieties" of epilepsy ... as each points to a "discharging lesion" of this or that part of the cerebral cortex.[23]

---

[20] Anderson 1886, pp.385–386.

[21] Anderson 1886, p.389; Anderson's parentheses, my square brackets.

[22] Anderson 1886, pp.394–395; my underlining. The uncinate gyrus (uncus) is cortex in the most medial part of each temporal lobe.

[23] Jackson 1888c, p.61; Jackson's parentheses. He also gave preliminary notice of his case with Beevor in Jackson 1888e, p.179, footnote 1.

Also in July 1888 Jackson said, 'I have notes of about fifty cases of the variety of Epilepsy I am about to speak of'. And he went on to describe, 'A particular variety of epilepsy ("intellectual aura"), one case with symptoms of organic brain disease'. He explained that he had diagnosed many autopsy-proven intracranial tumors,

> But one of the cases … is the only one I have seen in my own practice in which this variety of epilepsy ["intellectual aura"] was … associated with marked symptoms of local gross organic brain disease … necropsy was forbidden … the so-called "intellectual aura" … is a striking symptom … Along with this voluminous mental state, there is frequently a "crude sensation" ("warning") of (a) smell or (b) taste … or (c) the "epigastric" or some other "systemic" sensation … the "dreamy state" sometimes occurs without any of the crude sensations mentioned … and … sometimes those crude sensations and movements occur without the "dreamy state" … [24]

To localize the dreamy state Jackson needed to find autopsied cases who also had crude sensations *and* well-defined, single lesions clearly associated with crude sensations. That set of events would correlate with his physiological conception.

> … I do not consider the "dreamy state" to be a "warning" ("aura") … [it is] not … of the same order as the crude sensations of smell, &c. Hence my objection to the term "intellectual aura," and adoption of the less question-begging adjective "dreamy" … It is very important … to distinguish mental states according to their degree of elaborateness … in order that we may infer the … [localization] proper to each. The crude sensations are properly called warnings; they occur during *epileptic* … discharges; the elaborate state I call "dreamy state" arises during … slightly increased discharges … of healthy nervous arrangements. [25]

The conceptual statement is in the last sentence. That is, if the dreamy state is only a release phenomenon it would not have its own epileptic focus. The relevant localization would be the focus of the crude sensation whose malfunction released the dreamy state. This appears to confirm the idea that *déjà vu* and elaborate behaviors are parts of the same spectrum, although Jackson did not say it that way. For him *déjà vu* and more complex dreamy states, such as the cocoa affair, are similar because of their quasi-cognitive qualities, as distinct from 'crude' sensations, which should be easier to localize.

At the Medical Society of London in February 1889 Jackson and Beevor presented a detailed report of the autopsied tumor case they had mentioned briefly in July 1888.[26] The patient was a cook who experienced 'a very horrid smell', and 'she saw a strange little black woman flitting about the kitchen'.[27] Her case appeared to meet the requisite criteria, except that her tumor, although smaller than Anderson's, was still too large and infiltrative to allow precise localization.

> … the right temporo-sphenoidal lobe was the seat at its most anterior extremity of a tumour of the size of a tangerine orange. The growth was seen to involve the extreme tip of

---

[24] Jackson 1888e, pp.179–180; Jackson's parentheses, my square brackets.
[25] Jackson 1888e, pp.180–181; Jackson's parentheses and italics, my square brackets.
[26] Jackson 1889c and Jackson 1889k. The earlier mentions were in Jackson 1888c, p.61, and in Jackson 1888e, p.179, footnote 1; see above in this chapter.
[27] Jackson 1889c, p.381.

the temporo-sphenoidal lobe, and especially the part of it which is in front of the uncus of the hippocampal or uncinate convolution, and which contains the structure known as the nucleus amygdalæ.[28]

This was still not fully definitive, but it pointed toward that happy state. In effect, Jackson and his colleagues were steadily removing more and more kinds of epileptic phenomena from the murky status of 'neuroses', but the term was still applied to genuine epilepsy.

Epilepsy Among the Neuroses in the 1880s

A medical dictionary of 1890 defined 'neurosis' simply as 'A nervous disease, more especially one in which no definite lesions are found'.[29] In the same year Jackson said: 'I now use the term epilepsy for that <u>neurosis</u>, which is often called "genuine" or "ordinary" epilepsy, and for that [kind] only'.[30] About the absence of pathology for the neuroses, he said:

> ... it is quite a legitimate hypothesis that the neuroses are nervous diseases in the sense that nervous elements are primarily in fault. But as we *know* nothing of their pathology, it is an hypothesis only. It is equally legitimate for me to put forward another hypothesis as to one of them – epilepsy proper. That hypothesis is that, in most cases of this disease, the pathology is primarily arterial ... and only secondarily nervous ... it is plugging of small cerebral arteries ...[31]

Despite the seeming commonality of the term 'neurosis' for both epilepsy proper and insanity, Jackson denied that they have a common etiology—and he did it with an expression that is more puzzling than illuminating.

> It follows from the hypothesis I hold as to the physiology and pathology of epilepsy that I do not entertain the hypothesis ... that there is *any relation of community of character* between epilepsy proper and insanity. There is, I think, no such relation between the pathological and physiological state of the brain in epilepsy and the pathological and physiological state of it in insanity. There is *a relation of sequence* often enough; not rarely there is temporary mania after a fit, and sometimes chronic mental failure occurs in epileptics ...[32]

I think '*community of character*' meant common pathophysiology, and '*relation of sequence*' referred to similarity of clinical presentation. Jackson's statement about the respective etiologies of epilepsy and insanity clearly separated the two categories of disease. In the paragraph before the above he described the discharging lesion in the highest centers as a 'hyperphysiological parasite', so I conclude that he kept epilepsy detached from insanity because there is no discharging focus to explain 'ordinary', non-epileptic insanity.

---

[28] Jackson 1889k, p.350. In the histological terminology of that time her tumor was called 'a small round celled sarcoma' (Jackson 1889k, p.351). It was likely a malignant glioma. The 'microscopic examination' was done by 'Dr. [Walter S.] Colman [1864–1934], the resident medical officer to the [National] hospital'. On the multiple duties of the resident house physician see Holmes 1954, pp.42–43; and Shorvon et al. 2019, pp.108–109.

[29] Billings 1890, vol.2, p.210.

[30] Jackson 1890c, p.704, footnote 5; my square brackets and underlining.

[31] Jackson 1888d, p.115; Jackson's italics. We do now attribute some epileptic seizures to strokes.

[32] Jackson 1888d, p.116; Jackson's italics.

Three Major Lectures, February 1888–March 1890

Table 11.4 lists eight titles that constituted Jackson's major papers in 1888–1890. Among those eight, five were limited to specific topics, and they have already been discussed. The remaining three presented large parts of Jackson's entire paradigm. They will now be taken up in the order of their public presentations.

An Address at the Medico-Psychological Association, London, on Postictal and Other Insanities, February 1888, Published October 1888 and January 1889

On February 24, 1888, Jackson read an invited paper 'On Post-Epileptic States' at 'The Quarterly Meeting of the Medico-Psychological Association ... at Bethlem Hospital'.[33] Apparently it was quite a *tour de force*, because the President of the Association started the discussion by remarking that

> ... a study of such complexity and elaborateness ... was calculated almost to take away one's power of expression if not power of thought. He must profess himself quite incapable of offering criticism ... but this did not preclude him from saying ... how gratified he was that Dr. Hughlings Jackson had consented to read it.[34]

An expanded version of the paper was published in two installments in the Association's *Journal of Mental Science*.[35] Jackson intended his comparative contribution to be a model for analysis of ordinary insanity, which others might use in their efforts to understand it scientifically. Such efforts were sorely needed. Looking back at some nosological conceptions of insanity at that time, they were rather a hodgepodge. Daniel Hack Tuke's famous *Dictionary of Psychological Medicine* (1892) has a full-page 'Definition of Insanity', which reaches no succinct conclusion.[36] Concerning the 'Forms of Insanity', Charles Mercier said perceptively:

> The number of different classifications of insanity is the same as the number of writers on the subject ... Most of these classifications are founded upon a general principle, but it has not been found possible to apply any one principle uniformly throughout. At some point it fails, and another principle has to be brought in; so that the classification comprises, as separate and mutually exclusive, such groups as Mania, Epileptic Insanity, General Paralysis of the Insane, Puerperal Insanity, Dementia, Idiocy, &c.[37]

[33] Jackson 1888b; Jackson's audience was about 50 people (p.145). The Association is now the Royal College of Psychiatrists; see Howells 1991, Renvoise 1991, and Bewley 2008, pp.23–40.
[34] Jackson 1888b, p.145. The President was a Yorkshireman, Frederick Needham (1836–1924). He was a progressive medical superintendent successively at York Hospital for the Insane (Bootham Park) and at Barnwood House, Hospital for the Insane, Gloucester. See [Needham, Sir Frederick] (Obituaries). Most of the discussion was about criminal responsibility.
[35] Jackson 1888g and Jackson 1889a. Jackson (Jackson 1888g, p.349, footnote) said this was 'an expansion' of his actual address. In the footnote he again acknowledged Spencer, and he recommended [John] 'Fiske's very valuable book, "Cosmic Philosophy"' of 1874.
[36] Tuke 1892, vol.1, pp.330–331; On Tuke's *Dictionary* see Bynum 1991.
[37] Mercier 1890, p.283. By 1890 he was much involved in asylum work.

Box 12.1 Section headings extracted from '*On Post-Epileptic States: A Contribution to the Comparative Study of Insanities*', October (1888g) and January (1889a).

    I.   *Difficulties of the Subject.*

    II. *Need of Psychological Knowledge.*

    III. *Remarks on the Anatomy, Physiology, and Pathology of Diseases of the Nervous System – the three Elements of a Clinical Problem.*

    IV. *On the Duplex Condition of Nervous Symptomatologies – Positive and Negative Elements in Symptomatologies.*

    V. *The Three Levels of Evolution of the Central Nervous System. Evolutionary Differences between the Lowest and Highest Levels. Movements v. Muscles. Positive and Negative Movements.*

    VI. *On Degrees of Detachment and Degrees of Independence of Levels of Evolution.*

    VII. *Evolution of the Physical Basis of Consciousness.*

    VIII. *Need of Wide Clinical Knowledge.*

    IX. *Limitation of the Inquiry into Mental Disorders of Epileptics.*

    X. *Degrees of Post-Epileptic States.*

    XI. *Three Depths of Dissolution: Shallows of Evolution Corresponding.*

    XII. *The Comparative Study of Insanities.*

    XIII. *On the Significance of Positive Mental Symptoms*[a]

---

[a] At the end of Jackson 1889a, p.500, it says '(*To be continued.*)', but it wasn't. Taylor, in Jackson 1931, vol.1, p.384, also notes this shortfall.

Given Mercier's relationship with Jackson, we might expect that his 'one principle' would be evolution/dissolution, but apparently he found it insufficient. This would actually be consistent with Jackson's view of his own efforts. He wasn't dealing with mental disease *per se*. In 1881 he had denied that he had 'put forward the Hypothesis of Dissolution as a basis for classification of cases of Insanity <u>for clinical purposes</u> …' He had refused a request to go to an asylum and show the alienists how to classify their patients' disorders.[38] In effect, for *scientific* analysis Jackson was saying to the alienists: 'Here's how I have approached my problems. You're welcome to copy my method to address your problems, but I can't tell you exactly how to do that.' What he did offer was the idea of three evolutionary levels. In Box 12.1 we see that what he submitted was a review of his nearly mature paradigm.

At the beginning Jackson laid out his problem with the '*Difficulties of the Subject*'.

> I find that I have not made my opinions as to the nature of Post-Epileptic States clear to many of my medical brethren … as the subject involves consideration of Psychology, the Anatomy and Physiology of the Nervous System, and Clinical Medicine, it is not easily presented in a simple way. It would be an absurdity to attempt to simplify it by ignoring its difficulties …[39]

The first difficulty was: 'The confusion of the Anatomy and Physiology of the Nervous System … with Psychology [which] is the bane both of Neurology and Psychology. It leads to superficial simplifications, and to crude popular "explanations", most of which are merely

---

[38] Jackson 1881h, p.329; my underlining. See Chapter 10, footnote 109.
[39] Jackson 1888g, p.349.

verbal.'[40] The antidote for this affliction was concomitance. The comparison that Jackson proposed was between the neurological basis of cerebration on the physical side and the psychological basis of mentation on the other. Relishing the opportunity to deal with the difficulties, he launched into his comparative neurological approach to 'the most difficult of all diseases – insanity ...' About the sensori-motor composition of the entire neuraxis, he said:

> ... I urge that unless the comparison and contrast ... be between *paralysis* resulting from the negative lesion of the highest centres, *signified by the loss of consciousness*, and the paralysis resulting from the negative lesion in the case of hemiplegia, we do not really enter upon the proper Comparative Study of the two Dissolutions ...
>
> It is one of the chief aims of this Address to show that a negative lesion of the highest centres (implied by the negative affection of consciousness which exists in every case of insanity) causes some paralysis, sensory or motor, or both.[41]

Once again it is difficult to know which side of concomitance Jackson was assuming at any particular moment. In the above passage I think he was implying that, given the effect on consciousness of negative lesions (hemiplegia) in the middle cerebral level, there must be corresponding negative effects in a hypothetical, middle psychological level. However, he never said this plainly, apparently because he felt some constraint on how far he could push the comparison to the middle level. Later in the paper he cautioned:

> ... I must speak here in detail of the evolutionary differences of the Lowest and Highest Levels of the central nervous system. I neglect the Middle Level ... one reason being that, so far as I know, no one agrees with me in dividing the brain proper into Middle and Highest Centres. But I take it for granted that at least two levels of the central nervous system will be admitted by all.[42]

Here Jackson remained on the neurological side of concomitance. With or without the middle level, he defended and extended his thoughts about the highest centers.

> I have never held the hypothesis that any part of the cerebral cortex is either purely sensory or purely motor ... I suppose that in the fore part of the prefrontal lobes sensory representation is [at] a vanishing point, and that motor representation in the occipital lobes is [at] a vanishing point. Hence I consider that from a negative lesion of any part of the cortex there is both sensory and motory [*sic*] paralysis, although the proportions of the two may be enormously different in differently seated lesions.
>
> On the basis that all centres are sensori-motor the *Comparative Study of Insanities* with diseases of lower centres can be instituted.[43]

---

[40] Jackson 1888g, pp.349–350; my square brackets. Jackson's usage of 'Psychology' seems to include psychiatry. The dictionary definitions of 'psychology' and 'psychiatry' were largely the same as ours—study and treatment respectively—but not as terms for professions; see Billings 1890, vol.2, p.403.

[41] Jackson 1888g, pp.351–352; Jackson's italics and parentheses.

[42] Jackson 1888g, p.360.

[43] Jackson 1888g, p.352, my square brackets and underlining.

Regardless of how many levels may be postulated, the principles of representation are the same in all motor and sensory centers.

> … motor nervous centres represent movements of muscles, not … muscles in their individual character. The simplest movement is not the arithmetical sum of the contractions of all the muscles engaged in effecting it; it is the algebraicle [*sic*] sum of the co-operating and antagonizing contractions of those muscles. (The same, *mutatis mutandis*, for sensory centres and impressions.) Paralysis from negative lesions of motor nervous centres is always loss of movements.
>   There are differences of evolutionary rank of movements of the same muscles.[44]

By 'arithmetical sum' Jackson meant only simple addition, whereas 'algebraicle sum' meant the summation of positive and negative (inhibitory) signals. Although he had not previously expressed the idea of an 'evolutionary rank of movements', it follows from his hierarchical view of the nervous system. That is, the same muscles can be directed by different levels of the nervous system to participate in the same or different movements, so what matters is the organization of the movements, not the individual muscles or their combinations into particular movements. He admitted that most of his narrative was concerned with the highest level, but in a footnote he offered an interesting speculation about integration among the lowest.

> In another article I shall try to show that in the fore part of the Lowest Level there is a rudimentary highest centre; I mean a centre co-ordinating all parts of this lowly evolved level in a simple way. This hypothetical highest centre will be very rudimentary in man. One would suppose that the amphioxus must have such a centre to give some degree of unity to its simple self.[45]

Moving on to the second installment of Jackson's paper '*On Post-Epileptic States*', in his opening section on '*Need of Wide Clinical Knowledge*' he went back to one of the difficulties that he had discussed at the beginning.

> For the scientific study of insanities a very wide clinical knowledge is necessary. It would never do to confine attention to cases described in text-books by Alienist Physicians, to what I may call "orthodox" cases of insanity … Not being an Alienist Physician … I should not presume to address … [them] on their special subject had I not the hope that from a long study of simpler diseases of the Nervous System, I might contribute something of at least indirect value for the elucidation of the most complex problems they have to deal with.[46]

This was his real proposal to the psychiatrists—with emphasis on 'indirect'. He would explain his ideas about the behavioral phenomena in epileptics, especially in the postictal state, so they could compare that to their observations of the mentally ill. In the course of his explanation he brought up some new points about epilepsy. Concerning the pathophysiology of the dreamy state he lamented, 'I may here express my surprise that I have not succeeded in making evident that my belief is that elaborate actions during unconsciousness in Epileptics occur after paroxysms.'[47] However, 'I believe I may assume that the majority of Alienist

---

[44] Jackson 1888g, p.359; Jackson's italics and parentheses, my square brackets.
[45] Jackson 1888g, p.361. Amphioxi are fish-like pre-vertebrates.
[46] Jackson 1889a, p.490; my square brackets and underlining.
[47] Jackson 1889a, p.493.

physicians admit that *suddenly* occurring *temporary* abnormal elaborate actions during un-consciousness in Epileptics ... are in most instances preceded by a fit, although not, as my hypothesis is, in all instances ...[48]

That said, Jackson proceeded to elaborate on '*Degrees of Post-Epileptic States*' and their correlative '*Three Depths of Dissolution: Shallows of Evolution Corresponding*'. That is, the '*Shallows*' were what was left to the patients in '*Post-Epileptic States*'. He had discussed those ideas in 1881,[49] but his discussion here in 1889 included a footnote with an interesting re-mark: 'In former papers ... I have spoken of what is known as the Intellectual Aura (I call it "dreamy state") as being the positive element in some cases of the first degree of post-epileptic states ... I now feel <u>uncertain</u> as to the exact <u>symptomatological nature</u> of the "dreamy state." '[50] Since 'symptomatology' meant the same thing then as now,[51] it would ap-pear that Jackson was not happy with his understanding of which symptoms would con-stitute a diagnosis of 'dreamy state'. What was causing his uncertainty was not evident in the rest of his paper. For the present I can only remain alert to its possibilities and go on to another Jacksonian footnote. At the end of his section on '*Three Depths of Dissolution*', he remarked: 'We are at present neglecting the important fact that post-epileptic Dissolution is ... Compound.*' And in the footnote he said:

> * ... Evolution and Dissolution ... are processes, respectively, of increase and decrease in Compound Order. I have long been possessed by this notion ...[52] It may be that in the sen-sory sphere Compound Order is analogous to Weber's Law ... An increase of the strength of a nervous discharge produces a compound effect. This applies to normal and abnormal discharges of sensory and of motor elements. The principle is exceedingly important with regard to differences in the physical processes during faint and vivid states of object con-sciousness, ideation and perception for example.[53]

In the penultimate section of Jackson's paper he gave some methodological suggestions for implementing '*The Comparative Study of Insanities*':

> ... by regarding all "Mental Diseases" ... as Dissolutions beginning in the highest (cerebral) centres of a great sensori-motor mechanism. Such a study is of three kinds.
>
> (1) We may consider different kinds of insanity in comparison and contrast to one an-other ... as they are physically owing to Dissolutions beginning ... in different divisions of the highest centres ... we might compare and contrast cases of melancholia with cases of general paralysis; hypothetically in the former there is Dissolution beginning in the pos-terior, in the latter beginning in the anterior lobes of the cerebrum.
>
> (2) We may compare and contrast different degrees of the same kind of insanity ... as each is a different depth of Dissolution of the same division of the highest centres ...
>
> (3) We may consider insanities (as they are diseases of the highest centres) in comparison and contrast with diseases of lower centres, with aphasia and hemiplegia, for example.[54]

---

[48] Jackson 1889a, p.493; Jackson's italics.
[49] Jackson 1881b; see Chapter 10.
[50] Jackson 1889a, p.494; my underlining. He cited 'April, 1887', which was Jackson 1887e.
[51] See Billings 1890, vol.2, p.632: 'The science of symptoms. Diagnosis, semeiology.'
[52] Here he referred back to Jackson 1868v, where he had stated 'details of the sequence of spasm in a case of epileptiform fits'. See Chapter 5 and Table 5.1.
[53] Jackson 1889a, p.496. Weber's Law is a fundamental of modern psychophysics.
[54] Jackson 1889a, p.496; Jackson's parentheses.

Here it appears that Jackson's advice to the psychiatrists was given entirely on the physical side of concomitance, and that is confirmed in his next paragraph.

> The comparisons and contrasts we mean are (1) of the *physical* conditions of different insanities with one another; (2) of degrees of the *physical* conditions of the same kind of insanity, and (3) of the *physical* conditions in insanities with those which are lesions of lower centres.[55]

This '*physical*' offering to the psychiatrists was consistent with Jackson's promise to avoid telling them how to conduct their practices, but at the same time it put his advice at a remove from their practicalities. What was not stated was his assumption that on the mental side of concomitance there will be parallel correlates to the physical side. Although he had always denied any interaction between the two, it is tempting to see here an immanence of interaction. Presumably his explanation would be that he was simply offering an analogy.

In his final section, '*On the Significance of Positive Mental Symptoms*', Jackson slid past an old ambiguity, perhaps intentionally: 'the negative symptoms of a patient's insanity alone answer to it. Positive Mental symptoms in all cases of insanity answer to activities of healthy nervous arrangements on the level of evolution remaining.'[56] The ambiguity is in the seemingly simple verb 'answer to'. It contains and conceals the Cartesian dilemma, including concomitance.[57] On that note we go on to another lecture later in the same year.

The Address in Medicine at the BMA, Leeds, 'On the Comparative Study of Diseases of the Nervous System', Presented and Published August 1889[58]

The British Medical Association (BMA) was founded in 1832 as the Provincial Medical and Surgical Association. Its name declared part of its original purpose—to be a counterweight to the concentration of medical power in London and Oxbridge. The BMA has long advocated for the interests of the general practitioners.[59] The now-prestigious *British Medical Journal* (*BMJ*), founded in 1832–1840, is its official organ.[60] We don't know when Jackson joined, but we do know that he first presented a published paper at the annual meeting in Plymouth in August 1871, and he gave other presentations occasionally over the years.[61] The BMA's Address in Medicine was a distinct honor, which he appreciated and acknowledged.[62] The fact that the meeting was held in Leeds (West Yorkshire) was doubtless an added incentive to his participation—he liked to go home.

---

[55] Jackson 1889a, pp.496–497; Jackson's italics.

[56] Jackson 1889a, p.497; my underlining.

[57] Jackson 1889a, p.498. A little later Jackson ignored the mind-brain conundrum when he made a pithy remark that we would call a reality check: 'although we speak … of defect of consciousness as if it were a something, it is a nothing; it is so much consciousness eliminated, got rid of'.

[58] Jackson 1889d (*BMJ*), which I have used mainly; also published as an 'Abstract' in *The Lancet* (Jackson 1889e) and in the New York *Medical Record* (Jackson 1889g).

[59] See Little [1933], pp.1–40; and more succinctly: Porter 1997, p.354.

[60] See Bartrip 1990, pp.1, 6–12; and Chapter 9.

[61] Jackson 1871g. Other BMA presentations are found in Jackson 1873p, Jackson 1882c, and Jackson 1882d, including his paper at the provincial branches in July 1888 (Jackson 1888c, Jackson 1888d; see Chapter 11).

[62] In his opening acknowledgements Jackson referred to 'this great Medical Association'. His use of the adjective 'great' in this context was unusual.

The main theme of Jackson's Address is given in his title, 'On the comparative study of diseases of the nervous system'. The bases of the comparisons, of course, were evolution and dissolution. At the outset he emphasized the importance of having 'general doctrines bearing on the science of medicine'. The need for such doctrines, he said, arises from the reality that: 'We have multitudes of facts, but we require, as they accumulate, organisations of them into higher knowledge; we require generalisations and working hypotheses.'[63] He had sounded this theme in July 1888.[64] What he added here was a personal *apologia*.

> The man who puts two old facts in new and more realistic order deserves praise as certainly as does the man who discovers a new one. There is an originality of method. Gaskell has found out much that is new in his recent well-known researches on the nervous system; but I imagine that the greatest merit of his work is that he has made fruitful generalisations, and has set many things long ill assorted in realistic order.[65]

The impression that Jackson recognized himself in this passage is hard to resist. On another aspect of his thought, moreover, he was quite explicit. After briefly mentioning aphasia and 'word-blindness'(alexia), which can involve issues about mentation and intelligence, he explained his views on race and intelligence in evolutionary terms, trying to be objective about 'the evolutionist's measure of mind'.

> Opinions will differ vastly as to who are the men of greatest mental elevation. Some would put Napoleons highest, others Shakespeares and Goethes. But evolution … supplies us with a scientific measure, which ignores superior and inferior … This measure is according to the intellectual and emotional differences between lower and higher races of mankind, and those between children and adults. Higher races of men and adults have the latest acquired faculties, and these, according to Spencer, are, intellectually, the power of abstract reasoning, and emotionally, the sentiment of justice. So that, instead of saying that a person is superior or inferior to most other men, we may say that he has more or less of the latest faculties of the race than most other men … I by no means think that to have the latest intellectual faculties most highly developed is the same thing as being most endowed intellectually … the poet inherits in some ways more of the earlier acquired faculties of the race, and has less of the latest than the scientific man … yet no one would say that poets are mentally inferior to scientific men.[66]

For his time and place Jackson was relatively liberal on the race/intelligence issue, trying to see the value in all (male) men. Still, he was an upper middle class, English Victorian. In other respects, there were persisting cultural attitudes that he sensed to be inimical to his work.

> I carry the doctrine of sensori-motor constitution of the nervous system further than anyone else … no one denies that very many, if not all, parts of the body are represented sensorily in the "organ of mind." But to their representation <u>motorily</u> in that organ there seems to be great objection. It is not many years since the ascription of motor representation of

---

[63] Jackson 1889d, p.355.
[64] Jackson 1888c, 1888d; see Chapter 11.
[65] Jackson 1889d, p.355. On the physiologist Walter H. Gaskell see Chapter 11.
[66] Jackson 1889d, p.357.

any part of the cerebrum proper was denied. It is agreed upon now that some convolutions (Rolandic region) contain motor elements – and, according to some, nothing else. The præ-frontal lobes ... are said to be ... the "mental centres" ... Ferrier, who agrees with me in thinking that these lobes are motor, finds that, after their ablation in monkeys, there is degeneration of fibres "descending" as low as the medulla oblongata ... this is proof positive that the præ-frontal lobes are, at least to some extent, motor.[67]

It was critical for Jackson to keep trying to establish the presence of motor functions in the prefrontal lobes, because he expected that some cases of generalized epilepsy would eventually be localized there. The clinical phenomena of *petit mal* served his argument as one kind of generalized seizure. In it 'the effects are ... crude, but this does not invalidate them as witnesses to the representation of parts of the body in the highest cerebral centres ... the "epileptic discharge" differs from normal discharges in being sudden, excessive, and rapid; and also ... in starting in some small part of the highest centres ...'[68]

In addition to his colleagues' resistance to motor functions in the highest centers, they still needed to be persuaded that the cerebral cortices are not organized into 'abruptly demarcated centres'. Referring to his Croonian Lecture of March 1884, he said:

... I then spoke of centres for Will, Memory, Reason, and Emotion, the artificially distinguished elements of consciousness. It was a mere artifice to imagine such centres. The evolutionist does not try to localise volition or any other mental faculty in the brain ... there are not in the cortex-cerebri any <u>abruptly demarcated centres</u> for any kind of representation. The recent researches of Beevor and Horsley on the mid-cortex seem to me to show that the current hypothesis as to localization is untenable.[69]

Here 'the current hypothesis' meant 'abruptly demarcated centres', which was Ferrier's tendency. Beevor and Horsley had agreed with Jackson when they concluded 'That there is no *absolute* line of demarcation between the area of localisation in the cortex of one movement and that of another; each movement having a centre of maximum representation, this <u>gradually shading off</u> into the surrounding cortex'.[70]

In Jackson's Address his clinically based, careful reasoning attracted another admiring editorial in the *BMJ*. Presumably it was written by the editor, Ernest Hart, who was a Jackson *aficionado*.[71] The editorial's title was 'The evolutionary theory in modern medicine', but it would have been more accurately 'The *Jacksonian* evolutionary theory *and method* in modern medicine'. The first two sentences set the tone: 'The Address in Medicine ... displays in a high degree both the profundity of thought and the intricacy of expression which are characteristic of its author. The peculiarity of Dr. Hughlings Jackson's work has always been its aim ... not so much to collect and register facts, as to elucidate them by organizing them into knowledge'.[72]

The substance of the editorial in the *BMJ* picked up on Jackson's earlier statement about 'The man who puts two old facts in new and more realistic order ...'[73] It gave a good

---

[67] Jackson 1889d, pp.357–358; my underlining. Further on he said: 'I fear the doctrine of sensori-motor constitution of the "mental centres" will be a hard one to many of my medical brethren.'

[68] Jackson 1889d, p.358; Jackson's internal quotation marks.

[69] Jackson 1889d, p.359, footnote 16; my underlining. He was referring back to Jackson 1884g.

[70] Beevor and Horsley 1887, p.166; Jackson's italics, my underlining.

[71] [Jackson, J.H.] 1889. On Hart see Chapters 9 and 10; his earlier editorial was Jackson 1882f.

[72] [Jackson, J.H.] 1889, p.385.

[73] Jackson 1889d, p.355.

summary of Jackson's method, including the remark that: 'The principle by virtue of which Dr. Hughlings Jackson performs his most remarkable feats of grouping superficially-unlike things, and the one which underlies all his explanations, is the principle of evolution.' In conclusion the editorial said that as a result of his great 'clinical industry' Jackson had achieved 'results which have won for him the universal admiration of his contemporaries, and will command the admiration of posterity'.[74] There will be more to say about posterity in Chapter 13. For now we go on to Jackson's Lumleian Lectures, 1890.

'On Convulsive Seizures', the Lumleian Lectures at the Royal College of Physicians, March 1890, Published March–April 1890

The Lumleian Lectures began in the sixteenth century as a continuing tenure.[75] When William Harvey (1578–1657) published *De Motu Cordis* in 1628 he had held the Lumleian lectureship since 1615.[76] In the nineteenth century the College sponsored four lecture-ships, all with more limited tenures. Jackson had already given the Gulstonian (1869) and the Croonian (1884), and now he was about to deliver the Lumleian in 1890.[77] His three Lumleians were given in March–April 1890. In his title, '*Convulsive*' was essentially a synonym for 'motor'. Thus his Lumleians can be considered largely definitive for his mature ideas about the motor aspects of epilepsy, but not for more than that—better information about the dreamy state was still to come.

Lumleian Lecture I

The main theme of Jackson's first Lumleian was his conception of three levels in the brain and the different clinical manifestations of seizures that originate from each level. At the outset he stated what he meant by 'nervous discharge'.

> Convulsions and other paroxysms are owing to (1) sudden, (2) excessive, and (3) tem-porary nervous discharges … The term "nervous discharge" (used before me by Spencer) has been much objected to; when I say that it is used synonymously with "liberation of energy by nervous elements," it will mislead no one. There are nervous discharges in all the operations of health.[78]

From there he again defined his three levels, because, he said, abnormal discharges can occur in any level: 'I speak briefly of what I suppose to be the hierarchy of centres of the nervous system as a basis for the classification of fits.'[79] Most of his descriptions of the levels and their susceptibilities to seizures were of long standing, but along the way he clarified some details.

---

[74] [Jackson, J.H.] 1889, p.386.

[75] See Clark 1964, p.150: 'In February 1581/2 the College accepted a gift of £40 a year offered by Lord Lumley and … Richard Caldwell for the stipend of a lecturer on surgery.'

[76] Clark 1964, p.250.

[77] Jackson never gave the College's Harveian Oration, although the requirement for its delivery in Latin ended in 1865; see Hurst 1937, p.783.

[78] Jackson 1890c, p.703. In citing Spencer's use of 'discharge' Jackson was apparently referring to Jackson 1870g, p.165, where he had cited Spencer 1870, vol.1, p.25. That volume of Spencer 1870, pp.79–96, has a chapter on 'Nervous Stimulation and Nervous Discharge'. In fact, Jackson had used 'discharge' without citing Spencer in Jackson 1867h, p.643, and in Jackson 1869c, p.345.

[79] Jackson 1890c, p.703.

To see them I will break the single paragraph in his text into headings for the definition of each level, using his actual words:

> (1) The lowest or first level is roughly and incompletely defined as consisting of cord, medulla, and pons[3] ...
> (2) The middle or second level ... is composed of centres of the Rolandic region (so-called "motor region" of the cerebral cortex), and, possibly, of the ganglia of the corpus striatum ...
> (3) The highest or third level ... is made up of centres of the præfrontal lobes (highest motor centres, motor division of the 'organ of mind') ...[80]

In his discussion Jackson said that the distinction between the middle level and the prefrontal lobes had been denied by some. He admitted that it was questionable whether there could be epileptic foci in the prefrontals, because they were not experimentally excitable to observable motor actions. In his defense he cited anatomical connections of the prefrontal lobes to lower motor levels in animals, as recently shown by Wallerian degeneration. Nonetheless, about the distinction between the middle and highest levels he said: 'Of course, this is speculative. I am not aware that anyone pretends to know the seat or the pathology of cases of "genuine epilepsy." I do not use the term "cortical epilepsy," because both epileptic and epileptiform seizures are, to my thinking, cortical fits.'[81] In another footnote he explained his broader conception of epilepsy and its terminology.

> I formerly used the term epilepsy generically for all excessive discharges of the cortex and their consequences. At that time I did not think there were any fits ... depending on excessive discharges beginning in any part of the ponto-bulbar centres ... So that under the term epilepsy used generically there were epilepsy proper, epileptiform seizures, and migraine (the last ... being then spoken of as a sensory epilepsy), and, indeed, any paroxysmal symptoms attributable to sudden excessive discharges of any part of the cortex. I now use the term epilepsy for that neurosis, which is often called "genuine" or "ordinary" epilepsy, and for that only.[82]

This footnote was inserted in the midst of Jackson's discussion about his use of the generic term 'fits'. It leaves the nomenclature for *chronic* middle level fits in abeyance. In his narrative he went on to define 'lowest level fits'.

> These are fits produced by excessive discharges beginning in parts of the lowest level ... which is common to the cerebral and the cerebellar systems. I suppose that most of them are owing to excessive discharges beginning in centres of the bulbar and pontal regions of the level, hence I sometimes use the term "ponto-bulbar fits."[83]

Accordingly, he asked:

> "What effects do excessive discharges beginning in ponto-bulbar centres produce?" This question is ... only to be replied to by experimenters who artificially produce fits in lower

---

[80] Jackson 1890c, p.703; Jackson's internal quotation marks and parentheses. In his footnote 3 Jackson said, 'I do not pretend to be able to define the upper limit of this level'. But his statement in section (2), about the striatum, removed it from the lowest level.
[81] Jackson 1890c, p.704; Jackson's italics.
[82] Jackson 1890c, p.704, footnote 5.
[83] Jackson 1890c, p.704. He explicitly ignored the cerebellar part; see p.707.

animals. I should be ... astonished if it turns out that excessive discharges beginning in any centres of the lowest level do produce convulsions having the same character as those produced by such discharges beginning in centres of the higher levels.[84]

Clinically, what Jackson meant by his prediction of different manifestations of lowest level fits was exemplified in their 'rough arrangement into three groups': (1) '*Respiratory fits ... beginning from primary discharge of the main (medulla) respiratory centre*'; (2) '*Fits produced by convulsant poisons ... from nitrous oxide and curara ...*'; and (3) '*A condition for fits consequent on certain injuries of the cord or sciatic nerve* in guinea-pigs (Brown-Séquard)'.[85] None of these phenomena would now be considered epileptic. Underlying all of this was Jackson's assumption that there must be unstable foci somewhere in the lowest level to account for the clinically observed, motor manifestations. Furthermore,

> In all severe lowest level fits it is supposed that the primary discharge of ponto-bulbar centres not only induces discharge of other lowest motor centres, but also that by intermediation of sensory ("ascending") fibres it discharges centres of higher levels. (I never thought of implication of higher centres in these or any other fits by intermediation of sensory nerves until after consideration of the researches of Victor Horsley and Binswanger.)[10][86]

In other words, Jackson now saw the possibility that epileptic discharges in the lowest level might spread to higher levels by causing discharge of their adjacent afferent pathways. This was a truly new element in his conception of how seizure discharges spread, which he had been trying to figure out since at least 1874.[87] This possibility of seizure spread by 'intermediation of sensory nerves' served to broaden his conception of epilepsy's pathophysiology.

> In recapitulation, the primary discharge in all kinds of fits is of some part of but one of the levels. And now I add that in epileptic and epileptiform seizures ... the excessive discharge begins in some part of one half (lateral) of a level ... If the discharging lesion be ... of but a few cells, very little of a convulsion is directly due to it. Most of the convulsion is produced by intermediation of fibres between the cells of the discharging lesion and other cells of its own level and of other levels; there are induced, consecutive discharges of normal stable cells. Hence the interconnecting fibres of each level and the fibres connecting the several levels with one another, and the fibres connecting the lowest level with all parts of the body ... have to be considered.[88]

In short, he was saying that a knowledge of how the normal brain's activities are integrated is required in order to have a full understanding of the phenomena of epileptic seizures.

> I am straining the meaning of the word fibre, making it stand for any kind of nervous pathway ensuring physiological union ... the study of the interconnections of the levels

---

[84] Jackson 1890c, p.704.

[85] Jackson 1890c, p.705; Jackson's italics, my parenthetical numerals.

[86] Jackson 1890c, p.705; my underlining. In his footnote 10 Jackson cited Horsley 1886c but nothing for Otto Binswanger (1852–1929).

[87] See Chapter 8, section on *Consciousness and the Spread of the Discharge*.

[88] Jackson 1890c, p.705.

is a necessary preliminary to the comparison and contrast of the effects of "discharging lesions" and of "destructive lesions", an essential thing in the scientific investigation of diseases of the nervous system...[89]

This realization about integration ('physiological union') is one of Jackson's most fundamental contributions to neurology and neuroscience, albeit not entirely unique—Charcot and others thought likewise. Jackson had been pursuing such knowledge since he published the *Suggestions* in 1863,[90] but here in 1890 the advances of a quarter-century's blossoming neuroscience could be brought to bear on it. An example would be the symmetrical and asymmetrical bilaterality of the nervous system ('twin series').

> There are connections (commissures) between "identical" [homologous] centres and between "non-identical" [non-homologous] centres of its two halves – presumably between the centres of the two halves as they correspond for co-operation of the parts of the body they represent in joint operations by the two sides of the body.[91]

For such interhemispheric considerations Jackson invented a classification of 'Intrinsic' and 'Extrinsic' fibres, where the former are fibers within each level and the latter are 'those interconnecting levels'. He considered both types to be part of the 'kinetic route', which included all motor pathways within and among the three levels.[92] Thence he postulated the existence of three 'sets of motor fibres, kinetic lines of the second segment, uniting all ... [unilateral] motor centres to all lowest motor centres...'. For the existence of each of the three sets of motor fibers he cited current work by Charcot, Sherrington, and many others.[93] And finally, toward the end of his first Lumleian he expressed his view of contemporary brain science: 'The distinction between muscles and movements of muscles is exceedingly important all over the field of neurology; I think the current doctrine of "abrupt" localisation would not be so much in favor if it were made.'[94]

Lumleian Lecture II

The main theme in Jackson's second Lumleian was the pathophysiology of motor seizures at the cellular and metabolic levels. To begin he restated his tripartite method: 'I have often urged that the Clinical Problem in every nervous malady is of three elements: (1) Anatomical, (2) Physiological, (3) Pathological.'[95] Here his nomenclature was more modern, but the underlying ideas were the same as a quarter century before.[96]

To explain his conception of normal and deranged function in motor cortex Jackson postulated the existence of a purely hypothetical 'Buttoning Centre'—an area of cortex which would coordinate the various movements that are required to carry out that common

---

[89] Jackson 1890c, p.705; my underlining.

[90] Jackson 1863a.

[91] Jackson 1890c, p.705; my square brackets.

[92] Jackson 1890c, p.705. In his footnote 11 Jackson again accepted Gower's theory of what we now call upper and lower motor neurons; see Chapter 11, and see Scott et al. 2012, pp.100–101. They called the neurons 'segments' because they did not yet have the neuron theory. Citing Gowers 1886, vol.1, p.116, Jackson said, 'Dr. Gowers ... gives a diagram of the "motor path". He makes two segments, "cerebro-spinal" and "spino-muscular". The kinetic route is a modification of his [Gowers'] scheme.' See also Phillips and Landau 1990.

[93] Jackson 1890c, pp.705–706.

[94] Jackson 1890c, p.706.

[95] Jackson 1890e, p.766.

[96] See Jackson 1864h, pp.146–147, and Chapter 3.

maneuver. Normally there is 'a harmony and a melody of the different movements of the hand and arm by which the button is got into its hole'.[97] Relying on the reader's imagination, he never said how impossible that task would be in the presence of excessive discharges of some of the involved cells. Rather, he went on to define 'physiological fulminate': 'I use it in almost a literal sense; the discharging lesion is supposed to be a detonator of collateral stable cells, just as a fulminate (in the artillerist's use of the term) is of the comparatively stable gunpowder in a cannon'.[98] And about those fulminating cells:

> If the few highly explosive cells, those of the discharging lesion, could be destroyed, the patient would be rid of his fits ... It is a pity that [the patient] ... cannot be rid of these worse than useless cells; but I know of no way of effecting this riddance. There is the surgical question of cutting out part of the cortex.[99]

To try to understand 'hyper-physiological discharges' that are 'excessive' and convulsions that are 'severe', Jackson fell back on the basics.

> I regret greatly that my ignorance of physics renders me unable to deal with it adequately.
>   With regard to nervous discharges ... as ... liberations of energy by nervous elements, we have to consider two aspects – quantity of energy liberated, and the rate of its liberation ... But the force of the more rapid but shorter liberation of energy will be greater than that of the slower and longer liberation. Force only exists while it lasts; there is no doctrine of conservation of force. The more rapid the liberation of energy by a discharging lesion the greater resistance will be overcome, the more numerous collateral stable elements will be compelled to discharge, and thus the more the amount of convulsion and the greater its range.[100]

Jackson's 'regret' notwithstanding, he understood the difference between energy and force. From there his discussion of seizure pathogenesis included brief use of his *xyz* theory to explain the 'Compound Order' of normal and abnormal movements, and there was another mention of the role of 'sensory (upward) fibres'. Despite his years of effort to understand seizure spread, he said: 'The process of universalisation of epileptiform seizures is a very intricate one, and deserves more precise analysis than I am capable of making'.[101] And then he asked *the* fundamental question:

> ... regarding all cases of epileptiform seizures (and epileptic too), we put the question: "How are local persistent discharging lesions established and kept up?"
>   The first question is: "What is the most general nature of the abnormal nutritive process of cells of discharging lesions in epileptiform seizures?"[102]

---

[97] Jackson 1890e, p.767.
[98] Jackson 1890e, p.768; my square brackets. Another reference to 'ammunition' is on p.771.
[99] Jackson 1890e, p.768. Early in Lumleian II Jackson said (Jackson 1890e, p.765): 'It is in epileptiform seizures that operations have been done by Macewen, Godlee, Horsley, Barker, and others. Hence, very precise study of fits of this kind is necessary.' 'Barker' probably refers to Gowers and Barker 1886, but that report says nothing about any kind of seizure.
[100] Jackson 1890e, p.768.
[101] Jackson 1890e, p.769; Jackson's parentheses.
[102] Jackson 1890e, p.769; Jackson's parentheses.

Jackson tried to answer the latter question with a long speculation about neural metabolism ('nutritive process'). It was based on the neurochemistry of the day, which was inadequate to the task, although the importance of nitrogen was recognized.[103] At the end of his second Lumleian he attempted to put 'the several hypotheses' together in an inclusive, histological–physiological speculation about epileptogenesis. The histological part—about small cells for small voluntary muscles—goes back to 1876.[104] Here in 1890 he reiterated:

> Epileptiform seizures begin most often in parts of the body having "small movements;" these movements are represented by nervous arrangements having many small cells.[27] Small cells present a more extensive surface to nutrient fluid than the small quantity of grey matter in large cells, and will be more quickly nourished than large ones are.[105]

We might say that Jackson had ventured out the wrong branch of the right tree. His conceptualization of cellular metabolism had elements of intracellular–extracellular relationships, and again it was necessary to have information about the normal in order to understand the abnormal.

> Small cells become highly unstable more readily than large ones do; thus discharging lesions are supposed to be especially of small cells. A rapid liberation of energy overcomes greater and more numerous resistances than a slower liberation of an equal quantity of energy. Small cells liberate their energy in a shorter time than large ones; hence the currents developed by fulminates of small cells overcome greater and thus more numerous resistances than would fulminates of large cells, and hence produce more convulsion and greater range of convulsion.[106]

Nowadays we would not think about the differences between small and large neurons in this way, but the main ideas in Jackson's third lecture followed logically from his second.

Lumleian Lecture III

At the start of his third Lumleian Jackson defined its theme: 'the After Effects of excessive nervous discharges in cases of epileptiform seizures'. His first order of business was to try to understand the pathophysiology of postictal phenomena. Temporary paralysis, he said, 'has been ascribed to cerebral congestion consequent on arrest of respiration in the preceding seizure'.[107] He argued against that idea—another one had to be considered.

> Gowers believes that discharges in epileptic fits sometimes inhibit; he thinks that temporary paralysis is found in some cases after a purely sensory discharge which does not next discharge motor centres, but inhibits them ... I express no decided opinion as to the validity of the inhibition hypotheses.[108]

---

[103] In Jackson 1890e, p.770, where Jackson used the term 'metabolism', and in his footnote 21 he gave a quotation from 'Foster, *Physiology*, pt. ii, p.828', which also includes 'metabolism', but I don't know which edition of Michael Foster's textbook he was using.

[104] See Jackson 1876o, p.146, footnote *a*. This paper is discussed in Chapter 8.

[105] Jackson 1890e, p.771. Jackson's footnote 27 included some ideas about the role of the cerebellum in motor control.

[106] Jackson 1890e, p.771.

[107] Jackson 1890g, p.821.

[108] Jackson 1890g, p.821. On Gowers and inhibition see Eadie 2011.

To illustrate his own point of view Jackson offered some hypothetical scenarios of patients with very limited postictal paralyses, e.g., 'loss of a few most special movements of the hand'.[109] Then he deduced the clinical status—the specific motor losses and reflex findings—based on which segments of the kinetic route were exhausted. All of this was done in exquisite detail, which I will not try to follow. However, I do wonder how well his audience followed him, even remembering that the published version was longer than the presentation.

Jackson's interest in postictal phenomena was old, of course, but he hinted at something new when he said there was 'sometimes aphasia with it'. In the latter part of Lecture III he discussed postictal aphasia extensively. About this, the first question that comes to my mind is why he returned to aphasia in 1890, after neglecting it for so long. His views on aphasia had last received substantial treatment in 1880.[110] Partly, I think, he was simply expanding his coverage of postictal phenomena, but his consideration of aphasia also gave him an opportunity to address other issues: 'in some cases of epileptiform seizures there may be permanent defect of speech and a temporary increase of that defect after a paroxysm'.[111] To avoid misunderstanding, he tried to explain his use of 'defect' in 'defect of speech'.

> I have not observed post-epileptiform *loss* of speech, but only defect of speech ("partial aphasia") ... The term "defect of speech" is equivocal, as is also the term "partial aphasia;" it really covers two opposite elements, negatively, loss of some speech, and positively retention of the rest of speech.[16][112]

In his footnote 16 Jackson used his dynamic conception of cerebral function at the cellular level to explain both the negative and the positive aspects of defect of speech.

> [16] ... I do not suppose that there are fixed nervous arrangements – some for these words or syllables (properly movements corresponding to syllables) only and some for those only. I would[,] rather than hold this mechanical doctrine[,] go to the other extreme, and say that there are no nervous arrangements for movements in any centres except at the time when these and those motor nervous elements are functioning together in a particular temporary grouping.[113]

In this passage there are two things that require exposition: (1) 'syllables' and (2) 'temporary grouping'. Concerning syllables, a few years later Jackson said:

> A word is a psychical thing, but of course there is a physical process correlative with it. I submit that this physical process is a discharge of cerebral nervous arrangements representing articulatory muscles in a particular movement, or, if there be several syllables, in a series of particular movements.
> ... the physical basis of a word, or rather syllable, is a sensori-motor, an audito-articulatory, nervous arrangement.[114]

---

[109] Jackson 1890g, p.823
[110] Jackson 1880e and Jackson 1880f.
[111] Jackson 1890g, p.824.
[112] Jackson 1890g, p.825; Jackson's parentheses and quotation marks.
[113] Jackson 1890g, p.825; Jackson's parentheses, my square brackets and underlining.
[114] Jackson 1893b, p.205, my underlining.

Given Jackson's theory of the motor origin of word recognition, the motor arrangements for the internal revival or external pronunciation of two syllables in a single word would be different for each syllable. How or why he came to this realization, or when, I don't know. Did he realize this on his own, or did someone point it out to him? The latter is unlikely because he would have acknowledged the source of the correction if he had been cognizant of it. In any case, the idea of a 'temporary grouping' plays into this point. In discussing it Jackson said, again:

> It is one thing to locate the negative lesion which destroys speech (renders a person unable to speak aloud), and quite another thing to say that "speech resides" in any particular part of the cortex . . . I submit that the highest centres ("organ of mind") must be engaged during speech, whether [the speech is] external or internal, notwithstanding that a negative lesion of a part of a middle motor level produces aphasia.[115]

The precept in the first sentence of this passage has become iconic. In 1874 Jackson had said: 'To locate the damage which destroys speech and to locate speech are two different things.'[116] Here, in 1890, he was also at pains to distinguish aphasia from any kind of defect of speech due to 'bulbar paralysis', although the muscles and movements in both are largely the same.[117] Throughout he emphasized the importance of staying on the physical side of concomitance: 'It is only the *physical bases* of words (or properly of syllables) which I assert to be sensori-nervous arrangements representing complex movements of the muscles of the tongue, etc., in association with complex combinations of auditory impressions.'[118] About the 'popular' psychological explanation of aphasia as loss of memory for words, he was dismissive.

> If it is admitted that the psychological statements as to the aphasic conditions are correct descriptions, those who make them are just as much bound as any one else to seek the abnormal material conditions of the several phenomena of "amnesic aphasia" . . . If any one says that he cannot understand how activities of motor nervous arrangements can correspond to words, I would remind him that, except the popular psychologist, no one pretends to understand how any material conditions correspond to any psychical states.[119]

In a word, *Vive* Concomitance!

Continuing Contributions, 1891–1894

The Lumleian Lectures of 1890 were Jackson's last major address to a large general medical audience, but he continued to publish original papers to the turn of the century,[120] and he continued to speak to smaller, local groups. An interesting example of the latter was a presentation at the Hunterian Society in March 1891. Jackson and his young colleague W.H.R.

---

[115] Jackson 1890g, p.825, footnote 17; Jackson's parentheses, my square brackets.
[116] Jackson 1874b, p.19; see Chapter 7.
[117] Jackson 1890g, p.826.
[118] Jackson 1890g, p.825; Jackson's italics.
[119] Jackson 1890g, p.827.
[120] E.g., Jackson 1892b, which was 'a case of syringomyelus', by Jackson and James Galloway (1862–1922); the latter had had junior appointments at the London. In Jackson 1867m Lockhart Clarke and Jackson had published the 'First important account of syringomyelia' (Morton 1961, p.410; but see McHenry 1969, p.433).

Rivers (1864–1922) 'showed a phonogram recording the abnormal talking of a patient the subject of disseminated sclerosis'.[121] Thomas Edison had invented the phonograph in 1877, and various versions were quickly commercialized.

'Neurological Fragments', Started March 1892

In February 1892 Jackson had 'the honourable task of giving the Hunterian Society's Lecture' for that year. His title was 'Lecture on Neurological Fragments'.[122] Thereafter he continued to publish another 21 installments with the same running title, 'Neurological Fragments'. They were among his last publications in 1909, before he died in 1911.[123] In each Fragment there were usually multiple subjects. Early on, his topics were often neuro-ophthalmological, and there were also discussions of reflexes, epilepsy, etc. The initial lecture itself was fragmentary. That is, it goes loosely from one subject to another, so the introductory lecture was really just the first of the Fragments. Among them was a new-found interest in spinal cord injuries,[124] which was directly related to Jackson's prior interest in the diagnostic utility of the knee jerk.

From a later source we have some interesting information about Jackson's behavior when he was publishing the Fragments. In James Taylor's memoir of Jackson he says that Jackson was always courteous, but at the same time very impatient: 'when he took anything to be typewritten it had always to be done at once, so that he might have it at the earliest possible moment!' Taylor went on to quote from a letter written by Squire Sprigge, the assistant editor of *The Lancet*.[125] He too remarked on Jackson's courteousness, and then he said:

> I am very glad to know the Neurological Fragments are to be published. I cannot forget how they used to be given to us 25 or 30 years ago. He generally used to bring them at about tea-time on Wednesday: He brought them himself by hand, and gave them to me personally. He arrived in a large barouche [four-wheeled carriage] with a pair of horses: he asked to see a proof the same day, and was told that would be impossible: he was quite pleased to leave the correction of the proof to us, but was desirous that the note should appear the same week, which generally entailed hacking half a column out of the pages which were already made up![126]

The fact that Sprigge was willing to hack up half a column speaks to his estimation of the readership that Jackson would bring to *The Lancet*. Getting back now to 1893, the list of Jackson's writings for that year contains only two items. It raises the suspicion that he may have been ill. If so, he recovered well in 1894, which saw a total of 14 items.[127] Before we leave 1893, however, we must consider the second item.

---

[121] Jackson 1891b; also Jackson 1891c. Rivers had a junior post at Queen Square; see Rivers 1922.

[122] Jackson 1892c (*British Medical Journal*) and Jackson 1892d (*Lancet*). They have different paragraphing but their substance is essentially the same. I will summarize Jackson 1892d because all subsequent Fragments were published only in the *Lancet*. All of the *Neurological Fragments* were published together by James Taylor (in Jackson 1925a).

[123] Fragment 'XXI' (Jackson 1909a) was dated February 6, 1909. Jackson 1909b, dated March 27, 1909, was not labeled 'Fragment', but it continued his intense interest in neuro-ophthalmology. About Neurological Fragments, Chance (1937, p.283) says that he was 'not a little proud' of them.

[124] Jackson 1892d, pp.513–514.

[125] (Samuel) Squire Sprigge (1860–1937) became assistant editor of *The Lancet* in 1893 and editor in 1909 [Oxford DNB online (May 18, 2018)]. The letter was written to Ernest Hodder-Williams (1876–1927), a publisher and author [Oxford DNB, same].

[126] Jackson 1925a, p.19; my square brackets.

[127] See York and Steinberg 2006, pp.123–126.

'Words and Other Symbols in Mentation', August 1893

The stated theme of this article was the issue of whether thought is possible without words or other symbols, such as pantomime.[128] For this, of course, Jackson's raw material was aphasia. When he wrote his discussion of postictal aphasia for his third Lumleian, that could have been an impetus to go back to studying language more generally. But there was another, more obvious factor in his professional environment. In 1886 Charlton Bastian published a well-regarded book on neurological diagnosis. It included detailed instructions for testing language,[129] and in 1887 he authored a long paper in the *BMJ*, 'On different kinds of aphasia, with special reference to their classification and ultimate pathology'.[130] At the least, Bastian's views on aphasia would have been the subject of informal discussions at Queen Square and beyond. In fact, he had begun to write about aphasia in an original way in 1869, and in 1887 he reminded his colleagues about that.

> It has of late been the fashion to suppose that <u>Wernicke</u> (*Der Aphasische Symptomen Complex*, Breslau, 1874) was the first to call attention to sensory aphasia ... but five years previously I had fully recognized the sensory nature of such defects (On the Various Forms of Loss of Speech in Cerebral Disease' ... 1869) ... [131]

Despite Bastian's prickly disposition, Jackson had a high regard for his opinions. According to John Marshall, Bastian's

> ... most famous aphasia-diagram (Bastian 1887) is presented as an abstract psychological model without commitment as to the anatomical loci where the functions of the centres and tracts are realized. That is, the diagram is *not* drawn on a schematic representation of the left hemisphere ...[132]

Marshall's latter point is technically correct—there was no anatomical background in that figure. However, the diagram was drawn with the visual and auditory areas to the right and the motor ('kinæsthetic') areas to the left, so the diagram is presented *as if* it were viewed from the left. Moreover, in the continuation of Bastian's paper, his Fig. 2 is an anatomical cartoon of what we now call Wernicke's and Broca's areas and their (then-theoretical) connecting 'commissure'. It is drawn on an outline of the left hemisphere.[133] This is critical, because Jackson was invoking a major role for the right hemisphere. In his paper on 'Mentation' he gave his assessment of the accepted pathophysiology of aphasia.

> Strictly, no doubt, the physical basis of a word, or rather syllable, is a sensori-motor, an audito-articulatory, nervous arrangement. But in speech, [which is] the objective part of verbalising, our main concern is with the motor element of the physical basis of words. It is <u>current doctrine</u> that the part of the brain destroyed in cases of loss of speech (aphasia) is

---

[128] Jackson 1893b.

[129] Bastian 1886; see Lorch 2013, pp.2632–2633.

[130] Bastian 1887a; throughout he mentioned Jackson only briefly. See also Lorch 2013. For an introduction to Bastian's neurological ideas see Marshall 1994, pp.103–111.

[131] Bastian 1887a, p.934, referring to Bastian 1869b; his parentheses, my underlining.

[132] Marshall 1994, p.106. '(Bastian 1887)' refers to Bastian 1887a, p.933.

[133] Bastian 1887a, p.968.

motor, and that it is a part of cortex cerebri (Broca's region) representative of movements of the tongue, palate, lips, &c.[134]

This ignores the sensory sides of Bastian and Wernicke.[135] Jackson apparently regarded Wernicke as a Johnny-come-lately, after Bastian. This is seen in the heading for Jackson's Fragment XI of August 1894.

CEREBRAL PAROXYSMS (EPILEPTIC ATTACKS) WITH AN AUDITORY WARNING; IN SLIGHT SEIZURES THE SPECIAL IMPERCEPTIONS CALLED "WORD-DEAFNESS" (WERNICKE) AND "WORD-BLINDNESS" (KUSSMAUL) ...[136]

Here Jackson considered Wernicke's aphasia to be a form of agnosia ('imperception')—a view that was not without its adherents. To my knowledge, it is the only place in Jackson's entire published corpus where he used the name 'Wernicke', and it is the first place where he used 'Kussmaul' in reference to alexia ('word-blindness').[137] Indeed, those names were not mentioned in the text for which the above is the heading. Since Jackson usually acknowledged predecessors, I suspect he did not mention Wernicke more often because he felt that Bastian's priority claim was well established. In any case, he was expressing his conception of how words function by using what was, for him, a new nomenclature.

> ... there are at least two ways in which words serve; they serve not only in speaking, but in the <u>reception</u> of the speech of others. In a case of aphasia with word-deafness (a special imperception) there is a loss of <u>receptivity</u> of words, but this is ... because, speaking now of the physical, the nervous arrangements for articulatory movements in the <u>right half of the brain</u> cannot be reached.[138]

We still use the terms 'reception' of auditory language and 'receptive' (Wernicke's) aphasia. Those words have a sensory implication, including a notion of language comprehension. But Jackson viewed comprehension as a motor-based process, beginning in the right hemisphere. In his view, Wernicke's aphasia is a special case of Broca's aphasia ('loss of speech'), explicable by defective motor processing. This is seen in the hypothetical case of Broca's aphasia that he postulated for discussion: 'I am supposing a case of speechlessness without that complication [of poor reception]; in this case the patient understands what we say to him, on simple matters at any rate, he receives our speech, has that service of words (b).'[139] Jackson's footnote (b) emphasized the point: 'Of course one does not take the expression "receiving speech of others" literally. We understand a speaker because he arouses our words.' And then he continued:

> Further, the damage to the left cerebral hemisphere in a case of speechlessness, is ... [in] a part of the middle motor centres of the cerebral sub-system, the highest motor centres ...

---

134 Jackson 1893b, p.205; my square brackets and underlining.
135 Marjorie Lorch (personal communication) emphasizes Jackson's relative lack of interest in sensory phenomena.
136 Jackson 1894m, p.252.
137 For 'Alexia and Agrapha', 1856–1900, see Henderson 2010; also Barrière and Lorch 2004.
138 Jackson 1893b, p.205, my underlining. Bastian used 'reception' (Bastian 1887a, p.933) only sparingly. I don't know by whom or when the term was first applied to linguistic phenomena.
139 Jackson 1893b, p.205; my square brackets.

(præ-frontal lobes) being intact. I think then that cases of loss of speech do not give proof that thought is possible without words. As, however, I am not aware that anyone agrees with me in thinking that the right half of the brain is "educated in words," and as I fear I am alone in making the distinction into middle and highest (cerebral) motor centres, I have no right to claim acceptance of the opinion that such a case of aphasia ... does not give proof that thought is possible without words.[140]

Clearly John Hughlings Jackson was not at all fearful of being alone about any of his opinions. That was a good thing, because his conception of three cerebral levels was not universally accepted, and I have never seen any evidence that any of his colleagues accepted Jackson's ideas as expressed in my Fig. 7.1, especially the role of the right hemisphere in language. According to his theory, the words in a proposition are initially received in the right hemisphere. 'Word-deafness' results when the information in the right side cannot get to the left. So he was postulating a disconnection, but without specifying its location, which would have to be on the physical side of concomitance. To explain the psychical side, he offered the example of the phantom limb phenomenon in amputees: 'I submit that all entire [intact] men have not only movements of their hands, but also actions—psychical states—correlative with activities of the cerebral nervous arrangements effecting these movements. When a man's arm is cut off, he finds this out. (d).'[141] And in the footnote he said:

> (d) I do not mean that these actions, psychical things, are "ideas of movements;" we have ... no ideas of any parts of our bodies ... it would surely be erroneous to speak of subject-consciousness (self-consciousness or self) as being a consciousness of the whole organism or of the highest centres. No doubt, a very different thing, subject consciousness is correlative with activities of nervous arrangements representing all parts of the body as one whole.[142]

I have struggled to understand this passage, especially the first sentence, but I can't. It seems to be internally inconsistent. I present it here because in Chapters 7 and 8 we saw that in the 1870s Jackson proposed his own idiosyncratic usages of subject and object consciousness. Here in 1893 he was again employing subject consciousness, apparently as he had used it before. Perhaps the issue hinges on the meaning of 'ideas' in 'ideas of movements'. Does he mean it in the associationists' sense of 'ideas', which itself is not well defined? In an Appendix titled *Ideation and Perception: their Resemblances and Differences*, Jackson explained those conceptions using the subjective–objective distinction and associationism's notion of weak and strong signals: 'I believe that ideation is commonly regarded as a subjective process; of course perception is recognized as an objective process. I submit that both ideation and perception are objective, two degrees of objectivisation.'[143] And on the physical side of concomitance:

> The cerebral centres for ideation and perception are one and the same; during ideation there are only central (cerebral) activities and these are slight; during perception the activities are periphery-cerebral and centro-peripheral and are strong. In ideation there is a slight discharge of the same cerebral nervous arrangements which are strongly discharged

---

[140] Jackson 1893b, p.205; Jackson's parentheses, my square brackets and underlining.
[141] Jackson 1893b, p.206; my square brackets.
[142] Jackson 1893b, p.206; Jackson's parentheses, my underlining.
[143] Jackson 1893b, p.208.

during perception ... Ideation always precedes perception; perception does not always follow ideation.[144]

The last two sentences in this passage are clear enough on the physical side, and he tried to keep to the physical in an often-cited paper on insanity.

'The Factors of Insanities', June 1894

In this well-organized paper Jackson once again tried to help the psychiatrists unravel the complexities of mental disease by applying dissolution on the physical side of concomitance.[145] In that regard, he said: 'we must also take into account the undamaged remainder – the evolution still going on in what is left intact of a nervous system mutilated by disease'.

> In every insanity more or less of the highest cerebral centres is out of function, temporarily or permanently, from some pathological process ... it matters little what that process may be. It only matters as the pathological processes produce loss of function, that is Dissolution, of more or less of the highest centres ...[146]

With that background, Jackson listed his four factors in a single narrative paragraph. For heuristic clarity I have put the individual sentences in outline form:

'There are four Factors (*a*) in insanity.'[147]
'(1) There are different <u>Depths</u> of Dissolution of the highest cerebral centres.'
'(2) There are different <u>Persons</u> who have undergone that Dissolution.'
'(3) There are different <u>Rates</u> with which the Dissolution is effected.'
'(4) There is the Influence of different <u>Local Bodily States</u> and of different <u>External Circumstances</u> on the persons who have undergone that Dissolution.'[148]

And in the highest centers there is an additional complexity.

> Although I speak of Dissolution of the highest cerebral centres ... as if all the divisions of these centres were "evenly" affected ... there are local Dissolutions of those centres ... Different regions of the highest cerebral centres undergo dissolution in different *kinds* of insanity. I shall nevertheless ... ignore *local* dissolutions of the highest cerebral centres and speak of different degrees as if the Dissolutions of those centres producing them were uniform. If we did consider local dissolutions of the highest cerebral centres we should have to say that there are <u>five factors</u> in insanities (*b*).[149]

---

[144] Jackson 1893b, p.208.
[145] Jackson 1894j; my square brackets. There is nothing to indicate that this paper was a lecture.
[146] Jackson 1894j, p.615.
[147] Footnote (*a*) cited Jackson 1874ii, where he said he had 'for the first time' stated 'what I suppose to be the factors of insanities'.
[148] Jackson 1894j, p.616; my underlining.
[149] Jackson 1894j, p.616; my underlining. Footnote (*b*) contained an important generalization: 'We rarely, if ever, meet with a dissolution from disease which is the exact reversal of evolution. Probably healthy senescence is the dissolution most nearly the exact reversal of evolution.' There was no mention of a fifth factor in Jackson 1874ii, because he had not then extended his analysis to the hypothetical 'layers' of the highest centers.

From there Jackson went on to discuss the four factors in detail. He started with a theoretical premise of four 'imaginary' layers in the highest centers: 'for simplicity of illustrations I shall <u>imagine</u> that the highest cerebral centres are in four layers, A.B.C.D. (*c*) In accord with this I make ... four depths of dissolution of these centres, and ... four degrees of insanity.'[150] In his discussion of the first (top) depth, loss of layer A, he was at pains to remind his readers that there are negative and positive phenomena, the latter resulting from the activities of surviving layers B, C, and D. In the process he harked back to the subjective–objective distinction, trying to be clear about nomenclature: '(*b*) Mind, Mentation and Consciousness are in the text used synonymously. I am ignoring Subject-consciousness and deal only with Object-consciousness.'[151] In the next footnote he tried to clarify his position about a common conception of consciousness.

> (*c*) ... the statements in the text imply that there is a sort of homogeneous consciousness, and that in the first depth of dissolution ... there is a certain quantity lost, corresponding to abrogation of layer A ... I repudiate the implication [about homogeneous consciousness] ... looking on it as an absurdity ... in the first depth of Dissolution there is loss of the most complex, &c., and retention of the next most complex, &c.... the deeper the Dissolution the less elaborate is the mentation remaining possible.[152]

This conception of the abnormal led to an explanation of how evolution and dissolution function cooperatively in the normal state.

> (*a*) ... There is a big rhythm of evolution and dissolution in healthy people, being awake in the day and asleep at night. Some of the "uses" of sleep are that the highest ranges of the highest centres may be "swept clean" of trivial acquirements made during the day, and that "internal evolution" (evolution going on without interference by or reaction upon the environment) of the lower ranges may be facilitated.[153]

Jackson had stated similar views on internal evolution and memory consolidation in his third Croonian of 1884.[154] Here in 1894 his use of the term 'evolution' was broadened toward a connotation of ongoing, adaptive ontogenesis, which gave a cerebral basis for psychiatric phenomena. Violating his promise to ignore local dissolutions in the highest centers, he said:

> I now take for further illustration a case of insanity from what I suppose to be a Local dissolution of the highest centres. When a general paralytic [third stage syphilitic] believes he is Emperor of Europe, I submit that this delusion ... arises during activity of perfectly healthy nervous arrangements, presumably those of the posterior lobes and those left intact of the anterior. The disease of the anterior lobes is responsible for his not knowing that he is X.Y., a clerk in the City.

---

[150] Jackson 1894j, p.616; my underlining. In Jackson 1894j, p.616, column 1, footnote (*c*), he said: 'Of course I am not speaking of what are morphologically called layers of cells of the cortex, but of imaginary anatomico-physiological layers.'

[151] Jackson 1894j, p.616, column 2.

[152] Jackson 1894j, p.616, column 2, footnote (*c*); my square brackets.

[153] Jackson 1894j, p.617, footnote (*a*); Jackson's parentheses.

[154] Jackson 1884g, pp.705–706; see Chapter 10.

Illusions, delusions, extravagant conduct and abnormal emotional states in an insane person signify evolution, not Dissolution; they signify evolution going on in what remains intact of the mutilated highest centres ...[155]

In summary, Jackson said: 'In the first depth of Dissolution the negative mental state is slight, the dissolution being very shallow; the positive mental state is very elaborate, the range of evolution remaining being very high.'[156] In the second and third depths of dissolution, the 'negative element' becomes greater and greater, until, in the fourth depth, 'the negative mental affection is greatest; is indeed total; there is dementia. There are no positive mental symptoms; there is no mind or consciousness.'[157]

Jackson's discussion of his second factor (Persons) was short. He simply listed the elements of an individual's age, gender, education, intelligence, occupation, etc., but then he raised

... the question of heredity of insanity. I submit that no one inherits a tendency to insanity in the sense that he inherits a tendency to disease ... of any part of his brain. He inherits a healthy brain, but a smaller one than the average ... smaller in the anatomico-physiological sense that he has fewer functional elements in the highest ranges of his highest cerebral centres. He inherits a brain that will "give out" more easily under unfavourable influences than the brain of the average man.[158]

This passage recognizes the primacy of what we call neural 'connectivity', which is exactly what Jackson meant. What the passage does not contain, however, is any reference to his earlier views on the heredity of disease. In 1874 he had discussed the hereditary 'transmission' of epilepsy, invoking 'transmission (1) of a tendency to diseases of tissues; and ... (2) transmission of imperfect Organs'.[159] Here in 1894 his conception of the heredity of insanity fits quite well with his earlier idea about 'Imperfect Organs', although he was silent about the mechanism of that genetic inheritance.

Jackson's discussions of his third and fourth factors were similarly brief. About the third factor, rate of dissolution, he explained: 'The more rapidly the Dissolution is effected the greater is the activity on the range of Evolution remaining... The [quiet] senile dement undergoes Dissolution very slowly. The post-epileptic maniac has undergone dissolution with extreme rapidity.'[160] His treatment of the fourth factor (bodily states and external circumstances) consisted of only two short clinical scenarios. At the end of the paper the text said: '(Here is given a qualification of the statements on heredity of insanity when speaking of the Second Factor [different persons])',[161] but we are left without specifics of the 'qualification'. Our disappointment would be enduring, because 'The Factors of Insanities' of June 1894 was Jackson's last major statement on the subject of insanity.

[155] Jackson 1894j, p.617; my square brackets.
[156] Jackson 1894j, p.617.
[157] Jackson 1894j, p.617; 'dementia' was then used narrowly, for a final stage.
[158] Jackson 1894j, p.618.
[159] Jackson 1874aa, p.351; already quoted and discussed in Chapter 8.
[160] Jackson 1894j, p.618; my square brackets.
[161] Jackson 1894j, p.619; Jackson's parentheses, my square brackets.

A Sincere Testimonial, October 1895

The Lancet of December 8, 1894, gave notice of a planned 'TESTIMONIAL TO DR. HUGHLINGS JACKSON' on the occasion of his retirement from the active staff of the London Hospital at age 60.[162] The announcement proclaimed that 'the increased precision in the diagnosis of diseases of the brain and the success of modern cerebral surgery are owing to Dr. Hughlings Jackson's work ...' So 'inasmuchas [*sic*] the clinical work upon which his discoveries have been founded was largely done in the wards of the great hospital with which he has been connected for over thirty years the movement will especially recommend itself to all London Hospital men.'[163] This can be translated to mean that all London Hospital men should defend the honor of the London in its claim on Jackson, without actually mentioning Queen Square. In fact, subscriptions were received from an international group of Jackson's admirers.

> Amongst the contributors to the Testimonial were Mr. Herbert Spencer, Sir Joseph Lister, Sir James Paget, Sir William Broadbent, Sir William Rogers, Sir F. Grainger Stewart, Sir Henry Acland, Professor Pierre Marie of Paris, Professor William Osler, Sir F. Spencer Wells, Professor Hitzig of Halle, Professor Bäumler of Freiburg, Sir B.W. Richardson and Professor Burdon Sanderson.[164]

With 'a sum of about £300 ... an oil portrait was painted by Mr. Lance Calkin, an artist of much distinction ...'[165] At the ceremony on October 1, 1895, the audience included Paget, Sanderson, Wells, Broadbent, 'Dr. [Thomas] Barlow, Dr. Buzzard, and others'.[166] The presentation and leading remarks were made by Paget—a Barts man! Recall that he had mentored Jackson at St. Bartholomew's Hospital in 1855–1856.[167] At age 81 he was still famously eloquent. About Jackson's work Paget confessed: 'I never have been able to follow him in all the minuteness and completeness of his work in neurology and diseases of the nervous system ...'[168]

The tone of the event that made it sincere was expressed in the anonymous report in *The Lancet*: 'Dr. Hughlings Jackson is one of the least demonstrative members of the profession, but this quality only increases the singular ... affection with which he is regarded, not only by his colleagues, but by the profession in every part of the United Kingdom and of the world.'[169] And Paget added, 'I wish I could express half the good feelings that have been said or written by those who have contributed to this testimonial.'[170] In Jackson's reply, he said: 'the honour was very much enhanced by the fact that the presentation had been made by Sir James Paget. He rejoiced to have the opportunity of declaring how much he had been indebted to Sir James, not only for scientific aid, but also by a bright example of uprightness of conduct.'[171]

---

[162] My description of this event is based on Jackson 1894n, Jackson 1895d, Jackson 1895e, and Jackson 1895f.
[163] Jackson 1894n.
[164] Jackson 1895f, p.35.
[165] Jackson 1895f, pp.34–35. 'In addition to the portrait, a silver claret jug and salver were presented to Dr. Jackson.' Jackson's will left the portrait to the Royal College of Physicians (Jackson 1911a, p.2). The Calkin portrait is the front cover of this book.
[166] Jackson 1895e; my square brackets. The venue was the Library of the London Hospital Medical College (Jackson 1895d, p.861).
[167] See Chapter 2.
[168] Jackson 1895d, p.862.
[169] Jackson 1895e.
[170] Jackson 1895d, p.861.
[171] Jackson 1895d, p.862. This is a reporter's paraphrase of Jackson's remarks.

By the time of Jackson's Testimonial his neurological paradigm had largely reached its final form—to the extent that anything was final in Jackson's mind. In his last publications (1894–1909) he tried to strengthen his theory of levels in the central nervous system, especially the lowest level, which had been relatively neglected.[172]

Exploring the Lowest Level, 1894–1897

This section will follow the development of Jackson's ideas about the lowest level in the years 1894–1897.[173] This was just before his extensive Hughlings Jackson Lecture of December 1897, which dealt with his theory of levels more broadly.[174] In February 1894 Jackson published 'A clinical study of a case of cyst of the cerebellum',[175] which included an autopsy. He thought the findings implied the existence of direct efferent fibers from the cerebellum to the spinal cord. This idea was supported by his junior author J.S. Risien Russell.[176] Risien Russell had done experiments on dogs and monkeys which 'seem to prove the existence of motor paresis as one factor in the causation of the inability on the part of the animal to walk or stand after ablation of parts or the whole of the cerebellum …'[177] However, Jackson acknowledged contradictory evidence, and a year later he named several investigators who were unable to confirm the existence of direct cerebellar-to-spinal-cord fibers.[178] About his lowest level, he said, it is 'much the same as Marshall Hall's "True Spinal System."'[179] Actually, Hall's 'excito-motory system' was independent of any connection to higher levels,[180] whereas Jackson's lowest level was explicitly connected. And then he made a broader statement.

I divide the central nervous system into two Sub-systems – Cerebral and Cerebellar. The lowest level of the cerebral sub-system is also … the lowest level of the cerebellar sub-system … However, no motor connexions … between the cerebellum and the spinal cord … have been yet proved to exist … I shall, for the most part, ignore the cerebellar sub-system in this and in subsequent notes, and shall speak of the lowest level *as if* it were the lowest level of the cerebral sub-system.[181]

Once again the cerebellum was disowned, but regarding the whole enterprise Jackson stressed: 'The foregoing and what is to follow on the hierarchy of nervous centres is, of course, hypothetical.'[182] Then he made it less hypothetical by giving it some anatomical boundaries.

Each of the three levels of the cerebral sub-system is sensori-motor … but I shall limit illustration to the motor provinces of the levels … (1) The anterior horns of the cord and the

---

[172] This statement disregards several papers on the knee-jerk, which is within the lowest level. Jackson's continuing interest in it was for its diagnostic specificity.

[173] Encompassing Jackson 1894g, Jackson 1895b, Jackson 1895c, Jackson 1896a, and Jackson 1897a.

[174] Jackson 1898a, Jackson 1898b.

[175] Jackson 1894g.

[176] John (variously James) Samuel Risien Russell (?1861–1939), usually known as Risien Russell, was appointed Pathologist to Queen Square in 1896 and Physician in 1898. See [Russell] 1939; [Russell] 1939a; Holmes 1954, pp.96 and 98; and Shorvon et al. 2019, p.104.

[177] Jackson 1894g, p.393.

[178] Jackson 1895b, p.394, footnote 2.

[179] Jackson 1895b.

[180] On Hall's 'excito-motory system' see Clarke and Jacyna 1987, pp.114–124.

[181] Jackson 1895b, p.394; Jackson's italics.

[182] Jackson 1895b, p.394.

motor nuclei of cranial nerves ... make up the ... motor province of the lowest level ... it extends from the tuber cinereus to the conus medullaris ... (2) The centres of the Rolandic regions of the cortex make up the motor province of the middle level. (3) The centres of the præ-frontal lobes make up the motor province of the highest level ...[183]

Again Jackson cautioned: 'The foregoing account of the constitution of the lowest level ... is in mere outline.'[184] Within the lowest level, he designated some nuclei as 'Superior Centres', in a way that is reminiscent of his postulating 'layers' in the highest levels.[185] Then he clarified his usage of a critical term: 'Although I use the words "connexion by fibres" that expression is not to be taken literally; it is to be taken as standing for any sort of junction, definite or indefinite, or ... for any contrivance by which different nervous elements can influence one another.'[186] The rest of the paper consisted of an extensive application of the four Spencerian factors of evolution to specific nuclei of the lowest level and thence to disease.[187] Those themes were continued in Jackson's next Fragment, whose implications he summarized at the end.

> ... the lowest level is, for organic duties ("menial work"), by itself very efficient, and ... it is *for those duties* considerably independent of the motor ... influence of the higher levels, although much under their negative (inhibitory) influence. Another general doctrine is that the centres of the lowest level which serve in organic ("industrial") duties can be compelled by higher levels to suspend those duties in order that the higher levels may act on animal centres of the level in "voluntary" operations. All of this seems to me to be but an application of Herbert Spencer's doctrines on analogies between an individual organism and a social organism ...[188]

To understand the quasi-independent function of the lowest level, Jackson enlisted the neurological phenomena of injury to the cervical spinal cord.[189] In discussing 'the symptomatology of fracture-dislocations of the spine – crushing the cervical cord completely across below the emergence of the phrenic nerves ...' he asserted: 'We have to attempt an answer to the question "How does the central nervous system ... 'get along' after it has been cut in two at the critical part mentioned?" '[190] His investigation of this question involved 'the four

---

[183] Jackson 1895b, p.394. This summary leaves out the basal ganglia, which he usually assigned to the middle level. The tuber cinereus (part of the hypothalamic–pituitary axis) is the rostral end of his lowest level, and the conus medullaris (lower end of the spinal cord) is the distal end.

[184] Jackson 1895b, p.394.

[185] 'I imagine that the corpora quadrigemina are superior centres of the lowest level ...' (Jackson 1895c, p.478).

[186] Jackson 1895b, p.394, footnote 4. Since the neuron theory was instantiated by Cajal, Waldeyer et al. in 1891 (see Shepherd 1991, pp.177–193, and Definition Section 1 in Chapter 3), I wonder if that is what Jackson had in mind here in 1895.

[187] Jackson 1895b, p.395.

[188] Jackson 1895c, p.478; Jackson's italics and parentheses. His use of Spencer's 'menial' and 'industrial' is repeated from his ideas about representation of the heart (Jackson 1887m); see Chapter 11. By the end of the nineteenth century, Spencer 'no longer attracted sophisticated readers' (Francis 2007, p.329).

[189] About this effort, Jackson (Jackson 1897a, p.19, footnote 6) said: 'We should have a scheme of the lowest level so that in fracture-dislocation cases and in other cases we might be helped in our analyses of the complex symptomatologies produced. I have made such a scheme, but it is too poor a thing to publish.'

[190] Jackson 1896a, p.1662. The 'X-ray' was invented by Wilhelm Roentgen in 1895, so in 1896 the location of *spinal fractures* was generally known only from autopsies. *Cervical spinal cord injuries* cause paralysis of intercostal muscles. In addition, the phrenic nerves that innervate the diaphragm originate from the spinal cord at the C4 level. Therefore spinal cord transections at and above the C4 level cause nearly total cessation of respiration and death.

systems', thermal, circulatory, respiratory, and digestive. All are affected by cervical cord injuries, and he added a fifth, 'Sexual system, priapism'.[191] In his next Fragment he postulated a crush injury of the cord at C5 and then analyzed its sequelae.[192] In these exhaustive discussions Jackson cited the literature widely. Nonetheless, he expressed a sense of falling behind in his knowledge of rapidly advancing biomedical science.

> For the proper analysis of so complex a symptomatology, a vastly greater knowledge of physiology than I possess is required ... If the symptomatology of the cervical fracture-dislocation case were thoroughly and correctly analysed a valuable contribution would be made to neurology. Were it right to suggest work for other people to do, I would commend the study of this complex neurological problem to well-trained physiologists.[193]

The Hughlings Jackson Lecture, December 1897

When the Neurological Society was founded in 1886 it was an immediate success. A decade later, 'On 15th October 1897, at a meeting of the Neurological Society and at the suggestion of Dr. W.S. Colman, it was decided to institute a Hughlings Jackson Lecture, to be delivered every three years, and that Jackson himself should be invited to give the first of these addresses'.[194] Colman's motivation was the example of the Bowman Lecture at the Ophthalmological Society.[195]

Jackson's inaugural Hughlings Jackson Lecture was delivered on December 8, 1897, 'On the Relations of Different Divisions of the Central Nervous System to One Another and to Parts of the Body'. It was published in the *BMJ* (short version) and *The Lancet* (long version).[196] I think he viewed the Lecture as an opportunity to consolidate his legacy, but that does not mean there were no new elements in it. There were clarifications that furthered older ideas, as well as acknowledgments of uncertainties. To set the stage he said, 'I divide the central nervous system into two Sub-systems – Cerebral and Cerebellar. The two have ... the Lowest Level in common ...'[197] This was followed by an anatomical definition that repeated his parameters of the lowest level from 1895,[198] but he added: 'There are also Superior levels of the lowest level itself ...'[199] This idea of 'Superior levels' within levels recalls Jackson's earlier idea of 'layers' within the highest centers.[200]

---

[191] Jackson 1896a, p.1663. Priapism is sometimes seen in acute cervical spinal cord injuries.
[192] Jackson 1897a, pp.19–23; the respiratory system was omitted and the sexual was included.
[193] Jackson 1897a, pp.19–20.
[194] Critchley and Critchley 1998, p.158; also Hunting 2002, p.264, and Casper 2014, p.45. Walter S. Colman was appointed Registrar and Pathologist at Queen Square in 1889 and again to both positions in 1893. He was appointed Physician in 1896 but he resigned in 1898 to join the staff at St. Thomas's Hospital. See Holmes 1954, pp.96 and 98; also [Colman] 1934.
[195] Casper 2014, pp.45 and 199, note 82. When the Society was amalgamated into the Royal Society of Medicine in 1907 it became the Section of Neurology (now Clinical Neurosciences), which has maintained the triennial Hughlings Jackson Lecture; see also Hunting 2002, pp.263–265.
[196] Jackson 1898a (*Lancet*) and Jackson 1898b (*BMJ*). The *BMJ*'s version must have been the report of Jackson's original presentation, because the *Lancet*'s version was twice the length of the *BMJ*'s. Jackson 1898a is reprinted in his *Selected Writings* (Jackson 1932, vol.2, pp.422–443), but Jackson 1898b is not. York and Steinberg 2006, p.131 (in ID column) describe Jackson 1898b in the *Selected Writings* with the same volume and page numbers as Jackson 1898a; apparently they assumed that the texts are the same.
[197] Jackson 1898b, p.65; my underlining.
[198] Jackson 1895b, p.394; see above in this section.
[199] Jackson 1898b, p.65; my square brackets.
[200] Jackson 1884d, p.660; and see Chapter 10.

Going on to the middle and highest levels, Jackson added a caveat on the sensory side: 'I have formerly spoken of the occipital lobes as the highest sensory centres of the cerebral sub-system, but I now find it difficult to conclude with any confidence as to what are the sensory provinces of the middle and highest levels of this sub-system.'[201] He had expressed similar reservations in 1887,[202] and it is important to remember that Ferrier was having difficulties with the auditory and visual systems.[203] Also, although cerebellar function was not well understood, there was an extensive comparison and contrast of cerebral versus cerebellar clinical phenomena.[204] In this Jackson assumed a state of normal antagonism between the cerebrum and the cerebellum, based on his conception of how each represents its corresponding body parts.

> I have now to restate an old hypothesis on dynamical relations of the two Sub systems by intermediation of motor centres of the lowest level. Speaking very roughly ... the cerebellum represents movements of the skeletal muscles in the order trunk, leg, arm, preponderatingly extensor-wise; the cerebrum represents movements of the same muscles in the order arm, leg, trunk, preponderatingly flexor-wise. [205]

This idea was derived from Jackson's observation that midline cerebellar lesions can be associated with abnormal truncal movements, which he interpreted as epileptic. He theorized that motor integration is achieved by interactions of the two systems, thus leading to explanations of pathological conditions. In hemiplegia 'there is cerebellar, "influx" into the parts which the cerebrum *has abandoned*'.[206] He had been trending toward this way of thinking for a long time,[207] and the same was true of his '*Scale of Fits*', which was clearly expressed in this Lecture: 'There are ... Lowest Level Fits, Middle Level [epileptiform] Fits ... and Highest Level Fits (so-called idiopathic epilepsy)[17]'. In the lowest level there are 'ponto-bulbar' fits,[208] and Jackson's footnote 17 raised another uncertainty.

> [17] I do not say that all fits *called* epileptic (so-called idiopathic) are owing to discharge-lesions of parts of the highest level. There are seizures *called* epileptic depending on discharges beginning in parts of the temporo-sphenoidal lobe; convolutions of these lobes may not be parts of the highest level.[209]

After this statement about the temporal lobe as a source of 'genuine' epileptic seizures, Jackson turned to the four factors in Spencerian evolution, which he had already explained in 1885.[210] This was background for his further discussion of the Scale of Fits: 'I now attempt a comparison and contrast between middle level and highest level fits as depending on discharges of levels of the cerebral sub-system of different evolutionary grades', but 'I have nothing to say as to the comparison and contrast of lowest level with middle level fits'. The

[201] Jackson 1898b, p.65.
[202] Critchley and Critchley 1998, pp.58–59. They refer to Jackson 1887e, pp.30–31, where he cited Gowers 1885, pp.22 and 74, which were parts of Gowers' discussions of the visual system.
[203] See Glickstein 1985; Heffner 1987; and Fishman 1995.
[204] Jackson 1898a, pp.80–81.
[205] Jackson 1898b, p.65.
[206] Jackson 1898b, p.65; Jackson's italics.
[207] In Jackson 1888e, pp.182–183, footnote 2, Jackson discussed 'three 'classes' of fits.
[208] Jackson 1898a, p.82; Jackson's italics and parentheses, my square brackets.
[209] Jackson 1898a, p.82; Jackson's italics and parentheses.
[210] Jackson 1898a, pp.82–83 (also Jackson 1898b, p.67), referring to Jackson 1885f, p.945.

'Rolandic' localization of epileptiform seizures was well settled, he said, but he was thinking about localization of epileptic seizures in the prefrontal cortices: 'Highest level fits are those of the so-called idiopathic epilepsy ... they are "ordinary epileptic fits;" I suppose that most of these seizures depend on a discharge-lesion of some part of the præ-frontal lobe ... of one half of the brain.'[211] Regarding epileptiform and epileptic seizures:

> The two kinds of fits are examples of *Dissolution being effected*. I submit that the differences in the paroxysms of the two kinds are such as might be expected if the evolutionary differences between ... the motor province of the middle level and that of the highest level are such as were suggested when the Process of Evolution was considered ... it is an error to suppose that an epileptiform seizure at first partial has, when become universal, "turned into" an epileptic seizure.[212]

So the principle is that the classification of a seizure is determined by its characteristics at its onset, not by manifestations later in its course. On the other hand:

> In accord with the foregoing hypothesis is the fact that the difference between the two kinds of fits is not absolute ... a very rapidly developing epileptiform seizure approaches an epileptic fit in character and ... a very slowly developed epileptic fit approaches an epileptiform seizure in character; if so the hypothesis is further supported.[213]

But the question is, which hypothesis? It's not entirely clear, but I think he meant the idea of a common pathophysiology for all epileptic seizures: 'I suppose that in cases of epilepsy and of epileptiform seizures there is a very local discharge-lesion ... of a few highly unstable cells of one half of the brain.'[214] Then something truly new appeared. Beginning with some remarks about phantom limb, he brought up a question about the physiology of dreams: 'In this connexion I draw attention to a very interesting paper by Mr. F.H. Bradley ... [who] asks: "Why, when we strive to move in dreams do we not always move?" Perhaps this inability accords with the hypothesis that large movements (those especially engaged in locomotion) are but little represented in the highest level ("mental centres") ...'[215]

Francis Herbert Bradley (1846–1924) was a Hegelian philosopher at Oxford, who had criticized the association psychology.[216] In effect, Jackson was offering an empiricist answer to Bradley's interesting question.

> I believe the physical side of this inability to act in a dream is partly because locomotor movements ... of large muscles, are little represented in the highest level and partly because the discharges of the highest level corresponding to the ideation of the dreamer (incipient action) are not strong enough to overcome the resistance of the motor centres of the middle level; when they become strong enough to do so the patient awakes, or perhaps there is somnambulism.[217]

---

[211] Jackson 1898a, p.83.
[212] Jackson 1898a, p.83; Jackson's italics.
[213] Jackson 1898a, p.83; my underlining.
[214] Jackson 1898a, p.83; my underlining.
[215] Jackson 1898a, p.86; Jackson's parentheses, my square brackets. The title in Jackson's citation to Bradley 1894 says 'Dreams', but in the actual article it is singular, 'Dream'.
[216] www.britannica.com/biography/F-H-Bradley, accessed September 27, 2018.
[217] Jackson 1898a, p.86; Jackson's parentheses.

Regarding dreams, Jackson went on to compare their concomitant physiological discharges with those of epileptic seizures and elaborate postictal actions.

> When speaking of dreams we are dealing with … normal discharges of nervous elements perhaps <u>slightly greater than in waking</u>; when speaking of an epileptic paroxysm we are dealing with a *suddenly occurring* and *excessive* discharge beginning in *part* of the highest level … *After* an epileptic fit there may be elaborate actions and these result … from discharges that are very much slighter in degree than the excessive discharges productive of the prior paroxysm …[218]

This implies a hierarchy of heightened discharges: (1) in dreams the normal discharges are only slightly exaggerated and unable to overcome the resistance of lower levels; (2) in postictal complex behaviors the discharges are greater than in normal dreams, so they overcome the resistance of lower centers; and (3) in major convulsions the discharges are overwhelming. Thus, Jackson thought that truly epileptic discharges must be overwhelming by definition. This expansion of his pathophysiological framework for epileptic seizures in 1898 was directly relevant to his contemporaneous thoughts about the dreamy state.

Localizing the Dreamy State, Part 2, 1894–1900

In Part 1, covering 1874–1889, we saw that Jackson was searching for evidence that the dreamy state could be localized to the medial temporal lobe and to the uncus in particular. His hunch was based on Ferrier's experimental induction of gustatory phenomena from stimulation of homologous areas in monkeys.[219] In a survey of the titles of Jackson's writings from November 1889 through 1897[220] it appears that the dreamy state was on his back burner during that entire period, but the reality was more complicated. The 'back burner' does appear to be true for 1890 through 1893. However, the dreamy state was very much on his mind in *January 1894*, when *Quærens died and came to autopsy*. Although the report was not published until January 1899 or later,[221] the postmortem findings would have been resonating in Jackson's mind while he was otherwise focused mainly on the lowest level in 1894–1897. Accordingly, I will discuss the postmortem findings as of 1894, using Jackson's name for the patient, 'Z'.[222]

---

[218] Jackson 1898a, p.86; Jackson's italics, my underlining. On slightly raised discharges see also Jackson 1885f, p.946.

[219] Jackson gave no detailed citations to Ferrier for this—only Ferrier's name. Apparently he assumed that his audience would know whereof he spoke, because Ferrier's Croonian Lectures to the Royal College of Physicians were published in the *BMJ* (Ferrier 1890) and as a book (Ferrier 1890a). These Croonians are not to be confused with Ferrier's Croonian at the Royal Society (Ferrier 1875c); see Chapter 8.

[220] York and Steinberg 2006, pp.119–130.

[221] York and Steinberg 2006, p.131, list Jackson 1898c as published in 1898, which is the date on the title page of that volume (21) of *Brain*. However, on p.586 of Jackson 1898c, referring to Jackson 1899a, Jackson said, 'In the *Lancet*, January, 14, 1899, I published a note …' Therefore Jackson 1898c was actually published in or after January 1899.

[222] There are *three names for the same person*: (1) Quærens, (2) Jackson's Z, and (3) A.T. Myers. About Jackson's Z see Jackson 1898c, p.580, footnote 2, which cites Jackson 1888e, p.200, *et seq*. In 1980 Taylor and Marsh identified Quærens/Z as Arthur Thomas Myers (1851–1894). Taylor and Marsh 1980 and the Critchleys 1998 use 'Dr Z'. I've not seen 'Dr Z' in Jackson's writings, although he may have used it informally. The Critchleys misspell Myers as 'Meyers'.

The Lesion in the Brain of Z (Quærens), January 1894

Z's death and autopsy occurred in the home of his physician, Dawtrey Drewitt (1848–1942), who was Jackson's neighbor in Manchester Square.[223] Responsibility for performing the autopsy fell to Walter Colman, who was then both Registrar and Pathologist to the National Hospital.[224] Before the autopsy Jackson 'begged Dr. Colman to call on me before he went to make the necropsy on Z, in order to ask him to search the taste region of Ferrier on each half of the brain ... Dr. Colman ... found a very small focus of softening in that region (in the uncinate gyrus) of the left half of the brain'.[225] About this Colman said:

> ... in the left uncinate gyrus ... there was a patch of softening beneath the surface ...
> [Fig. 12.1] ... it was found to be a small cavity ... with indefinite walls, situated in the uncinate gyrus ... below the surface just in front of the curved tip of the uncus ... The existence of the patch and its position were verified in the fresh specimen by Dr. Hughlings Jackson, Dr. Dawtrey Drewitt, Dr. James Taylor, and Dr. Guy Wood. The cavity was like those seen long after softening from thrombosis or embolism.[226]

Colman searched for evidence of vascular disease but found none. Moreover, 'the uncinate region became so soft and friable during the hardening process that it was impossible to make satisfactory sections, and the microscope did not throw any further light on the cause of the lesion'.[227] Nonetheless, for Jackson Z was the crucial case that validated his idea about localization of the dreamy state in the uncus—there was no other lesion to explain it. As usual, he applied his new knowledge slowly and carefully—there was, after all, only one validating case.

Two Complex Cases Without Autopsies, July–August 1894

In July–August 1894—half a year after he knew about Z's lesion—Jackson reported two clinical cases with complex epileptic phenomena.[228] They shared many features, including: 'an auditory warning; in slight seizures the special imperceptions called "word-deafness" (Wernicke) and "word-blindness" (Kussmaul); inability to speak and spectral words ...'[229] In our terms, both patients were experiencing ictal Wernicke's aphasia and alexia, and each one also had some unique features. In the July report of the first patient *déjà vu* was described but not named. Jackson localized that patient's focus to 'some part of the [cortical] auditory centre of Ferrier and of that part alone ...'[230] Nothing was said about the uncus in either report. About the second patient Jackson lamented: 'This case is a very

---

[223] Taylor and Marsh 1980, p.765. On Drewitt see [Drewitt, F. Dawtrey] 1942.

[224] See Holmes 1954, pp.96 and 98; also [Colman] 1934, and above in this chapter.

[225] Jackson 1898c, p.586; Jackson's parentheses.

[226] Jackson 1898c, pp.587–589; my square brackets and underlining. Guy Wood 'was then Jackson's house physician at Queen Square' (Taylor and Marsh 1980, p.764).

[227] Jackson 1898c, p.589.

[228] Jackson 1894l (July) and Jackson 1894m (August). My discussion will commingle them. In both he gave further details of the patient reported earlier in Jackson 1888e, pp.191–193.

[229] Jackson 1894m, p.252; Jackson's parentheses. On Kussmaul's role in the history of alexia see Henderson 2010, p.589.

[230] Jackson 1894l, p.182; my square brackets. On 'Ferrier and the study of auditory cortex' see Heffner 1987.

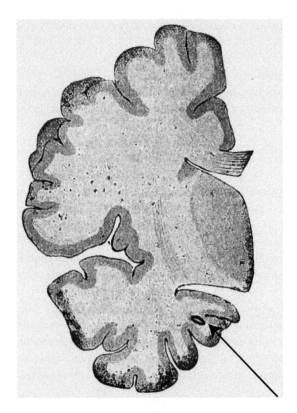

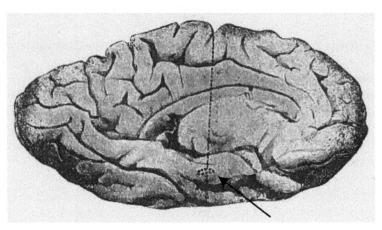

Fig. 12.1 Case of epilepsy with tasting movements and 'dreamy state'—very small patch of softening in the left uncinate gyrus. (Patient Z in Jackson 1898c, p.588, Figs 1 and 2.) Medial surface (lower) and coronal slice (upper) of left hemisphere. Arrows point to the small lesion in each view. The vertical dotted line in part *a* shows the plane of the coronal slice for *b*.

(Reproduced from Brain, Case of epilepsy with tasting movements and "dreamy state"–very small patch of softening in the left uncinate gyrus. 21:580–590, 1898.) [98-03]

complicated one. For the present I refrain from an attempt to analyse its symptomatology.'[231] He had even tried an unorthodox approach.

> Those who have <u>pondered</u> over <u>diagrams</u> intended to illustrate the cerebral mechanism of speaking, reading, and writing, and of reception of the speech of others will see what is here meant. Probably in this case several of the phenomena mentioned were the after-effects of the discharge ...[232]

To understand the significance of 'diagrams' a little fast-forwarding is in order. We have been dealing with events in 1894. In 1906 the Parisian neurologist Pierre Marie (1853–1940) launched a full-blown attack on those who tried to analyze brain-based behavioral syndromes by constructing diagrams of cerebral centers and their connecting tracts,[233] thus to explain the production of normal 'speaking, reading, and writing, and of reception of the speech of others ...' Then they postulated lesions in those circuits, and the resulting models predicted many details of actual clinical syndromes. Marie's counterpart in Britain was Jackson's disciple <u>Henry Head</u>, the archetypical holist. He used 'diagram-makers' as a pejorative.[234] Head claimed that Jackson was the embodiment of holism, although Jackson always tried to be neutral about such things.

With that background, Jackson's remark about 'diagrams' can be seen as his indication of possible credibility for the diagram-makers, who were represented by Bastian. On the other hand, Jackson said 'pondered', which does not indicate finality. If he had found diagrams to be satisfying he would have said so, but he did not want to delegitimatize them. They might be useful.

The 'Uncinate Group of Fits', 1894–1899

Fast-forward again.[235] In the mid-twentieth century the international epileptology community was intensely interested in temporal lobe epilepsy (TLE), whose clinical phenomena were largely but not entirely localized to the temporal lobe.[236] Other names for it were 'psychomotor' seizures and 'limbic' seizures.[237] To Jackson goes much of the credit for the recognition of that common form of epilepsy. That is why the lesions in Z and the others now loom so large. Jackson's name for this heterogeneous syndrome was 'Uncinate Group of epileptic fits'. Presumably he began to use that term informally *circa* 1894, but its first published appearance was in *The Lancet* of January 14, 1899.[238]

In the 4 years from September 1894 through 1898 Jackson published only one paper on epilepsy, and that was about another physician's old case from 1874.[239] In 1899, after his

---

[231] Jackson 1894m, p.253.
[232] Jackson 1894l, p.182; my underlining.
[233] See Lebrun 1994; and Clarac and Boller 2010.
[234] See Jacyna 2008, pp.137–138; and Eling and Whitaker 2010, pp.578–579.
[235] Jackson 1900a was an editorial report about Jackson 1899c in *The Lancet*, February 17, 1900.
[236] See Thornton 1976, p.36: 'Temporal lobe epilepsy became the subject of great international congresses in the fifties when neurologists from all over the world gathered to discuss this new form of epilepsy.' It was new only in the sense of having been ignored.
[237] See Engel 2013, pp.14–17.
[238] Jackson 1899a, p.79; also in *Brain* of the same year, Jackson 1899c, p.538.
[239] Jackson 1895a. Recall that Jackson 1898c was actually published in or after January 1899. Jackson's second author on Jackson 1898c was 'Purves Stewart ... *Assistant-Physician to the Westminster Hospital*'. James Purves-Stewart (1869–1949) was 'a resident house-physician at the National Hospital for Nervous Diseases', 1897–1899; see [Stewart, J.P.] 1949.

introduction of 'Uncinate Group', he began to struggle with its boundaries, which were not easily defined. He signaled his intention to do something about the unsatisfactory state of its semiology when he said, 'I hope soon to be able to write more fully on the uncinate group of epileptic fits. I shall then consider exceptions ... and shall re-enquire particularly as to the relation in slight epileptic paroxysms of crude auditory sensations to the dreamy state.'[240] Unfortunately, it never happened, presumably due to illness.

This paper of 1899 was Jackson's last publication on the uncinate group. To the end he remained discomfited by uncertainties about the dreamy state and the uncus. About this he said, 'the dreamy state does not occur in the paroxysms of every case of the uncinate group, and ... [it] may ... occur ... without the chewing, &c., movements.'[241] From there he extended his perspective to point out the biological system to which the crude sensations are related: 'much of the symptomatology of uncinate fits refers very especially to the <u>digestive system</u>; the crude sensations, smell, taste, and the epigastric sensation are ... developments of "digestive sensations".'[242] Another way to approach it was from the psychical side of concomitance, although he did not say it exactly that way.

It is quite evident that in ... slight epileptic paroxysms ... there is a kind of double consciousness – a "mental diplopia" ... I think, too, that there is probably some defect of consciousness in every paroxysm with the dreamy state ... The psychical condition, therefore, is a very complex one. There is defect of consciousness, so far negatively. Positively, there is (1) the quasi-parasitical state of consciousness (dreamy state), and (2) there are remains of normal consciousness; and thus (1 and 2) there is double consciousness. To discover the physical conditions correlative with this complex psychical condition is a very complex task.[243]

The rub is in the final sentence. Albeit incomplete, Jackson did leave us some last thoughts about the complex 'physical conditions' associated with the uncinate group. His patient 'A.B.' was a physician who had a crude sensation of smell and a dreamy state.[244] Jackson and Gowers suspected 'tumour, of one temporo-sphenoidal lobe', but surgery was not advised, and 'necropsy was not permitted'.[245] Jackson said that he had

... suggested for these cases the name of Uncinate Group of Fits ... on the hypothesis that the discharge-lesions in these cases are made up ... not of the uncinate gyrus alone, but of some cells of different parts of a region of which this gyrus is part ... In cases of this group there is at the onset ... a crude sensation of smell, or one of taste, or there are movements of chewing, smacking of the lips, &c.... In some cases ... there is a warning by ... epigastric sensation ... Different varieties of this group of cases depend ... on discharge-lesions of different parts of ... the uncinate region ... it is supposed that especially in this cortical region, not confined to this region, are the physical bases of some of the systemic sensations ... especially ... to the digestive system.[246]

---

[240] Jackson 1899c, p.539.

[241] Jackson 1899c, p.539, footnote 1; my square brackets.

[242] Jackson 1899c, p.541; my underlining.

[243] Jackson 1899c, p.540; on pp.541–545 Jackson quoted extensively in the original French from case descriptions by Théodore Herpin (1799–1865), saying: 'I have long known his valuable work, *Du Pronostic et du Traitement Curatif de l'Epilepsie*, 1852, but I have only recently heard of his still more valuable work, *Des Accès Incomplets d'Epilepsie*, 1867.' On Herpin see Temkin 1971, pp.324–327; and Eadie 2002.

[244] Jackson 1899c, pp.534–535.

[245] Jackson 1899c, p.538. Here 'tumour' was generic for mass lesion.

[246] Jackson 1899c, pp.538–539.

In the last part of this passage Jackson made a clear statement to the effect that cerebral areas beyond the uncinate region are involved in the uncinate group, but those outlying areas were not specified. And there the matter rested—at least, that was as far as Hughlings Jackson could take it. In his last years, however, he did produce some further thoughts about lowest level fits.

The Last Years, 1900–1911

With the turn of the new century Jackson turned 65. We have already seen that he retired from the active staff of the London at age 60. At Queen Square, in 1900 Jackson and Buzzard were 'appointed consulting physicians, and as they had been associated with the Hospital since its early days each was requested to continue the care of ten beds',[247] which allowed them to continue teaching. Apparently Jackson did so for at least a few more years, but his deafness progressed and his health deteriorated. He resigned from the active staff in 1906.[248] After 1899 his rate of publication diminished, although he continued to produce one or two papers in some years. One of his publications in 1900 was unusual because it was not clinical or theoretical. It was related to other, uncomfortable professional matters.

Revolt of the Medical Staff of the National Hospital, August 1900

Long before 1900 there was escalating tension between the medical staff and the Board of Management of the National Hospital, but in 1900 it came to a head. The Board was represented by the secretary-director B. Burford Rawlings (1840–1916). He had come to Queen Square in 1866, at the ripe old age of 26, when the Hospital was in its seventh year of existence. That he was efficient and effective was not disputed, but neither was the fact of his autocratic outlook. Sometimes he admitted or discharged patients without consulting the responsible staff. For those and other reasons the medical staff asked for two seats (of 12) on the Board of Management, which was the general practice at most other metropolitan hospitals. This was repeatedly refused. At one point the entire medical staff were 'prepared to resign in a body'.[249]

All of this spilled into public view on July 27, 1900, when *The Times* of London published an item about it, including direct quotations from medical staff communications to the Board and Rawling's tart reply.[250] On August 4 *The Lancet* carried a long letter-to-the-editors that set out the staff's position,[251] concluding with the 'desire only to reaffirm our view that the affairs of the hospital need a searching inquiry and its constitution thorough reform. We are unanimous in our resolve to put an end to the evils of the present system of administration.'[252] Since Jackson's name was listed *first* among 18 signatories, we can assume that

---

[247] Holmes 1954, p.46.

[248] Holmes 1954, p.96.

[249] Holmes 1954, pp.43–45. Since Holmes 'came to the National Hospital … as a junior house officer in 1902 …' ([Holmes] 1966), he would have experienced the immediate aftermath of the controversy. See also Shorvon et al. 2019, pp.43–50.

[250] 'National Hospital For Paralyzed and Epileptic.' *The Times* [London, England] July 27, 1900:10. *The Times Digital Archive*, accessed March 25, 2018.

[251] Jackson 1900b.

[252] Jackson 1900b, p.352.

he agreed about the 'evils'. It is important to note that the order of the signatures was not alphabetical. It was by seniority of appointment, so Jackson and Buzzard were listed first as Consulting Physicians. As portrayed by Ferrier, this was the time when Buzzard's Nestorian qualities were 'exhibited in striking manner in the long-continued dissensions which occurred ... between the medical staff and the then board of management. It was largely owing to Buzzard's judicious leadership, aided by the skilful advocacy of Dr. Ormerod, that the staff triumphed and harmony was established. Buzzard had a quiet, genial manner and catholic sympathies.'[253]

Buzzard's 'genial manner' notwithstanding, the letter to *The Lancet* contained some strong language—much more than Jackson ordinarily used. Eventually, 'in 1901 a commission appointed by the governors ... issued their report. This led to the resignation of the Board and the retirement of the secretary-director.'[254] In Jackson's medical writings of this period there was no hint of those difficulties. Nor was there any notice of Queen Victoria's death in 1901 and the ascension of Edward VII, bringing Britain and the world into the Edwardian era. Medical politics aside, his attention was on an unsettled part of his paradigm for seizures and epilepsy

Back to Lowest Level Fits: Respiratory Movements, Normal and Abnormal, 1899 and 1902

In Chapter 11 we saw that in the 1880s Jackson returned to the idea that some seizures could arise from foci in the lowest level. For many years previously he had thought that they are always cortical. In accordance with his own principles, if lowest level fits were to be diagnosed it would have to be done by finding the foci through clinical observation of initial symptoms. From 1886 through 1899 the symptoms that he tried to recruit for this purpose were mainly patterns of respiratory movements, normal and abnormal. No surprise, it turned out to be difficult. In 1902 he complained that 'The state of the respiratory apparatus in "epileptic" paroxysms has received little special attention ...'[255] He pointed out that he had previously suggested that

> ... besides what are commonly called epileptic fits, there occur ... bulbo-pontal (lowest level) fits, analogous to those experimentally produced in some lower mammals ... it is ... particularly important to note where the first spasm is, or what the very first symptoms are. Are there seizures, such as would be commonly called epileptic, which *begin by* fixation of the chest, or in which the chest is involved before the limbs ... or ... more generally, are there fits which begin by convulsion of respiratory muscles?[256]

Table 12.2 is an overview of Jackson's efforts to understand epileptic respiratory patterns. It starts with laryngismus stridulus as 'respiratory convulsions' because that appears to be what aroused his renewed interest in lowest level fits in the 1880s. Since many of the earlier

---

[253] Ferrier 1919, p.59. Joseph A. Ormerod (1848–1925) was assistant physician to the National Hospital 1880–1900 and physician 1900–1913 (Brown 1955, p.304).

[254] Holmes 1954, p.45; see also Shorvon et al. 2018, pp.43–50.

[255] Jackson 1902b, p.122.

[256] Jackson 1902b, pp.122–123.

Table 12.2 Jackson's writings on respiratory phenomena in the lowest level, 1886–1902.

Month/year	Main subject	Respiratory detail	Citation
April 1886	Laryngismus stridulus	'Respiratory convulsions'	Jackson 1886b, pp.1–2
March 1890	Lowest (ponto-bulbar) level	'Respiratory fits'	Jackson 1890c, p.705
February 1895	Lowest level/tabes	Respiration as one of the 'organic' duties	Jackson 1895b, p.395
February 1895	Lowest level	Control of normal respiration	Jackson 1895c
January 1897	Cord injury	'Inefficient respiration'	Jackson 1897a, pp.18, 22[a]
January 1899	Asphyxia in slight fits	Cortical respiratory arrest center	Jackson 1899a
December 1899	Hemiplegia	Asymmetrical chest movements	Jackson 1899b
Brain 1899	Anesthesia and recovery	Intercostals vs. diaphragm	Jackson 1899d
March 1902	Laryngeal crises in tabes	Crises are epileptic	Jackson 1902a
Brain 1902	Trunk seizures	Case of lowest level fits	Jackson 1902b
Brain 1902	Trunk seizures (continued from Jackson 1902b)	Same	Jackson 1902c

[a] This is a continuation of Jackson 1896a, where the subject of cord injury was first raised.

items in the table have already been discussed I will comment mainly on those published after 1897.

The idea of a cortical respiratory 'arrest centre' was proposed in 1894 by the surgeon Walter George Spencer (1858–1940), who had worked with Horsley at the Brown Institution.[257] There was a tie-in to Jackson's interest in uncinate fits. As quoted by Jackson, Spencer said: 'It has ... been shown that the respiration can be slowed and arrested by excitation of a certain spot and a limited area around it. This spot is situated ... to the outer side of the olfactory tract just in front of the junction of the tract with the uncinate.'[258] About this proposed 'arrest' area, Jackson said, 'I presume that the arrest is by great cortical inhibition of the respiratory (medulla) centre...'[259]

In his pursuit of information about respiratory patterns Jackson enlisted assistance from several colleagues. In his later years his coauthors often were his juniors. However, in the Fragments he never listed other authors, although he mentioned people who had given assistance. An example is Fragment XIX, where he tried to find side-to-side asymmetries of respiratory movements in hemiplegic patients, but he had to admit that the differences were 'trifling, sometimes trivial'.[260] In the text he mentioned having evaluated '28 cases of old

---

[257] Spencer, W.G. 1894. See also [Spencer, W.G.] 1940; and Power and Lefanu 1953, pp.730–732. There is no statement that Horsley took any part in this work, although he communicated it to the Royal Society on January 5, 1894, and probably he did contribute to it.

[258] Jackson 1899a, p.79, wherein Jackson quoted W.G. Spencer 1894, p.629.

[259] Jackson 1899a, p.79; Jackson's parentheses.

[260] Jackson 1899b, p.1660.

hemiplegia' with the assistance of Dr. W.H. Stoddart.[261] About this, in a previous Fragment of 1895, he had said, 'Most of the observations were made by Dr. Stoddart'.[262]

By contrast, in an article in *Brain* in 1899 about 'loss of movements of the intercostal muscles in some cases of surgical anæsthesia ...', Jackson named his second author, James S. Collier (1870–1935).[263] In this paper he was trying to understand the physiological difference between ordinary, brainstem-mediated breathing versus 'voluntary' chest movements, which presumably are mediated at cortical levels. That is, 'drawing in the breath prior to vocalization is a "voluntary"... cerebral movement ...'.[264] Thus he 'suggested to Dr. Collier a further research on the respiratory condition during anesthesia by ether and chloroform'. Collier said that he had 'examined the respiratory movements in sixty patients, before and during the administration of anæsthetics for surgical purposes'. His findings were detailed but not otherwise significant.[265]

After a few years' interval, in 1902 Jackson returned to the lowest level with a discussion of laryngeal crises in tabetics, which he interpreted as epileptic. In that condition there is abductor paralysis of one or both vocal cords, leaving the cords closed or nearly so. Here the unstated logic was: since there is medullary representation of adductors, which are unrestrained, there can be abnormal discharges from that center. By Jackson's definition such centers are epileptic or at least epileptiform.[266] He was combining substantive physiological data (innervation and normal activity of vocal cord muscles) with a supposition about their abnormal actions in tabetic crises. To strengthen his pathophysiology, he prevailed upon Horsley to do some experiments.

> Mr. Victor Horsley was so good as to make for me some experiments ... on the condition of the vocal cords during artificially produced asphyxia ... It is of importance with regard to the asphyxia occurring in severe laryngeal crises to know what goes on in the larynx in the asphyxia of otherwise healthy animals in which abductor as well as adductor movements of the cords are possible.[267]

For Jackson the significant point was that, 'In the [normal] animals ... the abductor muscles and their centres were intact and thus there was inspiratory activity of the vocal cords in asphyxia, a thing impossible in the asphyxia of a tabetic with paralysis of the abductors'.[268] In tabetic laryngeal crises with asphyxia,

> The limbs are, it is said, convulsed in some severe attacks. But perhaps in some of these attacks there occur only writhings of the limbs as an indirect consequence of arrest of respiration; these writhings ... ought not to be confounded with convulsion proper ... If the limbs were the subject of such an intense discharge as produces convulsion there could not

---

[261] Jackson 1899b, p.1659. William Henry Butter Stoddart (1868–1950) was a junior house officer at Queen Square *circa* 1895; he became a prominent psychiatrist (Brown 1955, p.495).

[262] Jackson 1895c, p.477.

[263] Jackson 1899d. Collier was a house officer at Queen Square *circa* 1895, registrar in 1899, and assistant physician in 1902 (Brown 1955, p.446).

[264] Jackson 1899d, p.552.

[265] Jackson 1899d, p.556; on pp.560–562 they thanked Risien Russell for performing similar experiments on animals, again with marginally significant results.

[266] Jackson 1902a, pp.727–728. He cited some French authors in agreement, including Charcot.

[267] Jackson 1902a, p.730.

[268] Jackson 1902a, p.730; my square brackets

be movements even so little elaborate as those of writhing: there would be tonic or clonic spasm ... and not movements properly so called.[269]

So the idea of an epileptic focus in tabetic laryngeal crises was called into question. The reasoning in the last sentence of this passage was from purely theoretical premises, but it was the best he could do. He had no EEG. The basic question—are laryngeal crises epileptic?—remained unanswered. And that same state of uncertainty plagued his other efforts to define lowest level fits. Of course, he kept trying. In successive issues of *Brain* in 1902, and in conjunction with two younger colleagues, he published two extensive reports about the two admissions of a 17-year-old girl who had two episodes of apparently symmetrical status epilepticus of the neck and trunk muscles bilaterally. About the patient's 'severe fits', he asked the crucial question:

Where is the lesion ... which, on its occasional 'intense' discharge, produces a convulsion *beginning* in the muscles of the trunk (that is, in muscles of two sides of the body, the normal action of which may be and often is bilateral) and beginning in those muscles of the two sides of the body simultaneously ...[?][270]

Jackson's coauthors in the two reports were H. Douglas Singer (1875–1940) and Arthur Stanley Barnes (1881–1956), respectively.[271] Both papers contained information from both admissions. There were significant findings, but not about laterality. 'The first change observed in these attacks was a sudden and complete fixation of the thorax with arrest of all respiratory movement ...'. Most significant was '*the order in which the muscles of the arms were involved* [which] *was from the large thoraco-humeral muscles to the smaller forearm and hand muscles*'.[272] In the second episode 'the limbs were affected, but after the trunk; Dr. Barnes carefully describes a "march" of the spasm *down* the arms ...'.[273] In the end, Jackson said cautiously, 'I think now, considering especially the observations Dr. Stanley Barnes made on the "inspiratory cry" in a certain part of the march of some of the patient's attacks, that her fits are probably Lowest Level (Ponto-Bulbar) Fits and not fits of ordinary Epilepsy (Higher Level Fits)'.[274] And there the matter rested in 1902, never to be further resolved by Jackson.

Midline Cerebellar Tumors Revisited, 1906

The fact that Jackson published nothing in 1904 and 1905 was probably due to his worsening health status, but if so he rallied somewhat in 1906. In the last part of *Brain* for that year there was a special message: 'This number of 'Brain' is dedicated as a tribute of respect and affection to John Hughlings Jackson, M.D., F.R.S., on the 50th year of his medical practice

---

[269] Jackson 1902a, p.731.

[270] Jackson 1902b, p.124; Jackson's parentheses, my square brackets. Krumholz et al. 1994 have suggested that Jackson was actually seeing myoclonic phenomena, which were not then understood as such.

[271] Jackson 1902b. Singer had 'three years' post-graduate training under Hughlings Jackson and Sir Richard Gowers at the National Hospital' (Trail 1968, p.381). He became a prominent American psychiatrist. In 1901–1903 Barnes 'was resident medical officer at the National Hospital ...' He became a prominent neurologist in Birmingham ([Barnes, S.] 1955).

[272] Jackson 1902b, p.132; Jackson's italics, my square brackets.

[273] Jackson 1902c, p.286; Jackson's italics.

[274] Jackson 1902c, pp.286–287; Jackson's parentheses.

by the Neurological Society of the United Kingdom.'[275] The first two papers were by Jackson himself—to be discussed shortly. They were followed by Horsley's Hughlings Jackson Lecture for 1906, whose title was 'On Dr. Hughlings Jackson's views of the functions of the cerebellum as illustrated by recent research'.[276] Other contributors included Sherrington,[277] Beevor, Edinger (Frankfurt), Farquhar Buzzard, the young Gordon Holmes (1876–1965), and Henry Head.

Jackson's papers in his *festschrift* were reprints of cases that he had published in 1871 and 1872, with intercalated comments in 1906.[278] Both patients had midline cerebellar tumors. During his original presentations of the patients at the London Jackson had passed around sketches of the patients' postures, but the sketches were not included when the papers were published.[279] Now, in 1906, he was redressing those omissions.[280] In 1871–1872 he had said nothing about the place of the cerebellum in a hierarchy of levels, because he had not then formulated his three-level theory. In 1895 he had postulated separate cerebral and cerebellar 'subsystems', which shared the lowest level.[281] But there was no mention of that in 1906. Rather, his attention was on the similarities between the postures of patients in tetanus and the postures of cerebellar tumor patients, because both pathologies can be associated with opisthotonus.

Referring to opisthotonus, Jackson called it '*Convulsive seizures* ... I now call such seizures ... "tetanus-like seizures." '[282] This was followed by a description of the first patient in opisthotonus, as seen in the accompanying sketch (Fig. 12.2): 'the opisthotonus in tetanus-like seizures is a gross exaggeration of the activity of the extensor muscles of the spine in swift running ... In this connection I beg the reader's attention to the position of the arms in a *severe* seizure of *surgical* tetanus.'[283] Then he made an offer which, in reality, he did not fulfill.

I hope shortly to publish an article on the comparisons and contrasts which may be made between (1) degrees of locomotion from walking to swiftest running; (2) degrees of tetanus-like seizures in some cases of cerebellar tumour, and (3) degrees of paroxysms of ordinary surgical tetanus. The order of development of movement in 2 and 3 is but a brutal caricature of the order of development in 1.[284]

Despite his infirmities, in 1906 Jackson could still generate an original approach to a difficult problem. Underlying this proposal was a basic assumption about pathophysiology: 'Tetanus-like seizures ... owing to changes of instability, set up in nerve cells near the tumour – are owing to a cerebellar discharge lesion; the tetanus-like seizures are owing to occasional intense discharges of this persisting discharge lesion.'[285] This was Jackson's final pronouncement on this issue, i.e. , the cerebellar cortex can harbor discharging foci that are

---

[275] *Brain*, vol.29, after p.420 and after frontispiece. At the top of Jackson 1906a, p.425, it says '[March 1907]', so vol.29 was *for* 1906.

[276] Horsley 1906 (in *Brain*, March 1907) and 1907 (in *BMJ*, April 6). Probably Horsley obtained Jackson's agreement to reprint his old papers of 1871–1872, but Jackson's intercalated comments were as much as he could provide in the face of poor health.

[277] Sherrington 1906a.

[278] Jackson 1906a reprinted Jackson 1871j, and Jackson 1906b reprinted Jackson 1872l and Jackson 1872m.

[279] The sketches were made by Stephen Mackenzie (1844–1909), who was then a medical student. See [Mackenzie] 1909 and [Mackenzie] 2019. He worked with Jackson at the London and at Moorfields.

[280] Note that Jackson still had the sketches *and* he could find them, despite the 'apparently hopeless disorder' of his books and papers, as described by Head (in Kennard and Swash 1989, p.32; also in Jacyna 2008, pp.101–102).

[281] Jackson 1895b, p.394; see above in this chapter.

[282] Jackson 1906a, p.429; Jackson's italics.

[283] Jackson 1906a, p.430, Jackson's italics.

[284] Jackson 1906a, p.432.

[285] Jackson 1906b, p.442.

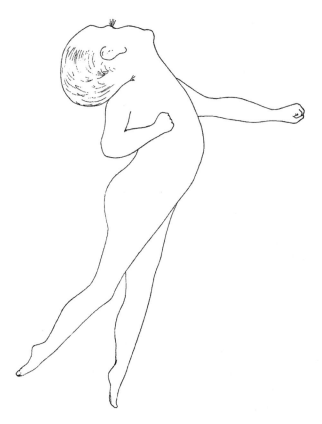

Fig. 12.2 Case of tumor of middle lobe of cerebellum—cerebellar paralysis with rigidity (cerebellar attitude)—occasional tetanus-like seizures (Jackson 1906a).

(Reproduced from Brain, Case of tumour of middle lobe of cerebellum–cerebellar paralysis with rigidity (cerebellar attitude)–occasional tetanus-like seizures (1871). 29:425–440. From Jackson 1906a, p.431.) [06-01].

physiologically the same as those in the cerebral cortices. This whole idea of 'cerebellar fits' is not currently accepted.[286] About Jackson's place in the long tradition of frustrating cerebellar research, *circa* 1907, we have Horsley's Conclusion: 'all research, ancient and modern, tends to confirm the view of Flourens, Luciani, Jackson, and Edinger, that the cerebellar cortex is the first chief station of representation of the afferent basis of movements of all the skeletal muscles.'[287] By our current standards, Horsley's Conclusion is simplistic.

Visitors, 1905 and 1906

Jackson spent his last years largely in isolation in his home in Manchester Square, partly due to deafness and vertigo.[288] However, we do have records of visits by two younger colleagues,

---

[286] Engel (2013, p.461; italics in original) states that so-called ' "*cerebellar fits*" ... are now known to reflect brief episodes of decerebrate posturing due to fluctuating increased intracranial pressure ...'

[287] Horsley 1907, p.465; he listed citations for three of the individuals mentioned by Jackson, except Flourens.

[288] Critchley and Critchley 1998, pp.187–188.

Henry Head and Samuel Alexander Kinnier Wilson (1874–1937). When Head recorded a visit to Jackson he said Jackson was then 'nearly 70'. Since Jackson's 70th birthday was April 4, 1905, Head's visit was probably a few months earlier. Head was then 49, well established at the London and well along in his studies of human sensation. The door was 'opened by a very old butler', who said of Jackson, 'he has not been well lately but is better now'. In a large room, 'Roundabout, in apparently hopeless disorder, lie innumerable books, pencilled journals and scraps of typewritten manuscript'. Jackson rose from a large chair, almost ghost-like, and they plunged immediately into a scientific conversation.

> At first he is somewhat shy for his life during many years has been lonely … Although nearly 70 years old he is still full of ideas and has maintained a wonderful freshness of interest. But he has a curious and embarrassing habit of assuming, in his great modesty, that fundamental principles enunciated by him a quarter of a century ago are still unknown to me, to whom they have been elemental steps in intellectual training …
>
> Under his shyness he hungers for affection and has been the fairy godfather to a multitude of children, many of them are grown up, some are married, and a host of photographs fill the mantelpiece.[289]

In the summer of 1906 another young companion recorded his impressions of Jackson. Kinnier Wilson was only 28 at the time and a house physician at Queen Square. This was 6 years before his classic description of the disorder of copper metabolism that is still known as 'Wilson's disease'.[290] Wilson made notes of conversations with Jackson while they were driving to outlying hospitals in his open landau.[291] There were no unusual revelations during those outings. Sometimes Jackson spoke about clinical cases and about his basic theories. Sometimes he made amusing remarks—in one instance about Titus Oates, a seventeenth-century Anglican priest who fabricated the claim of a Catholic Plot. For Jackson, Wilson said, 'Titus Oates was his favourite scamp. If Titus Oates is not in hell, then they had better get a new devil who knows his business.'[292] Probably Wilson's most important observation was his warning about assessments of Jackson by the 'younger generation'. 'Those who knew him when he was old, and beginning to show signs of failing vigor … saw him after his best was over, and had little genuine opportunity of judging for themselves in regard to those qualities which had so impressed their seniors.'[293]

The Saga of the Bust: A Still Unsolved Whodunit, November 1907 to Present

We have already seen abundant evidence for Jackson's deep impression on his contemporaries, and there was another at Queen Square in 1907. When Jackson retired, the medical staff commissioned a bust of his likeness. About this, Kinnier Wilson recalled, 'I asked him whether it was tiring to sit for his bust … and he said he much preferred driving about to having his hair cut. It is hard work doing nothing. Sitting still is being under restraint, and

---

[289] Henson 1989, p.32; also in Critchley and Critchley 1998, pp.180–181, and Jacyna 2008, pp.101–102.
[290] Martin 1975; also [Wilson] 1937. He was usually known as 'Kinnier Wilson'.
[291] Critchley and Critchley 1998, p.182, note that after he 'had completed a ward round, Jackson often invited the house physician to join him in his carriage for a ride'.
[292] Martin 1975, p.314. Martin was usually known as Purdon Martin.
[293] Wilson 1935, p.882.

that is an active inhibitory process.'[294] In the event, 'a small ceremony [was] held in the front hall on 28 November 1907 ... when Sir William Gowers pulled aside the drapery and exposed the bust he said "Our Master!" and turned toward Jackson. Gowers was not ordinarily given to compliments.'[295] Eight decades later the bust was stolen and the original was never recovered, but international cooperation filled the void: 'through the generosity of colleagues at the Montreal Neurological Institute, a copy was made of their own copy of the original bust.'[296]

Death and Funeral, October 1911

Jackson died on October 7, 1911, at his home. He was buried on October 12 in London's Highgate Cemetery (West), next to his wife. His death certificate[297] stated:

> When and where died – Seventh October 1911. 3 Manchester Square
>   Cause of death – Arterio Sclerosis Cerebral Thrombosis Coma. Certified by J. Taylor M.D.
>   Signature, description and residence of informant – C.S. Jackson Cousin Present at Death 25 Nightingale Place Woolwich

There was nothing about an autopsy. In his memorial of Ferrier, Sherrington recorded a remark by Ferrier at Jackson's funeral: 'Walking from the cemetery on the day of Hughlings-Jackson's funeral in 1911 it is told of him [Ferrier] that after silent occupation with his own thoughts for some minutes he turned quickly to the younger friend beside him and said: Well, when I cease to take interest in things it will be time for me to go.'[298]

Retrospect: Jackson as a Teacher—in the Lecture Hall and at the Bedside

The next chapter will attempt to assess the total effect of Jackson's achievement on subsequent generations—his legacy—at least to the mid-twentieth century. Here it will be appropriate to appraise his characteristics as a teacher, since that was the principal means by which his legacy was carried through. For present purposes, there are two kinds of lecture halls—one for teaching medical students and another for large invited lectures for one's colleagues. About the student lectures, Charles Mercier (1852–1911) would have known Jackson at the London because he was a student there in the early 1870s.

> Dr. Jackson had a weak voice, and his lectures were not well attended. Conscious of his tendency to talk over the heads of his audience, he would, when lecturing to a mixed class, be almost too elementary. Courteous and retiring as his manner was, he knew how to keep order, and could draw blood from a boisterous student by a cutting sarcasm.[299]

[294] Martin 1975, p.315.
[295] Martin 1975, p.316; my square brackets. See also Critchley and Critchley 1998, pp.181–182; and Shorvon 2019, pp.133–134.
[296] Critchley and Critchley 1998, p.182.
[297] General Registration Office, Application Number 3391101-1.
[298] Sherrington 1928, p.xvi; my square brackets. Probably the 'younger friend' was Sherrington himself.
[299] Mercier 1912, p.85.

With regard to Jackson's performances in prestigious lectures, and in more ordinary presentations, the published versions would indicate that his lectures were often over the heads of senior listeners. This is seen in some editorial comments about them.[300] Nonetheless, it has to be the case that most trustees of such honors were not going to deliberately invite themselves to hours of unremitting tedium. I think Jackson's attractiveness as a lecturer was attributable to his intellectual audacity, which was sometimes quite dazzling. For those who could follow his mental gymnastics it was a highly wrought form of entertainment, which was heightened when he politely but firmly took exception to the opinions of other neurologists.

Jackson's allure as a teacher was seen best in the clinic and at the bedside. A perspective of Jackson as a clinical teacher is given by Frederick Lucien Golla (1878–1968), who qualified in medicine at St. George's Hospital in 1904 and 'became a resident at the National Hospital, Queen Square, where he found Gordon Holmes as a [fellow trainee]'.[301]

> Former residents at the National Hospital will remember the thrill occasioned on many a busy Wednesday afternoon by the news that Dr. Jackson was in the hospital. Happy the youngster whose chief had already left, so he could join his still more fortunate colleague, Jackson's house physician, in attending the master through the wards! It is not too much to say that to anyone who had once listened to some of Jackson's marvellous expositions neurology could never be quite the same thing again.[302]

This kind of praise cannot be disingenuous. It can arise only from reality. Part of Jackson's allure was explained by Farquar Buzzard: 'There was always something "left over" after one of Jackson's visits to the hospital, something provocative of further inquiry.'[303] Indeed, that was Jackson's legacy. After his sojourn in neurology the field was never 'quite the same thing again' because he was constantly pushing its boundaries.

---

[300] See e.g. J85-08; J88-02, p.145; and above in this chapter.

[301] Golla 1968a, p.367; my square brackets. Despite some inexact dates, it is reasonably clear that Golla was a trainee with Jackson in the latter's last days at Queen Square, where 'Hughlings Jackson quietly strode the corridors of the National Hospital ...' (Golla 1968).

[302] Golla 1932, p.204.

[303] Buzzard, E.F. 1934, p.912.

13

Conclusion

Defining a Paradigm and Its Legacy

This final chapter will begin with a synopsis of Jackson's paradigm for analyzing the nervous system in health and disease. For this we will need to identify: (1) which parts of the paradigm became parts of his received legacy (see Table 13.2), and (2) which parts did not survive (see Table 13.3). To do that it is necessary to have a proximate time limit. In the later twentieth century there were truly revolutionary developments in molecular neurobiology and computerized imaging. Accordingly, I have chosen to limit my estimation of the reach of Jackson's legacy only into the mid-twentieth century. In 1961 Sir Francis Walshe (1885–1973) published a review of the 'Contributions of John Hughlings Jackson to neurology'.[1] His article can be enlisted to represent the mid-twentieth century's understanding of Jackson's contributions.

The Surviving Components of Jackson's Paradigm: His Legacy

Table 13.1 reproduces the section headings from Walshe's article. It will serve as a partial list of Jackson's ideas that came through in his legacy. As such it was the opinion of an astute observer, who was qualified as both a clinical neurologist and as a neurophysiologist.[2] However, Walshe was also famous for having his own points of view, so he was not comprehensively representative of his own time—probably no single individual could be. I will not follow his order of presentation, and this chapter will not be arranged with strict adherence to chronology. Thus Table 13.2 contains some Jacksonian ideas whose inclusion is the result of my retrospection. It is presented 'bottom-up', in the sense of level of abstraction. That is, it begins at the cellular level and ends with Jackson's approach to the mind-brain conundrum. *Inter alia*, it advances progressively, but only roughly, to more and more abstract levels of analysis. It is also important to note that Table 13.2 is not primarily a list of priority claims. Jackson's theories had complex origins, and surely their whole was greater than the sum of its parts.

The origins and functions of these precepts have been explored extensively in the preceding chapters, so here my comments will be limited to historical perspectives. In the process we will find that some of Jackson's paradigmatic theories have remained viable without his exact details, which is no surprise.

---

[1] Walshe 1961. He trained at Queen Square 1911–1915. For biographies see Landau and Aring 1973, Phillips 1974, and Shorvon et al. 2019, pp.232–239.

[2] About Walshe, Landau and Aring (1973, p.355) said: 'No contemporary knew better the works of John Hughlings Jackson, and his training under Sherrington peculiarly fitted him to weave their concepts into modern clinical neurology.'

Table 13.1 Section headings in Walshe 1961, listing the main parts of Jackson's legacy to neurology and neuroscience, as assessed by Walshe in the mid-twentieth century.

   I. On the Nature of the Relationship Between Mind and Brain

  II. On Movements and Their Organization

     1. Convulsions Beginning Unilaterally

     2. Hemiplegia

     3. The Plan of Representation (Localization) of Movements in the Cortex

 III. On Speech and Speechlessness

 IV. The Duality of Symptoms

  V. The Hierarchy of Levels in the Nervous System

 VI. The Meaning of the Term 'Representation'

VII. Evolution and Dissolution of the Nervous System

VIII. The Contrast Between the Nineteenth and Twentieth Century Approaches and Languages

---

Table 13.2 Summary of Jacksonian principles that survived into the mid-twentieth century, incorporating Walshe's (1961) list, and presented roughly 'bottom-up'.

Analysis at the cellular/histological level (Lockhart Clarke)

Neural cells in 'units' (Spencer)

Jacksonian seizures

The 'duality' of symptoms: positive and negative

Neural representation is for movements, not individual muscles

xyz theory of localization

Seizure focus

Common pathophysiological etiology of all epileptic seizures

Three hierarchical levels of the central nervous system: representation, re-representation, and re-re-representation

Release of function

Evolution and dissolution (Spencer)

Aphasia and language

Dreamy state/uncinate group: temporal lobe epilepsy (TLE)

Pre-Sherringtonian integration (Jackson's 'co-ordination')

The mind-body conundrum: psycho-physical parallelism ('Concomitance')

Table 13.3 Jackson's ideas and theories that did not survive into his legacy as received in the mid-twentieth century.

Lowest level fits as epileptic: actually decerebrate posturing (Sherrington)

Cerebellar physiology

Etiology of migraine (Chapter 8) and vertigo (Chapter 9) as epileptic

Constants: cardiac cycle as fiducial (Chapter 11)

The theory behind Fig. 7.1: auditory language processing

The theory behind Fig. 8.1: the neurology of subjective-objective

Relatively precise anatomical boundaries of the three-levels theory of brain organization

Compensation stated as such

The mind-body conundrum: psycho-physical parallelism ('Concomitance')

Analysis at the Cellular/Histological Level (Lockhart Clarke) and Neural Cells in 'Units' (Spencer)

This has been Jackson's least recognized and most basic contribution, because it is so fundamental to how we think. From early on, in the 1860s, he began to think about groups of cells and fibers as dynamically functional units—in the sense that individual cells can be parts of different units at different times for different functions. At that time most physicians thought about the pathophysiology of epileptic discharges at a more macroscopic level, involving events in the whole brain or large parts of it. This latter idea (whole brain) helps to explain why focal seizures were not considered 'genuine'. Doubtless other people were beginning to think at the cellular level as Jackson did—it was an idea whose time had come.[3] But again, priority is not the issue. The issue is independence. After the instantiation of the neuron theory by Cajal and Sherrington in the late nineteenth century, it was more widely understood that individual neurons normally discharge in controlled ways as components of dynamically changing units. When those units discharge excessively they produce exaggerated manifestations of their normal functions.

Jacksonian Seizures

Jackson's early instinct to try to understand (what we now call) Jacksonian seizures also began in the 1860s, simultaneously with his interest in neural histology. It might appear to be a fortunate happenstance, but chance favors the prepared mind. Jackson's mind was prepared by his comparative method, which sought to understand: (1) the *'compound sequence'* of the march of the seizure (see Chapter 6); and (2) the observation that seizures can occur in otherwise paralyzed parts of the body. From all of this and more he derived several basic precepts.

---

[3] Most famously, Rudolph Virchow's *Cellularpathologie* of 1858.

The 'Duality' of Symptoms: Positive and Negative

If we think about the possible conditions of neural cells ('neurons' in our terms) in health and disease, they can be: (1) alive and intact, thus producing 'positive', normal phenomena; (2) alive but injured and malfunctioning—either unstable and hyperfunctional and hence 'positive' or hypoactive and hence 'negative'; or they can be (3) dead, resulting in absence of function, that is, 'negative'. I believe that Jackson's conception of an injured cell being sometimes hyperfunctional, thus producing exaggerated phenomena, was unique in his time.

Neural Representation in Brain Is for Movements, Not Individual Muscles

This insight was also unique to Jackson, to the best of my knowledge. In Chapter 4 we saw that he understood it in the middle 1860s. Apparently the idea arose in his mind *de novo*. There is nothing in his writings to clarify its origin any further—except perhaps that it was another product of thinking at the histological level. In retrospect it was a form of integration.

xyz Theory of Localization

Using Jackson's notation system in Chapter 3, I gave the name '*xyz* theory' to his clinically derived conception of cerebral localization, which he first introduced in his 'Study' of 1870. It is striking that so few of his commentators have plumbed its depths.[4] Even Ferrier seems to have missed the subtleties. Walshe was an exception. He used the descriptors 'graded' and 'overlapping' to characterize the essence of Jackson's theory.[5]

Seizure Focus: Horsley's Name for Jackson's Conception

The word 'focus' was first applied to Jackson's idea of a group of abnormally firing cells by Horsley, and Jackson was happy to adopt the term. In Horsley's formulation it was essentially Jackson's conception of events at the microscopic level. We still use the word and its conception as Horsley and Jackson intended them.

Common Pathophysiological Etiology of all Epileptic Seizures

This paradigm-changing proposition was also based on Jackson's idea of the microscopic seizure focus. Even for initially generalized ('genuine') seizures Jackson explicitly assumed that there is a focus somewhere, although he was never able to support that presumption with robust clinical data.

---

[4] But see Walshe 1961, p.120; Greenblatt 1988; and York and Steinberg 1994 and 1995.
[5] Walshe 1961, p.124.

Three Hierarchical Levels of the Central Nervous System: Representation, Re-representation, and Re-re-representation

Many details of Jackson's three-levels theory of brain organization have not come through into modern neuroscience as such. In particular, his postulated anatomical boundaries for each level are mainly of historical interest. Hence, the same fate befalls his meaning of representation, re-representation, etc. Nonetheless, the general idea of hierarchical levels, and their interactions, is still very much with us, as seen in the following fundamental conceptions.

Release of Function

Jackson named his predecessors for this idea (i.e., Anstie, De Quincey, and others; see Chapters 7 and 8), but he was unique in applying it within his hierarchical view of brain function and dysfunction. We still use the idea of release in analyzing lower level dysfunctions, as in Gowers' idea of upper and lower level segments. Its use in our current conception of brain dysfunction is less straightforward than Jackson's.

Evolution and Dissolution (Spencer)

The ubiquitous influence of Herbert Spencer's highly wrought theories on Jackson's clinical thinking needs no further elaboration. The question is, if Spencer's associationist theories were deeply embedded in Jackson's ideas, and if we are direct heirs of Jackson, how much of Spencer is embedded in us? Dissolution is an example of theorizing that still resonates. It probably sees more use in psychiatry than in neurology, but the latter is not without its examples.[6]

Aphasia and Language

The most important effect of Jackson's early work on aphasia in the 1860s was the reputation that it gained for him in London's medical community, just before his 'Study' of epilepsy in 1870. Henry Head was correct to observe that later in Jackson's life his ideas about language were relatively neglected by his contemporaries and by himself. Still, Head's efforts to restore Jackson's conceptions were partly successful for a time in the mid-century. In short, Jackson's theory, as represented in Fig. 7.1, has not weathered well. In 1961 Walshe complained about the then-current nosologies of aphasia:

> The present terminology, empirical and redundant as it is . . . is certainly unsatisfactory and cannot endure.
> In the matter of the localization of the speech function, we may not be able to make more convincing proposals than those Jackson made, and yet find his division of function between the two hemispheres – the left representing speech movements,

---

[6] See e.g., Plum and Posner 1966, and later editions.

and the right subserving the understanding of speech movements, not wholly satisfying.[7]

Walshe's characterization of Jackson's speech localization in such stark left–right terms is not actually consistent with Jackson's more complex view, as cartooned in Fig. 7.1. On the other hand, Walshe was probably representative of how Jackson was understood by many people in the mid-century—remembering that he was discussing auditory speech comprehension, not language more generally. Jackson had a comprehensive view of the latter.

Dreamy State/Uncinate Group: Temporal Lobe Epilepsy (TLE)

In Chapter 12 we saw that Jackson continued to publish on the dreamy state as late as 1899, when he first named the 'Uncinate Group of epileptic fits' in print. However, his observations lay fallow in clinical neurology until the mid-twentieth century, when they were resurrected, initially by Wilder Penfield (1891–1976) and Herbert Jasper (1906–1999). They suggested the term *'temporal lobe epilepsy'*, while recognizing that some foci may lie outside the temporal lobe.[8] In neurology and neurosurgery, TLE was a hot topic in the mid-century.[9] An explication of its fascination was given by medical historian Elizabeth M. Thornton in 1976.

> Temporal lobe epilepsy became the subject of great international congresses in the fifties when neurologists from all over the world gathered to discuss this new form of epilepsy. The proceedings of these gathering records the unique fascination held by the subject for so many investigators who realized its potential to reveal something of the 'mysterious link between mind and body which had perplexed so many philosophers and historians through the centuries'.[10]

Through several different classifications, and with various names, TLE has retained its fascination.

Pre-Sherringtonian Integration (Jackson's 'Co-ordination')

A major theme of this book has been the proposition that Jackson had to create his own neuroscience of the normal, because the science of his day was inadequate.[11] By the end

---

[7] Walshe 1961, p.126. He was, in effect, criticizing the treatment of aphasia in his own textbook (Walshe 1963, pp.47–54). Note that his statement of dissatisfaction was made only 4 years before the publication of Norman Geschwind's paradigm-changing monograph on 'Disconnexion syndromes in animals and man' (1965). Geschwind trained at Queen Square 1952–1955 (Galaburda 1985). Walshe retired in 1955 (Shorvon et al. 2019, p.238).

[8] Penfield and Jasper 1954, p.528; italics in original. They said that William Feindel (1918–2014) 'took for analysis 37 cases of patients who were subject to attacks of automatism and who were suffering from what may be called *temporal lobe epilepsy*'. The phrase 'may be called' implies that the term *'temporal lobe epilepsy'* was invented there.

[9] Temkin 1971, p.vii, said: 'the modern concern with temporal lobe epilepsy has made much of the work done in the later part of the nineteenth century appear in a new light'.

[10] Thornton 1976, p.36. Another popular name for TLE in the mid-century was 'psychomotor epilepsy'.

[11] Feuerwerker et al. 1985 argue that Spencer had a major impact on Sherrington's conception of integration. They acknowledge Jackson's writings on integration, but his direct impact on Sherrington's view is little explored.

of the nineteenth century that was no longer the case. There was a growing cadre of experimental physiologists in the Western world, although most of them still had medical training.[12] That was certainly true of Sherrington, who trained at St. Thomas's Hospital (London) and Cambridge in the 1880s. His classic lectures, on *The Integrative Action of the Nervous System* (1906), set the paradigm for much of experimental neurophysiology in the twentieth century. Since Sherrington was so central to basic neuroscience, his relationship to Jackson can serve as a rough measure of Jackson's influence on it.

Jackson was senior to Sherrington by 22 years, but they knew each other from many professional interactions. Both, for example, were active in the Neurological Society, and they cited each other in their publications. In a section on decerebrate rigidity in *The Integrative Action*, Sherrington referred to Jackson's 'characteristic penetration of thought', and he quoted Jackson's expression, 'a cooperation of antagonism'.[13] In the book's lecture on 'The physiological position and dominance of the brain', Sherrington said: 'The "three levels" of Hughlings Jackson is an expressive figure of this grading of rank in nerve-centres.'[14] The neurohistorical literature contains many suggestions about direct connections between Jackson and Sherrington. Often it seems to have been assumed. Walshe thought that way,[15] and two seminal books by Penfield were dedicated to Jackson and Sherrington together. For Jackson they said: 'The dedication of this book to Hughlings Jackson is prompted by the knowledge that many of the conclusions reported here were long ago the surmise of the founder of the English School of Neurology.'[16]

The Mind-Body Conundrum: Psycho-Physical Parallelism ('Concomitance')

This part of Jackson's paradigm belongs on the list of things that made it through to his legacy (Table 13.2) *and*, at the same time, on the list of those parts that did not (Table 13.3). As a highly respected clinician he addressed the issue and therefore brought it to his colleagues' attention. Specifically, he used a version of psycho-physical parallelism that was derived from the associationist tradition and his own clinical thinking. Those origins of Jackson's 'Concomitance' were explored in Chapter 10. However, the term itself has not been carried through among neurologists. Even Walshe did not use that word, although he did use 'psychophysical parallelism'.[17]

The Discarded Parts of the Paradigm

Table 13.3 is an attempt to identify those of Jackson's ideas that were largely ignored in the mid-century. It includes only items that have been discussed in the preceding chapters.

---

[12] Bynum et al. 2006, p.113: 'Before the Great War, the Ph.D. was still a rare degree, and most professors of the medical sciences had qualified in medicine.'

[13] Sherrington 1906 (1923), pp.303–304.

[14] Sherrington 1906 (1923), p.314.

[15] Walshe 1961, especially p.127, and throughout.

[16] Penfield and Erickson 1941, p.v., and Penfield and Jasper 1954, p.viii. In both books the dedications used the same wording.

[17] Walshe 1961, p.121.

Lowest Level Fits as Epileptic: Actually Decerebrate Posturing
(Sherrington)

It was Sherrington whose experiments on the midbrain-lesioned cat showed that what looks like 'lowest level' seizures are better understood as stereotypical posturing, i.e., as release phenomena.[18]

Cerebellar Physiology

In Chapter 9 I said: 'The cerebellum has been torturing its investigators for a very long time.' To avoid my suffering a similar historical victimhood, I will say only that Jackson's views of the cerebellum have since been supplanted by the results of more than a century of increasingly sophisticated research.

Etiology of Migraine (Chapter 8) and Vertigo (Chapter 9)
as Epileptic

Given Jackson's effort to unify the pathophysiology of all paroxysmal neurological disorders, it made sense that migraine and vertigo are 'epileptic', using the term broadly. When EEGs were applied to those patients in the 1930s there was nothing definitive, while for epilepsy more narrowly defined the EEG was paradigm-changing.

Constants: Cardiac Cycle as Fiducial (Chapter 11)

Jackson presented this idea as only an inference, but it was a theory taken too far—without a discernable bridge to physiological reality. It died an early death by neglect.

The Theory Behind Fig. 7.1: Auditory Language Processing

Early on in Jackson's studies of aphasia, in 1868, a medical reporter said that his patients' 'involuntary utterances are, the author [Jackson] supposes the result of action of the *right* side. In other words, he thinks that the left is the leading side, and the right the automatic'.[19] In most of his subsequent work on aphasia Jackson maintained that basic functional distinction about the lateralities of the components of auditory language. In the 1890s he acknowledged Bastian's and Wernicke's ideas about speech reception in or near (what is now called) Wernicke's area, but it was only an acknowledgment.[20] He did not modify his theory (Fig. 7.1) to try to integrate their data into his paradigm—at least not in print.

---

[18] In Horsley's Hughlings Jackson Lecture for 1904 (Horsley 1906, pp.455–456), he cited Sherrington's 'decerebrate rigidity'. He also mentioned that in 1904 he had 'made a few [similar] experiments on dogs at Dr. Jackson's suggestion'.

[19] Jackson 1868p, p.238; my square brackets. See discussion of this passage in Chapter 5.

[20] Jackson 1894m, p.252. See Chapter 12.

The Theory Behind Fig. 8.1: The Neurology of Subjective-Objective

Remembering that Figs 7.1 and 8.1 are only my efforts to cartoon Jackson's narratives, the analogy between them is incomplete because their theories are likewise. Although some of Jackson's aphasiology survived into the mid-century, the same cannot be said for his treatment of subjective-objective. Indeed Jackson himself made little use of his theory about this recondite subject, and his posterity have ignored it.

Relatively Precise Anatomical Boundaries of the Three-Levels Theory of Brain Organization

See Table 13.2 and discussion in the section 'Three hierarchical levels'.

Compensation

Jackson's theory of neurological Compensation is derived directly from his *xyz* theory, but its potential power in that respect has been largely ignored.[21]

The Mind-Body Conundrum: Psycho-Physical Parallelism ('Concomitance')

See Table 13.2 and discussion in the section 'The mind-body conundrum'; see also next section regarding Freud.

Jackson's Legacy Beyond Neurology and Neuroscience

Neurosurgery

Separating Jackson's legacies in neurology and in neurosurgery is artificial. Macewen did his own neurology. Godlee worked with Bennett, and Horsley worked with Jackson and Ferrier, so the two specialties evolved together. They had the objective of localization in common. Nonetheless, for the early history of neurosurgery it is worth emphasizing the centrality of Jackson's conception of the seizure focus. Until Dandy's invention of ventriculography and pneumoencephalography in 1918–1919 (see Chapter 11), the only ways to localize brain lesions without external stigmata were by neurological examination and/or by the focality of seizures—and the latter was often more precise. Localization of brain tumors or other epileptogenic lesions, and their related surgical techniques, were among the main interests of early modern neurosurgery. Given Cushing's leading position after World War I and his intense interest in tumors, that remained the case into the mid-century and beyond.

---

[21] But see Greenblatt 1988, and York and Steinberg 1995.

Psychiatry

Jackson's influence on psychiatry was real but often poorly appreciated. Fortunately, an appraisal of *Hughlings Jackson on Psychiatry* (1982) by the psychiatrist Kenneth Dewhurst (1919–1984) is a valuable source on its subject. However, in the several decades since Dewhurst's publication there has been additional scholarship. Surveying that sizeable literature is far beyond the scope of this book, so herewith a few historical highlights.

The first thing to mention is Dewhurst's acerbic assessment of why Jackson's contributions to British psychiatry were not very substantial. He blames it on the institutional alienists: 'Why were Hughlings Jackson's ideas ignored by British psychiatrists? He practiced during the high noon of the Victorian asylum system when these medically administered institutions slumbered on, undisturbed in their siestas by the criticisms of a lack of progress in alleviating mental illness.'[22] Despite Dewhurst's complaint, in Chapter 12 we saw that Jackson interacted with some alienists, and some of Jackson's trainees became prominent psychiatrists.

In France Dewhurst nominated Henri Ey (1900–1977) as a significant Jacksonian force.[23] In America there were two major figures who invoked Jackson in the early and mid-twentieth century. James Jackson Putnam (1846–1918) was a neurologist-psychoanalyst at Harvard, and Adolf Meyer (1866–1950) was the first chief of psychiatry at Johns Hopkins.[24] Of course, in the first half of the twentieth century it was the founder of psychoanalysis, Sigmund Freud (1856–1939),[25] whose medical and cultural influence outpaced all the others. Within the enormous historical literature on Freud there are well substantiated claims that Jackson had a significant impact on Freud's early thinking.[26] The main topics in the assessments of Jackson's influence on Freud are aphasia, dissolution-release, and concomitance.

Freud studied with Charcot for 6 months in 1885–1886.[27] Given Charcot's admiration for Jackson, it is reasonable to think that Freud could have been introduced to Jackson's writings by Charcot, for whom aphasia was a critical interest.[28] Aphasia was also an early interest of Freud. In 1953 Erwin Stengel (1902–1973), a neuropsychiatrist and psychoanalyst, published his English translation of Freud's *Zur Auffassung der Aphasien. Eine Kritische Studie* (1891), which was rendered as *On Aphasia. A Critical Study*. Freud's book was broadly critical of contemporary concepts of aphasia. In his translator's Introduction, and in a subsequent paper, Stengel emphasized the then largely unnoticed significance of the book for Freud's subsequent development of psychoanalysis.[29]

> Here … we find for the first time in Freud's writings the principle of regression which underlies the genetic propositions of psycho-analysis. Freud had become acquainted with that principle in some form or other before … But it was in his studies in the literature on the aphasias that he found the concept of regression applied to mental processes of the

---

[22] Dewhurst 1982, pp.129–130. But see Sulloway 1979, pp.272–273; also Stengel 1963, p.352.

[23] Dewhurst 1982, pp.117–120. See Ey 1962.

[24] Critchley and Critchley 1998, pp.138–140.

[25] See Amacher 1965.

[26] The psychiatrist-historian Stanley W. Jackson (1969, p.751) said: 'From Freud's *On Aphasia* it is clear that, by 1891, he was thoroughly familiar with the writings of J. Hughlings Jackson which employed the notion of dissolution in the same way as Freud came to employ the notion of temporal regression.' See also Greenberg 1997, and D.L. Smith 1999, pp.71–80.

[27] Amacher 1965, p.55.

[28] Goetz et al. 1995, pp.127–134.

[29] Stengel 1954. Stengel 1963 also discusses Jackson's influence on Bleuler and Ey.

highest level. The author who introduced him to that concept was Hughlings Jackson, who himself had adopted it from Herbert Spencer . . .[30]

In Stengel's translation Freud had said:

In assessing the functions of the speech apparatus under pathological conditions we are adopting as a guiding principle Hughlings Jackson's doctrine that all these modes of reaction represent instances of functional retrogression (dis-involution) of a highly organized apparatus, and therefore correspond to the earlier states of its functional development.[31]

And about Freud's aphasia book as a whole Stengel said:

There are many more passages in the book which bear out the deep impression which Jackson had made on Freud. While none of the leading authorities in the field of aphasia escaped his criticism, he had nothing but praise for Hughlings Jackson, whom he pronounced his guiding spirit in the study of speech disorders. As far as I am aware, this was the last time in his career that Freud submitted to someone else's leadership.[32]

Since Jackson was not a strict localizationist, and his formulations of brain activity were 'dynamic', Stengel called him a 'holist', but we have seen that Jackson repeatedly resisted such designations. Jackson claimed to be restricting himself to the physical side of concomitance, and in Freud's view:

The relationship between the chain of physiological events in the nervous system and the mental processes is probably not one of cause and effect. The former do not cease when the latter set in; they tend to continue, but, from a certain moment, a mental phenomenon corresponds to each part of the brain, or to several parts. The psychic is, therefore, a process parallel to the physiological, "a dependent concomitant."[33]

Now a word of caution. The expression 'a dependent concomitant' is used *in English* in the original German book, as well as in Stengel's English translation of this passage.[34] Freud's insertion of quotation marks would seem to imply that he took the expression from somewhere else—presumably from Jackson. But Jackson never used 'dependent' with 'concomitant'. Although the above passage is otherwise consistent with Jackson's use of 'concomitant', he would not have used 'dependent' in this connection, because he considered the two streams of reality to be completely independent—forever parallel. Freud seemed to understand this in a footnote on the next page, when he said, approvingly, 'Hughlings Jackson has most emphatically warned against such a confusion of the physical with the psychic in

---

[30] Stengel 1954, p.2.
[31] Freud 1953, p.87.
[32] Stengel 1954, pp.2–3.
[33] Freud 1953, p.55. On 'dependent concomitant' see Sulloway 1979, pp.50–51. While discussing Spencer's role in all of this, Young (1970, p.196, footnote 3) says: 'His [Spencer's] theory of psychophysical parallelism, through Jackson's "Law of Concomitance", provided the form of Freud's psychoanalytic theory and ... the position which Freud held on the mind-body problem from his first work (*On Aphasia*, 1891) to his last (*Outline of Psychoanalysis*, 1940).'
[34] See Freud 1891/2019, p.57; and Freud 1953, p.55.

the study of speech ...' And then he quoted Jackson's warning against the idea that 'physical states in lower centres fine away into psychical states in higher centres ...'[35]

In sum, Jackson's influence on the development of psychoanalysis is clear for dissolution as regression. At the least, Jackson contributed significantly to Freud's reasoning about the mind-brain problem.

Other Specialist Fields: And Victorian Culture in General

One could make an argument that Jackson's influence spread beyond neurology, neurosurgery, and psychiatry—into (neuro)linguistics, (neuro)psychology, and perhaps into other cognate fields. Limitations of space and knowledge make such explorations impractical at this point in this book. However, in Chapters 2, 6, 9, and 11 I discussed the historical phenomenon of cultural secularization, which loosened the theological constraints on the work of Jackson and his colleagues. If we accept the reality of this cultural influence on Jackson's thought, the question arises, did Jackson have any perceptible influence on Victorian culture? In view of his connections to Spencer, Lewes, Eliot, and others, the question is legitimate, and surely interesting, but it must remain in abeyance.

A Balanced Assessment

In a short summary of Jackson's life and contributions, as of 1954, Gordon Holmes gave an appropriately balanced assessment.

> Much of his teaching is embodied in the corpus of modern neurology, but since there is no finality in science, not all of what he taught and wrote is of the same validity as it possessed half a century ago.
>
> It is easy to lapse into a kind of ancestor worship of Jackson, but those who know his thought best know that it has a life and pertinence to modern problems in neurology that justify the admiration of the most critical, and we can salute his genius without believing that all he said is final and forever adequate ... Yet if all he taught were to be replaced by wider and more perfect generalizations, we should still remain deeply in his debt for the lessons in method and in philosophic thinking which his writings provide ...[36]

What Jackson offered that so intrigued his colleagues was new ways of thinking about old problems. I hope this book has provided some new ways of thinking about Hughlings Jackson.

---

[35] Freud 1953, p.56, quoting Jackson 1878g, p.306; on the latter see Chapter 8. Sulloway 1979, pp.50–51, cites some of these passages with the statement that they are 'dualist'.

[36] Holmes 1954, p.33.

Published Writings of John Hughlings Jackson

BMJ—British Medical Journal
MPC—Medical Press and Circular
MTG—Medical Times and Gazette

For further descriptions see 'Bibliographies and Formatting' in Chapter 1. Square brackets contain identification numbers in York and Steinberg 2006

1861

1861a. Cases of abscess in the brain. *MTG* 1:196–200 (Feb. 23) [61–01].

1861b. Syphilitic affections of the nervous system. Cases of epilepsy associated with syphilis. *MTG* 1:648–652 (Jun. 22) [61–02].

1861c. Syphilitic affections of the nervous system. Cases of epilepsy associated with syphilis. *MTG* 2:59–60 (Jul. 20) [61–03].

1861d. Syphilitic affections of the nervous system. Cases of paralysis associated with syphilis. *MTG* 2:83–85 (Jul. 7) [61–04].

1861e. Syphilitic affections of the nervous system. Cases of paralysis associated with syphilis. *MTG* 2:133–135 (Aug. 10) [61-05].

1861f. Cases of reflex (?) amaurosis with colored vision. *Royal London Ophthalmic Hospital Reports* 3:286–291 (Oct.) [61–06].

1861g. Syphilitic affections of the nervous system. Cases of paralysis associated with syphilis. *MTG* 2:456 (Nov. 2) [61–07].

1861h. Syphilitic affections of the nervous system. Cases of amaurosis in connexion with syphilis. *MTG* 2:502–503 (Nov. 16) [61–08].

1861i. Cases of deafness associated with syphilis. *MTG* 2:530–531 (Nov. 23) [61–09].

1861j. Cases of paralysis of the portio dura. *MTG* 2:606–608 (Dec. 14) [61–10].

1862

1862a. Apoplexy of the pons Varolii–recovery–"fit" (nineteen years ago) followed by paralysis of the external recti and of the face and trunk both motion and sensation–gradual recovery–clinical remarks (case under the care of Dr. Brown-Séquard.) *MTG* 1:429–430 (Apr. 26) [62–01].

1862b. Cases of diseases of the cerebellum. *MTG* 2:221–226 (Aug. 30) [62–02].

1862c. Cases of diseases of the cerebellum. *MTG* 2:407–409 (Oct. 10) [62–03].

1862d. Cases of injury of the spine and of diseases of the spinal cord. *MTG* 2:463–465 (Nov. 1) [62–04].

1862e. Metropolitan Free Hospital. Sequelae of scarlet fever. (Under the care of Dr. Hughlings Jackson.) *MTG* 2:575 (Nov. 29) [62–05].

1862f. The ophthalmoscope, as an aid to the study of diseases of the brain. *MTG* 2:598–601 (Dec. 12) [62–06].

1863

1863a. Suggestions for studying diseases of the nervous system on Professor Owens' Vertebral Theory. London: H.K. Lewis. "[Printed for private circulation]" and therefore listed in York and Steinberg 2006, p.140, as pamphlet A3.

1863b. Testimonials of Dr. J. Hughlings Jackson M.D., Member of the Royal College of Physicians of London. London: Privately printed.

1863c. Cases of injury of the spine and of diseases of the spinal cord. *MTG* 1:31–33 (Jan. 10) [63–01].

1863d. Hospital for the Epileptic and Paralysed. Convulsive spasms of the right hand and arm preceding epileptic seizures. (Case under the care of Dr. Hughlings Jackson.) *MTG* 1:110–111 (Jan. 31) [63–02].

1863e. Metropolitan Free Hospital. Syphilis, followed by unilateral convulsions four months afterwards–temporary hemiplegia–paralysis of the sixth nerve on the same side–recovery. (Under the care of Dr. Hughlings Jackson.) *MTG* 1:111 (Jan. 31) [63–03].

1863f. Cases of disease of the pons Varolii. *MTG* 1:210–215 (Feb. 28) [63–04].

1863g. Hospital for the Epileptic and Paralysed. Severe pain at the back of the head, and frequent vomiting, followed in a few months by complete amaurosis–epileptiform convulsions and partial paralysis. (Under the care of Dr. Brown-Séquard.) [Communicated by Dr. Hughlings Jackson, Assistant-Physician at the Hospital.] *MTG* 1:533 (May 23) [63–05].

1863h. Hospital for the Epileptic and Paralysed. Vomiting and headache followed by amaurosis and epileptiform seizures–increase in size of the head. (Under the care of Dr. Hughlings Jackson.) *MTG* 1:533 (May 23) [63–06].

1863i. Hospital for the Epileptic and Paralysed. Unilateral epileptiform seizures, attended by temporary defect of sight. (Under the care of Dr. Hughlings Jackson.) *MTG* 1:588 (Jun. 6) [63–07].

1863j. Metropolitan Free Hospital. Epileptiform seizures – aura from the thumb – attacks of coloured vision. (Under the care of Dr. Hughlings Jackson.) *MTG* 1:589 (Jun. 6) [63–08].

1863k. Hospital for the Epileptic and Paralysed. Hemiplegia in an old man–recovery–spasm of the face. (Under the care of Dr. Hughlings Jackson.) *MTG* 2:11–12 (Jul. 4) [63–09].

1863l. Hospital for the Epileptic and Paralysed. Epilepsy following some months after injury to the head. (Under the care of Dr. Hughlings Jackson.) *MTG* 2:65 (Jul. 18) [63–10].

1863m. Hospital for the Epileptic and Paralysed. Epileptiform convulsions (unilateral) after an injury to the head. (Under the care of Dr. Hughlings Jackson.) *MTG* 2:65–66 (Jul. 18) [63–11].

1863n. An experimental inquiry into the effect of application of ice to the back of the neck on the retinal circulation. *MTG* 2:90–91 (Jul. 25) [63–12].

1863o. Hospital for the Epileptic and Paralysed. Notes on the use of the ophthalmoscope in affections of the nervous system. (Communicated by Dr. Hughlings Jackson, Assistant-Physician to the Hospital.) *MTG* 2:359 (Oct. 3) [63–13].

1863p. Unilateral chorea, interstitial keratitis; slow recovery under the use of iodide of potassium. (Under the care of Dr. Hughlings Jackson.) *MTG* 2:407–408 (Oct. 17) [63–14].

1863q. The London Hospital. Giddiness, pain in the head, and vomiting coming on suddenly–amaurosis–no paralysis–death eleven weeks after the first seizure–autopsy–apoplexy in middle cerebral lobe. (Under the care of Dr. Hughlings Jackson.) *MTG* 2:588–589 (Dec. 5) [63–15].

1863r. Observations on defects of sight in brain disease. *Royal London Ophthalmic Hospital Reports* 4:10–19 [63–16].

1863s. Ophthalmoscopic examination during sleep. *Royal London Ophthalmic Hospital Reports* 4:35–37 [63–17].

1864

1864a. Hospital for Epilepsy and Paralysis. Clinical remarks on hemiplegia, with loss of speech–its association with valvular diseases of the heart. (Cases under the care of Dr. Hughlings Jackson.) *MTG* 1:123 (Jan. 30) [64–01].

1864b. Hospital for Epilepsy and Paralysis. Clinical remarks on defects of sight in diseases of the nervous system. (Cases under the care of Dr. Hughlings Jackson.) *MTG* 1:480–482 (Apr. 30) [64–02].

1864c. Hemiplegia on the right side, with loss of speech. *BMJ* 1:572–573 (May 21) [64–03].

1864d. Note on amaurosis in hemiplegia. *MTG* 2:87 (Jul. 23) [64–04].

1864e. The London Hospital. Loss of speech, with hemiplegia on the left side–valvular disease–epileptiform seizures, affecting the side paralysed. (Under the care of Dr. Hughlings Jackson.) *MTG* 2:166–167 (Aug. 13) [64–05].

1864f. Hospital for Epilepsy and Paralysis. Epileptic aphemia with epileptic seizures on the right side. (Under the care of Dr. Hughlings Jackson.) *MTG* 2:167–168 (Aug. 13) [64–06].

1864g. Unilateral epileptiform seizures beginning by a disagreeable smell. *MTG* 2:168 (Aug. 13) [64–07].

1864h. On the study of diseases of the nervous system. A lecture delivered June, 1864. *Clinical Lectures and Reports by the Medical and Surgical Staff of the London Hospital* 1:146–158 (between Jun. and Nov. 1864) [64–08].

1864i. Illustrations of diseases of the nervous system. *Clinical Lectures and Reports by the Medical and Surgical Staff of the London Hospital* 1:337–387 (before Nov. 5) [64–09].

1864j. Loss of speech: its association with valvular disease of the heart, and with hemiplegia on the right side – defects of smell – defects of speech in chorea – arterial regions in epilepsy. *Clinical Lectures and Reports by the Medical and Surgical Staff of the London Hospital* 1:388–471 (before Nov. 5) [64–10].

1864k. Reviews and Notices. *Clinical Lectures and Reports by the Medical and Surgical Staff of the London Hospital. BMJ* 2:524 (Nov. 5) [64–11].

1864l. National Hospital for Epilepsy and Paralysis. Clinical remarks on cases of defects of expression (by words, writing, signs, etc.) in diseases of the nervous system. (Under the care of Dr. Hughlings Jackson.) *Lancet* 2:604–605 (Nov. 26) [64–12].

1864m. The London Hospital. Chorea, with paralysis, affecting the right side; difficulty in talking. (Under the care of Dr. Hughlings Jackson.) *Lancet* 2:606 (Nov. 26) [64–13].

1865

1865a. The London Hospital. Involuntary ejaculations following fright–subsequently chorea. (Under the care of Dr. Hughlings Jackson.) *MTG* 1:89 (Jan. 28) [65–01].

1865b. On a case of disease of the posterior columns of the cord-locomotor ataxy (?). *Lancet* 1:617–620 (Jun. 10) [65–02]. By-line: J. Lockhart Clarke and Jackson.

1865c. The London Hospital. Tumour at the base of the brain–death–autopsy–clinical remarks. (Under the care of Dr. Hughlings Jackson.) *MTG* 1:626–627 (Jun. 17) [65–03].

1865d. Affections of cranial nerves in locomotor ataxy. *Lancet* 2:247–248 (Aug. 26) [65–04].

1865e. Hospital for the Epileptic and Paralysed. Hemiplegia on the right side, with deficit of speech–death–autopsy. (Under the care of Dr. Hughlings Jackson.) *MTG* 2:283–284 (Sep. 9) [65–05].

1865f. Lectures on hemiplegia. *Clinical Lectures and Reports by the Medical and Surgical Staff of the London Hospital* 2:297–332 [65–06].

1865g. Observations on defects of sight in diseases of the nervous system. *Royal London Ophthalmic Hospital Reports* 4:389–446 [65–07].

1865h. Observations on defects of sight in diseases of the nervous system. *Royal London Ophthalmic Hospital Reports* 5:51–78 [65–08].

1866

1866a. The London Hospital. Clinical remarks on emotional and intellectual language in some cases of disease of the nervous system. (Under the care of Dr. Hughlings Jackson.) *Lancet* 1:174–176 (Feb. 17) [66–01].

1866b. Note on lateral deviation of the eyes in hemiplegia and in certain epileptiform seizures. *Lancet* 1:311–312 (Mar. 24) [66–02].

1866c. The London Hospital. A case of progressive locomotor ataxy: loss of smell and hearing: defect of sight with atrophy of the optic discs variocele and atrophy of the testis. (Under the care of Dr. Hughlings Jackson.) *Lancet* 1:345–346 (Mar. 31) [66–03].

1866d. National Hospital for the Epileptic and Paralysed. Clinical remarks on cases of temporary loss of speech and power of expression (epileptic aphemia? aphrasia? aphasia?) and on epilepsies. (Under the care of Dr. Hughlings Jackson.) *MTG* 1:442–443 (Apr. 28) [66–04].

1866e. National Hospital for the Epileptic and Paralysed. Clinical remarks on the occasional occurrence of subjective sensations of smell in patients who are liable to epileptiform seizures, or who have symptoms of mental derangements, and in others. (Under the care of Dr. Hughlings Jackson.) *Lancet* 1:659–660 (Jun. 16) [66–05].

1866f. Notes on the physiology and pathology of language. Remarks on those cases of disease of the nervous system in which defect of expression is the most striking symptom. *MTG* 1:659–662 (Jun. 23) [66–06].

1866g. On a case of loss of power of expression; inability to talk, to write, and to read correctly after convulsive attacks. *BMJ* 2:92–94 (Jul. 28) [66–07].

1866h. Hemiplegia on the left side, with defect of speech. *MTG* 2:210 (Aug. 25) [66–08].

1866i. Tobacco smoking in diseases of the nervous system. Sex in diseases of the nervous system. The form of amaurosis complicating locomotor ataxy. *MTG* 2:219–222 (Sep. 1) [66–09].

1866j. Aphasia. *BMJ* 2:258–261 (Sep.1). Unsigned editorial; not in York and Steinberg 2006.

1866k. On a case of loss of power of expression; inability to talk, to write, and to read correctly after convulsive attacks. *BMJ* 2:326–330 (Sep. 22) [66–10].

1866l. The London Hospital. Case of disease of cerebral arteries (syphilitic?); softening of the brain; clinical remarks. (Under the care of Dr. Hughlings Jackson.) *Lancet* 2:467–468 (Oct. 27) [66–11].

1866m. Reports of Societies. Harveian Society of London. Oct. 18th, 1866. *BMJ* 2:586–590 (Nov. 24) [66–12].

1866n. The National Hospital for the Epileptic and Paralyzed. The electrical room. *MTG* 2:583–585 (Dec. 1) [66–13].

1866o. The London Hospital. Case of disease of the left side of the brain, involving corpus striatum, etc.; the aphasia of Trousseau; clinical remarks on psychico-physical symptoms. (Under the care of Dr. Hughlings Jackson.) *Lancet* 2:605–606 (Dec. 1) [66–14].

1866p. A physician's notes on ophthalmoscopy–cases of disease of the nervous system in which there were defects of smell, sight and hearing. *Royal London Ophthalmic Hospital Reports* 5:251–306 [66–15].

1866q. A lecture on cases of cerebral haemorrhage. *Clinical Lectures and Reports by the Medical and Surgical Staff of the London Hospital* 3:237–255 [66–16].

1866r. Note on the functions of the optic thalamus. *Clinical Lectures and Reports by the Medical and Surgical Staff of the London Hospital* 3:373–377 [66–17].

1866s. Amaurosis. Tumour at the base of the brain–death–autopsy–clinical remarks. *Ophthalmic Review* 2:288–290 [66–18].

1867

1867a. Note on the comparison and contrast of regional palsy and spasm. *Lancet* 1:205 (Feb. 16) [67–01].

1867b. Note on the comparison and contrast of regional palsy and spasm. *Lancet* 1:295–297 (Mar. 9) [67–02].

1867c. The London Hospital. Choreal movements of the right arm and leg in a man seventy-four years of age: clinical remarks on cases of chorea. (Under the care of Dr. Hughlings Jackson.) *BMJ* 1:570–572 (May 18) [67–03].

1867d. The ophthalmoscope in physicians' practice. *BMJ* 1:722 (Jun. 25) [67–04].

1867e. Remarks on the occasional utterances of "speechless" patients. *Lancet* 2:70–71; not in York and Steinberg 2006.

1867f. National Hospital for the Epileptic and Paralysed. Notes on cases of diseases of the nervous system. (Under the care of Dr. Hughlings Jackson.) *BMJ* 2:472–474 (Nov. 23) [67–05].

1867g. National Hospital for the Epileptic and Paralysed. Notes on cases of diseases of the nervous system. (Under the care of Dr. Hughlings Jackson.) *BMJ* 2:499–500 (Nov. 30) [67–06].

1867h. Remarks on the disorderly movements of chorea and convulsion. *MTG* 2:642–643 (Dec. 24) [67–07].

1867i. Remarks on the disorderly movements of chorea and convulsion, and on localization. *MTG* 2:669–670 (Dec. 21) [67–08].

1867j. Note on regional palsy and spasm. *BMJ* 2:587 (Dec. 28) [67–09].

1867k. Notes of hospital cases. *Royal London Ophthalmic Hospital Reports* 6:50–53 [67–10].

1867l. Cases of disease of the nervous system. *Clinical Lectures and Reports by the Medical and Surgical Staff of the London Hospital* 4:314–394 [67–11].

1867m. On a case of muscular atrophy, with disease of the spinal cord and medulla oblongata. *Medico-Chirurgical Transactions published by the Medical and Chirurgical Society of London* 32:489–499 (Jun. 25) [67–12]. By-line: Clarke and Jackson.

1868

1868a. On latency of optic neuritis in cerebral disease. *MTG* 1:143 (Feb. 8) [68–01].

1868b. The London Hospital. Case of occasional loss of consciousness, with subjective sensations of smell. (Under the care of Dr. Hughlings Jackson.) *MTG* 1:231 (Feb. 29) [68–02].

1868c. The London Hospital. Aphasia with hemiplegia of left side. (Under the care of Dr. Hughlings Jackson.) *Lancet* 1:316 (Mar. 7) [68–03].

1868d. Hospital for the Epileptic and Paralysed. The ophthalmoscope in physicians' practice: clinical remarks on cases of optic neuritis in brain-disease. (Under the care of Dr. Hughlings Jackson.) *BMJ* 1:300 (Mar. 28) [68–04].

1868e. Defect of intellectual expression (aphasia) with left hemiplegia. *Lancet* 1:457 (Apr. 4) [68–05].

1868f. The London Hospital. Case of severe brain disease with double optic neuritis. (Under the care of Dr. Hughlings Jackson.) *MTG* 1:392 (Apr. 17) [68–06].

1868g. National Hospital for the Epileptic and Paralysed. Case of convulsive attacks arrested by stopping the aura. (Under the care of Dr. Hughlings Jackson.) *Lancet* 1:618–619 (May 16) [68–07].

1868h. The London Hospital. Clinical remarks on cases of convulsions beginning unilaterally with double optic neuritis. (Under the care of Dr. Hughlings Jackson.) *MTG* 1:524–525 (May 16) [68–08].

1868i. Syphilitic affections of the nervous system. *MTG* 1:551–553 (May 23) [68–09].

1868j. The ophthalmoscope in pyaemia. *MTG* 1:653 (Jun. 13) [68–10].

1868k. Reports of Societies. Obstetrical Society of London. Wednesday July 1, 1868. Chorea in pregnancy. *MTG* 2:137–138 (Aug. 1) [68–11].

1868l. Notes on the physiology and pathology of the nervous system. *MTG* 2:177–179 (Aug. 15) [68–12].

1868m. Notes on the physiology and pathology of the nervous system. *MTG* 2:208–209 (Aug. 22) [68–13].

1868n. Dr. Hughlings Jackson, F.R.C.P., on the physiology of language. *MTG* 2:275–276 (Sep. 5) [68–14].

1868o. Reports of Societies. British Association for the Advancement of Science. Section II. Biology: Department of anatomy and physiology. The physiology of language. *BMJ* 2:259 (Sep. 5) [68–15].

1868p. The physiology of language. *MPC* 6:237–239 (Sep. 9) [68–16].

1868q. Notes on the physiology and pathology of the nervous system. *MTG* 2:358–359 (Sep. 26) [68–17].

1868r. Observations on the physiology and pathology of hemi-chorea. *Edinburgh Medical Journal* 14:294–303 (Oct.) [68–18].

1868s. Chorea in pregnancy. *MTG* 2:410 (Oct. 3) [68–19].

1868t. National Hospital for the Epileptic and Paralysed. Syphilitic disease of the brain; optic neuritis; convulsions beginning unilaterally. (Under the care of Dr. Hughlings Jackson.) *Lancet* 2:539–540 (Oct. 24) [68–20].

1868u. Notes on the physiology and pathology of the nervous system. *MTG* 2:526–528 (Nov. 7) [68–21].

1868v. Notes on the physiology and pathology of the nervous system. *MTG* 2:696 (Dec. 19) [68–22].

1868w. Cases of disease of the nervous system in patients the subjects of inherited syphilis. *St. Andrews Medical Graduates' Association Transactions 1867*:146–160 [68–23].

1868x. A case of epileptiform amaurosis. *Royal London Ophthalmic Hospital Reports* 6:131–135 [68–24].

1868y. Convulsions. *A System of Medicine* 2:217–250 [68–25].

1868z. On apoplexy and cerebral hemorrhage. *A System of Medicine* 2:504–543 [68–26].

1869

1869a. Abstract of the Gulstonian lectures on certain points in the study and classification of diseases of the nervous system. Delivered at the Royal College of Physicians. *Lancet* 1:307–308 (Feb. 27) [69–01].

1869b. Gulstonian lectures on certain points in the study and classification of diseases of the nervous system. Delivered at the Royal College of Physicians. *BMJ* 1:184 (Feb. 27) [69–02].

1869c. Abstract of the Gulstonian lectures on certain points in the study and classification of diseases of the nervous system. Delivered at the Royal College of Physicians. *Lancet* 1:344–345 (Mar. 6) [69–03].

1869d. Gulstonian lectures on certain points in the study and classification of diseases of the nervous system. Delivered at the Royal College of Physicians. *BMJ* 1:210 (Mar. 6) [69–04].

1869e. Notes on the physiology and pathology of the nervous system. *MTG* 1:245–246 (Mar. 6) [69–05].

1869f. Abstract of the Gulstonian lectures on certain points in the study and classification of diseases of the nervous system. Delivered at the Royal College of Physicians. *Lancet* 1:379–380 (Mar. 13) [69–06].

1869g. Gulstonian lectures on certain points in the study and classification of diseases of the nervous system. Delivered at the Royal College of Physicians. *BMJ* 1:236 (Mar. 13) [69–07].

1869h. Cases of diseases of the nervous system in patients the subjects of inherited syphilis. *Lancet* 1:498 (Apr. 10) [69–08].

1869i. Notes on the physiology and pathology of the nervous system. *MTG* 1:600 (Jun. 5) [69–09].

1869j. Hospital for the Epileptic and Paralysed. Epileptic or epileptiform seizures occurring with discharge from the ear. (Cases under the care of Dr. Hughlings Jackson.) *BMJ* 1:591 (Jun. 26) [69–10].

1869k. Report of a case of disease of one lobe of the cerebrum, and of both lobes of the cerebellum. *Medical Mirror* 6:126–127 (Sep. 1) [69–11].

1869l. The function of the cerebellum. *Medical Mirror* 6:138–140, 147 (Oct. 1) [69–12].

1869m. Notes on the physiology and pathology of the nervous system. *MTG* 2:481–482 (Oct. 23) [69–13].

1869n. The London Hospital. Death by haemorrhage from cerebral tumours. (Under the care of Dr. Hughlings Jackson.) *Lancet* 2:571–572 (Oct. 23) [69–14].

1869o. The London Hospital. Lateral deviation of the eyes in cases of hemiplegia. *Lancet* 2:672 (Nov. 13) [69–15].

1869p. National Hospital for the Epileptic and Paralysed. Remarks on an association of nervous symptoms which frequently depends on intra-cranial syphilitic disease. *Lancet* 2:803 (Dec. 11) [69–16].

1869q. The periscope. Dr. Hughlings Jackson on cerebral disease in connection with ophthalmic symptoms. *Royal London Ophthalmic Hospital Reports* 6:240 [69–17].

1869r. On chorea in pregnancy. *Transactions of the Obstetrical Society of London* 10:147–195 [69–18].

1870

1870a. Hospital for Epilepsy and Paralysis. Digitalis with bromide of potassium in epilepsy. *BMJ* 1:32 (Jan. 8); written by anonymous reporter; not in York and Steinberg 2006.

1870b. The London Hospital. Cases of palsies of several cranial nerves, including the nerves to the larynx, all on the left side–weakness of limbs on right side. (Under the care of Dr. Hughlings Jackson and Dr. Morell Mackenzie.) *MTG* 1:34–35 (Jan. 8) [70–01].

1870c. Reports of Societies. Clinical Society. *MTG* 1:480–481 (Apr. 30) [70–02].

1870d. Remarks on tongue-biting in convulsions. *BMJ* 1:409 (Apr. 23) [70–03].

1870e. Reports of Societies. Clinical Society of London. Friday April 8th. *BMJ* 1:482 (Apr. 30) [70–04].

1870f. Hospital for the Epileptic and Paralysed. Notes on cases of disease of the nervous system. (Under the care of Dr. Hughlings Jackson.) *BMJ* 2:459–460 (Oct. 29) [70–05].

1870g. A study of convulsions. *St. Andrews Medical Graduates' Association Transactions* 1869:162–204 (before Nov. 12) [70–06].

1870h. Reviews and notices of books. A study of convulsions. *Lancet* 2:674 (Nov. 12) [70–07].

1871

1871a. The London Hospital. Notes from the out-patient practice of Dr. Hughlings Jackson. *Lancet* 1:376–377 (Mar. 18) [71–01].

1871b. Case illustrating difficulties in the diagnosis of cerebral haemorrhage and drunkenness. *MTG* 1:360–361 (Apr. 1) [71–02].

1871c. Defect of hearing in diphtherial paralysis. *Lancet* 1:728 (May 27) [71–03].

1871d. On the routine use of the ophthalmoscope in cases of cerebral disease. *MTG* 1:627–629 (Jun. 3) [71–04].

1871e. Reports of Societies. Clinical Society of London. *MTG* 1:702–703 (Jun. 17) [71–05].

1871f. Lecture on optic neuritis from intracranial disease. Delivered at the London Hospital. *MTG* 2:241–243 (Aug. 26) [71–06].

1871g. Tumour of the middle lobe of the cerebellum. *BMJ* 2:241–243 (Aug. 26) [71–07].

1871h. Lecture on optic neuritis from intracranial disease. Delivered at the London Hospital. *MTG* 2:341–342 (Sep. 16) [71–08].

1871i. Singing by speechless (aphasic) children. *Lancet* 2:430–431 (Sep. 23); not in York and Steinberg 2006.

1871j. The London Hospital. Case of tumour of the middle lobe of the cerebellum. *BMJ* 2:528–529 (Nov. 4). [71–09]

1871k. Lecture on optic neuritis from intracranial disease. Delivered at the London Hospital. *MTG* 2:581 (Nov. 11) [71–10].

1871l. Hospital for the Epileptic and Paralysed. Notes on cases of disease of the nervous system. (Under the care of Dr. Hughlings Jackson.) *BMJ* 2:641–642 (Dec. 2) [71–11].

1871m. The London Hospital. Case of epileptiform seizure, beginning in the right hand. (Under the care of Dr. Hughlings Jackson.) *MTG* 2:767–769 (Dec. 23) [71–12].

1871n. Case of hemiplegia in a syphilitic subject. Read May 26, 1870. *Clinical Society of London Transactions* 4:183–187 [71–13].

1872

1872a. On partial convulsive seizures, with plugging of cerebral veins. *MTG* 1:4–5 (Jan. 6) [72–01].

1872b. On a case of defect of speech following right-sided convulsion. *Lancet* 1:72–73 (Jan. 20) [72–02].

1872c. On partial convulsive seizures, with plugging of cerebral veins. *MTG* 1:94 (Jan. 27) [72–03].

1872d. The London Hospital. Remarks on a case of chorea in a dog. *Lancet* 1:148 (Feb. 3) [72–04].

1872e. Abstract of the oration delivered before the Hunterian Society of London, February 7th, 1872. The physiological aspect of education. *BMJ* 1:179–181 (Feb. 17) [72–05].

1872f. Abstract of the Hunterian oration, delivered before the Hunterian Society, Feb. 17th, 1872. The physiological aspect of education. *Lancet* 1:260 (Feb. 24) [72–06].

1872g. The London Hospital. Remarks on difficulties in the diagnosis of the causes of apoplexy. *Lancet* 1:505 (Apr. 13) [72–07].

1872h. The London Hospital. Case of disease of the brain–left hemiplegia–mental affection. (Under the care of Dr. Hughlings Jackson.) *MTG* 1:513–514 (May 4) [72–08].

1872i. National Hospital for Epileptics. Notes of cases under the care of Dr. Hughlings Jackson. *BMJ* 1:526 (May 18) [72–09].

1872j. The London Hospital. Remarks on affections of hearing in cases of disease of the nervous system. *MTG* 2:37–39 (Jul. 13) [72–10].

1872k. Corrigendum. *MTG* 2:84 (Jul. 20) [72–11].

1872l. The London Hospital. Remarks on cases of intracranial tumour. (Under the care of Dr. Hughlings Jackson.) *BMJ* 2:67–68 (Jul. 20) [72–12].

1872m. The London Hospital. Sequel of a case of supposed tumour of the middle lobe of the cerebellum. (Under the care of Dr. Hughlings Jackson.) *BMJ* 2:125 (Aug. 3) [72–13].

1872n. On auditory vertigo (Ménière's disease). *MTG* 2:169–170 (Aug. 17) [72–14].

1872o. The London Hospital. A series of cases illustrative of cerebral pathology. Cases of intra-cranial tumour. (Under the care of Dr. Hughlings Jackson.) *MTG* 2:541–542 (Nov. 16) [72–15].

1872p. The London Hospital. A series of cases illustrative of cerebral pathology. Cases of intra-cranial tumour. (Under the care of Dr. Hughlings Jackson.) *MTG* 2:568–569 (Nov. 23) [72–16].

1872q. The London Hospital. A series of cases illustrative of cerebral pathology. Cases of intra-cranial tumour. (Under the care of Dr. Hughlings Jackson.) *MTG* 2:597–599 (Nov. 30) [72–17].

1872r. On a case of paralysis of the tongue from haemorrhage in the medulla oblongata. *Lancet* 2:770–773 (Nov. 30) [72–18]. By-line: Jackson and Clarke.

1872s. The London Hospital. A series of cases illustrative of cerebral pathology. Cases of intra-cranial tumour. (Under the care of Dr. Hughlings Jackson.) *MTG* 2:625–626 (Dec. 7) [72–19].

1872t. The London Hospital. A series of cases illustrative of cerebral pathology. Cases of intra-cranial tumour. (Under the care of Dr. Hughlings Jackson.) *MTG* 2:698–699 (Dec. 28) [72–20].

1872u. Jackson, J.H. 1872–1873. Double optic neuritis, in which vision was perfect. *Proceedings of the Medical Society of London* 1:131–132; not in York and Steinberg 2006.

1873

1873a. On the anatomical & physiological localisation of movements in the brain. *Lancet* 1:84–85 (Jan. 18) [73–01].

1873b. On palsy of vocal cord from intra-cranial syphilis. *BMJ* 1:86 (Jan. 25) [73–02].

1873c. On the anatomical & physiological localisation of movements in the brain. *Lancet* 1:162–164 (Feb. 1) [73–03].

1873d. On the anatomical & physiological localisation of movements in the brain. *Lancet* 1:232–234 (Feb. 15) [73–04].

1873e. Observations on defects of sight in diseases of the nervous system. *Royal London Ophthalmic Hospital Reports* 7:513–527 (Feb.) [73–05].

1873f. The London Hospital. A series of cases illustrative of cerebral pathology. Cases of intra-cranial tumour. (Under the care of Dr. Hughlings Jackson.) *MTG* 1:223–225 (Mar. 1) [73–06].

1873g. The London Hospital. A series of cases illustrative of cerebral pathology. Cases of intra-cranial tumour. (Under the care of Dr. Hughlings Jackson.) *MTG* 1:329–330 (Mar. 29) [73–07].

1873h. The London Hospital. Abscess in the left lobe of the cerebellum from suppurative disease of the ear; double optic neuritis. (Under the care of Mr. Maunder.) *Lancet* 1:443–444 (Mar. 29) [73–08].

1873i. Abscess in the right lobe of the cerebellum from aural disease: no optic neuritis. (Under the care of Dr. Hughlings Jackson.) *Lancet* 1:444–445 (Mar. 29) [73–09].

1873j. The London Hospital. A series of cases illustrative of cerebral pathology. Cases of intra-cranial tumour. (Under the care of Dr. Hughlings Jackson.) *MTG* 1:493–495 (May 10) [73–10].

1873k. On the anatomical investigation of epilepsy and epileptiform convulsions. *BMJ* 1:531–533 (May 10) [73–11].

1873l. The London Hospital. Notes on cases of disease of the nervous system. *BMJ* 1:560–561 (May 17) [73–12].

1873m. The London Hospital. A series of cases illustrative of cerebral pathology. Cases of intra-cranial tumour. (Under the care of Dr. Hughlings Jackson.) *MTG* 2:33–35 (Jul. 12) [73–13].

1873n. Remarks on the double condition of loss of consciousness and mental automatism following certain epileptic seizures. *MTG* 2:63–64 (Jul. 19) [73–14].

1873o. Lectures on diagnosis of tumours of the brain. *MTG* 2:139–140 (Aug. 9) [73–15].

1873p. Forty-first meeting of the British Medical Association. Demonstrations on patients. *BMJ* 2:239–240 (Aug. 23) [73–16].

1873q. Lectures on diagnosis of tumours of the brain. *MTG* 2:195–197 (Aug. 23) [73–17].

1873r. On a case of local softening of the brain from thrombosis of syphilitic arteries. *BMJ* 2:254 (Aug. 30) [73–18].

1873s. The London Hospital. Remarks on cases of vertigo, reeling and vomiting, from ear disease. *Lancet* 2:334–335 (Sep. 6) [73–19].

1873t. On hemiplegia, with paralysis of the third nerve. *Lancet* 2:335 (Sep. 6) [73–20].

1873u. Pulmonary apoplexies (haemorrhagic infarctions) in cases of cerebral apoplexy. *BMJ* 2:483–484 (Oct. 25) [73–21].

1873v. Lectures on diagnosis of tumours of the brain. *MTG* 2:541–543 (Nov. 15) [73–22].

1873w. The London Hospital. Remarks on limited convulsive seizures and on the after-effects of strong nervous discharges. *Lancet* 2:840–841 (Dec. 13) [73–23].

1873x. Observations on the localisation of movements in the cerebral hemispheres, as revealed by cases of convulsion, chorea and 'aphasia.' *West Riding Lunatic Asylum Medical Reports* 3:175–195 [73–24].

1873y. On the anatomical, physiological, and pathological investigations of epilepsies. *West Riding Lunatic Asylum Medical Reports* 3:315–349 [73–25].

1874

1874a. Hospital for the Epileptic and Paralysed. A series of cases illustrative of cerebral pathology. Cases of intra-cranial tumour. (Under the care of Dr. Hughlings Jackson.) *MTG* 1:6–7 (Jan. 3) [74–01].

1874b. On the nature of the duality of the brain. *MPC* 17:19–21 (Jan. 14) [74–02].

1874c. On the nature of the duality of the brain. *MPC* 17:41–44 (Jan. 21) [74–03].

1874d. Hospital for the Epileptic and Paralysed. A series of cases illustrative of cerebral pathology. Cases of intra-cranial tumour. (Under the care of Dr. Hughlings Jackson.) *MTG* 1:96 (Jan. 24) [74–04].

1874e. On the nature of the duality of the brain. *MPC* 17:63–65 (Jan. 28) [74–05].

1874f. The London Hospital. A series of cases illustrative of cerebral pathology. Cases of intra-cranial tumour. (Under the care of Dr. Hughlings Jackson.) *MTG* 1:151–153 (Feb. 7) [74–06].

1874g. Ophthalmoscopic examination during an attack of epileptiform amaurosis. *Lancet* 1:193–194 (Feb. 7) [74–07].

1874h. Hospital for the Epileptic and Paralysed. Remarks on coloured vision preceding epileptic attacks. *BMJ* 1:174 (Feb. 7) [74–08].

1874i. Hospital for the Epileptic and Paralysed. On the after-effects of severe epileptic discharges: speculations as to epileptic mania. *BMJ* 1:174 (Feb. 7) [74–09].

1874j. Hospital for the Epileptic and Paralysed. Remarks on systemic sensations in epilepsies. *BMJ* 1:174 (Feb. 7) [74–10].

1874k. The London Hospital. A series of cases illustrative of cerebral pathology. Cases of intra-cranial tumour. (Under the care of Dr. Hughlings Jackson.) *MTG* 1:234–235 (Feb. 24) [74–11].

1874l. Charcot and others on auditory vertigo (Ménière's disease). *London Medical Record* 2:238–240 (Apr. 22) [74–12].

1874m. Charcot and others on auditory vertigo (Ménière's disease). *London Medical Record* 2:254–256 (Apr. 29) [74–13].

1874n. Temporary affection of speech (aphasia): "aphasic" writing. *BMJ* 1:574 (May 2) [74–14].

1874o. The London Hospital. On a case of recovery from hemiplegia. (Under the care of Dr. Hughlings Jackson.) *Lancet* 1:618–619 (May 2) [74–15].

1874p. The comparative study of drunkenness. *BMJ* 1:652–653 (May 16) [74–16].

1874q. The comparative study of drunkenness. *BMJ* 1:685–686 (May 23) [74–17].

1874r. A case of right hemiplegia and loss of speech from local softening of the brain. *BMJ* 1:804–805 (Jun. 20) [74–18].

1874s. Clinical lecture on a case of hemiplegia. *BMJ* 2:69–71 (Jul. 18) [74–19].

1874t. Clinical lecture on a case of hemiplegia. *BMJ* 2:99–101 (Jul. 25) [74–20].

1874u. Two cases of intra-cranial syphilis. *Journal of Mental Science* 20:235–243 (Jul.) [74–21].

1874v. The London Hospital. A series of cases illustrative of cerebral pathology. Cases of intra-cranial tumour. (Under the care of Dr. Hughlings Jackson.) *MTG* 2:118–119 (Aug. 1) [74–22].

1874w. Jackson on syphilitic disease within the cranium. *London Medical Record* 2:635–666 (Oct. 7) [74–23].

1874x. Jackson on hemiplegia. *London Medical Record* 2:648–650 (Oct. 14) [74–24].

1874y. On the scientific and empirical investigations of epilepsies. *MPC* 18:325–327 (Oct. 14) [74–25].

1874z. Hospital for the Epileptic and Paralysed. A series of cases illustrative of cerebral pathology. Cases of intra-cranial tumour. (Under the care of Dr. Hughlings Jackson.) *MTG* 2:441–442 (Oct. 17) [74–26].

1874aa. On the scientific and empirical investigations of epilepsies. *MPC* 18:347–352 (Oct. 21) [74–27].

1874bb. The London Hospital. A series of cases illustrative of cerebral pathology. Cases of intra-cranial tumour. (Under the care of Dr. Hughlings Jackson.) *MTG* 2:471–472 (Oct. 24) [74–28].

1874cc. The London Hospital. Remarks on loss of smell and taste. *Lancet* 2:622 (Oct. 31) [74–29].

1874dd. Periscope. *Royal London Ophthalmic Hospital Reports* 8:88–102 (Oct.) [74–30].

1874ee. On the scientific and empirical investigations of epilepsies. *MPC* 18:389–392 (Nov. 4) [74–31].

1874ff. On the scientific and empirical investigations of epilepsies. *MPC* 18:409–412 (Nov. 11) [74–32].

1874gg. The London Hospital. Attacks of giddiness and vomiting, with deafness and ear disease. (Under the care of Dr. Hughlings Jackson.) *Lancet* 2:727–728 (Nov. 21) [74–33].

1874hh. On the scientific and empirical investigations of epilepsies. *MPC* 18:475–478 (Dec. 2) [74–34].

1874ii. On the scientific and empirical investigations of epilepsies. *MPC* 18:497–499 (Dec. 9) [74–35].

1874jj. On the scientific and empirical investigations of epilepsies. *MPC* 18:519–521 (Dec. 16) [74–36].

1874kk. On a case of recovery from hemiplegia. Much damage of motor tract and convolutions remaining. Remarks on chorea. *St. Andrews Medical Graduates' Association Transactions 1872 and 1873*:60–68 [74–37].

1874ll. On a case of recovery from double optic neuritis. *West Riding Lunatic Asylum Medical Reports* 4:24–29 [74–38].

1875

1875a. Clinical and physiological researches on the nervous system. No. 1. London: J. and A. Churchill. Listed by York and Steinberg 2006, p.141, as Pamphlet A30.

1875b. Psychology and the nervous system. *BMJ* 2:400–401, 432–433, 462–463, 499–500; not listed in York and Steinberg 2006. The first three installments are labeled parts 'I', 'II', and 'III'; the fourth (pp.499–500, not so labeled), apparently also written by Jackson, was in response to a reader's letter to the editor. Jones 1972, p.306, states that Bastian attributed this piece to Jackson in *Brain* 10:107–109, 1887, but there is no such direct statement in those pages of Bastian's paper.

In first two sentences: 'Some of those who are sceptical as to there being representation of movements in the cerebral hemispheres seem to us to altogether overlook several kinds of evidence in favour of it. This evidence has recently been presented in a pamphlet [York and Steinberg A30], of which this article is in great part a summary.'

In 1881h, p.330, Jackson said, 'In earlier papers I used the term "Reduced to a More Automatic Condition."' He did that in 1875p, 1875q. (see my Chapter 8).

1875c. The London Hospital. Clinical observations on cases of disease of the nervous system. *Lancet* 1:85 (Jan. 16) [75–01].

1875d. The London Hospital. Cases of nervous disease; with clinical remarks. (Under the care of Dr. Hughlings Jackson.) *Lancet* 1:161 (Jan. 30) [75–02].

1875e. Nervous symptoms in cases of congenital syphilis. *Journal of Mental Science* 20:517–527 (Jan.) [75–03].

1875f. On the scientific and empirical investigation of epilepsies. *MPC* 19:353–355 (Apr. 26) [75–04].

1875g. The London Hospital. Cases illustrative of cerebral pathology. Cases of intracranial tumour. (Under the care of Dr. Hughlings Jackson.) *MTG* 1:468–469 (May 1) [75–05].

1875h. The London Hospital. Remarks on difficulties in the diagnosis of causes of apoplexy. *MTG* 1:498–499 (May 8) [75–06].

1875i. On the scientific and empirical investigation of epilepsies. *MPC* 19:397–400 (May 12) [75–07].

1875j. On choreal movements and cerebellar rigidity in a case of tubercular meningitis. *BMJ* 1:636–637 (May 15) [75–08].

1875k. On automatic actions during coma from cerebral haemorrhage. *MTG* 1:522 (May 15) [75–09].

1875l. On the scientific and empirical investigation of epilepsies. *MPC* 19:419–421 (May 19) [75–10].

1875m. Hospital for the Epileptic and Paralysed. Autopsy on a case of hemianopia with hemiplegia and hemianaesthesia. *Lancet* 1:722 (May 22) [75–11].

1875n. Hospital for the Epileptic and Paralysed. Remarks on cases of hemianopsia with hemiplegia. *Lancet* 1:722 (May 22) [75–12].

1875o. The London Hospital. Cases of partial convulsion from organic brain disease, bearing on experiments of Hitzig and Ferrier. *MTG* 1:578–579 (May 29) [75–13].

1875p. The London Hospital. Cases of partial convulsion from organic brain disease, bearing on experiments of Hitzig and Ferrier. *MTG* 1:606–607 (Jun. 5) [75–14].

1875q. Hughlings Jackson on nervous dissolution, as illustrated by epileptic mania. *London Medical Record* 3:349–350 (Jun. 9) [75–15].

1875r. The London Hospital. Clinical memoranda of a series of interesting cases of nerve-disorder now in hospital. (Under the care of Dr. Hughlings Jackson.) *BMJ* 1:773–774 (Jun. 12) [75–16].

1875s. Hughlings Jackson on cases of nervous disease. *London Medical Record* 3:367–368 (Jun. 16) [75–17].

1875t. On nervous dissolution. *London Medical Record* 3:379–380 (Jun. 16) [75–18].

1875u. The London Hospital. Cases of partial convulsion from organic brain disease, bearing on experiments of Hitzig and Ferrier. *MTG* 1:660–661 (Jun. 19) [75–19].

1875v. Hughlings Jackson on difficulties in the diagnosis of the causes of apoplexy. *London Medical Record* 3:398–399 (Jun. 30) [75–20].

1875w. Hemikinesis. *BMJ* 2:43 (Jul. 10) [75–21].

1875x. The London Hospital. Cases of partial convulsion from organic brain disease, bearing on experiments of Hitzig and Ferrier. *MTG* 2:94 (Jul. 24) [75–22].

1875y. On a case of nearly complete deafness following apoplexy. *MTG* 2:118 (Jul. 31) [75–23].

1875z. On syphilitic affections of the nervous system. *Journal of Medical Science* 20:207–225 (Jul.) [75–24].

1875aa. The London Hospital. Observations of Mèniére's disease. *MTG* 2:161–162 (Aug. 7) [75–25].

1875bb. Hospital for the Paralysed and Epileptic. Case illustrating the relation betwixt certain cases of migraine and epilepsy. *Lancet* 2:244–245 (Aug. 14) [75–26].

1875cc. The London Hospital. Cases of partial convulsion from organic brain disease, bearing on experiments of Hitzig and Ferrier. *MTG* 2:264–266 (Sep. 4) [75–27].

1875dd. A lecture on softening of the brain. *Lancet* 2:335–339 (Sep. 4) [75–28].

1875ee. The London Hospital. Cases of partial convulsion from organic brain disease, bearing on experiments of Hitzig and Ferrier. *MTG* 2:330–331 (Sep. 18) [75–29].

1875ff. A periscope of contemporary ophthalmic literature. *Royal London Ophthalmic Hospital Reports* 8:318–343 (Sep.) [75–30].

1875gg. Editorial comment. *Lancet* 2:497–498 (Oct. 2) [75–31].

1875hh. On the scientific and empirical investigation of epilepsies. *MPC* 20:313–315 (Oct. 20) [75–32].

1875ii. Royal Medical and Chirurgical Society. On the pathology of chorea. *MTG* 2:481–483 (Oct. 23) [75–33].

1875jj. On the scientific and empirical investigation of epilepsies. *MPC* 20:355–358 (Nov. 3) [75–34].

1875kk. On the scientific and empirical investigation of epilepsies. *MPC* 20:487–489 (Dec. 15) [75–35].

1875ll. On temporary mental disorders after epileptic paroxysms. *West Riding Lunatic Asylum Medical Reports* 5:105–129 [75–36].

1876

1876a. The London Hospital. Cases of partial convulsion from organic brain disease, bearing on experiments of Hitzig and Ferrier. *MTG* 1:8–10 (Jan. 1) [76–01].

1876b. Jackson on temporary mental disorders after epileptic paroxysms. *London Medical Record* 4:22–23 (Jan. 15) [76–02].

1876c. Clinical and physiological researches on the nervous system. No. 1. *London Medical Record* 4:43–44 (Jan. 15) [76–03].

1876d. On the scientific and empirical investigation of epilepsies. *MPC* 21:63–65 (Jan. 26) [76–04].

1876e. On the scientific and empirical investigation of epilepsies. *MPC* 21:129–131 (Feb. 16) [76–05].

1876f. Les troubles intellectuels momentanées qui suivant les accès épileptiques. *La Revue Scientifique de la France et de l'Etranger* 34:169–178 (Feb. 19) [76–06].

1876g. On the scientific and empirical investigation of epilepsies. *MPC* 21:173–176 (Mar. 1) [76–07].

1876h. Notes on cases of disease of the nervous system. *Medical Examiner* 1:170–171 (Mar. 2) [76–08].

1876i. Hospital for the Epileptic and Paralysed. On cases of epileptic seizures, with auditory warning. *Lancet* 1:386–387 (Mar. 11) [76–09].

1876j. The London Hospital. Epilepsy–automatic and unconscious performance of complex actions in epilepsy. (Under the care of Dr. Hughlings Jackson.) (Reported by Mr. R. Atkinson.) *MTG* 1:304 (Mar. 18) [76–10].

1876k. On the scientific and empirical investigation of epilepsies. *MPC* 21:313–316 (Apr. 19) [76–11].

1876l. Case of large cerebral tumour without optic neuritis and with left hemiplegia and imperception. *Royal London Ophthalmic Hospital Reports* 8:434–444 (May) [76–12].

1876m. A case of double optic neuritis without cerebral tumour. *Royal London Ophthalmic Hospital Reports* 8:445–455 (May) [76–13].

1876n. On the scientific and empirical investigation of epilepsies. *MPC* 21:479–481 (Jun. 14) [76–14].

1876o. On the scientific and empirical investigation of epilepsies. *MPC* 22:145–147 (Aug. 23) [76–15].

1876p. On the scientific and empirical investigation of epilepsies. *MPC* 22:185–187 (Sep. 6) [76–16].

1876q. Clinical and physiological researches on the nervous system. *Journal of Psychological Medicine and Mental Pathology n.s.* 2 (1):150–155 (before Oct.) [76–17].

1876r. On the scientific and empirical investigation of epilepsies. *MPC* 22:475–477 (Dec. 13) [76–18].

1876s. On the gravity of cerebral lesions. *Medical Examiner* 2:890–891 (Dec. 21) [76–19].

1876t. Note on the "embolic theory" of chorea. *BMJ* 2:813–814 (Dec. 23) [76–20].

1876u. The London Hospital. Notes on cases of disease of the nervous system. (Under the care of Dr. Hughlings Jackson.) *MTG* 2:700–702 (Dec. 23) [76–21].

1876v. On epilepsies and the after-effects of epileptic discharges. (Todd and Robertson's hypothesis). *West Riding Lunatic Asylum Medical Reports* 6:266–309 [76–22].

1877

1877a. On nervous symptoms with ear disease. *Lancet* 1:415–417 (Mar. 24) [77–01].

1877b. On nervous symptoms with ear disease. *BMJ* 1:349–351 (Mar. 24) [77–02].

1877c. On nervous symptoms with ear disease. *MTG* 1:308–310 (Mar. 24) [77–03].

1877d. The London Hospital. Cases of tumour of the middle lobe of the cerebellum. (Under the care of Dr. Hughlings Jackson.) *BMJ* 1:354 (Mar. 24) [77–04].

1877e. The London Hospital. Hemiplegia coming on without loss of consciousness; autopsy; atheromatous and syphilitic disease of cerebral arteries. (Under the care of Dr. Hughlings Jackson.) *Lancet* 1:457–458 (Mar. 31) [77–05].

1877f. On unconscious and automatic actions after epileptic fits. 1. *BMJ* 1:393–395 (Mar. 31) [77–06].

1877g. Remarks on rigidity in hemiplegia. *Medical Examiner* 2:271–272 (Apr. 5) [77–07].

1877h. On unconscious and automatic actions after epileptic fits. 2. *BMJ* 1:431–432 (Apr. 7) [77–08].

1877i. Ophthalmology in its relation to general medicine. *Medical Examiner* 2:365–367 (May 10) [77–09].

1877j. An address on ophthalmology in its relation to general medicine. *BMJ* 1:575–577 (May 12) [77–10].

1877k. Ophthalmology in its relation to general medicine. *Lancet* 1:674–678 (May 12) [77–11].

1877l. Ophthalmology in its relation to general medicine. *MTG* 1:496–500 (May 12) [77–12].

1877m. Ophthalmology in its relation to general medicine. *Medical Examiner* 2:388–390 (May 17) [77–13].

1877n. An address on ophthalmology in its relation to general medicine. *BMJ* 1:605–606 (May 19) [77–14].

1877o. Ophthalmology in its relation to general medicine. *Medical Examiner* 2:427–429 (May 31) [77–15].

1877p. An address on ophthalmology in its relation to general medicine. *BMJ* 1:672–674 (Jun. 2) [77–16].

1877q. Ophthalmology in its relation to general medicine. *Medical Examiner* 2:448–40 (Jun. 7) [77–17].

1877r. An address on ophthalmology in its relation to general medicine. *BMJ* 1:703–705 (Jun. 9) [77–18].

1877s. Ophthalmology in its relation to general medicine. *Medical Examiner* 2:467–468 (Jun. 14) [77–19].

1877t. The London Hospital. Case of suspected "discharging lesion" of the hinderpart of the uppermost right frontal convolution–illustration of Ferrier's researches. (Under the care of Dr. Hughlings Jackson.) *Lancet* 1:876 (Jun. 16) [77–20].

1877u. Ophthalmology in its relation to general medicine. *Medical Examiner* 2:509–510 (Jun. 28) [77–21].

1877v. An address on ophthalmology in its relation to general medicine. *BMJ* 1:804–805 (Jun. 30) [77–22].

1877w. Clinical notes on nervous disease: case of convulsions from syphilitic disease of the brain. *Medical Examiner* 2:1018–1019 (Dec. 13) [77–23].

1878

1878a. On cerebral paresis or paralysis with cerebellar tremor or rigidity. *Medical Examiner* 3:266–277 (Mar. 28) [78–01].

1878b. The London Hospital. Remarks on non-protrusion of the tongue in some cases of aphasia. *Lancet* 1:716–717 (May 18) [78–02].

1878c. Buzzard on blepharospasm. *Brain* 1:285–286 (Jul.) [78–03].

1878d. Remarks on comparison and contrast betwixt tetanus and a certain epileptiform seizure. *MTG* 2:484–485 (Oct. 26) [78–04].

1878e. Remarks on the cerebellum. *MTG* 2:485–486 (Oct. 26) [78–05].

1878f. The London Hospital. Case of temporary hemiplegia after localized epileptiform convulsion. (Under the care of Dr. Hughlings Jackson.) *Lancet* 2:581–582 (Oct. 26) [78–06].

1878g. On affections of speech from disease of the brain. *Brain* 1:304–330 (Oct.) [78–07].

1878h. The London Hospital. Tetanus-like seizures with double optic neuritis–no autopsy. (Under the care of Dr. Hughlings Jackson.) *MTG* 2:596–597 (Nov. 23) [78–08].

1879

1879a. Lectures on the diagnosis of epilepsy. *MTG* 1:29–33 (Jan. 11) [79–01].

1879b. Abstract of lectures on the diagnosis of epilepsy. *Lancet* 1:42–43 (Jan. 11) [79–02].

1879c. Lectures on the diagnosis of epilepsy. Delivered before the Harveian Society. *BMJ* 1:33–36 (Jan. 11) [79–03].

1879d. Lectures on the diagnosis of epilepsy. *MTG* 1:85–88 (Jan. 25) [79–04].

1879e. Abstract of lectures on the diagnosis of epilepsy. *Lancet* 1:110–112 (Jan. 25) [79–05].

1879f. Lectures on the diagnosis of epilepsy. Delivered before the Harveian Society. *BMJ* 1:109–112 (Jan. 25) [79–06].

1879g. Lectures on the diagnosis of epilepsy. Delivered before the Harveian Society. *BMJ* 1:141–143 (Feb. 1) [79–07].

1879h. Lectures on the diagnosis of epilepsy. *MTG* 1:141–143 (Feb. 8) [79–08].

1879i. Abstract of lectures on the diagnosis of epilepsy. *Lancet* 1:184–185 (Feb. 8) [79–09].

1879j. Lectures on the diagnosis of epilepsy. *MTG* 1:223–226 (Mar. 1) [79–10].

1879k. Auditory vertigo. *Brain* 2:29–38 (Mar.) [79–11].

1879l. Remarks on the routine use of the ophthalmoscope in cerebral disease. *MPC* 27:439–441 (Jun. 4) [79–12].

1879m. Remarks on the routine use of the ophthalmoscope in cerebral disease. *MPC* 27:459–461 (Jun. 11) [79–13].

1879n. Remarks on the routine use of the ophthalmoscope in cerebral disease. *MPC* 27:479–480 (Jun. 18) [79–14].

1879o. On affections of speech from disease of the brain. *Brain* 2:203–222 (Jul.) [79–15].

1879p. Note on Dr. J. Hughlings Jackson's case of auditory vertigo in April no. of 'Brain'. *Brain* 2:273–274 [79–16].

1879q. Psychology and the nervous system. *MPC* 28:199–201 (Sep. 3) [79–17].

1879r. Psychology and the nervous system. *MPC* 28:239–241 (Sep. 17) [79–18].

1879s. Psychology and the nervous system. *MPC* 28:283–285 (Oct. 1) [79–19].

1879t. On affections of speech from disease of the brain. *Brain* 2:323–356 (Oct.) [79–20].

1879u. Psychology and the nervous system. *MPC* 28:409–411 (Nov. 12) [79–21].

1879v. Psychology and the nervous system. *MPC* 28:429–430 (Nov. 19) [79–22].

1880

1880a. On tumours of the cerebellum. *Lancet* 1:122–124 (Jan. 24) [80–01].

1880b. Remarks on tumours of the cerebellum. *BMJ* 1:196–198 (Feb. 7) [80–02].

1880c. Remarks on tumours of the cerebellum. *Lancet* 1:275–277 (Feb. 21) [80–03].

1880d. Lecture on a case of intracranial syphilis. *Lancet* 1:357–359 (Mar. 6) [80–04].

1880e. On affections of speech. *MPC* 29:253–255 (Mar. 31) [80–05].

1880f. On aphasia, with left hemiplegia. *Lancet* 1:637–638 (Apr. 24) [80–06].

1880g. Remarks on diseases of the cerebellum. *MPC* 29:448–449 (Jun. 2) [80–07].

1880h. Remarks on diseases of the cerebellum. *MPC* 29:469–471 (Jun. 9) [80–08].

1880i. Case illustrating the value of the ophthalmoscope in the investigation and treatment of diseases of the brain. *Lancet* 1:906 (Jun. 12) [80–09].

1880j. On right or left-sided spasm at the seat of epileptic paroxysms and on crude sensation-warnings and elaborate mental states. *Brain* 3:192–206 (Jul.) [80–10].

1880k. Buzzard on certain points in tabes dorsalis. *Brain* 3:266–268 (Jul.) [80–11].

1880l. Part of a lecture on auditory vertigo. *Lancet* 2:525–528 (Oct. 2) [80–12].

1880m. On a case of recovery from organic brain-disease. *BMJ* 2:654–656 (Oct. 23) [80–13].

1880n. National Hospital for the Paralysed and Epileptic. Peculiar phenomena after epileptic seizures. (Under the care of Dr. Hughlings Jackson.) *BMJ* 2:776–777 (Nov. 13) [80–14].

1880o. Eye symptoms in locomotor ataxy. *Lancet* 2:968–969 (Dec. 18) [80–15].

1880p. Ophthalmological Society of the United Kingdom. Eye-symptoms in locomotor ataxy. *BMJ* 2:980–981 (Dec. 18) [80–16].

1881

1881a. On a case of temporary left hemiplegia, with foot-clonus and exaggerated knee-phenomenon, after an epileptiform seizure beginning in the left foot. *MTG* 1:183–186 (Jan. 12) [81–01].

1881b. On temporary paralysis after epileptiform and epileptic seizures; a contribution to the study of dissolution of the nervous system. *Brain* 3:433–451 (Jan.) [81–02].

1881c. Buzzard on transfer-phenomena in epilepsy produced by encircling blisters. *Brain* 3:554–555 (Jan.) [81–03].

1881d. Harveian Society of London. A case of temporary hemiplegia after localised convulsion. *Lancet* 1:335 (Feb. 26) [81–04].

1881e. On optic neuritis in intracranial disease. *MTG* 1:311–317 (Mar. 19) [81–05].

1881f. Ophthalmological Society of Great Britain. Optic neuritis in intracranial disease. *BMJ* 1:472–474 (Mar. 26) [81–06].

1881g. Ophthalmological Society. *MTG* 1:434 (Apr. 16) [81–07].

1881h. Remarks on dissolution of the nervous system, as exemplified by certain post-epileptic conditions. *MPC* 31:329–332 (Apr. 20) [81–08].

1881i. The discussion on optic neuritis at the ophthalmological society. *MTG* 1:460–461 (Apr. 23) [81–09].

1881j. Ophthalmological Society of Great Britain. Cases illustrating the condition of the discs ten years after optic neuritis. *BMJ* 1:645–646 (Apr. 23) [81–10].

1881k. Remarks on dissolution of the nervous system, as exemplified by certain post-epileptic conditions. *MPC* 31:399–400 (May 11) [81–11].

1881l. Remarks on dissolution of the nervous system, as exemplified by certain post-epileptic conditions. *MPC* 32:68–70 (Jul. 27) [81–12].

1881m. Buzzard on the affection of bones and joints in locomotor ataxy, and its association with gastric crises. *Brain* 4:276–27 (Jul.) [81–13].

1881n. Buzzard on acute anterior polio-myelitis in infants and adults. *Brain* 4:278–280 (Jul.) [81–14].

1881o. Buzzard on tendon reflex in the diagnosis of diseases of the spinal cord. *Brain* 4:280–82 (Jul.) [81–15].

1881p. Epileptiform convulsions from cerebral disease. *BMJ* 2:322–333 (Aug. 20) [81–16].

1881q. Ophthalmological Society of Great Britain. The relation between the apparent movement of objects and the rotation of the eyes. *BMJ* 2:667–668 (Oct. 22) [81–17].

1881r. Remarks on dissolution of the nervous system, as exemplified by certain post-epileptic conditions. *MPC* 32:380–382 (Nov. 2) [81–18].

1881s. Remarks on dissolution of the nervous system, as exemplified by certain post-epileptic conditions. *MPC* 32:399–401 (Nov. 9) [81–19].

1881t. Remarks on dissolution of the nervous system, as exemplified by certain post-epileptic conditions. *MPC* 32:421–422 (Nov. 16) [81–20].

1881u. Discussion on the relation between optic neuritis and intracranial disease. *Transactions, Ophthalmological Society of the United Kingdom* 1:60–115 [81–21].

1881v. On eye symptoms in locomotor ataxy. *Transactions, Ophthalmological Society of the United Kingdom* 1:139–154 [81–22].

1881w. Epileptiform convulsions from cerebral disease. *Transactions of the International Medical Congress. Seventh Session* 2:6–15 [81–23].

1881x. Epileptiform convulsions from cerebral disease. *Transactions of the International Medical Congress. Seventh Session* 2:21–22 [81–24].

1881y. Contribution to discussion on connection between optic neuritis and intracranial disease. *Transactions of the International Medical Congress. Seventh Session* 3:61 [81–25].

1881z. On tumours of the cerebellum. *Proceedings, Medical Society of London* 5:48–56 [81–26].

1881aa. A case of recovery from symptoms of brain disease. *Proceedings, Medical Society of London* 5:175–178 [81–27].

1882

1882a. Critical Digests and Notices of Books. A Treatise on the Diseases of the Nervous System. By James Ross, M.D. Two vols. J. and A. Churchill. *Brain* 4:519–524 (January); not in York and Steinberg 2006.

1882b. Medical Society of London. Cortical tumour of brain. *Lancet* 1:441 (Mar. 18) [82–01].

1882c. Epidemiological Society. South-eastern branch: East and West Surrey districts. Observations on migraine. *BMJ* 1:464 (Apr. 1) [82–02].

1882d. An address delivered at the opening of the section of pathology at the annual meeting, British Medical Association, in Worcester, August 1882. *BMJ* 2:305–308 (Aug. 19) [82–03].

1882e. Address delivered at the opening of the section of pathology. At the Annual Meeting of the British Medical Association, in Worcester, August 1882. *MTG* 2:239–242 (Aug. 26) [82–04].

1882f. The study of pathology. *BMJ* 2:494–495 (Sep. 9) [82–05].

1882g. Localised convulsions from tumour of the brain. *Brain* 5:364–374 (Oct.) [82–06].

1882h. On some implications of dissolution of the nervous system. *MPC* 34:411–414 (Nov. 15) [82–07].

1882i. On some implications of dissolution of the nervous system. *MPC* 34:433–434 (Nov. 22) [82–08].

1882j. On the relation between the apparent movements of objects and the rotation of the eyes. *Transactions, Ophthalmological Society of the United Kingdom* 2:213–217 [82–09]. By-line: Professor [F.C.] Donders and Jackson.

1883

1883a. Comment on a case of paralysis of the third nerve, with cerebral symptoms, by David Lees. *MTG* 1:80 (Jan. 20); not in York and Steinberg 2006.

1883b. Commentary. *Transactions, Ophthalmological Society of the United Kingdom* 3:229–232 (Jan.) [83–01].

1883c. On ocular movements, with vertigo, produced by pressure on a diseased ear. *Transactions, Ophthalmological Society of the United Kingdom* 3:261–265 (Jan.) [83–02].

1883d. Movements of the eyes provoked by pressure on a diseased ear. *BMJ* 1:113 (Jan. 20) [83–03].

1883e. The Ophthalmological Society. Movements of the eyes provoked by pressure on a diseased ear. *MTG* 1:80–81 (Jan. 20) [83–04].

1883f. Buzzard on diseases of the nervous system. *Brain* 5:382–388 (Jan.); not in York and Steinberg 2006.

1883g. Ophthalmological Society of the United Kingdom. Eye symptoms in spinal disease. *BMJ* 1:1180–1182 (Jun. 16) [83–05].

1883h. The Ophthalmological Society. The relation of eye symptoms to diseases of the spinal cord. *MTG* 1:684–685 (Jun. 16) [83–06].

1883i. On some implications of dissolution of the nervous system. *MPC* 36:64–66 (Jul. 25) [83–07].

1883j. On some implications of dissolution of the nervous system. *MPC* 36:84–86 (Aug. 1) [83–08].

1884

1884a. Croonian lectures on evolution and dissolution of the nervous system. Delivered at the Royal College of Physicians. *Lancet* 1:555–558 (Mar. 29) [84–01].

1884b. The Croonian lectures on evolution and dissolution of the nervous system. Delivered at the Royal College of Physicians, March, 1884. *BMJ* 1:591–593 (Mar. 29) [84–02].

1884c. Croonian lectures on evolution and dissolution of the nervous system. Delivered at the Royal College of Physicians. *MTG* 1:411–413 (Mar. 29) [84–03].

1884d. The Croonian lectures on evolution and dissolution of the nervous system. Delivered at the Royal College of Physicians, March, 1884. *BMJ* 1:660–663 (Apr. 5) [84–04].

1884e. Croonian lectures on evolution and dissolution of the nervous system. Delivered at the Royal College of Physicians. *MTG* 1:445–447 (Apr. 5) [84–05].

1884f. Croonian lectures on evolution and dissolution of the nervous system. Delivered at the Royal College of Physicians. *Lancet* 1:649–652 (Apr. 12) [84–06].

1884g. The Croonian lectures on evolution and dissolution of the nervous system. Delivered at the Royal College of Physicians, March, 1884. *BMJ* 1:703–707 (Apr. 12) [84–07].

1884h. Croonian lectures on evolution and dissolution of the nervous system. Delivered at the Royal College of Physicians. *MTG* 1:485–487 (Apr. 18) [84–08].

1884i. The Croonian lectures. *MTG* 1:529–530 (Apr. 19) [84–09].

1884j. Croonian lectures on evolution and dissolution of the nervous system. Delivered at the Royal College of Physicians. *Lancet* 1:739–744 (Apr. 26) [84–10].

1884k. Evolution and dissolution of the nervous system. *Popular Science Monthly* 25:171–180 (Nov.) [84–11].

1884l. A case of convulsive seizure beginning in the right foot owing to cortical tumour of the left cerebral hemisphere. *Proceedings, Medical Society of London* 6:151–152 [84–12].

1885

1885a. Discussion of Bennett and Godlee 1885. *BMJ* 1:988–989 (May 16); not in York and Steinberg 2006.

1885b. Royal Medical and Chirurgical Society. The experimental production of chorea and other results of capillary embolism. *MTG* 1:730–731 (May 30) [85–01].

1885c. Reviews and notices of books. A treatise on the diseases of the nervous system. By James Ross. *Brain* 5:423–425 (Oct.) [85–02].

1885d. Medical Society of London. The clinical significance of the deep tendon reflexes. *BMJ* 2:867–870 (Nov. 7) [85–03].

1885e. The Bowman Lecture. Ophthalmology and diseases of the nervous system. Delivered before the Ophthalmological Society, Nov. 13th, 1885. *Lancet* 2:935–938 (Nov. 21) [85–04].

1885f. The Bowman Lecture. Ophthalmology and diseases of the nervous system. Delivered before the Ophthalmological Society, Friday November 13th, 1885. *BMJ* 2:945–949 (Nov. 21) [85–05].

1885g. The Bowman lecture. *BMJ* 2:980–981 (Nov. 21) [85–06].

1885h. The Bowman Lecture. Ophthalmology and diseases of the nervous system. Being the Bowman lecture, delivered before the Ophthalmological Society of the United Kingdom, Friday November 13th, 1885. *MTG* 2:695–701 (Nov. 21) [85–07].

1885i. The Bowman Lecture. *MTG* 2:743 (Nov. 28) [85–08].

1886

1886a. Harveian Society. Paralysis of tongue, palate and vocal cord. *Lancet* 1:689-690 (Apr. 10). [86–01].

1886b. A contribution to the comparative study of convulsions. *Brain* 9:1–23 (Apr.) [86–02].

1886c. Comment on case of Horsley at BMA annual meeting. *Lancet* 2:347 (Aug. 21); not in York and Steinberg 2006.

1886d. Brain-surgery. *BMJ* 2:670–675 (Oct. 9) [86–03].

1886e. Medical Society of London. A rare case of epilepsy. Epileptic guinea-pigs. *Lancet* 2:975–976 (Nov. 20) [86–04].

1886f. On a case of fits resembling those artificially produced in guinea-pigs. *BMJ* 2:962–963 (Nov. 20) [86–05].

1886g. Harveian Society. Paraplegia in Pott's disease. *BMJ* 2:977 (Nov. 20) [86–06].

1886h. The Bowman Lecture. Ophthalmology and diseases of the nervous system. Being the Bowman lecture, delivered before the Ophthalmological Society of the United Kingdom, Friday November 13th, 1885. *Transactions, Ophthalmological Society of the United Kingdom* 6:1–22 [86–07].

1886i. Graves's disease. *Transactions, Ophthalmological Society of the United Kingdom* 6:58–59 [86–08].

1887

1887a. Case of left crural monoplegia with subcortical disease: fracture of left femur, which was cancerous. *Transactions, Clinical Society of London* 20:134–136 [87–01].

1887b. Clinical Society of London. Paralysis of the left leg from sub-cortical disease, with cancer and fracture of the left femur. *BMJ* 1:510 (Mar. 5) [87–02].

1887c. Medical Society of London. Random association of nervous symptoms with syphilis. Facial monoplegia. *Lancet* 1:680–681 (Apr. 2) [87–03].

1887d. Medical Society of London. A case of hemianopsia, and of wasting and paralysis on one side of the tongue in a syphilitic patient. *BMJ* 1:729 (Apr. 2) [87–04].

1887e. Remarks on evolution and dissolution of the nervous system. *Journal of Mental Science* 23:25–48 (Apr.) [87–05].

1887f. The 'muscular sense'; its nature and cortical localisation. *Brain* 10:107–109 (Apr.) [87–06].

1887g. Remarks on the psychology of joking, delivered at the Medical Society of London, October 17th, 1887. *Lancet* 2:800–801 (Oct. 22) [87–07].

1887h. An address on the psychology of joking, delivered at the opening of the Medical Society of London, October, 1887. *BMJ* 2:870–871 (Oct. 22) [87–08].

1887i. Medical Society of London. Removal of cerebral tumour. *BMJ* 2:997–998 (Nov. 5) [87–09].

1887j. Remarks on evolution and dissolution of the nervous system. *MPC* 95:461–462 (Nov. 16) [87–10].

1887k. Remarks on evolution and dissolution of the nervous system. *MPC* 95:491–492 (Nov. 23) [87–11].

1887l. Remarks on evolution and dissolution of the nervous system. *MPC* 95:511–513 (Nov. 30) [87–12].

1887m. Remarks on evolution and dissolution of the nervous system. *MPC* 95:586–588 (Dec. 21) [87–13].

1887n. Remarks on evolution and dissolution of the nervous system. *MPC* 95:617–620 (Dec. 28) [87–14].

1887o. On a case of fits resembling those artificially produced in guinea-pigs. *Proceedings, Medical Society of London* 10:78–85 [87–15].

1888

1888a. Muscular hypertonicity in paralysis. *Brain* 10:312–318 (Jan.) [88–01].

1888b. The medico-psychological association. *Journal of Mental Science* 34:145–147 (Apr.) [88–02].

1888c. Remarks on the diagnosis and treatment of diseases of the brain. *BMJ* 2:59–63 (Jul. 14) [88–03].

1888d. Remarks on the diagnosis and treatment of diseases of the brain. *BMJ* 2:111–117 (Jul. 21) [88–04].

1888e. On a particular variety of epilepsy ("intellectual aura"), one case with symptoms of organic brain disease. *Brain* 11:179–207 (Jul.) [88–05].

1888f. Inhibition. *Brain* 11:386–393 (Oct.) [88–06].

1888g. On post-epileptic states: a contribution to the comparative study of insanities. *Journal of Mental Science* 34:349–365 (Oct.) [88–07].

1888h. Malposition of the left scapula. *Lancet* 2:1236. Patient shown at the Medical Society of London, December 17; not in York and Steinberg 2006, but same case in *BMJ* (Jackson 1888i).

1888i. Medical Society of London. Monday December 27, 1888. Case of paralysis of the lower part of the trapezius. *BMJ* 2:1393–1394 (Dec. 22) [88–08].

1888j. Opening address. *Proceedings, Medical Society of London* 11:1–7 [88–09].

1888k. Case in which a cerebral tumour had been removed. *Proceedings, Medical Society of London* 11:298 [88–10].

1889

1889a. On post-epileptic states: a contribution to the comparative study of insanities. *Journal of Mental Science* 34:490–500 (Jan.) [89–01].

1889b. Malposition of the scapula from paralysis of the lower part of the trapezius. *Illustrated Medical News* 2:100–101 (Feb. 2) [89–02].

1889c. Medical Society of London. Epilepsy with olfactory aura. *Lancet* 2:381–381 (Feb. 23) [89–03]. By-line: Jackson and Beevor.

1889d. Address in medicine by J. Hughlings Jackson. On the comparative study of diseases of the nervous system. *BMJ* 2:355–362 (Aug. 17) [89–04].

1889e. Abstract of the address in medicine delivered at the meeting of the British Medical Association, Leeds, by J. Hughlings Jackson. On the comparative study of diseases of the nervous system. *Lancet* 2:355–357 (Aug. 17) [89–05].

1889f. Editorial, presumably by Ernest Hart. The evolutionary theory in modern medicine. *BMJ* 2:385–386 (Aug. 17); not in York and Steinberg 2006.

1889g. On the comparative study of diseases of the nervous system. *Medical Record* 38:225–232 (Aug. 31) [89–06].

1889h. Presidential address on ophthalmology and general medicine, delivered before the Ophthalmological Society of the United Kingdom. *Lancet* 2:837–839 (Oct. 26) [89–07].

1889i. Ophthalmological Society. Presidential address. *Lancet* 2:854–855 (Oct. 26) [89–08].

1889j. Presidential address on ophthalmology and general medicine, delivered before the Ophthalmological Society of the United Kingdom. *BMJ* 2:911–913 (Oct. 26) [89–09].

1889k. Case of tumour of the right temporo-sphenoidal lobe bearing on the localisation of the sense of smell and on the interpretation of a particular variety of epilepsy. *Brain* 12:346–357 (Oct.) [89–10]. By-line: Jackson and Charles E. Beevor.

1889l. Ophthalmological Society of the United Kingdom. Note on a case of hereditary tendency to cataract in early childhood. *BMJ* 2:1895 (Dec. 31) [89–11].

1889m. Paralysis of trapezius. *Proceedings, Medical Society of London* 12:285–286 [89–12].

1890

1890a. On rigidity with exaggerated tendon reactions, and cerebellar influx. *BMJ* 2:541 (Mar. 8) [90–01].

1890b. The Lumleian Lectures on convulsive seizures. *Lancet* 1:685–688 (Mar. 29) [90–02].

1890c. The Lumleian Lectures on convulsive seizures,. delivered before the Royal College of Physicians of London. *BMJ* 1:703–707 (Mar. 29) [90–03].

1890d. The Lumleian Lectures on convulsive seizures. *Lancet* 1:735–738 (Apr. 5) [90–04].

1890e. The Lumleian Lectures on convulsive seizures, delivered before the Royal College of Physicians of London. *BMJ* 1:765–771 (Apr. 5) [90–05].

1890f. The Lumleian Lectures on convulsive seizures. *Lancet* 1:785–788 (Apr. 12) [90–06].

1890g. The Lumleian Lectures on convulsive seizures, delivered before the Royal College of Physicians of London. *BMJ* 1:821–827 (Apr. 12) [90–07].

1890h. Convulsive seizures, in Wood's Medical and Surgical Monographs, vol. 6, no. 3 (June). New York: William Wood and Company. Not in York and Steinberg 2006, but this is a reprinting of Jackson's Lumleian Lectures of 1890; see 1890b to 1890h.

1890i. Presidential address, delivered at the first meeting of the session, October 17th, 1889. *Transactions, Ophthalmological Society of the United Kingdom* 10:xliv–lix [90–08].

1891

1891a. Medical Society of London. Treadler's cramp. *Lancet* 1:434–435 (Feb. 21) [91–01]. By-line: Jackson and W.H.R. Rivers.

1891b. Hunterian Society. Phonographic illustration of disease. *BMJ* 1:644–645 (Mar. 21) [91–02]. By-line: Jackson and Rivers.

1891c. Hunterian Society. Phonographic illustration of disease. *Lancet* 1:884–885 (Apr. 18) [91–03]. By-line: Jackson and Rivers.

1891d. Clinical Society of London. Pseudohypertrophic paralysis. *Lancet* 1:988 (May 2) [91–04]. By-line: Jackson and James Taylor.

1891e. Remarks on a case of return of knee-jerks after hemiplegia in a tabetic. *BMJ* 2:57–58 (Jul. 11) [91–05]. By-line: Jackson and Taylor.

1891f. A case of treadler's cramp. *Brain* 14:110–111 [91–06]. By-line: Rivers and Jackson.

1892

1892a. Note on the knee-jerk in the condition of super-venosity. *BMJ* 1:326 (Feb. 13) [92–01].

1892b. A case of syringomyelus. *Lancet* 1:408–411 (Feb. 20) [92–02]. By-line: Jackson and James Galloway.

1892c. Lecture on neurological fragments. Delivered before the Hunterian Society. *BMJ* 1:487–492 (Mar. 5) [92–03].

1892d. Lecture on neurological fragments. Delivered before the Hunterian Society. *Lancet* 1:511–514 (Mar. 5) [92–04].

1892e. A case of double hemiplegia with bulbar symptoms. *Lancet* 2:1320–1322 (Dec. 10) [92–05]. By-line: Jackson and Taylor.

1892f. Case of Friedreich's ataxy. *Transactions, Medical Society of London* 15:462 [92–06].

1893

1893a. Neurological fragments. No. I. Two cases of ophthalmoplegia externa with paresis of the orbicularis palpebrarum (illustrations of Mendel's hypothesis). *Lancet* 2:128–129 (Jul. 15) [93–01].

1893b. Words and other symbols in mentation. *MPC* 107:205–208 (Aug. 30) [93–02].

1894

1894a. Neurological fragments. No. II. Congenital ptosis-innervation of the upper eyelid. *Lancet* 1:11 (Jan. 6) [94–01].

1894b. Neurological fragments. No. III. On the use of cocaine in the investigation of certain abnormal motorial conditions of the eyes. *Lancet* 1:11–12 (Jan. 6) [94–02].

1894c. Neurological fragments. No. IV. On the pupil and eyelids in cases of paralysis of the cervical sympathetic nerve. *Lancet* 1:12 (Jan. 6) [94–03].

1894d. Neurological fragments. No. V. Dr. Risien Russell's researches on the knee-jerks during artificially induced asphyxia in dogs and rabbits. *Lancet* 1:134–135 (Jan. 20) [94–04].

1894e. Neurological fragments. No. VI. The knee-jerks in two cases of opium poisoning. *Lancet* 1:135 (Jan. 20) [94–05].

1894f. Neurological fragments. No. VII. Temporo-sphenoidal (left) abscess from ear disease; right hemiplegia with lateral deviation of the eyes and aphasia; trephining; recovery. *Lancet* 1:390–392 (Feb. 17) [94–06].

1894g. A clinical study of a case of cyst of the cerebellum: weakness of spinal muscles: death from failure of respiration. *BMJ* 1:393–395 (Feb. 24) [94–07]. By-line: Jackson and J.S. Risien Russell.

1894h. Neurological fragments. No. VIII. Intensification of lateral deviation of the eyes in a case of hemiplegia during chloroform anaesthesia; Dr. Risien Russell's researches on reappearance under anaesthesia of lateral deviation of the eyes in dogs, recovered from that deviation which had been produced by ablation of part of the eye area of the cerebral cortex, and on lateral deviation of the eyes in intact dogs when under ether. *Lancet* 1:1052–1053 (Apr. 24) [94–08].

1894i. Neurological fragments. No. IX. Further remarks on lateral deviation of the eyes; Dr. Risien Russell's researches on representation of various ocular movements in the cerebral cortex; slight degrees of lateral deviation of the eyes; "punctuation" of motions of the eyeballs (trivial nystagmus) in some cases of hemiplegia. *Lancet* 1:1053–1054 (Apr. 28) [94–09].

1894j. The factors of insanities. *MPC* 108:615–619 (Jun. 13) [94–10].

1894k. A further note on the return of the knee-jerk in a tabetic patient after an attack of hemiplegia. *BMJ* 1:1350–1351 (Jun. 23) [94–11]. By-line: Jackson and Taylor.

1894l. Neurological fragments. No. X. On slight and severe cerebral paroxysms (epileptic attacks) with auditory warning; slight paroxysms with deafness and the slight imperception called "word-blindness;" spectral words (auditory); inability to speak and write. *Lancet* 2:182–183 (Jul. 28) [94–12].

1894m. Neurological fragments. No. XI. Cerebral paroxysms (epileptic attacks) with an auditory warning; in slight seizures, the special imperceptions called "word-deafness" (Wernicke) and "word-blindness" (Kussmaul); inability to speak and spectral words (auditory and visual). *Lancet* 2:252–253 (Aug. 8) [94–13].

1894n. Testimonial to Dr. Hughlings Jackson. *Lancet* 2:1362 (Dec. 8) [94–14].

1894o. Neurological fragments. No. XII. Absent knee-jerks in some cases of pneumonia–inaction of the intercostal muscles in respiration, and good voluntary action of the same muscles in a case of "latent pneumonia." *Lancet* 2:1472–1473 (Dec. 22) [94–15].

1895

1895a. Neurological fragments. No. XIII. Fits following touching the head – a case published by Dr. Dunsmure (1874). *Lancet* 1:274–275 (Feb. 2) [95–01].

1895b. Neurological fragments. No. XIV. The lowest level of the central nervous system–the study of tabes dorsalis and some other nervous maladies, as owing to disease of this level and its immediate connexions. *Lancet* 1:394–396 (Feb. 10) [95–02].

1895c. Neurological fragments. No. XV. Superior and subordinate centres of the lowest level. *Lancet* 1:476–478 (Feb. 23) [95–03].

1895d. The London Hospital. Presentation of testimonial to Dr. Hughlings Jackson, F.R.S., by Sir James Paget. *BMJ* 2:861–863 (Oct. 5) [95–04].

1895e. Presentation to Dr. Hughlings Jackson. *Lancet* 2:857 (Oct. 5) [95–05].

1895f. The testimonial to Dr. Hughlings Jackson, F.R.S. *London Hospital Gazette* 2:34–39 (Oct.) [95–06].

1895g. On imperative ideas. Being a discussion of Dr. Hack Tuke's paper (*Brain*, 1894). 1. – Dr. Hughlings Jackson. *Brain* 18:318–322 [95–07].

1896

1896a. Neurological fragments. No. XVI. The lowest level–negative and positive symptoms. The physiological element in symptomatologies. Remarks on the symptomatology of fracture-dislocations of the spine, crushing the cervical cord completely across below the emergence of the phrenic nerves. Charlton Bastian's researches on complete transverse lesions of the cord above the cervical enlargement; loss of the knee-jerks from these lesions; observations by Sherrington. *Lancet* 2:1662–1664 (Dec. 12) [96–01].

1897

1897a. Neurological fragments. No. XVII. Cervical fracture-dislocation cases. Destruction by complete transverse lesion of the cervical cord of intrinsic and extrinsic elements of the lowest level. Paralysis "at" and paralysis "below" the lesion. Mutilation of the nervous mechanisms of the "four systems" (thermal, circulatory, respiratory, digestive). Intracentral inhibition. *Lancet* 1:18–23 (Jan. 2) [97–01].

1898

1898a. The Hughlings Jackson lecture on the relation of different divisions of the central nervous system to one another and to parts of the body. Delivered before the Neurological Society, Dec. 8th, 1897. *Lancet* 1:79–87 (Jan. 8) [98–01].

1898b. Remarks on the relation of different divisions of the central nervous system to one another and to parts of the body. Delivered before the Neurological Society, December 8th, 1897. *BMJ* 1:65–69 (Jan. 8) [98–02].

1898c. Case of epilepsy with tasting movements and "dreamy state"–very small patch of softening in the left uncinate gyrus. *Brain* 21:580–590 [98–03]. By-line: Jackson and Walter S. Colman.

1899

1899a. Neurological fragments. No. XVIII. On asphyxia in slight epileptic paroxysms. On the symptomatology of slight epileptic fits supposed to depend on discharge-lesions of the uncinate gyrus. *Lancet* 1:79–80 (Jan. 14) [99–01].

1899b. Neurological fragments. No. XIX. A case of left hemiplegia with turning of the eyes to the right – slightly greater amplitude of movement of the left side of the chest in inspiration proper: and slightly less amplitude of movement of that side in voluntary expansion of the chest. *Lancet* 2:1659–1660 (Dec. 16) [99–02].

1899c. Epileptic attacks with a warning of a crude sensation of smell, and with the intellectual aura ("dreamy state") in a patient who had symptoms pointing to gross organic disease of the right temporo-sphenoidal lobe. *Brain* 22:534–549 [99–03]. By-line: Jackson and Purves Stewart.

1899d. Remarks on loss of movements of the intercostal muscles in some cases of surgical anaesthesia by chloroform and ether. *Brain* 22:550–562 [99–04]. By-line: Jackson and James S. Collier.

1899e. On certain relations of the cerebrum and cerebellum (on rigidity of hemiplegia and on paralysis agitans). *Brain* 22:621–630 [99–05].

1900

1900a. Epileptic attacks with crude sensations of smell and an intellectual aura. *Lancet* 1:477 (Feb. 17) [00–01]. By-line: Jackson and Stewart.

1900b. The medical staff and the management of the National Hospital for the Paralysed and Epileptic, Queen Square. *Lancet* 2:351–352 (Aug. 4) [00–02]. By-line: Jackson (first author) and medical staff.

1901

1901a. Sprengel's shoulder. *The Polyclinic* 3:102–104 (Oct.) [01–01].

1902

1902a. Neurological fragments. No. XX. Lowest level fits. Hypothesis on the mechanism of laryngeal crisis in tabes dorsalis. The physiological factor in symptomatologies. Remarks on some other lowest level fits. Terminal tonic spasms. *Lancet* 1:727–731 (Mar. 15) [02–01].

1902b. Observations on a case of convulsions (trunk fit or lowest level fit?). *Brain* 25:122–132 [02–02]. By-line: Jackson and Douglas Singer.

1902c. Further observations on a case of convulsions (trunk fit or lowest level fit?). *Brain* 25:286–292 [02–03]. By-line: Jackson and Stanley Barnes.

1903

1903a. On the study of diseases of the nervous system. A lecture delivered June, 1864. Reprinted from the London Hospital Reports, vol. I, 1864, at the special request of Sir William Broadbent. *Brain* 26:367–382 [03–01].

1903b. On aural vertigo. *The Polyclinic* 5:98–101 [03–02].

1906

1906a. Case of tumour of middle lobe of cerebellum–cerebellar paralysis with rigidity (cerebellar attitude)–occasional tetanus-like seizures (1871). *Brain* 29:425–440 (March) [06–01].

1906b. Case of tumour of middle lobe of cerebellum. Cerebellar attitude. No tetanus-like seizures. General remarks on the cerebellar attitude (1872). *Brain* 29:441–445 [06–02].

1907

1907a. Obituary. Sir William Broadbent. *BMJ* 2:180–181 (Jul. 20) [07–01].

1907b. Announcement. *Lancet* 2:1632–1633 (Dec. 7) [07–02].

1907c. Announcement. *BMJ* 2:1738 (Dec. 14) [07–03].

1909

1909a. Neurological fragments. No. XXI. Remarks on certain abnormalities of the sensations heat and cold.-Illustration of physiological antagonism. *Lancet* 1:377–378 (Feb. 6) [09–01].

1909b. On some abnormalities of ocular movements, with particular reference to "erroneous projection" in cases of paralysis of muscles of the eye-ball, especially in cases of paralysis of an external rectus-outgoing (centro-peripheral) v. In-going (periphero-central) currents. *Lancet* 1:900–904 (Mar. 27) [09–02]. By-line: Jackson and Leslie Paton.

1925

1925a. Neurological Fragments. With Biographical Memoir by James Taylor, M.D., F.R.C.P. [,] and Including the "Recollections" of the Late Sir Jonathan Hutchinson and the late Dr. Charles Mercier. London: Humphrey Milford. Oxford University Press.

1931–1932

1931–1932. Selected Writings of John Hughlings Jackson. 2 vols. Edited by James Taylor, Gordon Holmes, and F.M.R. Walshe. London: Hodder and Stoughton. Reprinted in 1958 by Basic Books, New York, and again in 1996 by Arts & Boeve, Nijmegen, The Netherlands. The page numberings of the main texts are consistent throughout all three printings. Thus, I have used all three printings, and I will refer to these Selected Writings as: 'Jackson 1931' for Vol. 1 and 'Jackson 1932' for Vol. 2. However, the Arts

& Boeve (1996) printing contains extra introductory sections and secondary bibliographies. They are added with capital Roman numeral paginations separate from and before the original lowercase Roman numerals of the original Introductions, which follow the original title pages. I will refer to these newer Introductions as N.J.M. Arts, Introduction, in Jackson 1931 or 1932.

1935

1935a. Hughlings Jackson memorial dinner. *Lancet* 1:872 (Apr. 13).
1935b. Hughlings Jackson Centenary. A Commemorative Dinner. *BMJ* 17:769–770 (Apr. 13).

General Bibliography

BHM—Bulletin of the History of Medicine
BMJ—British Medical Journal
JHN—Journal of the History of the Neurosciences
MTG—Medical Times and Gazette

For further description see 'Bibliographies and Formatting' in Chapter 1.

Ackerknecht, E.H. 1967. *Medicine at the Paris Hospital 1794–1848.* Baltimore: Johns Hopkins Press.

Ackerknecht, E.H. 1979. German Jews, English Dissenters, French Protestants: Nineteenth-century pioneers of modern medicine and science. In Rosenberg, C.E., ed. *Healing and History: Essays for George Rosen.* New York: Dawson Science History Publications, pp.86–96.

Ackerknecht, E.H., Vallois, H.V. 1956. *Franz Joseph Gall, Inventor of Phrenology and His Collection. Wisconsin Studies in Medical History*, No.1. Translated by C. St. Léon. Madison: Department of History of Medicine, University of Wisconsin Medical School.

[Adams, W. 1900]. Obituary. William Adams, F.R.C.S. *BMJ* 1:359.

Albert, D.M., Edwards, D.D. 1996. *The History of Ophthalmology.* Cambridge, MA: Blackwell Science.

Alexander, M.P. 1999. D. Frank Benson, M.D.: contributions to clinical aphasiology. *Aphasiology* 13:13–20.

Allbutt, T.F. 1871. *On the Use of the Ophthalmoscope in Diseases of the Nervous System and of the Kidneys; also in Certain Other General Disorders.* London: Macmillan.

Allen, R.C. 1999. *David Hartley on Human Nature.* Albany: State University of New York Press.

Amacher, M.P. 1964. Thomas Laycock, I. M. Sechenov, and the reflex arc concept. *BHM* 38:168–183.

Amacher, M.P. 1965. *Freud's Neurological Education and Its Influence on Psychoanalytic Theory. Psychological Issues 4* (no.4. Monograph 16). New York: International Universities Press.

Aminoff, M.J. 1993. *Brown-Séquard. A Visionary of Science.* New York: Raven Press.

Aminoff, M.J., ed. 1996. Special Issue. Brown-Séquard Centennial. *JHN* 5:5–42.

Aminoff, M.J. 2011. *Brown-Séquard: An Improbable Genius Who Transformed Medicine.* New York: Oxford University Press.

Andermann, A.A.J. 1997. Hughlings Jackson's deductive science of the nervous system: A product of his thought collective and formative years. *Neurology* 48:471–481.

Anderson, J. 1886. On sensory epilepsy. A case of basal cerebral tumour, affecting the left temporo-sphenoidal lobe, and giving rise to a paroxysmal taste-sensation and dreamy state. *Brain 9*: 385–395. Jackson 1888e, p.182, footnote 1, gives date of this as Oct. 1886.

[Anderson, J.] 1893. Obituaries. James Anderson, M.A., M.D., F.R.C.P. *BMJ* 1:494 (March 4); *Lancet* 1:560–562 (March 11).

Angel, R.W. 1961. Jackson, Freud and Sherrington on the relation of brain and mind. *American Journal of Psychiatry 118*:193–197.

Anstie, F.E. 1864. *Stimulants and Narcotics, Their Mutual Relations.* London: Macmillan.

Ashton, R. 1991. *G.H. Lewes: A Life.* New York: Oxford University Press.

Ashton, R. 2012. *Victorian Bloomsbury.* New Haven, CN: Yale University Press.

Austin, [S.] ed. 1855. *A Memoir of the Reverend Sydney Smith. By His Daughter, Lady Holland. with a Selection of his Letters*. 2 vols. London: Longman, Brown, Green, and Longmans.

Bailey, J.B. 1895. The medical institutions of London. The medical societies of London. *BMJ* 2:24–26, 100–103.

Bain, A. 1855. *The Senses and the Intellect*. London: John W. Parker. Reprinted 1998 by Thoemmes Press: Bristol.

Bain, A. 1859. *The Emotions and the Will*. London: John W. Parker. Reprinted 1998 by Thoemmes Press: Bristol.

Bain, A. 1861. *On the Study of Character, Including an Estimate of Phrenology*. London: Parker, Son, and Bourn.

Bain, A. 1864. *The Senses and the Intellect*. 2 ed. London: Longman, Green, Longman, Roberts, & Green.

Barfoot, M. 1995. "To ask the suffrages of the patrons": Thomas Laycock and the Edinburgh Chair of Medicine, 1855. *Medical History Supplement* 15:i–xv, 1–226.

Barfoot, M. 2009. David Skae: Resident asylum physician; scientific general practitioner of insanity. *Medical History* 53:469–488.

Barlow, T. 1919. William Allen Sturge, M.V.O., M.D. Lond., F.R.C.P. *BMJ* 1:468–469.

[Barnes, S.] 1955. Obituary. *BMJ* 2:567–568.

Barrett, P.H., Weinshank, D.J., Gottleber, T.T., eds. 1981. *A Concordance to Darwin's* Origin of Species. Ithaca, NY: Cornell University Press.

Barrett, P.H., Weinshank, D.J., Ruhlen, P., Ozminski, S.J., Berghage, B.N., eds. 1986. *A Concordance to Darwin's* The Expression of the Emotions in Man and Animals. Ithaca, NY: Cornell University Press.

Barrett, P.H., Weinshank, D.J., Ruhlen, P., Ozminski, S.J., eds. 1987. *A Concordance to Darwin's* The Descent of Man, and Selection in Relation to Sex. Ithaca, NY: Cornell University Press.

Barrière, I., Lorch, M.P. 2004. Premature thoughts on writing disorders. *Neurocase* 10:91–108.

Bartholow, R. 1874. Experimental investigations into the functions of the human brain. *American Journal of the Medical Sciences* 67:305–313.

Barton, R. 1998. "Huxley, Lubbock, and half a dozen others." Professionals and gentlemen in the formation of the X Club, 1851–1864. *Isis* 89:410–444.

Barton, R. 2018. *The X Club: Power and Authority in Victorian Science*. Chicago: University of Chicago Press.

Bartrip, P.W.J. 1990. *Mirror of Medicine: A History of the* British Medical Journal. Oxford: *BMJ* and Clarendon Press.

Bartrip, P. 1992. The *British Medical Journal*: a retrospect. In Bynum et al., pp.126–145.

Bastian, H.C. 1867. Case of "red softening" of the surface of the left hemisphere of the brain; with sudden loss of speech and hemiplegia. *BMJ* 2:544–546.

Bastian, H.C. 1869a. On the physiology of thinking. *Fortnightly Review* 5(new series):57–71 (January).

Bastian, H.C. 1869b. On the various forms of loss of speech in cerebral disease. *British and Foreign Medico-Chirurgical Review* 43:209–236 (January), 470–492 (April).

Bastian, H.C. 1886. *Paralysis, Cerebral, Bulbar and Spinal: A Manual of Diagnosis for Students and Practitioners*. London: H.K. Lewis.

Bastian, H.C. 1887. The "muscular sense"; its nature and cortical localisation. *Brain* 10:1–137. (Contains comments by several others, including Jackson 1887f, and reports of two operations in pp.27–32. Brown University's copy includes bound-in small brochure between p.4 and p.5: *Rules and List of Office Bearers and Members of the Neurological Society of London. 1887.*)

Bastian, H.C. 1887a. On different kinds of aphasia, with special reference to their classification and ultimate pathology. *BMJ* 2:931–936, 985–990.

Bateman, F. 1865. On aphasia, or loss of the power of speech; with remarks on our present knowledge of its pathology. *Lancet* 2:532–533.

Bateman, F. 1867. On the localisation of the faculty of speech. *BMJ* 2:419–421.

Bateman, F. 1869. On aphasia and the localisation of the faculty of speech. *MTG* 1:486–488.

Bateman, F. 1870. *On Aphasia, or the Loss of Speech, and the Localisation of the Faculty of Articulate Language.* London: John Churchill and Sons. Reprinted 2010 by Kessinger Publishing: Whitefish, MT.

Bazil, C.W. 2008. Sensory disorders. In Engel and Pedley, vol.3, pp.2779–2782.

Beale, L.S. 1870. *Protoplasm; or, Life, Matter, and Mind.* 2 ed. London: John Churchill and Sons.

Beale, L.S. 1875. Abstract of the Lumleian Lectures on life, and on vital action in health and disease. Lecture III. *BMJ* 1:600–603.

Beevor, C.E., Horsley, V.1887. A minute analysis (experimental) of the various movements produced by stimulating in the monkey different regions of the cortical centre for the upper limb, as defined by Professor Ferrier. *Philosophical Transactions of the Royal Society of London B 178*:153–167.

Behrman, S. 1982. Congestion of the brain. In Rose and Bynum, pp. 179–184.

Bell, S. 1981. George Henry Lewes: A man of his time. *Journal of the History of Biology* 14:277–298.

Bellon, R. 2011. Inspiration in the harness of daily labor. Darwin, botany, and the triumph of evolution, 1859–1868. *Isis 102*:393–420.

Bennett, A. H. 1888. Muscular hypertonicity in paralysis. *Brain* 10:289–332.

[Bennett, A.H.] 1901. Obituary. Alexander Hughes Bennett, M.D., F.R.C.P. Lond. *BMJ* 2:1444 (November 9).

Bennett, A.H., Godlee, R.J. 1884. Excision of a tumour from the brain. *Lancet* 2:1090–1091 (December 20).

Bennett, A.H., Godlee, R.J. 1885. Case of cerebral tumour. *BMJ* 1:988–989 (May 16).

Bennett, A.H., Godlee, R.J. 1885a. Case of cerebral tumour. *Medico-Chirurgical Transactions* 68:243–275 (read May 12 at the Royal Medical and Chirurgical Society).

Bennett, A.H., Godlee, R.J. 1885b. Excision of a tumour from the brain. *BMJ* 1:19 (January 3).

Bennett, A.H., Godlee, R.J. 1885c. Sequel to the case of excision of a tumour from the brain. *Lancet* 1:13 (January 3).

Bennett, A.H., Godlee, R.J. 1885d. Case of cerebral tumour. *Proceedings of the Royal Medical and Chirurgical Society 1*(new series):438–444.

[Bennett, A.H., Godlee, R.J.] 1885e. Excision of tumour of the brain. *BMJ* 1:1006–1007.

Benson, D.F. 1967. Fluency in aphasia: Correlation with radioactive scan localization. *Cortex* 3:373–394.

Benson, D.F., Ardila, A. 1996. *Aphasia. A Clinical Perspective.* New York: Oxford University Press.

Benton, A. 2000. *Exploring the History of Neuropsychology. Selected Papers.* New York: Oxford University Press.

Berg, A.T., Schaeffer, I.E. 2011. New concepts in classification of the epilepsies: Entering the 21 st century. *Epilepsia 52*:1058–1062.

Berker, E.A., Berker, A.H., Smith, A. 1986. Translation of Broca's 1865 report. Localization of speech in the third left frontal convolution. *Archives of Neurology* 43:1065–1072.

Berkowitz, A. 2018. You can observe a lot by watching: Hughlings Jackson's underappreciated and prescient ideas about brain control of movement. *The Neuroscientist* 24:448–455.

Bernard, C. 1865. *Introduction à l'Étude de la Médicine Expérimentale*. Paris: Bailliere.

Berrios, G.E. 1984. Epilepsy and insanity in the early 19th century. A conceptual history. *Archives of Neurology* 41:978–981.

Berrios, G.E. 1985. Positive and negative symptoms and Jackson. *Archives of General Psychiatry* 42:95–97.

Berrios, G.E., Freeman, H., eds. 1991. *150 Years of British Psychiatry, 1841–1991*. London: Royal College of Psychiatrists.

Betz, [V.] 1875. Distinction of two nerve-centres in the brain. *Quarterly Journal of Microscopical Science* 15:190–192.

Bewley, T. 2008. *Madness to Mental Illness: A History of the Royal College of Psychiatrists*. London: Royal College of Psychiatrists.

Billings, J.S. 1890. *The National Medical Dictionary*. 2 vols. Philadelphia: Lea Brothers & Co.

Billroth, T. 1878. *Lectures on Surgical Pathology and Therapeutics. A Handbook for Students and Practitioners*. Vol.2. Translated from the eighth [German] edition. London: New Sydenham Society.

Binder, D.K, Reynolds, E.H. 2017. Robert Bentley Todd's contributions to the structure and function of nerve tissue. *JHN* 26:336–337.

Binder, D.K., Rajneesh, K.F., Lee, D.J., Reynolds, E.H. 2011. Robert Bentley Todd's contribution to cell theory and the neuron doctrine. *JHN* 20:123–134.

Bing, R. 1939. *Textbook of Nervous Diseases*. Translated and enlarged by Webb Haymaker. St. Louis: C.V. Mosby.

Birken, W. 1995. The dissenting tradition in English medicine of the seventeenth and eighteenth centuries. *Medical History* 39:197–218.

Bladin, P.F. 1998. History of "epileptic vertigo": its medical, social, and forensic problems. *Epilepsia* 39:442–447.

Bladin, P.F. 2004. Murray Alexander Falconer and The Guy's–Maudsley Hospital seizure surgery program. *Journal of Clinical Neuroscience* 11:577–583.

Blair, J.S.G. 1987. *History of Medicine in the University of St Andrews*. Edinburgh: Scottish University Press.

Bland-Sutton, J. 1930. *The Story of a Surgeon*. Boston: Houghton Mifflin.

Bliss, M. 1999. *William Osler: A Life in Medicine*. Toronto: University of Toronto Press.

Bliss, M. 2012. Medical exceptionalism. *Perspectives in Biology and Medicine* 55:402–408.

Blume, W.T., Lüders, H.O., Mizrahi, E., et al. 2001. Glossary of descriptive terminology for ictal semiology: Report of the ILAE Task Force on Classification and Terminology. *Epilepsia* 42:1212–1218.

Bogen, J.E. 1997. The neurosurgeon's interest in the corpus callosum. In Greenblatt et al., pp.489–498.

Boling, W., Olivier, A., Fabinyi, G. 2002. Historical contributions to the modern understanding of function in the central area. *Neurosurgery* 50:1296–1310.

Bonin, G. von. 1960. *Some Papers on the Cerebral Cortex*. Springfield, IL: Charles C. Thomas.

Bonner, T.N. 1995. *Becoming a Physician. Medical Education in Great Britain, France, Germany, and the United States 1750–1945*. New York: Oxford University Press.

Bowler, P.J. 1988. *The Non-Darwinian Revolution. Reinterpreting a Historical Myth*. Baltimore: Johns Hopkins University Press.

Bowler, P.J. 1989. *The Invention of Progress. The Victorians and the Past*. Oxford: Basil Blackwell.

Bowler, P.J. 2005. Revisiting the eclipse of Darwinism. *Journal of the History of Biology* 38:19–32.

[Bowman, W.] 1892. Obituary. Sir William Bowman, Bart. F.R.C.S., F.R.S., L.L.D., M.D. *BMJ* 1:742–745.

Bracegirdle, B.1978. *A History of Microtechnique*. London: William Heinemann.

Bradbury, S. 1967. *The Evolution of the Microscope*. Oxford: Pergamon Press.

Bradley, F.H. 1894. On the failure of movement in dream. *Mind* 3:373–377.

Brain, W.R. 1935. Epilepsy. *Post-Graduate Medical Journal* 11:145–150.

Brain, W.R. 1964. *Clinical Neurology*. 2 ed. London: Oxford University Press.

Breidbach, O. 1997. *Die Materialisierung das Ichs. Zur Geschichte der Hirnforschung im 19. und 20. Jahrhundert*. Frankfurt: Suhrkamp.

British Association. 1868. British Association for the Advancement of Science. Meeting held at Norwich from 19th to 25th August. *Lancet* 2:291–294.

British Association. 1869. *Report of the Thirty-Eighth Meeting of the British Association for the Advancement of Science; Held at Norwich in August 1868*. London: John Murray.

Broadbent, M.E. 1909. *The Life of Sir William Broadbent, Bart., K.C.V.O.* London: John Murray.

Broadbent, W.H. 1866. An attempt to remove the difficulties attending the application of Dr. Carpenter's theory of the function of the sensori-motor ganglia to the common form of hemiplegia. *British and Foreign Medico-Chirurgical Review* 37:468–481.

Broadbent, W. 1903. Hughlings Jackson as pioneer in nervous physiology and pathology. *Brain* 26:305–366.

Broca, P. 1861. Remargues sur le siège de la faculté du langage articulé, suivies d'une observation d'aphémie. *Bulletin de la Société Anatomique de Paris* 2e serie, 6:330–357. Translated as 'Remarks on the seat of the faculty of articulate language, followed by an observation of aphemia' in Bonin 1960, pp.49–72.

Broca, P. 1863. Localisation des fonctions cerebrales. Siege de la faculte du langage articule. *Bulletin de la Société d'Anthropologie* 4:200–208.

[Broca, P.] 1864. Report of letter to Trousseau. *BMJ* 1:161.

Broca, P. 1865. Du siège de la faculté du langage articulé dans l'hemisphère gauche du cerveau. *Bulletin de la Société d'Anthropologie* 6:377–393.

Brown, G.H., ed. 1955. *Lives of the Fellows of the Royal College of Physicians of London 1826–1925* ("*Munk's Roll*", *vol.4*.) London: Royal College of Physicians.

Brown, J.W., Chobor, K.L. 1992. Phrenological studies of aphasia before Broca: Broca's aphasia or Gall's aphasia? *Brain and Language* 43:475–486.

Brown-Séquard, C.E. 1860. *Course of Lectures on the Physiology and Pathology of the Central Nervous System Delivered at the Royal College of Surgeons of England in May, 1858*. Philadelphia: Collins. Reprinted 1987 by The Classics of Neurology & Neurosurgery Library: Birmingham, AL.

Brown-Séquard, C.E. 1861. Lectures on the diagnosis and treatment of the various forms of paralytic, convulsive, and mental affections, considered as effects of morbid alterations of the blood, or of the brain or other organs. *Lancet* 2:1–2, 29–30, 55–56, 79–80,153–154, 199–200, 391–392, 415–416, 515–516, 611–613.

Brown-Séquard, C.E. 1878. Dual character of the brain. *Smithsonian Miscellaneous Collections* *15*:1–21.

Brunton, T.L. 1885. *A Text-Book of Pharmacology, Therapeutics and Materia Medica*. London: Macmillan.

Buchwald, J., Devinsky, O. 1988. J. Russell Reynolds and the study of interictal symptoms in epilepsy. *Archives of Neurology 45*:802–803.

Buckingham, H.W. 1984. Early development of association theory in psychology as a forerunner to connection theory. *Brain and Cognition 3*:19–34.

Buckingham, H.W. 2003. Walter Moxon and his thoughts about language and the brain. *JHN 12*:292–303.

Buckingham, H.W., Finger, S. 1997. David Hartley's psychobiological associationism and the legacy of Aristotle. *JHN 6*:21–37.

Burr, A.R. 1929. *Weir Mitchell. His Life and Letters*. New York: Duffield.

Burrow, J.W. 2000. *The Crisis of Reason. European Thought, 1848–1914*. New Haven, CN: Yale University Press.

Butler, S.V.A. 1988. Centers and peripheries: The development of British physiology, 1870–1914. *Journal of the History of Biology 21*:473–500.

Buzzard, E.F. 1934. Hughlings Jackson and his influence on neurology. *Lancet 2*:909–913.

Buzzard, T. 1874. *Clinical Aspects of Syphilitic Nervous Affections*. Philadelphia: Lindsay and Blakiston. Reprinted 2012 by General Books: Philadelphia.

Buzzard, T. 1878–1879. On some points in the diagnosis of spinal sclerosis. *Lancet 2*(1878): 111–112, 175–176, continued in *Lancet 1*(1879):74–76.

Buzzard, T. 1878a. On a prolonged first stage of tabes dorsalis: amaurosis, lightning, pains, recurrent herpes; not ataxia; absence of patellar tendon reflexes. *Brain 1*:168–181.

Buzzard, T. 1880. On "tendon-reflex" as an aid to diagnosis in diseases of the spinal cord. *Lancet 2*:842–844, 884–885.

Buzzard, T. 1882. *Clinical Lectures on Diseases of the Nervous System*. London: J. & A. Churchill. Reprinted 2014 by Repressed Publishing: Provo, UT.

[Buzzard, T]. 1919. Obituary. *BMJ 1*:59–60. Includes 'An appreciation by Sir David Ferrier, F.R.S.'

Bynum, W.F. 1991. Tuke's dictionary and psychiatry at the turn of the century. In Berrios and Freeman, pp.163–179.

Bynum, W.F. 1994. *Science and the Practice of Medicine in the Nineteenth Century*. New York: Cambridge University Press.

Bynum, W.F., Wilson, J.C. 1992. Periodical knowledge: medical journals and their editors in nineteenth-century Britain. In Bynum et al., 1992, pp.29–48.

Bynum, W.F., Lock, S., Porter, R., eds. 1992. *Medical Journals and Medical Knowledge. Historical Essays*. London: Routledge.

Cahan, D., ed. 2003. *From Natural Philosophy to the Sciences. Writing the History of Nineteenth-Century Science*. Chicago: University of Chicago Press.

Cant, R.G. 1970. *The University of St Andrews. A Short History*. Edinburgh: Scottish Academic Press.

Carpenter, W.B. 1855. *Principles of Human Physiology, with their Chief Applications to Psychology, Pathology, Therapeutics, Hygiène, and Forensic Medicine*. Philadelphia: Blanchard and Lea.

Carter, K.C. 1991. The development of Pasteur's concept of disease causation and the emergence of specific causes in nineteneth-century medicine. *BHM 65*:528–548.

Casper, S.T. 2014. *The Neurologists: A History of a Medical Speciality in Modern Britain, c.1789–2000*. Manchester: Manchester University Press.

Casper, S.T. 2014a. History and neuroscience: an integrative legacy. *Isis 105*:123–132.

Catani, M. 2011. John Hughlings Jackson and the clinico-anatomical correlation method. *Cortex 47*:905–907.

Catani, M., Ffytche, D.H. 2005. The rises and falls of disconnection syndromes. *Brain 128*:2224–2239.

Catani, M., Mesulam, M. 2008. The arcuate fasciculus and the disconnection theme in language and aphasia: History and current state. *Cortex 44*:953–961.

Chadwick, O. 1970. The established church under attack. In Symondson, pp.91–105.

Chadwick, O. 1975. *The Secularization of the European Mind in the Nineteenth Century*. Cambridge: Cambridge University Press.

Chamberlin, J.E., Gilman, S.L., eds. 1985. *Degeneration. The Dark Side of Progress*. New York: Columbia University Press.

[Chambers, R.] 1844. *Vestiges of the Natural History of Creation*. London: John Churchill.

Chance, B. 1937. Short studies on the history of ophthalmology. III. Hughlings Jackson, the neurologic ophthalmologist, with a summary of his works. *A.M.A. Archives of Ophthalmology 17*:241–289.

Charcot, J.-M. 1881. *Lectures on Diseases of the Nervous System. Delivered at La Salpêtrière*. Second Series. Translated by G. Sigerson. London: New Sydemham Society. Reprinted 1962 by Hafner: New York. From the original French edition of 1877.

Charcot, J.-M. 1887. *Lecons du Mardi à la Salpêtrière*. Paris: Delahaye & Lecrosnier.

Charcot, J.-M., Pitres, A.1883. *Etude Critique et Clinique de la Doctrine des Localizations Motrices dans l'Écorce des Hémisphères Cérébraux de l'Homme*. Paris: Alcan.

Cherry, S. 1996. *Medical Services and the Hospitals in Britain 1860–1939*. Cambridge: Cambridge University Press.

Chirimuura, M. 2017. Hughlings Jackson and the "doctrine of concomitance": mind-brain theorizing between metaphysics and the clinic. *History and Philosophy of the Life Sciences 39*(3), Article no.26 (September).

Chirimuura, M. 2019. Synthesis of contraries: Hughlings Jackson on sensory-motor representation in the brain. *Studies in History and Philosophy of Biology and Biomedical Sciences 75*:34–44.

Clarac, F., Boller, F. 1994. History of neurology in France. In Finger et al., pp.641–642.

Clark, G. 1964. *A History of the Royal College of Physicians of London*, vol.1. Oxford: Clarendon Press.

Clarke, E. 1971. Ferrier, David. In Gillispie, vol.4, pp.593–595.

Clarke, E., Jacyna, L.S. 1987. *Nineteenth-Century Origins of Neuroscientific Concepts*. Berkeley: University of California Press.

Clarke, E., O'Malley, C.D. 1996. *The Human Brain and Spinal Cord: A Historical Study Illustrated by Writings from Antiquity to the Twentieth Century*. 2 ed. San Franciso: Norman Publishing (1 ed., Berkeley: University of California Press, 1968).

Clarke, J.L. 1851. Researches into the structure of the spinal chord. *Philosophical Transactions of the Royal Society of London 141*:607–621.

Clarke, J.L. 1861. Notes of researches on the intimate structure of the brain. Second Series. *Proceedings of the Royal Society of London 11*(1860–1862):359–366.

Clarke, J.L. 1862. On the nature of volition, psychologically and physiologically considered. *The Medical Critic and Psychological Journal* ('*Winslow's Psychological Journal*') *2*:569–592 (no.8; nos 9 and 10 not obtained).

Clarke, J.L. 1863. Notes of researches on the intimate structure of the brain. Third Series. *Proceedings of the Royal Society of London 12*(1862–1863):716–722.

[Clarke, J.L.] 1880a. Obituary. *BMJ 1*:188.

[Clarke, J.L.] 1880b. Obituary. *Lancet 1*:189.

[Clarke, J.L.] 1880c. Obituary. *MTG 1*:189.

Clark-Kennedy, A.E. 1962–1963. *The London. A Study in the Voluntary Hospital System.* 2 vols. London: Pitman Medical.

Clark-Kennedy, A.E. 1979. *London Pride. The Story of a Voluntary Hospital.* London: Hutchinson Benham.

Coats, J. 1876. A study of two illustrative cases of epilepsy. *BMJ 2*:647–649.

[Coats, J.] 1899. Obituary. *BMJ 1*:317–319. Signed 'W.T.G.'.

Collins, E.T. 1929. *The History & Traditions of the Moorfields Eye Hospital. One Hundred Years of Ophthalmic Discovery & Development.* London: H.K. Lewis.

Collins, F.H. 1889. *An Epitome of the Synthetic Philosophy.* London: Williams and Norgate.

[Colman, W.S.] 1935. Obituary. *Lancet 1*:120–122.

Compston, A. 2015. The 'muscular sense'; its nature and cortical localization. By H. Charlton Bastian MD FRS. Professor of Clinical Medicine and of Pathological Anatomy in University College Hospital, London. *Brain* 1887; *10*:1–137. *Brain 138*:3449–3458.

Conlin, J. 2014. *Evolution and the Victorians. Science, Culture and Politics in Darwin's Britain.* London: Bloomsbury.

Cooke, A.M. 1972. *A History of the Royal College of Physicians of London.* vol. 3. Oxford: Clarendon Press.

Cooter, R. 1984. *The Cultural Meaning of Popular Science. Phrenology and the Organization of Consent in Nineteenth-Century Britain.* Cambridge: Cambridge University Press.

Cranefield, P.F. 1974. *The Way In and the Way Out. François Magendie, Charles Bell and the Roots of the Spinal Nerves.* Mt. Kisco, NY: Futura.

Crichton-Browne, J. 1926. *Victorian Jottings from an Old Commonplace Book.* London: Etchells & Macdonald.

Crichton-Browne, J. 1930. *What the Doctor Thought.* London: Ernest Benn.

[Crichton-Browne, J.] 1934. Brain surgery. Jubilee of pioneer operation. A veteran's memories. *The Times (London)*, November 28, p.16. *The Times* Digital Archive, accessed January 31, 2016.

Critchley, M. 1949. *Sir William Gowers, 1845–1915: A Biographical Appreciation.* London: William Heinemann.

Critchley, M. 1960. *Queen Square and the National Hospital 1869–1960.* London: Edward Arnold.

Critchley, M. 1960a. The contribution of Hughlings Jackson to neurology. *Cerebral Palsy Bulletin 2*:7–9. Reprinted 1964 with minor alterations in *The Black Hole and Other Essays.* London: Pitman, pp.133–136.

Critchley, M. 1960b. The beginnings of the National Hospital, Queen Square (1859–1860). *BMJ i*:1829–1837. Reprinted 1964 with minor alterations in *The Black Hole and Other Essays.* London: Pitman, pp.155–173.

Critchley, M. 1960c. Early days of the National Hospital, Queen Square. *Cerebral Palsy Bulletin 2*:5–6.

Critchley, M. 1960d. Jacksonian ideas and the future, with special reference to aphasia. *BMJ ii*:6–12. Reprinted 1970 in *Aphasiology and Other Aspects of Language.* London: Edward Arnold, pp.41–52.

Critchley, M. 1960e. Hughlings Jackson, the man; and the early days of the National Hospital. *Proceedings of the Royal Society of Medicine* 53:613–618. Reprinted 1964 with minor alterations in *The Black Hole and Other Essays*. London: Pitman, pp.124–132.

Critchley, M., Critchley, E.A. 1998. *John Hughlings Jackson: Father of English Neurology*. New York: Oxford University Press. Sometimes cited in my text as 'the Critchleys 1998'.

Crombie, C.M. 1875. Psychology and the nervous system. *BMJ* 2:514 (October 16). Letter to the Editor.

Cubelli, R., Montagna, C.G. 1994. A reappraisal of the controversy of Dax and Broca. *JHN* 3:215–226.

Cummings, J.L. 1999. D. Frank Benson, M.D.: biography and overview of contributions. *Aphasiology* 13:3–11.

Cushing, H. 1905. The special field of neurological surgery. *Bulletin of the Johns Hopkins Hospital* 16:77–87.

Cushing, H. 1926. *The Life of Sir William Osler*, 2 vols. Oxford: Clarendon Press.

Dacey, M. 2015. Associationism without associative links: Thomas Brown and the associationist project. *Studies in History and Philosophy of Science* 54:31–40.

Dalton, J.C. 1859. *A Treatise on Human Physiology Designed for the Use of Students and Practitioners of Medicine*. Philadelphia: Blanchard and Lea.

Dalton, J.C. 1867. *A Treatise on Human Physiology Designed for the Use of Students and Practitioners of Medicine*. 4 ed. Philadelphia: Henry C. Lea.

[Dalton, J.C.] 1968. Editorial. John C. Dalton, Jr (1825–1889). Experimental physiologist. *Journal of the American Medical Association* 203:155–156.

Damasio, A.R., Geschwind, N. 1984/1997. The neural basis of language. In Devinsky, O. and Schachter, S.C. eds. *Norman Geschwind. Selected Publications on Language, Epilepsy, and Behavior*. Boston: Butterworth-Heinemann, 1997. Reprinted from *Annual Review of Neuroscience* 7:127–147, 1984.

Daniels, E.A. 1972. *Jessie White Mario. Risorgimento Revolutionary*. Athens, OH: Ohio University Press.

Danziger, K. 1982. Mid-nineteenth-century British psycho-physiology: A neglected chapter in the history of psychology. In Woodward and Ash.

Daras, M.D., Bladin, P.F., Eadie, M.J., Millett, M. 2008. Epilepsy: historical perspectives. In Engel and Pedley, vol.1, pp.13–39.

Darwin, C. 1859. *On the Origin of Species*. London: John Murray.

Darwin, C. 1871. *The Descent of Man, and Selection in Relation to Sex*. 2 vols. London: John Murray. I have used the reprint with a New Introduction by J.T. Bonner and R.M. May, 1981, Princeton University Press: Princeton.

Darwin, C. 1872. *The Expression of the Emotions in Man and Animals*. London: John Murray. I have used the reprint from the Authorized Edition of D. Appleton, Introduction by K. Lorenz, 1965, University of Chicago Press: Chicago.

Darwin, C. 1874. *The Descent of Man, and Selection in Relation to Sex*. 2 ed. London: John Murray. I have used the printing of 1901, John Murray: London.

[Darwin, C.] 1994. *A Calender of the Correspondence of Charles Darwin, 1821–1882, with Supplement*. Cambridge: Cambridge University Press.

Daston, L.J. 1982. The theory of will versus the science of mind. In Woodward and Ash.

Davis, M. 2006. *George Eliot and Nineteenth-Century Psychology. Exploring the Unmapped Country*. Aldershot: Ashgate.

Dawson, G., Lightman, B., eds. 2014. *Victorian Scientific Naturalism: Community, Identity, Continuity.* Chicago: University of Chicago Press.

Dear, P., Jasanoff, S.A. 2010. Dismantling boundaries in science and technology studies. *Isis* 101:759–774.

Debru, C. 2006. Time, from psychology to neurophysiology. A historical view. *C.R. Biologies* 329:330–339.

DeFelipe, J., Jones, E.G. 1988. *Cajal on the Cerebral Cortex. An Annotated Translation of the Complete Writings.* New York: Oxford University Press.

DeLong, M.R. 2000. Basal ganglia. In Kandel et al., pp.853–867.

De Quincey (or Quincy), T. 2003. *Confessions of an English Opium-Eater and Other Writings.* Edited by B. Milligan. London: Penguin Books. Reprint of *Confessions* from *London Magazine* 1821 (p.xlii).

Dewhurst, K. 1982. *Hughlings Jackson on Psychiatry.* Oxford: Sandford Publications.

Dickson, J.T. 1873. On the dynamics of epilepsy and convulsions. *Guys Hospital Reports* 18:173–191.

Dictionary of National Biography. 1906. *The Concise Dictionary Part I. From the Beginnings to 1900.* Reprinted 1965 by Oxford University Press: London.

Dictionary of National Biography. 1961. *The Concise Dictionary Part II. 1901–1950.* Reprinted 1964 by Oxford University Press: London.

[Drewitt, F. Dawtrey]. 1942. Obituary. *BMJ* 2:174–175.

Duncan, D. 1908. *The Life and Letters of Herbert Spencer.* London: Methuen & Co. I have used the 'CHEAP RE-ISSUE' of 1911, Williams & Norgate: London.

Dunglison, R. 1860. *Medical Lexicon. A Dictionary of Medical Science.* Revised (2nd) ed. Philadelphia: Blanchard and Lea.

Dunglison, R. 1874. *Medical Lexicon. A Dictionary of Medical Science.* New edition revised by R.J. Dunglison. Philadelphia: Henry C. Lea. The copyright date on the inside of the title page says 1873.

Dunn, R. 1858. *An Essay on Physiological Psychology.* London: John Churchill.

Durante, F. 1887. Contribution to endocranial surgery. *Lancet* 2:654–655.

During, S. 2013. George Eliot and secularism. In Anderson, A., Shaw, H.E. eds. *A Companion to George Eliot.* Chichester: John Wiley & Sons, pp.428–441.

Eadie, M.J. 1990. The evolution of J. Hughlings Jackson's thought on epilepsy. *Clinical and Experimental Neurology* 27:29–41.

Eadie, M.J. 1999. The origin of the concept of partial epilepsy. *Journal of Clinical Neuroscience* 6:103–105.

Eadie, M.J. 2002. The epileptology of Théodore Herpin. *Epilepsia* 43:1256–1261.

Eadie, M.J .2005. Victor Horsley's contribution to Jacksonian epileptology. *Epilepsia* 46:1836–1840.

Eadie, M.J. 2007a. The neurological legacy of John Russell Reynolds (1828–1896). *Journal of Clinical Neuroscience* 14:309–316.

Eadie, M.J. 2007b. Cortical epileptogenesis—Hughlings Jackson and his predecessors. *Epilepsia* 48:2010–2015.

Eadie, M.J. 2007c. The philosopher of emerging clinical neurology. Essay-review of: York and Steinberg 2006. *Brain* 130:1968–1971.

Eadie, M.J. 2007d. The epileptology of John Thompson Dickson (1841–1874). *Epilepsia* 48:23–30.

Eadie, M.J. 2009. The role of focal epilepsy in the development of Jacksonian localization. *JHN* 18:262–282.

Eadie, M.J. 2011. William Gowers' interpretation of epileptogenic mechanisms: 1880–1906. *Epilepsia* 52:1045–1051.

Eadie, M.J. 2012. Sir Charles Locock and potassium bromide. *Journal of the Royal College of Physicians of Edinburgh* 42:274–279.

Eadie, M.J. 2012a. *Headache Through the Centuries*. New York: Oxford University Press.

Eadie, M.J. 2013. James Taylor (1859–1946): favourite disciple of Hughlings Jackson and William Gowers. *Journal of the Royal College of Physicians of Edinburgh* 43:361–365.

Eadie, M. 2015. William Henry Broadbent (1835–1907) as a neurologist. *JHN* 24:137–147.

Eadie, M. 2015a. Alexander Robertson (1834–1908): Glasgow's pioneer aphasiologist and epileptologist. *JHN* 24:292–302.

Eadie, M. 2018. Cortical epileptogenesis and David Ferrier. *JHN* 27:107–116.

Eadie, M.J., Bladin, P.F. 2001. *A Disease Once Sacred. A History of the Medical Understanding of Epilepsy.* Eastleigh: John Libbey.

Eadie, M.J., Bladin, P.F. 2010. The idea of epilepsy as a disease per se. *JHN* 19:209–220.

Ecker, A. 1873. *On the Convolutions of the Human Brain.* Translated by J.C. Galton. London: Smith, Elder.

Edelman, G.M. 1987. *Neural Darwinism. The Theory of Neuronal Group Selection.* New York: Basic Books.

Eling, P., ed. 1994. *Reader in the History of Aphasia. From [Franz] Gall to [Norman] Geschwind.* Amsterdam: John Benjamins.

Eling, P., Whitaker, H. 2010. History of aphasia: from brain to language. In Finger et al., pp.571–582.

Ellegård, A. 1990. *Darwin and the General Reader. The Reception of Darwin's Theory of Evolution in the British Periodical Press, 1859–1872.* Chicago: University of Chicago Press.

Ellis, H. 1993. Jonathan Hutchinson 1828–1913. *Journal of Medical Biography* 1:11–16.

Ellis, J. 1986. *L H M C 1785–1985. The Story of the London Hospital Medical College. England's First Medical School.* London: London Hospital Medical Club.

Elwick, J. 2007. *Styles of Reasoning in the British Life Sciences: Shared Assyumptions, 1820–1858.* London: Pickering & Chatty.

Engel, J. Jr. 2005. The emergence of neurosurgical approaches to the treatment of epilepsy. In Waxman, S., ed. *From Neuroscience to Neurology. Neuroscience, Molecular Medicine, and the Therapeutic Transformation of Neurology.* Amsterdam: Elsevier Academic Press, pp.81–105.

Engel, J. Jr. 2013. *Seizures and Epilepsy.* 2 ed. Oxford: Oxford University Press.

Engel, J. Jr., Pedley, T.A., eds. 2008. *Epilepsy. A Comprehensive Textbook.* 2 ed., 3 vols. Philadelphia: Lippincott Williams & Wilkins.

Engelhardt, H.T., Jr. 1975. John Hughlings Jackson and the mind-body relation. *BHM* 49:137–151.

[Erichsen, Sir John Eric] 1896. Obituary. *BMJ* 2:885–887.

Ey, H. 1932. *Des Idées de Jackson à un Modèle Organo-Dynamique en Psychiatrie.* Paris: Doin. Reprinted 1997 by L'Hartmattan: Paris.

Ey, H. 1962. Hughlings Jackson's principles and the organo-dynamic concept of psychiatry. *American Journal of Psychiatry* 118:673–682.

Eyler, J.M. 1992. The sick poor and the state: Arthur Newsholme on poverty, disease, and responsibility. In Rosenberg, C.E., Golden, J., eds. *Framing Disease. Studies in Cultural History.* New Brunswick, NJ: Rutgers University Press, pp.276–296. Reprinted 1997.

Feil, K. 2006. *Evolution and the Developmental Perspective in Medicine: The Historical Precedent and Modern Rationale for Explaining Disorder and Normality with Evolutionary Processes*. Unpublished Ph.D. thesis. University of Chicago.

Feiling, A. 1958. *A History of the Maida Vale Hospital for Nervous Diseases*. London: Butterworth.

Feindel, W., Leblanc, R. 2016. *The Wounded Brain Healed: The Golden Age of the Montreal Neurological Institute, 1934–1984*. Montreal: McGill-Queen's University Press.

Feindel, W., Leblanc, R., Villemure, J.-G. 1997. History of the surgical treatment of epilepsy. In Greenblatt et al., pp.465–488.

Feinsod, M. 2012. Neurognostic answer. The brilliant science and shadowy life of Ilia Fadeyevich Tsion, alias Elias Cyon, alias Elie de Cyon. *JHN 21*:337–342.

Feinstein, C.H., ed. 1981. *York 1831–1981. 150 Years of Scientific Endeavour and Social Change*. York: William Sessions.

Ferrier, D. 1873a. Experimental researches in cerebral physiology and pathology. *BMJ 1*:457.

Ferrier, D. 1873b. Experimental researches in cerebral physiology and pathology. *West Riding Lunatic Asylum Medical Reports 3*:30–96.

Ferrier, D. 1873c. Experimental researches in cerebral physiology and pathology. *Journal of Anatomy and Physiology 8*(second series vol.7):152–155 (published in 1874).

Ferrier, D. 1873d. The localisation of the functions in the brain. *Nature 8*:477–478.

Ferrier, D. 1874a. The localization of function in the brain. *Proceedings of the Royal Society of London 22*:229–232.

Ferrier, D. 1874b. On the localisation of the functions of the brain. *BMJ 2*:766–767.

Ferrier, D. 1874c. Pathological illustrations of brain function. *West Riding Lunatic Asylum Medical Reports 4*:30–62.

Ferrier, D. 1875a. Experiments on the brain of monkeys—No.I. *Proceedings of the Royal Society of London 23*:409–430.

Ferrier, D. 1875b. The Croonian Lecture: Experiments on the brain of monkeys (second series). [Abstract] *Proceedings of the Royal Society of London 23*:431–432.

Ferrier, D. 1875c. The Croonian Lecture – Experiments on the brain of monkeys (second series). *Philosophical Transactions of the Royal Society of London 165*:433–488.

Ferrier, D. 1876. *The Functions of the Brain*. London: Smith, Elder. Reprinted 1966 by Dawsons of Pall Mall: London.

Ferrier, D. 1878a. The Goulstonian Lectures on the localisation of cerebral disease. Delivered at the Royal College of Physicians of London. *BMJ 1*:399–402, 443–447, 471–476, 515–519, 555–559, 591–595.

Ferrier, D. 1878b. *The Localisation of Cerebral Disease: Being the Gulstonian Lectures of the Royal College of Physicians for 1878*. New York: G.P. Punam's Sons, 1879 (published in London in 1878 by Smith, Elder). Reprinted 2010 by Nabu Press: LaVergne, TN.

[Ferrier, D. 1881a]. Letter from London, dated "November 17, 1881". The prosecution or persecution of Professor David Ferrier, F.R.S., M.D., by the anti-vivisectionists. *Boston Medical and Surgical Journal 105*:552–554 (December 8).

[Ferrier, D. 1881b]. Editorial. Dr. Ferrier's localizations; for whose advantage? *BMJ 2*:822–824.

Ferrier, D. 1883. An address on the progress of knowledge in the physiology and pathology of the nervous system. Delivered at the first meeting of the session of the Royal Medical and Chirurgical Society. *BMJ 2*:805–808.

Ferrier, D. 1886. *The Functions of the Brain*. 2 ed. New York: G.P. Putnam's Sons. Reprinted 2015 by Facsimile: Delhi.

Ferrier, D. 1890. The Croonian Lectures on Cerebral Localization. Delivered at the Royal College of Physicians, June, 1890. *BMJ* 1:1289–1295, 1349–1355, 1413–1418, 1473–1479; 2:10–16, 68–75.

Ferrier, D. 1890a. *The Croonian Lectures on Cerebral Localization. Delivered at the Royal College of Physicians, June, 1890*. London: Smith, Elder. Reprinted from the BMJ; republished 2015 by Loeb Classical Library: Middletown, DE.

Ferrier, D. 1912. John Hughlings Jackson 1835–1911. *Proceedings of the Royal Society of London, Series B* 84:xviii–xxv.

Ferrier, D. 1919. An appreciation [of Thomas Buzzard]. In [Buzzard] Obituary, p.59.

Ferrier, D., Yeo, G.F. 1884. The effects of lesions of different regions of the cerebral hemispheres. *Proceedings of the Royal Society of London* 36:222–224.

Feuerwerker, E., Couillard, P., Gauthier, Y. 1985. Herbert Spencer's influence on the genesis of Sherrington's concept of the integrative action of the nervous system. *Canadian Bulletin of Medical History* 2:205–219.

Fields, W.S., Lemak, N.A. 1989. *A History of Stroke. Its Recognition and Treatment*. New York: Oxford University Press.

Fine, E.J., Darkhabani, M.Z. 2010. History of the development of the neurological examination. In Finger et al., pp.213–233.

Finger, S. 1994. *Origins of Neuroscience: A History of Explorations into Brain Function*. Oxford: Oxford University Press.

Finger, S. 2000. *Minds Behind the Brain: A History of the Pioneers and their Discoveries*. New York: Oxford University Press.

Finger, S., Roe, D. 1996. Gustave Dax and the early history of cerebral dominance. *Archives of Neurology* 53:806–813.

Finger, S., Stone, J.L. 2010. Landmarks of surgical neurology and the interplay of disciplines. In Finger et al., pp.189–202.

Finger, S., Boller, F., Tyler, K.L., eds. 2010. *History of Neurology*. (*Handbook of Clinical Neurology*, vol.95.) Amsterdam: Elsevier

Fish, F. 1965. David Skae, M.D., F.R.C.S., founder of the Edinburgh school of psychiatry. *Medical History* 9:36–53.

Fisher, R.B. 1977. *Joseph Lister 1827–1912*. Briarcliff Manor, NY: Stein and Day.

Fisher, R.S., Boas, W.v.E., Blume, W., et al. 2005. Epileptic seizures and epilepsy: definitions proposed by the International League Against Epilepsy (ILAE) and the International Bureau for Epilepsy (IBE). *Epilepsia* 46:470–472.

Fisher, R.S., Acevedo, C., Arzimanoglou, A., et al. 2014. ILAE official report: A practical clinical definition of epilepsy. *Epilepsia* 55:475–482.

Fishman, R.S. 1995. Ferrier's mistake revisited, or when it comes to the brain, nothing is simple. *Archives of Neurology* 52:725–730.

Fiske, J. 1874. *Outlines of Cosmic Philosophy Based on the Doctrine of Evolution, with Criticisms of the Positive Philosophy*. 2 Vols. Boston: Houghton, Mifflin.

Fiske, J. 1884. *The Destiny of Man Viewed in the Light of his Origin*. Boston: Houghton, Mifflin.

Fletcher, J.S. 1864. Case of embolism, following syncope from post partum hæmorrhage. *BMJ* 1:469–471 (April 30).

Flint, A. 1868. *A Treatise on the Principles and Practice of Medicine; Designed for the Use of Practitioners and Students of Medicine*. 3 ed. Philadelphia: Henry C. Lea.

Flourens, P. 1842. *Examen de la Phrénologie*. Paris: Paulin.

Foerster, O. 1936. The motor cortex in man in the light of Hughlings Jackson's doctrines. *Brain* 59:135–159.

Fournié, E. 1866. *Physiologie de la Voix et de la Parole*. Paris: Adrien Delahaye, 1866.

Francis, M. 2007. *Herbert Spencer and the Invention of Modern Life*. Ithaca, NY: Cornell University Press.

Franz, E.A., Gillett, G. 2011. John Hughlings Jackson's evolutionary neurology: a unifying framework for cognitive neuroscience. *Brain* 134:3114–3120.

Freud, S. 1891. *Zur Auffassung der Aphasien. Eine kritische Studie*. Leipzig: Franz Deuticke. Reprinted (on demand) 2019 by Wentworth Press.

Freud, S. 1953. *On Aphasia. A Critical Study*. Translated by E. Stengel. London: Imago.

French, R.D. 1975. *Antivivisection and Medical Science in Victorian Society*. Princeton, NJ: Princeton University Press.

Friedlander, W.J. 2001. *The History of Modern Epilepsy. The Beginning, 1865–1914*. Westport, CT: Greenwood Press.

Fritsch, G., Hitzig, E. 1870. Ueber die elektrische Erregbarkeit des Grosshirns. *Archiv für Anatomie, Physiologie und Wissenschaftliche Medizin* 37:300–332. Translated as 'On the electrical excitability of the cerebrum' in Bonin 1960, pp.73–96; and translated as 'The electrical excitability of the cerebrum' in Wilkins 1965 (1992), pp.16–27.

Fritz, E. 1864. Troubles du langage. *Gazette Hebdomadaire de Médecine et de Chirurgie* 1:873 (no.53, December 30).

F.R.S. [James Crichton-Browne] 1885. *The Times (London), December 16*, p.5, column 5.

Fulton, J.F. 1946. *Harvey Cushing: A Biography*. Springfield, IL: Charles C. Thomas.

F.W.M. 1920. Sir Victory Horsley, 1857–1916. *Proceedings of the Royal Society of London, Series B* 91:xliv–xlviii.

Galaburda, A.M. 1985. Norman Geschwind 1926–1984. *Neuropsychologia* 23:297–304.

Garrison, F.H. 1929. *An Introduction to the History of Medicine*. 4 ed. Philadelphia: W.B. Saunders. Reprinted 1966: Philadelphia: W.B. Saunders.

Gaskell, W.H. 1886. On the structure, distribution and function of the nerves which innervate the visceral and vascular systems. *Journal of Physiology* 7:1–80.

Gastaut, H. 1970. Clinical and electroencephalographical classification of epileptic seizures. *Epilepsia* 11:102–113.

Gastaut, H., Caveness, W.F., Landolt, H., et al. 1964. A proposed international classification of epileptic seizures. *Epilepsia* 5:297–306.

Gazzaniga, M.S., Bogen, J.E., Sperry, R.W. 1962. Some functional effects of sectioning the cerebral commissures in man. *Proceedings of the National Academy of Sciences* 48:1765–1769.

Geison, G.L. 1970. Beale, Lionel Smith. In Gillispie, vol.1. pp.539–541.

Geison, G.L. 1972. Social and institutional factors in the stagnancy of English physiology, 1840–1870. *BHM* 46:30–58.

Geison, G.L. 1978. *Michael Foster and the Cambridge School of Physiology. The Scientific Enterprise in Late Victorian Society*. Princeton, NJ: Princeton University Press.

Gelfand, T., Kerr, J., eds. 1992. *Freud and the History of Psychoanalysis*. Hillsdale, NJ: Analytic Press.

George, M.S., Trimble, M.R. 1992. The changing 19th century view of epilepsy as reflected in the West Riding Lunatic Asylum Medical Reports, 1871–1876, vols 1–6. *Neurology 42*:246–249.

Geschwind, N. 1964. The paradoxical position of Kurt Goldstein in the history of aphasia. *Cortex 1*:214–224. Reprinted 1997 in Devinsky, O., Schachter, S.C., eds., *Norman Geschwind: Selected Publications on Language, Epilepsy, and Behavior*. Boston: Butterworth-Heinemann, pp.53–61. I have used the latter source.

Geschwind, N. 1965. Disconnexion syndromes in animals and man. *Brain 88*:237–294, 585–644.

Ghez, C., Krakauer, J. 2000. The organization of movement. In Kandel et al., pp.653–673.

Ghez, C., Thach, W.T. 2000. The cerebellum. In Kandel et al., pp.832–852.

Gillispie, C.C., ed. 1970–1980. *Dictionary of Scientific Biography*, 16 vols. New York: Charles Scribner's Sons.

Glassman, R.B., Buckingham, H.W. 2007. David Hartley's neural vibrations and psychological associations. In Whitaker, H., Smith, C.U.M., Finger, S., eds., *Brain, Mind and Medicine: Essays in Eighteenth-Century Neuroscience*. New York: Springer, pp.177–190.

Glickstein, M. 1985. Ferrier's mistake. *Trends in Neuroscience 8*:341–344.

Gobo, D.J. 1997. Localization techniques: neuroimaging and electroencephalography. In Greenblatt et al., pp.223–246.

Godlee, R.J. 1918. *Lord Lister*. 2 ed. London: Macmillan.

[Godlee, R.J.] 2013. Godlee, Sir Rickman John (1849–1925). http:/livesonline.rcseng.ac.uk/biogs/E000221b.htm, accessed December, 26, 2013.

Goetz, C.G. 2010. Jean-Martin Charcot and the anatomo-clinical method of neurology. In Finger et al., pp.203–212.

Goetz, C.G., Bonduelle, M., Gelfand, T. 1995. *Charcot. Constructing Neurology*. New York: Oxford University Press.

Goldenberg, G. 2013. *Apraxia. The Cognitive Side of Motor Control*. Oxford: Oxford University Press.

Golla, F.L. 1932. Review of Jackson, J.H. 1931 (vol.1). *Journal of Mental Science 78*:204–206.

[Golla, F.L.] 1968. Obituary. *BMJ 1*:584.

[Golla, F.L.] 1968a. Obituary. *Lancet 1*:367–368.

Gooddy, W. 1964. Some aspects of the life of Dr C E Brown-Sequard. *Proceedings of the Royal Society of Medicine 57*:189–192.

Goodglass, H. 1986. Norman Geschwind (1926–1984). *Cortex 22*:7–10.

Goodman, J.H., Stewart, M., Drislane, F.W. 2008. Chapter 190. Autonomic disturbances. In Engel and Pedley, vol.2, p.2000.

Gowers, E. 1960. *Queen Square and the National Hospital 1860–1960*. London: Edward Arnold.

Gowers, W.R. 1874. Cases of convulsion from organic brain-disease. *BMJ 2*:398–400.

Gowers, W.R. 1879. *Manual and Atlas of Medical Ophthalmoscopy*. London: J. & A. Churchill.

Gowers, W.R. 1881a. Case of slight optic neuritis with paresis of sixth nerve, probably due to transient meningitis. *Transactions of the Ophthalmological Society of the United Kingdom 1*:115–117.

Gowers, W.R. 1881b. Case of intracranial disease with optic neuritis and paralysis of the upward movement of both eyes. *Transactions of the Ophthalmological Society of the United Kingdom 1*:117–119.

Gowers, W.R. 1885. *Lectures on the Diagnosis of Diseases of the Brain Delivered at University College Hospital*. London: J. & A. Churchill. Reprinted 2018 by BiblioLife: Charleston, SC.

Gowers, W.R. 1886–1888. *A Manual of Diseases of the Nervous System.* 2 vols. London: J. & A. Churchill. Reprinted 1995 by Arts & Boeve: Nijmegen.

Gowers, W.R., Barker, A.E. 1886. On a case of abscess of the temporo-sphenoidal lobe of the brain, due to otitis media, successfully treated by trephining and drainage. *BMJ* 2:1154–1156.

Granshaw, L. 1989. 'Fame and fortune by means of bricks and mortar': the medical profession and specialist hospitals in Britain, 1800–1848. In Granshaw, L., Porter, R., eds. *The Hospital in History.* London: Routledge, pp.199–220.

Greenberg, V.D. 1997. *Freud and his Aphasia Book. Language and the Sources of Psychoanalysis.* Ithaca, NY: Cornell University Press.

Greenblatt, S.H. 1964. *John Hughlings Jackson: The Development of his Main Ideas to 1864.* Unpublished M.A. thesis. Baltimore: Johns Hopkins University, Department of the History of Medicine.

Greenblatt, S.H. 1965a. *The English Neurologist, John Hughlings Jackson (1835–1911). American Philosophical Society Yearbook 1964.* Philadelphia: American Philosophical Society, pp.522–523.

Greenblatt, S.H. 1965b. The major influences on the early life and work of John Hughlings Jackson. *BHM* 39:346–376.

Greenblatt, S.H. 1970. Hughlings Jackson's first encounter with the work of Paul Broca: The physiological and philosophical background. *BHM* 44:555–570.

Greenblatt, S.H. 1974. Some philosophical and clinical background to Sherrington's concept of integrative action. *Proceedings of the XXIII International Congress of the History of Medicine*, London, 1972. London: Wellcome Institute for the History of Medicine, pp.58–61.

Greenblatt, S.H. 1977. The development of Hughlings Jackson's approach to the diseases of the nervous system 1863–1866: Unilateral seizures, hemiplegia and aphasia. *BHM* 52:412–430.

Greenblatt, S.H. 1984. The multiple roles of Broca's discovery in the development of the modern neurosciences. *Brain and Cognition* 3:249–258.

Greenblatt, S.H. 1988. Hughlings Jackson's theory of localization and compensation. In Finger, S., Levere, T.E., Almli, C.R., Stein, D.G., eds. *Brain Injury and Recovery. Theoretical and Controversial Issues.* New York: Plenum, pp.181–190.

Greenblatt, S.H. 1991. The development of modern neurological thinking in the 1860's. *Perspectives in Biology and Medicine* 35:129–139.

Greenblatt, S.H. 1995. Phrenology in the science and culture of the 19th century. *Neurosurgery* 37:790–805.

Greenblatt, S.H. 1997. The crucial decade: modern neurosurgery's definitive development in Harvey Cushing's early research and practice, 1900–1910. *Journal of Neurosurgery* 87:964–971.

Greenblatt, S.H. 1997a. Cerebral localization: from theory to practice. Paul Broca and Hughlings Jackson to David Ferrier and William Macewen. In Greenblatt et al., pp.137–152.

Greenblatt, S.H. 1999. John Hughlings Jackson and the conceptual foundations of the neurosciences. *Physis (Firenze)* 36:367–386.

Greenblatt, S.H. 2000. Book review of Critchley and Critchley 1998. *JHN* 9:223–225.

Greenblatt, S.H. 2002. Dialogues in historiography. Inclusiveness and coherency in the history of the neurosciences. *JHN* 11:185–193.

Greenblatt, S.H. 2003. Harvey Cushing's paradigmatic contribution to neurosurgery and the evolution of his thoughts about specialization. *BHM* 77:789–822.

Greenblatt, S.H. 2006. Broca, [Pierre] Paul. In Bynum, W.F., Bynum, H., eds., *Dictionary of Medical Biography*, vol.1. Westport, CT: Greenwood Publishing Group, pp.262–265.

Greenblatt, S.H. 2007. Owsei Temkin. October 6, 1902–July 18, 2002. *Biographical Memoirs of the National Academy of Sciences 89*:324–343.

Greenblatt, S.H. 2017. Book review of Raitiere 2012. *JHN 26*:339–340.

Greenblatt, S.H., Dagi, T.F., Epstein, M.H., eds. 1997. *A History of Neurosurgery in its Scientific and Professional Contexts*. Park Ridge, IL: American Association of Neurological Surgeons. Reprinted 2016 as ebook and 2017 in hardback by Thieme Medical Publishers: New York.

Gross, C.G. 2007. The discovery of motor cortex and its background. *JHN 16*:320–331.

Guenther, K. 2015. *Localization and its Discontents: A Genealogy of Psychoanalysis and the Neuro Disciplines*. Chicago: University of Chicago Press.

Guillain, G. 1959. *J.-M. Charcot. 1825–1893. His Life—His Work*. Translated by P. Bailey. New York: Paul B. Hoeber.

Guttmann, G., Scholz-Strasser, I. 1998. *Freud and the Neurosciences: From Brain Research to the Unconscious*. Vienna: Österreichischen Akademie der Wissenschaften.

Hagner, M. 1999. *Ecce Cortex. Beiträge zur Geschichte des Modernen Gehirns*. Göttingen: Wallstein.

Hagner, M. 2000. *Homo cerebralis. Der Wandel vom Seelenorgan zum Gehirn*. Frankfurt: Insel.

Hagner, M. 2003. Scientific medicine. In Cahan, pp.49–87.

Hagner, M. 2012. The electrical excitability of the brain: Toward the emergence of an experiment. *JHN 21*:237–249.

Haight, G.S. 1954–1978. *The George Eliot Letters*, 9 vols. New Haven, CT: Yale University Press.

Hakosalo, H. 2006. The brain under the knife: serial sectioning and the development of late nineteenth-century neuroanatomy. *Studies in the History and Philosophy of Biology and the Biomedical Sciences 37*:172–202.

Hall, M.B. 1986. Guerlac, Henry 10 June 1910–29 May 1985—Eloges. *Isis 77*:504–506.

Hannaway, C., La Berge, A., eds. 1998. *Clio Medica 50. Constructing Paris Medicine*. London: Wellcome Institute for the History of Medicine.

Harley, G., Brown, G.T. 1866. *Histological Demonstrations: A Guide to the Microscopical Examination of the Animal Tissues in Health and Disease*. London: Longmans, Green, and Co.

Harrington, A. 1987. *Medicine, Mind, and the Double Brain. A Study in Nineteenth-Century Thought*. Princeton, NJ: Princeton University Press.

Harrington, A. 1996. *Reenchanted Science. Holism in German Culture from Wilhelm II to Hitler*. Princeton, NJ: Princeton University Press.

Harrington, A. 2008. *The Cure Within. A History of Mind-Body Medicine*. New York: W.W. Norton.

Harris, L.J. 1991. Cerebral control for speech in right-handers and left-handers: An analysis of the views of Paul Broca, his contemporaries, and his successors. *Brain and Language 40*:1–50.

Harris, L.J. 1993. Broca on cerebral control for speech in right-handers and left-handers: A note on translation and some further comments. *Brain and Language 45*:108–120.

Harris, W. 1935. John Hughlings Jackson, 1835–1911. *Post-Graduate Medical Journal 11*(new series):131–134.

[Hart, E.] 1898. Obituary. Ernest Hart, M.R.C.S., D.C.L., Editor of the British Medical Journal. *BMJ 1*:175–186.

Hartley, D. 1749. *Observations on Man, his Frame, his Duty, and his Expectations*. 2 vols. London: Leake and Frederick.

Harveian Society of London. 1981. *Harveian Society of London 1831–1981*. London: Edward Collins.

Hawkins, J.E., Schacht, J., eds. 2008. *Sketches of Otohistory. A Series of Articles Originally Published in Audiology & Neurotology, Vols. 9–11, 2004–2006.* Basel: Karger.

Haymaker, W., Schiller, F., eds., 1970. *The Founders of Neurology.* 2 ed. Springfield, IL: Charles C. Thomas.

Head, H. 1915. Hughlings Jackson on aphasia and kindred affections of speech. *Brain* 38:1–27.

Head, H. 1918. President's address. Some principles of neurology. *Proceedings of the Royal Society of Medicine* 12:1–12. Delivered at the Section of Neurology, November 14, 1918.

Head, H. 1926. *Aphasia and Kindred Disorders of Speech.* 2 vols. Cambridge: Cambridge University Press.

Healey, E. 1978. *Lady Unknown. The Life of Angela Burdett-Coutts.* London: Sidgwick & Jackson.

Hearnshaw, L.S. 1964. *A Short History of British Psychology 1840–1940.* London: Methuen & Co.

Heffner, H.E. 1987. Ferrier and the study of auditory cortex. *Archives of Neurology* 44:218–221.

Heilman, K. 1997. Educator. In Schachter and Devinsky, pp.5–13.

Henderson, V.W. 1986. Paul Broca's less heralded contributions to aphasia research. *Archives of Neurology* 43:609–612.

Henderson, V.W. 1990. Alalia, aphemia, and aphasia. *Archives of Neurology* 47:85–88.

Henderson, V.W. 2010. Alexia and agraphia. In Finger et al., p.586.

Henson, R.A. 1989. The Hughlings Jackson tradition at the London Hospital. In Kennard and Swash, pp.31–36.

Herrnstein, R.J., Boring, E.G., eds. 1965. *A Source Book in the History of Psychology.* Cambridge, MA: Harvard University Press.

Heyck, T.W. 1982. *The Transformation of Intellectual Life in Victorian England.* Chicago: Lyceum Books.

Hierons, R. 1993. Charcot and his visits to Britain. *BMJ* 307:1589–1591.

Hitzig, [E.] 1865. Review of Clinical Lectures and Reports by the medical and surgical staff of the London Hospital 1864 [Vol.1]. *Berliner Klinische Wochenschrift* 2:173–174.

Hitzig, E. 1900. Hughlings-Jackson and the cortical motor centers in the light of physiological research. *Brain* 23:545–581.

Hogan, R.E., English, E.A. 2012. Epilepsy and brain function: common ideas of Hughlings-Jackson and Wilder Penfield. *Epilepsy & Behavior* 24:311–313.

Hogan, R.E., Kaiboriboon, K. 2003. The "dreamy state:" John Hughlings-Jackson's ideas of epilepsy and consciousness. *American Journal of Psychiatry* 160:1740–1747.

Hogan, R.E., Kaiboriboon, K. 2004. John Hughlings-Jackson's writings on the auditory aura and localization of the auditory cortex. *Epilepsia* 45:834–837.

Holmes, G. 1954. *The National Hospital, Queen Square, 1860–1948.* Edinburgh: E. & S. Livingstone.

[Holmes, G.] 1966. Obituary. Sir Gordon Holmes, C.M.G., C.B.E., M.D., F.R.C.P., F.R.S. *BMJ* 1:111–112.

Horsley, V. 1886. Brain-surgery. *BMJ* 2:670–675 (October 9).

Horsley, V. 1886a. Surgery. *Lancet* 2:346–347 (August 21).

Horsley, V. 1886b. Production of epilepsy in guinea-pigs. *BMJ* 2:976–977 (November 20).

Horsley, V.1886c. Abstract of the Brown Lectures. *Lancet* 2:1211–1213.

Horsley, V. 1887. Remarks on ten consecutive cases of operations upon the brain and cranial cavity to illustrate the details and safety of the method employed. *BMJ* 1:863–865 (April 23).

Horsley, V. 1887a. Demonstration of photographs of epileptic guinea-pigs, with remarks. *Proceedings of the Medical Society of London 10*:86.

Horsley, V. 1906. On Dr. Hughlings Jackson's views of the functions of the cerebellum as illustrated by recent research. The Hughlings Jackson Lecture, 1906. *Brain 29*:446–466 (published March 1907).

Horsley, V. 1907. On Dr. Hughlings Jackson's views of the functions of the cerebellum as illustrated by recent research. Being the Hughlings Jackson Lecture for 1906. *BMJ 1*:803–808 (April 6).

[Horsley, V.] 1916. Obituary. Sir Victor Horsley, C.B., F.R.S., M.B., F.R.C.S. *BMJ 2*:162–167.

Horsley, V., Schäfer, E.A. 1884. Experimental researches in cerebral physiology. *Proceedings of the Royal Society of London 36*:437–442.

Howarth, O.J.R. 1931. *The British Association for the Advancement of Science: A Retrospect 1831–1931*. Centenary (2nd) ed. London: British Association for the Advancement of Science.

Howells, J.G. 1991. The establishment of the Royal College of Psychiatrists. In Berrios and Freeman, pp.117–134.

Huhn, A. 1965. *Die Thrombosen der intrakraniellen Venen und Sinus*. Stuttgart: F.K. Schauttauer. Critchley and Critchley 1998, p.211, give the incorrect date as 1956.

Hunt, T., ed. 1972. *The Medical Society of London 1773–1973*. London: William Heinemann.

Hunting, P. 2002. *The History of the Royal Society of Medicine*. London: Royal Society of Medicine Press.

Hunting, P. 2003. *The Medical Society of London 1773–2003*. London: The Medical Society of London.

Hutchinson, H. 1946. *Jonathan Hutchinson. Life and Letters*. London: William Heinemann. Reprinted 1947.

Hutchinson, J. 1863. *A Clinical Memoir on Certain Diseases of the Eye and Ear, Consequent on Inherited Syphilis: With an Appended Chapter of Commentaries on the Transmission of Syphilis from Parent to Offspring, and its More Remote Consequences*. London: John Churchill.

Hutchinson, J. 1911. The late Dr. Hughlings Jackson: Recollections of a lifelong friendship. *BMJ 2*:1551–1554. Reprinted in Jackson 1925, pp.27–39.

Huxley, L. 1900. *Life and Letters of Thomas Henry Huxley*. 2 vols. London: Macmillan.

Huxley, T.H. 1874. On the hypothesis that animals are automata, and its history. *Nature 10*:362–366.

Huxley, T.H. 1887. Science. In Ward, pp.322–387.

Huxley, T.H. 1896. *Science and Christian Tradition. Essays*. New York: D. Appleton.

Huxley, T.H. 1904. *Method and Results. Essays*. London: Macmillan.

Isler, H. 1992. The roots of concomitance: The origin of Hughlings Jackson's psychophysical parallelism. In Boucher, M., Broussolle, E., eds. *History of Neurology. 3rd European Meeting, Veyrier-du-Lac, May 23–24, 1991*. Lyon: Fondation Marcel Mérieux, pp.199–203.

Isler, H. 1999. Laycock as the source of Hughlings Jackson's reflex and evolutionary theories. In Rose, pp.145–150.

Ivry, R.B., Schlerf, J.E. 2008. Dedicated and intrinsic models of time perception. *Trends in Cognitive Sciences 12*:273–280.

[Jackson, J.H.] 1911. Obituary (no byline). John Hughlings Jackson, M.D., F.R.C.P., F.R.S. *BMJ 2*:950–954 (Oct.14). Apparently written by James Taylor, with bylined contributions from Jonathan Hutchinson, Thomas Buzzard, Henry Head, Risien Russell, William Gowers, F.J.Smith. With portrait (Calkin).

[Jackson, J.H.] 1935. Hughlings Jackson centenary. A commemorative dinner. *BMJ 17*:769–770.

[Jackson, J.H.] 1935a. Hughlings Jackson memorial dinner. *Lancet 1*:872 (April 13).

Jackson, S.W. 1969. The history of Freud's concepts of regression. *Journal of the American Psychoanalytic Association* 17:743–784.

Jacyna, L.S. 1981. The physiology of mind, the unity of nature, and the moral order in Victorian thought. *British Journal for the History of Science* 14:109–132.

Jacyna, L.S. 1982. Somatic theories of mind and the interests of medicine in Britain, 1850–1879. *Medical History* 26:233–258.

Jacyna, L.S. 2000. *Lost Words. Narratives of Language and the Brain 1825–1926*. Princeton, NJ: Princeton University Press.

Jacyna, L.S. 2007. The contested Jacksonian legacy. *JHN* 16:307–317.

Jacyna, L.S. 2008. *Medicine and Modernism: A Biography of Sir Henry Head*. London: Pickering & Chatto.

Jacyna, L.S. 2009. The most important of all the organs: Darwin on the brain. *Brain* 132:3481–3487.

Jacyna, L.S. 2011. Process and progress: John Hughlings Jackson's philosophy of science. *Brain* 134:3121–3126.

Jacyna, L.S., Casper, S.T., eds. 2012. *The Neurological Patient in History*. Rochester, NY: University of Rochester Press.

James, F.E. 1998. Thomas Laycock, psychiatry and neurology. *History of Psychiatry* 9:491–502.

James, W. 1890. *The Principles of Psychology*. 2 vols. New York: Henry Holt and Company.

Jefferson, G. 1935. Jacksonian epilepsy. A background and a post-script. *Post-Graduate Medical Journal* 11:150–162

Jefferson, G. 1938. The tentorial pressure cone. *Archives of Neurology and Psychiatry* 40:857–876.

Jelliffe, S.E., White, W.A. 1935. *Diseases of the Nervous System. A Textbook of Neurology and Psychiatry*. 6 ed. Philadelphia: Lea & Febiger.

Jellinek, E.H. 2000. Dr H C Bastian, scientific Jekyll and Hyde. *Lancet* 356:2180–2183.

Jellinek, E.H. 2005. Sir James Crichton-Browne (1840–1938): pioneer neurologist and scientific dropout. *Journal of the Royal Society of Medicine* 98:428–430.

Jenkins, T.W. 1978. *Functional Mammalian Neuroanatomy*. Philadelphia; Lea & Febiger.

Jensen, J.V. 1988. Return to the Wilberforce–Huxley debate. *British Journal for the History of Science* 21:161–179.

[Johnson, M.] 1902. Obituary. *BMJ* 1:303.

Jones, C.H. 1870. *Studies on Functional Nervous Disorders*. London: John Churchill and Sons.

Jones, E.G. 1972. The development of the 'muscular sense' concept during the nineteenth century and the work of H. Charlton Bastian. *Journal of the History of Medicine* 27:298–310.

Jones, G. 2004. Spencer and his circle. In Jones and Peel, pp.1–16.

Jones, G., Peel, R.A., eds. 2004. *Herbert Spencer. The Intellectual Legacy*. London: Galton Institute.

Joynt, R.J. 1982. The great confrontation: The meeting between Broca and Jackson in 1868. In Rose and Bynum, pp.99–102.

Kaitaro T. 2001. Biological and epistemological models of localization in the nineteenth century: From Gall to Charcot. *JHN* 10:262–276.

Kandel, E.R., Schwartz, J.H., eds. 1981. *Principles of Neural Science*. New York: Elsevier/North Holland.

Kandel, E.R., Schwartz, J.H., Jessell, T.M., eds. 2000. *Principles of Neural Science*. 4 ed. New York: McGraw-Hill.

Kennard, C., Swash, M. 1989. *Hierarchies in Neurology. A Reappraisal of a Jacksonian Concept.* London: Springer.

Kennedy, J.G. 1978. *Herbert Spencer.* Boston: Twayne Publishers.

Kernohan, J.W., Woltman, H.W. 1929. Incisura of the crus due to contralateral brain tumor. *Archives of Neurology and Psychiatry 21*:274–287.

Kevles, B.H. 1997. *Naked to the Bone. Medical Imaging in the Twentieth Century.* New Brunswick, NJ: Rutgers University Press.

Kitchel, A.T. 1933. *George Lewes and George Eliot. A Review of Records.* New York: The John Day Company.

Koehler, P.J. 1994. Brown-Séquard's spinal epilepsy. *Medical History 38*:189–203.

Koehler, P.J. 1996. Brown-Séquard and cerebral localization as illustrated by his ideas on aphasia. *JHN 5*:26–33.

Koehler, P.J. 1999. The evolution of British neurology in comparison with other countries. In Rose, pp.58–74.

Koehler, P.J., Wijdicks, E.F.M. 2008. Historical study of coma: looking back through medical and neurological texts. *Brain 131*:877–889.

Koehler, P.J., Wijdicks, E.F.M. 2015. Fixed and dilated: the history of a classic pupil abnormality. *Journal of Neurosurgery 122*:453–463.

Koehler, P.J., Bruyn, G.W., Pearce, J.M.S. eds. 2000. *Neurological Eponyms.* New York: Oxford University Press.

Kotagal, P., Lüders, H.O. 2008. Simple motor seizures. In Engel and Pedley, p.522.

Krakauer, J., Ghez, C. 2000. Voluntary movement. In Kandel et al., pp.781–756.

Krumholz, A., Bergey, G.K., Nathanson, M. 1994. John Hughlings Jackson's observations on 'lower level', or 'pontobulbar', fits and their relevance to current concepts of seizures and myoclonus. *Neurology 44*:1527–1530.

Kuhn, P. 2017. *Psychoanalysis in Britain, 1893–1913. Histories and Historiography.* Lanham, MD: Lexington Books.

Kuhn, T.S. 1962. *The Structure of Scientific Revolutions.* Chicago: University of Chicago Press. 2 ed. 1970, 3 ed. 1996.

Kushchayev, S.V., Moskalenko, V.F., Wiener, P.C., et al. 2012. The discovery of the pyramidal neurons: Vladimir Betz and a new era of neuroscience. *Brain 135*:285–300.

Kushner, H.I. 1999. *A Cursing Brain? The Histories of Tourette Syndrome.* Cambridge, MA: Harvard University Press.

Kushner, H.I. 2015. Norman Geschwind and the use of history in the (re)birth of behavioral neurology. *JHN 24*:173–192.

Kussmaul, A., Tenner, A. 1859. On the nature and origin of epileptiform convulsions caused by profuse bleeding and also of those of true epilepsy. Translated by E. Bronner. Selected Monographs. London: New Sydenham Society, pp.1–109.

Lancet. 1868. Editorial. *Lancet 2*:386 (September 19).

Landau, W.M., Aring, C.D. 1973. [Obituary] Francis Martin Rouse Walshe 1885–1973. *Archives of Neurology 29*:355–357.

Lanska, D.J. 2010. The history of movement disorders. In Finger et al., pp.501–546.

Laporte, Y. 1992. Brown-Séquard and the discovery of the vasoconstrictor nerves. *JHN 5*:21–25.

Lardreau, E. 2011. An approach to nineteenth-century medical lexicon: the term "Dreamy State". *JHN* 20:34–41.

Lassek, A.M. 1979. *The Unique Legacy of Doctor Hughlings Jackson.* Springfield, IL: Charles C. Thomas.

Latham, R.G. 1856. *Logic in its Application to Language.* London: Walton and Maberly.

Lawrence, C. 1985. Incommunicable knowledge: science, technology and the clinical art in Britain 1850-1914. *Journal of Contemporary History* 20:503–520.

Lawrence, C., Weiss, G., eds. 1998. *Greater than the Parts: Holism in Biomedicine 1920–1950.* New York; Oxford University Press.

Laycock, T. 1845. On the reflex function of the brain. *British and Foreign Medical Review* 19 (January–April):298–311.

Laycock, T. 1846. A lecture on clinical observation; its value and nature, and the mode and means of practising it. Delivered at the York Medical School. *London Medical Gazette* 3:141–148.

Laycock, T. 1846a. An introductory lecture. Delivered October 1st, 1846, at the opening of the York Medical School. *London Medical Gazette* 3:613–617.

Laycock, T. 1855. Further researches into the functions of the brain. *British and Foreign Medico-Chirurgical Review* 16:155–187.

Laycock, T. 1856. *Lectures on the Principles and Methods of Medical Observation and Research for the Use of Advanced Students and Junior Practitioners.* Edinburgh: Adam and Charles Black.

Laycock, T. 1859. Phrenology. In *The Encyclopaedia Britannica*, 8 ed., vol.17. Boston: Little, Brown, & Co., pp.556–567.

Laycock, T. 1860. *Mind and Brain: or, the Correlations of Consciousness and Organisation; with their Applications to Philosophy, Zoology, Physiology, Mental Pathology, and the Practice of Medicine.* 2 vols. Edinburgh: Sutherland and Knox. Reprinted 1976 by Arno Press: New York.

Lazar, J.W. 2009a. Anglo-American interest in cerebral physiology. *JHN* 18:304–311.

Lazar, J.W. 2009b. Diffusion of electrical current in the experiments of Fritsch and Hitzig and Ferrier failed to negate their conclusion of the existence of cerebral motor centers. *JHN* 18:366–376.

Lazar, J.W. 2010. Acceptance of the neuron theory by clinical neurologists of the late-nineteenth century. *JHN* 19:349–364.

Lazar, J.W. 2015. A contextual analysis of nervous force in medico-scientific and literary writings in English of the nineteenth and early-twentieth centuries. *JHN* 24:244–267.

Leblanc, R. 2017. *Fearful Asymmetry: Bouillaud, Dax, Broca, and the Localization of Language, Paris, 1825–1879.* Montreal: McGill-Queen's University Press.

Lebrun, Y. 1994. Pierre Marie. In Eling, pp.219–229.

Lee, S. 1965. *The Dictionary of National Biography. The Concise Dictionary. Part 1.* 2 ed. Reprinted by Oxford University Press: London.

Lees, D.B., Bellamy, E. 1880. Case of traumatic epilepsy treated by trephining. *BMJ* 2:624.

Leff, A. 1991. Thomas Laycock and the cerebral reflex: a function arising from and pointing to the unity of nature. *History of Psychiatry* 2:385–407.

Lekka, V. 2015. *The Neurological Emergence of Epilepsy: The National Hospital for the Paralyzed and Epileptic (1870–1895) (Boston Studies in the Philosophy and History of Science 305).* Cham: Springer.

Lennox, W.G., Lennox, M.A. 1960. *Epilepsy and Related Disorders*, vol.1. Boston: Little, Brown and Company.

Lepore, F.E. 1982. Toward a definition of papilledema: A historical review, 1851–1911. *Surgical Neurology 17*:178–180.

Lesky, E. 1976. *The Vienna Medical School of the 19th Century*. Baltimore: Johns Hopkins University Press.

Leuret, F., Gratiolet, P. 1839–1857. *Anatomie Comparée du Système Nerveux, Considérée dans ses Rapports avec l'Intelligence*. 2 vols. (2nd vol. by Gratiolet alone). Paris: J.B. Baillière et Fils.

Lewes, G.H. 1853. *Comte's Philosophy of the Sciences: Being an Exposition of the Principles of the Cours de Philosophie Positive of Auguste Comte*. London: Henry G. Bohn.

Lewes, G.H. 1859–1860. *The Physiology of Common Life*, 2 vols. Edinburgh: William Blackwood and Sons (vol.1, 1859; vol.2, 1860).

Lewes, G.H. 1874. *Problems of Life and Mind. First Series. The Foundations of a Creed*, vol.1. London: Trübner & Co. Reprinted 2011.

Lewes, G.H. 1874–1879. *Problems of Life and Mind*. 5 vols. London; Trübner.

Lewes, G.H. 1875. *Problems of Life and Mind. First Series. The Foundations of a Creed*, vol.2. Boston: James R. Osgood & Co. Reprinted 2011.

Lewes, G.H. 1876. Book review of Ferrier 1876. *Nature 15*:73–74, 93–95.

Lewes, G.H. 1877. *The Physical Basis of Mind ... Being the Second Series of Problems of Life and Mind*. Boston: James R. Osgood & Co.

Lewes, G.H. 1879. *Problems of Life and Mind. Third Series. Problem the First. The Study of Psychology*. Boston: Houghton, Osgood & Co.

Lewes, G.H. *Manuscripts in George Eliot and George Henry Lewes Collection, Yale Collection of American Literature, Beinecke Rare Book and Manuscript Library*. New Haven, CT: Yale University. Visited October 12, 2006.

Lewis, B. 1878. On the comparative structure of the cortex cerebri. *Brain 1*:79–96.

Lightman, B. 1987. *The Origins of Agnosticism. Victorian Unbelief and the Limits of Knowledge*. Baltimore: Johns Hopkins University Press.

Lightman, B. 2007. *Victorian Popularizers of Science. Designing Nature for New Audiences*. Chicago: University of Chicago Press.

Lightman, B. 2017. On Tyndall's Belfast address. In Felluga, D.F. ed. *BRANCH: Britain, Representation and Nineteenth-Century History*. http://www.branchcollective.org/.

Linker, B. 2007. Resuscitating the 'Great Doctor': The career of biography in medical history. In Söderqvist, pp.221–239.

Little, E.M. [1933]. *History of the British Medical Association 1832–1932*. London: British Medical Association.

Lorch, M.P. 2004a. The unknown source of John Hughlings Jackson's early interest in aphasia and epilepsy. *Cognitive and Behavioral Neurology 17*:124–132.

Lorch, M.P. 2004b. Revisitng the great debate of 1868: Broca, Jackson and the seat of the language faculty. *JHN 13*:182–183.

Lorch, M.P. 2008. The merest logomachy: The 1868 Norwich discussion of aphasia by Hughlings Jackson and Broca. *Brain 131*:1658–1670.

Lorch, M.P. 2009. The Third Man: aphasia research in mid 19th century England. *JHN 18*:120–121.

Lorch, M. 2011. Re-examining Paul Broca's initial presentation of M. Leborgne: Understanding the impetus for brain and language research. *Cortex 47*:1228–1235.

Lorch, M.P. 2012. Speaking for yourself. The medico-legal aspects of aphasia in nineteenth-century Britain. In Jacyna and Casper, pp.63–80.

Lorch, M.P. 2013. Examining language functions: a reassessment of Bastian's contribution to aphasia assessment. *Brain* 136:2629–2637.

Lorch, M.P. 2016. The Third Man: Robert Dunn's (1799–1877) contribution to aphasia research in mid-19th-century England. *JHN* 25:188–203.

Lorch, M., Hellal, P. 2010. Darwin's 'Natural Science of Babies'. *JHN* 19:140–157.

Lorch, M., Hellal, P. 2016. The Victorian question of the relation between language and thought. *Publications of the English Goethe Society* 85:110–124.

[Lost Hospitals of London.] Maida Vale Hospital for Nervous Diseases. http://ezitis.myzen.co.uk/maidavale.html, accessed February 9, 2016.

Louis, E.D., ed. 2002. The neurological examination (with an emphasis on its historical underpinnings). *Seminars in Neurology* 22 (no.4, December).

Louis, E.D. 2002a. Erb and Westphal: simultaneous discovery of the deep tendon reflexes. In Louis, pp.385–389.

Loudon, J., Loudon, I. 1992. Medicine, politics and the medical periodical 1800-50. In Bynum et al., pp.49–69.

Lyle, H.W. 1935. *King's and Some King's Men: Being a Record of the Medical Department of King's College, London, from 1830–1909 and of King's College Hospital Medical School from 1909 to 1934.* London: Oxford University Press (Humphrey Milford).

Lyons, A.E. 1997. The crucible years 1880–1900: Macewen to Cushing. In Greenblatt et al., pp.153–166.

Lyons, J.B. 1966. *Citizen Surgeon. A Biography of Sir Victor Horsley.* London: Peter Dawnay.

Lyons, J.B. 1967. Sir Victor Horsley. *Medical History* 11:361–373.

Lyons, J.B. 1998. Some contributions of Robert Bentley Todd. *JHN* 7:11–26.

Lyons, J.B. 2000. Todd's paralysis. In Koehler et al., pp.100–105.

Mac Cormac, W., ed. 1881. *Transactions of the International Medical Congress, Seventh Session, Held in London, August 2nd to 9th, 1881.* 4 vols. London: J.W. Kolckmann.

Macewen, [W.] 1879a. Tumour of the dura mater—convulsions—removal of tumour by trephining—recovery. *Glasgow Medical Journal* 2:210–213.

Macewen, [W.] 1879b. Cases of trephining. *BMJ* 2:1022 (December 27).

Macewen, W. 1881. Intra-cranial lesions, illustrating some points in connexion with the localization of cerebral affections and the advantages of antiseptic trephining. *BMJ* 2:541–543, 581–583 (September 24, October 1).

Macewen, W. 1888. An address on the surgery of the brain and spinal cord. *BMJ* 2:302–309.

[Mackenzie, S.] 1909. Obituary. *BMJ* 2:732–733.

[Mackenzie, S.] 2019. Mackenzie, Sir Stephen (1844–1909). www.oxforddnb.com, accessed March 1, 2019.

Macklis, R.M., Macklis, J.D. 1992. Historical and phrenologic reflections on the nonmotor functions of the cerebellum: Love under the tent? *Neurology* 42:928–932.

Macmillan, M. 2004. Localization and William Macewen's early brain surgery. Part I: The controversy. *JHN* 13:297–325.

Macmillan, M. 2005. Localization and William Macewen's early brain surgery. Part II: The cases. *JHN* 14:24–56.

Mansel, H.L. 1866. *Metaphysics or the Philosophy of Consciousness Phenomenal and Real.* 2 ed. Edinburgh: Adam and Charles Black.

Marshall, J.C. 1994. Henry Charlton Bastian. In Eling, pp.99–111.

Martensen, R.L. 2004. *The Brain Takes Shape. An Early History.* Oxford: Oxford University Press.

Martin, J.P. 1973. Neurology in fiction: The Turn of the Screw. *BMJ* 4:717–721.

Martin, J.P. 1975. Kinnier Wilson's notes of conversations with Hughlings Jackson. *Journal of Neurology, Neurosurgery, and Psychiatry* 38:313–316.

Matthew, H.C.G., Harrison, B., eds. 2004. Oxford Dictionary of National Biography, in Association with the British Academy. From the earliest times to the year 2000. 60 vols. New York: Oxford University Press.

Maudsley, H. 1866. On some of the causes of insanity. *BMJ* 2:586.

Maurice-Williams, R.S. 1967. The achievement of Hughlings Jackson. *St. Thomas's Hospital Gazette* 65:43–51.

Mayr, E. 1982. *The Growth of Biological Thought. Diversity, Evolution, and Inheritance.* Cambridge, MA: Harvard University (Belknap) Press.

McComas, A.J. 2016. Hypothesis: Hughlings Jackson and presynaptic inhibition: Is there a big picture? *Journal of Neurophysiology* 116:41–50.

McHenry, L.C. 1969. *Garrison's History of Neurology.* Revised ed. Springfield, IL: Charles C. Thomas.

McWilliam, J.A. 1888. On the rhythm of the mammalian heart. *Journal of Physiology* 9:167–198 (nos.2–3, August).

Mercier, C. 1887. Coma. *Brain* 9:469–487 (January).

Mercier, C. 1888. Inhibition. *Brain* 11:361–405 (October).

Mercier, C. 1888a. *The Nervous System and the Mind. A Treatise on the Dynamics of the Human Organism.* London: Macmillan.

Mercier, C. 1890. *Sanity and Insanity.* London: Walter Scott.

Mercier, C. 1912. The late Dr. Hughlings Jackson. Recollections by Dr. Mercier. *BMJ* 1:85–86. Reprinted as 'Recollections' in Jackson 1925, pp.40–46.

[Mercier, C.A.] 1919. Obituary. Charles Arthur Mercier, M.D. Lond., F.R.C.P., F.R.C.S. *BMJ* 2:363–365. Includes appreciations by Sir Bryan Donkin and Sir William Osler.

Merrington, W.R. 1976. *University College Hospital and its Medical School: A History.* London: William Heinemann.

Merritt, H.H. 1963. *A Textbook of Neurology.* 3 ed. Philadelphia: Lea & Febiger.

Mesulam, M.-M. 1985. Norman Geschwind, 1926–1984. *Annals of Neurology* 18:98–100.

Mettler, C.C., Mettler, F.A. 1947. *History of Medicine. A Correlative Text, Arranged According to Subjects.* Philadelphia: The Blakiston Company.

Meyer, A. 1920. Herniation of the brain. *Archives of Neurology and Psychiatry* 4:387–400.

Meyer, A. 1971. *Historical Aspects of Cerebral Anatomy.* London: Oxford University Press.

Meyer, A. 1978. The concept of a sensorimotor cortex. Its early history, with special emphasis on two experimental contributions by W. Bechterew. *Brain* 101:673–685.

Meyer, A. 1982. The concept of a sensorimotor cortex: its later history during the twentieth century. *Neuropathology and Applied Neurobiology* 8:81–93.

Meynell, G.G. 1985. *The Two Sydenham Societies. A History and Bibliography of the Medical Classics Published by the Sydenham Society and the New Sydenham Society (1844–1911)*. Acrise, Kent: Winterdown Books.

Mill, J.S. 1851. *A System of Logic, Ratiocinative and Inductive*. 2 vols. 3 ed. London: John W. Parker.

Mill, J.S. 1872. *A System of Logic, Ratiocinative and Inductive*. 2 vols. 8 ed. London: Longman, Green, Reader, and Dyer.

Millett, D. 1998. Illustrating a revolution: An unrecognized contribution to the 'golden era' of cerebral localization. *Notes and Records of the Royal Society of London* 52:283–305.

Millett, D. 2001. Hans Berger. From psychic energy to the EEG. *Perspectives in Biology and Medicine* 44:522–542.

Millett, D. 2010. A history of seizures and epilepsy: from the falling disease to dysrhythmias of the brain. In Finger et al., pp.387–400.

Mitchell, S.W. 1873. The influence of rest in locomotor ataxia. *American Journal of the Medical Sciences* 66:113–115.

Mitchell, S.W. 1876. Rest in nervous disease. In Sequin, E.C. ed. *A Series of American Clinical Lectures*, vol.1, pp.83–102 (April). Contains the 12 issues published monthly in 1875.

Mitchell, S.W. 1881. *Lectures on Diseases of the Nervous System—Especially in Women*. Philadelphia: Henry C. Lea's Son and Co. Dedicated to Jackson.

Morabito, C. 1996. *La Cartografia del Cervello. Il Problema delle Localizzazioni Cerebrali nell'Opera di David Ferrier, fra Fisiologia, Psicologia e Folosophia*. Milan: FrancoAngeli. Privately translated as *Cerebral Cartography. The Localization of Brain Functions in David Ferrier's Work*.

Morabito, C. 2017. David Ferrier's experimental localization of cerebral functions and the antivivisection debate. *Nuncius* 32:146–165.

Morgan, J.P. 1982. The first reported case of electrical stimulation of the human brain. *Journal of the History of Medicine and Allied Sciences* 37:51–64.

Morris, E.W. 1910. *A History of the London Hospital*. London: Edward Arnold.

Morton, L.T. 1961. *Garrison and Morton's Medical Bibliography. An Annotated Check-List of Texts Illustrating the History of Medicine*. 2 ed. (1954, reprinted 1961). London: André Deutsch.

Morus, I.R. 2000. 'The nervous system of Britain': space, time and the electric telegraph in the Victorian age. *British Journal for the History of Science* 33:455–474.

Mott, F.W. 1894. The sensory motor functions of the central convolutions of the cerebral cortex. *Journal of Physiology, London* 15:464–487.

Mottolese, C., Richard, N., Harquel, S., et al. 2013. Mapping motor representations in the human cerebellum. *Brain* 136:330–342.

Moxon, W. 1866. On the connexion between loss of speech and paralysis of the right side. *British and Foreign Medico-Chirurgical Review* 37:481–489.

Moxon, W. 1870. On the necessity for a clinical nomenclature of disease. *Guy's Hospital Reports. Third Series* 15:479–500.

Müller, F. 1881. Zur Jackson'chen epilepsie und localisation des armcentrums (mit illustrationen eines falles von isolirter und circumscripter convexläsion). In Mac Cormac, vol.2, pp.15–20.

Müller, M. 1861. *Lectures on the Science of Language Delivered at the Royal Institution of Great Britain in April, May, and June, 1861*. London: Longman, Green, Longman, and Roberts (a fourth edition was published in 1864).

Müller, M. 1864. *Lectures on the Science of Language Delivered at the Royal Institution of Great Britain in February, March, April, & May, 1863*. Second Series. London: Longman, Green, Longman, Roberts, & Green.

Munk, W. 1878. *The Roll of the Royal College of Physicians of London; Comprising Biographical Sketches*, 2 ed., 3 vols ("Munk's Roll"). London: Royal College of Physicians. For continuation covering 1826–1925 ('vol.4'), see Brown 1955.

Murphy, G. 1949. *An Historical Introduction to Modern Psychology*. Revised ed. New York: Harcourt.

[Myers, A.T.] 1894. Obituary. *BMJ* 1:223 (January 27).

[Needham, Sir Frederick] 1924. Obituaries. *BMJ* 2:545–546 (September 20), and *Lancet* 2:627–628 (September 20).

Neuberger, M. 1981. *The Historical Development of Experimental Brain and Spinal Cord Physiology before Flourens*. Translated from the original German of 1897 by E. Clarke. Baltimore: Johns Hopkins University Press.

Neurological Society of London. 1887. *Rules and List of Office Bearers and Members of the Neurological Society of London*. Printed by George Fulman, Manchester Square. Bound into Brown University's copy of *Brain* 10 (1888), between pp.4 and 5.

Neve, M., Turner, T. 1995. What the doctor thought and did: Sir James Crichton-Browne (1840–1938). *Medical History* 39:399–432.

Newman, C. 1957. *The Evolution of Medical Education in the Nineteenth Century*. London: Oxford University Press.

Newsome, D. 1997. *The Victorian World Picture. Perceptions and Introspections in an Age of Change*. New Brunswick, NJ: Rutgers University Press.

Niemeyer, [F. von]. 1870. On aphasia, consequent on embolism of the left arteria fossae sylvii. *MTG* 1:29–30, 57–58, 87–88.

Niemeyer, F. von. 1876. *A Text-Book of Practical Medicine, with Particular Reference to Physiology and Pathological Anatomy*, vol.2. Translated from eighth German edition by G.H. Humphrey and C.E. Hackley. New York: D. Appleton. Reprinted 2014 by Kessinger Publishing: Whitefish, MT.

Noel, P.S., Carlson, E.T. 1970. Origins of the word "phrenology." *American Journal of Psychiatry* 127:694–697.

Nolte, J. 2002. *The Human Brain. An Introduction to Its Functional Anatomy*. 5 ed. St. Louis, MO: Mosby.

Nordlander, R.H., Egar, M.W., Bryant, S.V. 1995. In memoriam. A remembrance of Marcus Singer (1914–1994). *Developmental Biology* 169:v–vi.

OED Online. *Oxford English Dictionary*. Oxford: Oxford University Press.

Ojemann, G. 2003. In memoriam. Mark Rayport, M.D., C.M., Ph.D., F.A.C.S. *Epilepsia* 44:1262–1264.

Olson, R.G. 2004. *Science and Religion, 1450–1900. From Copernicus to Darwin*. Baltimore: Johns Hopkins University Press.

[Ophthalmological Society]. 1885. News item. The Ophthalmological Society. *BMJ* 2:981 (November 21).

[Ophthalmological Society]. 1975. Ophthalmological Society of the United Kingdom. Brief history of the Society. *Annals of the Royal College of Surgeons of England* 56:52–53.

Orchard, C.H. 2004. Ringer, Sydney (1835–1910). www.oxforddnb, accessed October 31, 2013.

Osler, W. 1881. The International Medical Congress. London, August 10, 1881. *Canada Medical and Surgical Journal* 10:121–125.

Osler, W. 1892. *The Principles and Practice of Medicine*. New York: D. Appleton. Reprinted 1978 by Gryphon Editions: Birmingham, AL.

Otis, L. 2007. *Müller's Lab*. New York: Oxford University Press.

Owen, C.M., Howard, A., Binder, D.K. 2009. Hippocampus minor, calcar avis, and the Huxley–Owen debate. *Neurosurgery* 65:1098–1105.

Pagenstecher, H., Genth, C. 1875. *Atlas der Pathologischen Anatomie des Augapfels/Atlas of the Pathological Anatomy of the Eyeball*. Wiesbaden: C.W. Kreidel. Parallel English translation by W.R. Gowers.

Paget, J. 1895. Presentation of testimonial to Dr. Hughlings Jackson, F.R.S., by Sir James Paget. *BMJ* 2:861–862.

Paget, J., Bennett, J.R., Bowman, W., Mac Cormac, W. 1880. International Medical Congress, 1881. *MTG* 2:159.

Paget, S. 1902. *Memoirs and Letters of Sir James Paget*. New Edition. London: Longmans, Green and Co.

Paget, S. 1919. *Sir Victor Horsley. A Study of his Life and Work*. London: Constable and Company.

Parsons, J.H. 1913. Edward Nettleship, F.R.S. Obituary. *Nature* 92:297.

Parsons, M. 2002. *Yorkshire and the History of Medicine*. York: William Sessions.

[Paton, L.J.] 1943. Obituary. *BMJ* 1:741.

Pearce, J.M.S. 1982. The first attempts at removal of brain tumors. In Rose and Bynum, pp.239–242.

Pearce, J.M.S. 2002. Armand Trousseau—some of his contributions to neurology. *JHN* 11:125–135.

Pearce, J.M.S. 2002a. Bromide, the first effective antiepileptic agent. *Journal of Neurology, Neurosurgery and Psychiatry* 72:412.

Pearce, J.M.S. 2003. *Fragments of Neurological History*. London: Imperial College Press.

Pearce, J.M.S. 2004. Positive and negative cerebral symptoms: the roles of Russell Reynolds and Hughlings Jackson. *Journal of Neurology, Neurosurgery and Psychiatry* 75:1148.

Pearce, J.M.S. 2009a. Sir Samuel Wilks (1824–1911): 'The most philosophical of English physicians.' *European Neurology* 61:119–123.

Pearce, J.M.S. 2009b. Sir Samuel Wilks (1824–1911): On epilepsy. *European Neurology* 61:124–127.

Pearce, J.M.S., Lees, A.J. 2013. Yorkshire's influence on the foundation of British neurology. *Journal of Neurology, Neurosurgery, and Psychiatry* 84:6–9.

Peel, J.D.Y. 1975. Spencer, Herbert. In Gillespie, C.C. ed. *Dictionary of Scientific Biography, Vol.12*. New York: Charles Scribner's Sons, pp.569–572.

Peel, J.D.Y. 2004. Galton Lecture 2003: Spencer in history: The second century. In Jones and Peel, pp.125–149.

Penfield, W. 1936. Epilepsy and surgical therapy. *Archives of Neurology and Psychiatry* 36:449–484.

Penfield, W. 1975. *The Mystery of the Mind*. Princeton, NJ: Princeton University Press.

Penfield, W. 1977. *No Man Alone. A Neurosurgeon's Life*. Boston: Little, Brown and Company.

Penfield, W., Erickson, T.C. 1941. *Epilepsy and Cerebral Localization. A Study of the Mechanism, Treatment and Prevention of Epileptic Seizures*. Springfield, IL: Charles C. Thomas.

Penfield, W., Jasper, H. 1954. *Epilepsy and the Functional Anatomy of the Human Brain*. Boston: Little, Brown and Company.

Penfield, W., Rasmussen, T. 1950. *The Cerebral Cortex of Man. A Clinical Study of Localization of Function*. New York: Macmillan.

Perrin, R.G. 1993. *Herbert Spencer. A Primary and Secondary Bibliography*. New York: Garland Publishing.

Peterson, M.J. 1978. *The Medical Profession in Mid-Victorian London*. Berkeley: University of California Press.

Phillips, C.G. 1974. Francis Martin Rouse Walshe. 1885–1973. *Biographical Memoirs of Fellows of the Royal Society 20*:457–481.

Phillips, C.G., Landau, W.M. 1990. Upper and lower motor neuron: The little old synecdoche that works. *Neurology 40*:884–886.

Piñero, J.M.L. 1973. *John Hughlings Jackson (1835–1911). Evolucionismo y Neurologia*. Madrid: Editorial Moneda y Credito.

Piñero, J.M.L. 2010. The work of John Hughlings Jackson: Parts I and II (translated by G.E. Berrios). *History of Psychiatry 21*:85–95.

Pitman, J. 1992. Out of the College Archives. Thomas Laycock. *Proceedings of the Royal College of Physicians of Edinburgh 22*:384–389.

Plum, F., Posner, J.B. 1966. *The Diagnosis of Stupor and Coma*. Philadelphia: F.A. Davis.

Porter, R. 1997. *The Greatest Benefit to Mankind. A Medical History of Humanity*. New York: W.W. Norton.

Posner, J.B., Saper, C.B., Schiff, N.D., Plum, F. 2007. *Plum and Posner's Diagnosis of Stupor and Coma*. 4 ed. New York: Oxford University Press.

Powell, M.P. 2016. Sir Victor Horsley at the birth of neurosurgery. *Brain 139*:631–634.

Powell, M., Kitchen, N. 2007. The development of neurosurgery at the National Hospital for Neurology and Neurosurgery, Queen Square, London, England. *Neurosurgery 61*:1077–1090.

Power, D'A., Le Fanu, W.R., eds. 1953. *Lives of the Fellows of the Royal College of Surgeons of England. 1930–1951*. London: Royal College of Surgeons.

Poynter, F.N.L., ed. 1968. *Medicine and Science in the 1860s*. London: Wellcome Institute for the History of Medicine.

Prevost, J.-L. 1868. *De la Déviation Conjuguée des Yeux: et de la Rotation de la Tête dans Certain Cas d'Hémiplegie*. Paris: Victor Masson et Fils.

Price, E.H. 2012. Do brains think? Comparative anatomy and the end of the Great Chain of Being in 19th-century Britain. *History of the Human Sciences 25*:32–50.

Price, E.H. 2014. George Henry Lewes (1817–1878): Embodied cognition, vitalism, and the evolution of symbolic perception. In Smith and Whitaker, pp.105–123.

Purves-Stewart, J. 1939. *Sands of Time. Recollections of a Physician in Peace and War*. London: Hutchinson & Co.

Pye-Smith, P.H. 1907. Lionel Smith Beale, 1828–1906. *Proceedings of the Royal Society of London 79B*:lvii–lxiii.

Quærens. 1874. A prognostic and therapeutic indication in epilepsy. *Practitioner 3*:284–285.

Quétel, C. 1990. *History of Syphilis*. Translated by J. Braddock and B. Pike. Baltimore: Johns Hopkins University Press.

Radick, G. 2000. Language, brain function, and human origins in the Victorian debates on evolution. *Studies in History and Philosophy of Biological and Biomedical Sciences 31*:55–75.

Radick, G. 2007. *The Simian Tongue. The Long Debate about Animal Language*. Chicago: University of Chicago Press.

Raitiere, M. 2008. Did Herbert Spencer have epilepsy? Some links involving John Hughlings-Jackson, G.H. Lewes, and George Eliot. *George Eliot—George Henry Lewes Studies. Issue 54–55*:107–147.

Raitiere, M. 2011. Did Herbert Spencer have reading epilepsy? *JHN 20*:357–367.

Raitiere, M. 2012. *The Complicity of Friends. How George Eliot, G.H. Lewes, and John Hughlings-Jackson Encoded Herbert Spencer's Secret.* Lewisburg, PA: Bucknell University Press.

Ramachandran, M., Aronson, J.K. 2012. Jacob Lockhart Clarke's and John Hughlings Jackson's first description of syringomyelia. *Journal of the Royal Society of Medicine 105*:60–65.

Ramskill, J.S. 1864. Cases of dilatation of the left ventricle of the heart, associated with difficulty of articulation, and with sub-occipital pain. *Clinical Lectures and Reports by the Medical and Surgical Staff of the London Hospital 1*:472–484.

Rapaport, D. 1974. *The History of the Concept of the Association of Ideas.* New York: International Universities Press.

Rawlings, B.B. 1884. Letter to the editor. National Hospital for the Paralysed and Epileptic. *BMJ 2*:494.

Rawlings, B.B. 1913. *A Hospital in the Making. A History of the National Hospital for the Paralysed and Epileptic (Albany Memorial) 1859–1901.* London: Sir Isaac Pitman & Sons.

Reed, E.S. 1997. *From Soul to Mind. The Emergence of Psychology from Erasmus Darwin to William James.* New Haven, CT: Yale University Press.

Renvoize, E. 1991. The Association of Medical Officers of Asylums and Hospitals for the Insane, the Medico-Psychological Association, and their Presidents. In Berrios and Freeman, pp.29–78.

Reynolds, E.H. 2001. Todd, Hughlings Jackson, and the electrical basis of epilepsy. *Lancet 358*: 575–577.

Reynolds, E.H. 2007. Jackson, Todd, and the concept of "discharge" in epilepsy. *Epilepsia 48*: 2016–2022.

Reynolds, E.H., Andrew, M. 2007. Hughlings Jackson's early education. *Journal of Neurology, Neurosurgery, and Psychiatry 78*:92.

Reynolds, J.R. 1861. *Epilepsy: Its Symptoms, Treatment, and Relation to Other Convulsive Diseases.* London: John Churchill. Reprinted 1981 by Abbott Laboratories: Chicago, IL.

Reynolds, J.R. ed. 1866–1879. *A System of Medicine,* 5 vols. London: Macmillan.

Reynolds, J.R. 1868. Epilepsy. In Reynolds, 1866–1879, vol.2, pp.251–284.

[Reynolds, J.R.] 1896. Obituary. *BMJ 1*:1422–1425.

Reynolds, J.R. 1998 [1858]. 'On the pathology of convulsions' by Sir J.R. Reynolds. Introduction by G.E. Berrios. *History of Psychiatry 9*:509–522.

Ribot, T. 1874. *English Psychology.* New York: D. Appleton.

Richards, R.J. 1987. *Darwin and the Emergence of Evolutionary Theories of Mind and Behavior.* Chicago: University of Chicago Press.

Rivers, W.H.R. 1922. Obituary. *BMJ 1*:936–937 (June 10).

Rivett, G. 1986. *The Development of the London Hospital System 1823–1982.* London: King Edward's Hospital Fund for London.

Roberts, M.J.D. 2009. The politics of professionalization: MPs, medical men, and the 1858 Medical Act. *Medical History 53*:37–56.

Rocca, J. 2003. *Galen on the Brain. Anatomical Knowledge and Physiological Speculation in the Second Century AD.* Leiden: Brill.

Roe, D., Finger, S. 1996. Gustave Dax and his fight for recognition: An overlooked chapter in the early history of cerebral dominance. *JHN 5*:228–240.

Rolleston, H.D. 1929. *The Right Honourable Sir Thomas Clifford Allbutt KCB. A Memoir*. London: Macmillan.

Rolleston, H. 1943. History of *The Practitioner. Practitioner* 150:321–328.

Rollin, H.R., Reynolds, E.H. 2018. Yorkshire's influence on the understanding and treatment of mental diseases in Victorian Britain: The golden triangle of York, Wakefield, and Leeds. *JHN* 27:72–84.

Román, G.C. 1987. Cerebral congestion. A vanished disease. *Archives of Neurology* 44:444–448.

Romberg, M.H. 1853. *A Manual of the Nervous Diseases of Man*. 2 vols. Translated by E.H. Sieveking. London: New Sydenham Society. Reprinted 1983 by Gryphon Editions: Birmingham, AL. Original German edition 1840–1846: *Lehrbuch der Nervenkrankheiten des Menschen*. Berlin: A. Dunker.

Rose, F.C., ed. 1989. *Neuroscience across the Centuries*. London: Smith-Gordon and Company.

Rose, F.C., ed. 1999. *A Short History of Neurology. The British Contribution 1660–1910*. Oxford: Butterworth-Heinemann.

Rose, F.C., Bynum, W.F., eds. 1982. *Historical Aspects of the Neurosciences. A Festschrift for Macdonald Critchley*. New York: Raven Press.

Rosenberg, C.E. 1997. *No Other Gods. On Science and American Social Thought*. Revised ed. Baltimore: Johns Hopkins University Press.

Rosenthal, M. 1879. *A Clinical Treatise on the Diseases of the Nervous System*, 2 vols. Translated by L. Putzel. New York: William Wood & Company.

Rowlette, R.J. 1939. *The Medical Press and Circular 1839–1939. A Hundred Years in the Life of a Medical Journal*. London: Medical Press and Circular.

Royle, E. 1981. Religion in York, 1831–1981. In Feinstein, pp.205–233.

Rupke, N.A. 1987. Pro-vivisection in England in the early 1880s: arguments and motives. In Rupke, N.A., ed. *Vivisection in Historical Perspective*. London: Croom Helm.

Rupke, N.A. 1993. Richard Owen's vertebrate archetype. *Isis* 84:231–251.

Rupke, N.A. 1994. *Richard Owen. Victorian Naturalist*. New Haven, CT: Yale University Press.

Ruse, M. 2005. The Darwinian revolution, as seen in 1979 and as seen twenty-five years later in 2004. *Journal of the History of Biology* 38:3–17.

Russell, J. 1864a. Hemiplegia on the right side, with loss of speech. *BMJ* 2:81–85.

Russell, J. 1864b. Hemiplegia, with loss of speech. *BMJ* 2:211–213, 239–241.

Russell, J. 1864c. Loss of speech, in conjunction with suspension of certain other functions of the brain, following an epileptiform attack. *BMJ* 2:408–411.

[Russell, J.S.R.] 1939. Obituary. J.S. Risien Russell, M.D., F.R.C.P. *BMJ* 1:645.

[Russell, J.S.R.] 1939a. Obituary. John Samuel Risien Russell *Lancet* 1:790.

Rylance, R. 1987. Vital intersections: G.H. Lewes and the meeting of physiology and philosophy in psychology in the 1860s. *Ideas and Production* 7:60–80.

Rylance, R. 2000. *Victorian Psychology and British Culture 1850–1880*. Oxford: Oxford University Press.

Sachs, E. 1952. *The History and Development of Neurological Surgery*. London: Cassell and Company.

Sachs, E. 1958. Victor Horsley. *Journal of Neurosurgery* 15:240–244.

Sacks, O.W. 1998. Sigmund Freud: the other road. In Guttmann and Scholz-Strasser, pp.11–22.

Sakula, A. 1982. Baroness Burdett-Coutts' garden party: The International Medical Congress, London, 1881. *Medical History* 26:183–190.

Sander, W.J.A.S., Barclay, J., Shorvon, S.D. 1993. The neurological founding fathers of the National Society for Epilepsy and of the Chalfont Centre for Epilepsy. *Journal of Neurology, Neurosurgery, and Psychiatry* 56:599–604.

Sanes, J.R., Jessell, T.M. 2000. The formation and regeneration of synapses. In Kandel et al., pp.1087–1114.

Saul, F.P., Saul, J.M. 1997. Trepanation: old world and new world. In Greenblatt et al., pp.29–35.

Savage, G. 1917. Dr. Hughlings Jackson on mental disorders. *Journal of Mental Science* 68:315–328.

Scarff, J.E. 1955. Fifty years of neurosurgery, 1905–1955. *Surgery Gynecology and Obstetrics, with International Abstracts of Surgery* 101:417–513 (see pp.418–419). Reprinted in Davis, L., ed. *Fifty Years of Surgical Progress 1905–1955.* Chicago: Franklin H. Martin Memorial Foundation, pp.303–399 (see pp.304–305).

Schachter, S.C., Devinsky, O., eds. 1997. *Behavioral Neurology and the Legacy of Norman Geschwind.* Philadelphia: Lippincott-Raven.

Schiller, F. 1970. Concepts of stroke before and after Virchow. *Medical History* 14:115–130.

Schiller, F. 1975. The migraine tradition. *BHM* 49:1–19.

Schiller, F. 1979. *Paul Broca. Founder of French Anthropology, Explorer of the Brain.* Berkeley: University of California Press.

Schmahmann, J.D., Pandya, D.N. 2007. Cerebral white matter—historical evolution of facts and notions concerning the organization of the fiber pathways of the brain. *JHN* 16:237–267.

Schorstein, G. 1895. Some notes on the contributions made by Dr. Hughlings Jackson to our knowledge of nervous disease. *London Hospital Gazette* 2:35–39. Contained in J95-06.

Schroeder van der Kolk, J.L.C. 1859. *Professor Schroeder van der Kolk on the Minute Structure and Functions of the Spinal Cord and Medulla oblongata, and on the Proximate Cause and Rational Treatment of Epilepsy. Translated by William Daniel Moore.* London: New Sydenham Society.

Schurr, P.H. 1985. Outline of the history of the Section of Neurology of the Royal Society of Medicine. *Journal of the Royal Society of Medicine* 78:146–148.

Scott, A., Eadie, M., Lees, A. 2012. *William Richard Gowers 1845–1915. Exploring the Victorian Brain: A Biography.* Oxford: Oxford University Press.

Scott, D.F. 1993. *A History of Epileptic Therapy: An Account of How Medication Was Discovered.* Carnforth: Parthenon Publishing Group.

Secord, J.A. 2000. *Victorian Sensation. The Extraordinary Publication, Reception, and Secret Authorship of Vestiges of the Natural History of Creation.* Chicago: University of Chicago Press.

Semon, F., Horsley, V. 1889. On the central motor innervation of the larynx. A preliminary communication. *BMJ* 2:1383–1384.

Semon, F., Horsley, V. 1890. An experimental investigation of the central motor innervation of the larynx. *Philosophical Transactions of the Royal Society of London B* 181:187–211.

Sengoku, A. 2002. The contribution of J.H. Jackson to present day epileptology. *Epilepsia* 43 (Suppl.9):6–8.

Sessions, W.K., Sessions, E.M. 1987. *The Tukes of York in the Seventeenth, Eighteenth and Nineteenth Centuries.* York: Sessions Book Trust.

Shafi, N. 2015. Aphasia secondary to tuberculosis: a review of a nineteenth century case report by Booth and Curtis (1893). *JHN* 24:58–78.

Shephard, J.A. 1972. Medical teaching at St. Andrews University 1413–1972. *BMJ* 3:38–41.

Shepherd, G.M. 1991. *Foundations of the Neuron Doctrine.* New York: Oxford University Press.

Sherrington, C.S. 1906. *The Integrative Action of the Nervous System*. New Haven, CT: Yale University Press. Delivered at Yale as the Silliman Lectures in 1904. I have used the seventh printing of 1923.

Sherrington, C.S. 1906a. On the proprio-ceptive system, especially in its reflex aspect. *Brain* 29:467–482.

Sherrington, C.S. 1928. Sir David Ferrier, 1843–1928. *Proceedings of the Royal Society of London* 103B:viii–xvi.

Sherrington, C.S. 1940. *Selected Writings of Sir Charles Sherrington*. Edited by D. Denny-Brown. New York: Paul B. Hoeber.

Sherrington, C.S. 1965. Inhibition as a coordinative factor. In *Nobel Lectures. Physiology or Medicine 1922–1941*. Amsterdam: Elsevier, pp.278–289. (Nobel Lecture delivered December 12, 1932.)

Shorvon, S.D. 2011. The causes of epilepsy: Changing concepts of etiology of epilepsy over the past 150 years. *Epilepsia* 52:1033–1044.

Shorvon, S.D. 2011a. The etiologic classification of epilepsy. *Epilepsia* 52:1052–1057.

Shorvon, S. 2014. The evolution of epilepsy theory and practice at the National Hospital for the Relief and Cure of Epilepsy, Queen Square between 1860 and 1910. *Epilepsy & Behavior* 31:228–242.

Shorvon, S., Weiss, G., Avanzini, G., et al. 2009. *The International League Against Epilepsy 1909–2009: Centenary History*. Chichester: Wiley-Blackwell.

Shorvon, S., Compston, A., Lees, A., et al. 2019. *Queen Square: A History of the National Hospital and its Institute of Neurology*. Cambridge: Cambridge University Press.

Sieveking, E.H. 1858. *On Epilepsy and Epileptiform Seizures*. London: John Churchill.

Singer, C. 1957. *A Short History of Anatomy from the Greeks to Harvey*. 2 ed. New York: Dover Publications.

Smith, C. 1998. *The Science of Energy. A Cultural History of Energy Physics in Victorian Britain*. Chicago: University of Chicago Press.

Smith, C.U.M. 1982. Evolution and the problem of mind: Part I. Herbert Spencer. *Journal of the History of Biology* 15:55–88.

Smith, C.U.M. 1982a. Evolution and the problem of mind: Part II. John Hughlings Jackson. *Journal of the History of Biology* 15:241–262.

Smith, C.U.M. 1987. David Hartley's Newtonian neuropsychology. *Journal of the History of the Behavioral Sciences* 23:123–136.

Smith, C.U.M. 1989. Neurology and mental atomism: some continuities and discontinuities. In Rose, pp.49–57.

Smith, C.U.M. 1992. The hippopotamus test: A controversy in nineteenth-century brain science. *Cogito I: Supplement to the Italian Journal of Neurological Sciences* 1:69–74.

Smith, C.U.M. 1997. Worlds in collision: Owen and Huxley on the brain. *Science in Context* 10:343–365.

Smith, C.U.M. 1999. Thomas Henry Huxley and neuroscience. *Physis (Firenze)* 36:355–365.

Smith, C.U.M. 2007. Evolution and the problem of mind in 19th century England. In Turrini, S.K., ed. *Consciousness and Learning Research*. New York: Nova Science Publishers.

Smith, C.U.M. 2010. Darwin's unsolved problem: the place of consciousness in an evolutionary world. *JHN* 19:105–120.

Smith, C.U.M. 2012. Philosophy's loss, neurology's gain. The endeavor of John Hughlings-Jackson. *Perspectives in Biology and Medicine* 55:81–91.

Smith, C.U.M. 2014a. Herbert Spencer: brain, mind, and the hard problem. In Smith and Whitaker, pp.125–145.

Smith, C.U.M. 2014b. The 'Hard Problem' and the Cartesian strand in British neurophysiology: Huxley, Foster, Sherrington, Eccles. In Smith and Whitaker, pp.255–272.

Smith, C.U.M., Whitaker, H., eds. 2014. *Brain, Mind and Consciousness in the History of Neuroscience*. Dordrecht: Springer.

Smith, C.U.M., Frixione, E., Finger, S., Clower, W. 2012. *The Animal Spirit Doctrine and the Origins of Neurophysiology*. New York: Oxford University Press.

Smith, D.L. 1999. *Freud's Philosophy of the Unconscious*. Dordrecht: Kluwer.

Smith, R. 1992. *Inhibition. History and Meaning in the Sciences of the Mind and Brain*. Berkeley: University of California Press.

Smith, R. 2013. *Free Will and the Human Sciences in Britain, 1870–1910*. London: Pickering & Chatto.

Snyder, P.J., Whitaker, H.A. 2013. Neurologic heuristics and artistic whimsy: the cerebral cartography of Wilder Penfield. *JHN 22*:277–291.

Söderqvist, T., ed. 2007. *The History and Poetics of Scientific Biography*. Aldershot: Ashgate Publishing.

Solms, M., Saling, M. 1986. On psychoanalysis and neuroscience: Freud's attitude to the localizationist tradition. *International Journal of Psycho-Analysis 67*:397–416.

Sourkes, T.L. 2006. On the energy cost of mental effort. *JHN 15*:31–47.

Sparrow, E.P., Finger, F. 2001. Edward Albert Schäfer (Sharpey-Schafer) and his contributions to neuroscience: Commemorating the 150th anniversary of his birth. *JHN 10*:41–57.

Spencer, H. 1851. *Social Statics*. London: Chapman.

Spencer, H. 1852. The development hypothesis. *The Leader 3*:280–281.

Spencer, H. 1855. *The Principles of Psychology*. London: Longman, Brown, Green, and Longmans. Reprinted 1970 by Gregg International Publishers: Farnborough.

Spencer, H. 1858. *Essays: Scientific, Political and Speculative*. London: Longman, Brown, Green, and Longmans, et al., pp.359–384.

Spencer, H. 1862/1864. *First Principles*. London: Williams and Norgate. I have used the first American edition 1864: *First Principles of a New System of Philosophy*. New York: D. Appleton.

Spencer, H. 1864, 1867. *The Principles of Biology*. 2 vols (vol.1, 1864; vol.2, 1867). London: Williams and Norgate. American edition, vol.1, 1870; vol.2, 1867. New York: D. Appleton. These American editions are not listed in Perrin 1993.

Spencer, H. 1867a. *First Principles*. 2 ed. London: Williams and Norgate. See Spencer 1867 in *The Principles of Biology* above.

Spencer, H. 1870, 1872. *The Principles of Psychology*. 2 ed. 2 vols. London: Williams and Norgate.

Spencer, H. 1876. *The Principles of Sociology, vol.1*. London: Williams and Norgate.

Spencer, H. 1880. *The Principles of Psychology*. 3 ed. 2 vols. London: Williams and Norgate. I have used the Authorized American edition by D. Appleton: New York, 1904, which has the same pagination.

Spencer, H. 1880a. *Appendix to First Principles, Dealing with Criticisms*. London: Williams and Norgate. This pamphlet was inserted into my copy of *First Principles* 1867 and closely (not pefectly) follows its pagination. The pamphlet is not listed in Perrin 1993.

Spencer, H. 1903. Last Will and Testament, June 19, 1903; probate granted to Charles Holme and Francis Edward Lott, executors, January 28, 1904. Copy obtained in July 1963, from Record Keeper, Principal Probate Registry, Somerset House, Strand, London, WC2.

Spencer, H. 1904. *An Autobiography*, 2 vols. London: Williams and Norgate.

Spencer, W.G. 1894. The effect produced upon respiration by faradic excitation of the cerebrum in the monkey, dog, cat and rabbit. *[Philosophical] Transactions of the Royal Society B 184*:609–657.

[Spencer, W.G.] 1940. Obituary. *Lancet 2*:638–639.

Stanley, M. 2014.Where naturalism and theism met: the uniformity of nature. In Dawson and Lightman, pp.242–262.

Star, S.L. 1989. *Regions of the Mind. Brain Research and the Quest for Scientific Certainty.* Stanford, CA: Stanford University Press.

Stein, J.F. 1989. Hierarchies in the cerebellum. In Kennard and Swash, pp.158–167.

Steinberg, D. 1999. What modern neuroscience can learn from Hughlings Jackson. In Rose, pp.165–177.

Steinberg, D.A. 2009. Cerebral localization in the nineteenth century—the birth of a science and its consequences. *JHN 18*:254–261.

Steinberg, D.A. 2013. The origin of scientific neurology and its consequences for modern and future neuroscience. *Brain 137*:294–300.

Stengel, E. 1954. A re-evaluation of Freud's book "*On Aphasia*". Its significance for psycho-analysis. *International Journal of Psycho-Analysis 35*:1–5.

Stengel, E. 1963. Hughlings Jackson's influence in psychiatry. *British Journal of Psychiatry 109*:348–355.

Stevenson, R.S. 1951. *In a Harley Street Mirror.* London: Christopher Johnson.

Stevenson, R.S., Guthrie, D. 1949. *A History of Oto-Laryngology.* Edinburgh: E. & S. Livingstone.

[Stewart, J.P.] 1949. Obituary. *BMJ 1*:1142–1143.

[Stewart, T.G.] 1900. Obituary. *BMJ 1*:355–359.

Stone, J.L. 1991. Paul Broca and the first craniotomy based on cerebral localization. *Journal of Neurosurgery 75*:154–159.

Storey, C.E., Pols, H. 2010. A history of cerebrovascular disease. In Finger et al., pp.401–415.

Stufflebeam, S.M., Liu, H., Sepulcre, J., et al. 2011. Localization of focal epileptic discharges using functional connectivity magnetic resonance imaging. *Journal of Neurosurgery 114*:1693–1697.

Sulloway, F.J. 1979. *Freud, Biologist of the Mind. Beyond the Psychoanalytic Legend.* New York: Basic Books.

Swanson, L.W. 2000. What is the brain? *Trends in Neuroscience 23*:519–527.

Swash, M. 1986. John Hughlings-Jackson: A sesquicentennial tribute. *Journal of Neurology, Neurosurgery, and Psychiatry 49*:981–985.

Swash, M. 2015. John Hughlings Jackson (1835–1911): An adornment to the London Hospital. *Journal of Medical Biography 23*:2–8.

Swash, M., Evans, J. 2006. Hughlings Jackson's clinical research: evidence from contemporary documents. *Neurology 67*:666–672.

Swerdlow, N.M. 2013. Thomas Samuel Kuhn. July 18, 1922–June 17, 1996. *Biographical Memoirs of the National Academy of Sciences.* http://www.nasonline.org/memoirs, accessed March 2014.

Sykes, A.H. 2000. Wallerian degeneration. In Koehler et al., pp.63–68.

Symonds, C., Bishop, W.J. 1960. Hughlings Jackson (1835–1911). *Cerebral Palsy Bulletin 2*:3–4.

Symondson, A., ed. 1970. *The Victorian Crisis of Faith.* London: Society for Promoting Christian Knowledge.

Taine, H. 1870. *De l'Intelligence.* Translated by T.D. Haye as *On Intelligence in 1871.* London: L. Reeve and Co.

Tansey, E.M. 1992. The science least adequately studied in England: Physiology and the G.H. Lewes studentship. *Journal of the History of Medicine and Allied Sciences* 47:163–186.

Taylor, C.S.R., Gross, C.G. 2003. Twitches versus movements: a story of motor cortex. *The Neuroscientist* 9:332–342.

Taylor, D.C., Marsh, S.M. 1980. Hughlings Jackson's Dr Z: the paradigm of temporal lobe epilepsy revealed. *Journal of Neurology, Neurosurgery, and Psychiatry* 43:758–767.

Taylor, J. 1915. The ophthalmological observations of Hughlings Jackson and their bearing on nervous and other diseases. *Brain* 38:391–417.

Taylor, J. 1925. Biographical memoir. In Jackson, pp.1–26.

Taylor, M.W. 2007. *The Philosophy of Herbert Spencer.* London: Continuum International Publishing Group.

Temkin, O. 1945. *The Falling Sickness. A History of Epilepsy from the Greeks to the Beginnings of Modern Neurology.* Baltimore: Johns Hopkins University Press.

Temkin, O. 1947. Gall and the phrenological movement. *BHM* 21:275–321. Reprinted in Temkin 2002, pp.87–130.

Temkin, O. 1951. The role of surgery in the rise of modern medical thought. *BHM* 25:248–259. Reprinted in Temkin 1977, pp.487–496.

Temkin, O. 1971. *The Falling Sickness. A History of Epilepsy from the Greeks to the Beginnings of Modern Neurology.* 2 ed. Baltimore: Johns Hopkins University Press.

Temkin, O. 1973. *Galenism. Rise and Decline of a Medical Philosophy.* Ithaca, NY: Cornell University Press.

Temkin, O. 1977. *The Double Face of Janus and Other Essays in the History of Medicine.* Baltimore: Johns Hopkins University Press.

Temkin, O. 2002. *"On Second Thought" and Other Essays in the History of Medicine and Science.* Baltimore: Johns Hopkins University Press.

Tesak, J., Code, C. 2008. *Milestones in the History of Aphasia. Theories and Protagonists.* New York: Routledge.

Thornton, E.M. 1976. *Hypnotism, Hysteria and Epilepsy. An Historical Analysis.* London: William Heinemann.

Todd, R.B., ed. 1847. *The Cyclopedia of Anatomy and Physiology*, vol.3. London: Sherwood, Gilbert, and Piper.

Todd, R.B. 1855. *Clinical Lectures on Paralysis, Diseases of the Brain, and Other Affections of the Nervous System.* Philadelphia: Lindsay & Blakiston.

Todd, R.B., Bowman, W. 1857. *The Physiological Anatomy and Physiology of Man.* Philadelphia: Blanchard and Lea.

Tomasello, F., Germanò, A. 2006. Francesco Durante: The history of intra cranial meningiomas and beyond. *Neurosurgery* 59:389–396.

Tomlinson, S. 2005. *Head Masters. Phrenology, Secular Education, and Nineteenth-Century Social Thought.* Tuscaloosa: University of Alabama Press.

Trail, R.R., ed. 1968. *Lives of the Fellows of the Royal College of Physicians of London, Continued to 1965.* (Munk's Roll, vol.5.) London: Royal College of Physicians.

Trimble, M.R. 2016. *The Intentional Brain: Motion, Emotion, and the Development of Modern Neuropsychiatry.* Baltimore: Johns Hopkins University Press.

Tröltsch, A. von, 1869. *Treatise on Diseases of the Ear: Including Anatomy of the Organ.* Translated and edited by D.B. St. John Roosa. New York: William Wood.

Trotter, W. 1934. A landmark in modern neurology. *Lancet 2*:1207–1210 (December 1).

[Trotter, W.] 1939. Obituary. Wilfred Trotter, M.S., F.R.S., L.L.D., M.D., D.Sc., F.R.C.S. *BMJ 2*:1117–1119 (December 2).

Trousseau, A. 1864. De l'aphasie, maladie décrite récemment sous le nom impropre d'aphémie. *Gazette des Hôpitaux Civils et Militaire 37*:13–14, 25–26, 37–39, 49–50.

Tuke, D.H. 1892. *A Dictionary of Psychological Medicine.* 2 vols. London: J. & A. Churchill.

Turner, F.M. 1975. Victorian scientific naturalism and Thomas Carlyle. *Victorian Studies 18*:325–343. Reprinted in Turner 1993, pp.131–150.

Turner, F.M. 1978. The Victorian conflict between science and religion: A professional dimension. *Isis 69*:356–376. Reprinted in Turner 1993, pp.171–200.

Turner, F.M. 1993. *Contesting Cultural Authority. Essays in Victorian Intellectual Life.* Cambridge: Cambridge University Press (paperback edition 2008).

Turner, M.R., Swash, M., Ebers, G.C. 2010. Lockhart Clarke's contribution to the description of amyotrophic lateral sclerosis. *Brain 133*:3470–3479.

Turner, W. 1866. The convolutions of the human cerebrum topographically considered. *Edinburgh Medical Journal 11*:1105–1122.

Uff, C., Frith, D., Harrison, C., et al. 2011. Sir Victor Horsley's 19th century operations at the National Hospital for Neurology and Neurosurgery, Queen Square. *Journal of Neurosurgery 114*:534–542.

van Elst, L.T., Trimble, M.R. 2008. Disorders of impulse control, episodic dyscontrol. In Engel and Pedley, vol.3, pp.2203–2207, 2811–2818.

Viets, H.R. 1938. West Riding, 1871–1876. *BHM 6*:477–487.

Virchow, R. 1860. *Cellular Pathology: As Based Upon Physiological and Pathological Histology. Translated from the second edition of the original by Frank Chance.* London: John Churchill. (Original German edition 1858.)

Vulpian, E.F.A. 1866. *Leçons sur la Physiologie Générale et Comparée du Systéme Nerveux: Fait au Muséum d'Histoire Naturelle.* Paris: Baillière.

Waddington, K. 2003. *Medical Education at St Bartholomew's Hospital 1123–1995.* Woodbridge: Boydell Press. Especially Chapter 3, 'Mid-Victorian medical education', pp.76–111.

Waitz, T. 1863. *Introduction to Anthropology*, edited by J.F. Collingwood. London: Longman, Green, Longman, and Roberts.

Wales, A.E. 1963. Sir Jonathan Hutchinson, 1828–1913. *British Journal of Venereal Disease 39*:67–86.

Walker, A.E., ed. 1951. *A History of Neurological Surgery.* Baltimore: Williams & Wilkins. Reprinted 1967 by Hafner: New York.

Walker, A.E. 1957. Stimulation and ablation. Their role in the history of cerebral physiology. *Journal of Neurophysiology 20*:435–449.

Walker, M.C., Kovac, S. 2015. Editorial. Seize the moment that is thine: how should we define seizures? *Brain 138*:1127–1128.

Wallesch, C.W. 1989. Hughlings Jackson and European neurology. In: Kennard and Swash, pp.17–23.

Walshe, F.M.R. 1943. On the mode of representation of movements in the motor cortex, with special reference to "convulsions beginning unilaterally" (Jackson). *Brain 66*:104–139. Reprinted 1948 in *Critical Studies in Neurology.* Edinburgh: Livingstone, pp.149–187.

Walshe, F.M.R. 1954. The contribution of clinical observation to cerebral physiology. *Proceedings of the Royal Society B 142*:208–224.

Walshe, F.M.R. 1958. Some reflections upon the opening phase of the physiology of the cerebral cortex. In: Poynter, F.N.L., ed. *The History and Philosophy of Knowledge of the Brain and its Functions*. Oxford: Blackwell (pp.223–234, mainly on Jackson).

Walshe, F.M.R. 1961. Contributions of John Hughlings Jackson to neurology. A brief introduction to his teachings. *Archives of Neurology 5*:119–131.

Walshe, F.M.R. 1963. *Diseases of the Nervous System Described for Practitioners and Students*. 10 ed. Edinburgh: E. & S. Livingstone.

Walter, R.D. 1970. *S. Weir Mitchell, M.D. Neurologist. A Medical Biography*. Springfield, IL: Charles C. Thomas.

Walton, J. 2014. The tardy development of UK neurology. Book review of Casper 2014. *Brain 137*:2868–2870.

Ward, T.H. 1887. *The Reign of Queen Victoria. A Survey of Fifty Years of Progress*. Vol.2. London: Smith, Elder & Co.

Warren, H.C. 1921. *A History of the Association Psychology*. New York: Charles Scribner's Sons.

Wechsler, I.S. 1963. *Clinical Neurology, with an Introduction to the History of Neurology*. Philadelphia: W.B. Saunders.

Weiner, D.B. 1994. "Le geste de Pinel": The history of a psychiatric myth. In: Micale, M.S., Porter, R., eds. *Discovering the History of Psychiatry*. New York: Oxford University Press, pp.232–247.

Weiner, W.J., Goetz, C.G., Shin, R.K., Lewis, S.L., eds. 2010. *Neurology for the Non-Neurologist*, 6 ed. Philadelphia: Lippincott Williams & Wilkins.

Weisz, G. 2006. *Divide and Conquer. A Comparative History of Medical Specialization*. New York: Oxford University Press.

Wernicke, C. 1874. *Der Aphasische Symptomencomplex. Eine Psychologische Studie auf Anatomischer Basis*. Breslau: Cohn & Weigert. Partial translations in Wilkins and Brody 1973, pp.142–144; and in Eling 1994, pp.69–98.

Werth, B. 2009. *Banquet at Delmonico's. Great Minds, the Gilded Age, and the Triumph of Evolution in America*. New York: Random House.

Wetherill, J.H. 1961. The York Medical School. *Medical History 5*:253–269.

Wilkes, A.L., Wade, N.J. 1997. Bain on neural networks. *Brain and Cognition 33*:295–305.

Wilkins, R.H. 1965. *Neurosurgical Classics*. New York: Johnson Reprint Corporation. Reprinted 1992 by American Association of Neurological Surgeons: Park Ridge, IL.

Wilkins, R.H., Brody, I.A. 1970. Jacksonian epilepsy. *Archives of Neurology 22*:183–188.

Wilkins, R.H., Brody, I.A. 1973. *Neurological Classics*. [New York:] Johnson Reprint Corporation. Reprinted 1997 by American Association of Neurological Surgeons: Park Ridge, IL.

Wilks, S. 1862. Abstract of lectures on pathology. Lecture I. On Virchow's theories. *MTG 2*:32–33.

Wilks, S. 1866. Observations on the pathology of some of the diseases of the nervous system. *Guy's Hospital Reports. Third Series 12*:152–244.

Williams, D. 1947. Jackson, 1835–1911. In Dumesnil, R., Bonnet-Roy, F., eds. *Les Médecins Célèbres*. Geneve: Mazenod, pp.244–247. The portrait facing p.244 is almost certainly not of Jackson.

Williams, D. 1983. *Mr George Eliot. A Biography of George Henry Lewes*. London: Hodder and Stoughton.

Williamson-Noble, F.A. 1935. Hughlings Jackson and the ophthalmoscope. *Post-Graduate Medical Journal 11*:163–166.

Wilson, L.G. 1996. The gorilla and the question of human origins: The brain controversy. *Journal of the History of Medicine and Allied Sciences 51*:184–207.

Wilson, S.A.K. 1920. On decerebrate rigidity in man and the occurrance of "tonic fits." *Proceedings of the Royal Society of Medicine 13*:89–92.

Wilson, S.A.K. 1935. The Hughlings Jackson centenary. *Lancet 1*:882–883.

[Wilson, S.A.K.] 1937. Obituary. S.A. Kinnier Wilson, M.D. *BMJ 1*:1094–1095.

Winslow, F. 1860. *On Obscure Diseases of the Brain, and Diseases of the Mind: Their Incipient Symptoms, Pathology, Diagnosis, Treatment and Prophylaxis*. Philadelphia: Blanchard & Lea.

Winslow, L.F. 1913. Obituary. *BMJ 1*:1302 (June 14).

Winter, A. 1997. The construction of orthodoxies and heterodoxies in the early Victorian life sciences. In Lightman, B., ed., *Victorian Science in Context*. Chicago: University of Chicago Press, pp.24–50.

Wolf, P., 2009. Development of the nosology and classification of epilepsy. In Shorvon et al., pp.131–142.

Woodward, W.R., Ash, M.G., eds. 1982. *The Problematic Science. Psychology in Nineteenth-Century Thought*. New York: Praeger Publishers.

Woolf, M. 1936. British Medical Societies: their early history and development. The Hunterian Society. *Medical Press and Circular 193*:304–308.

Wu, T., Hallett, M. 2013. The cerebellum in Parkinson's disease. *Brain 136*: 696–709.

Wyhe, J. van. 2004. *Phrenology and the Origins of Victorian Scientific Naturalism*. Aldershot: Ashgate.

York, G. K.1999. Hughlings Jackson's evolutionary neurophysiology. In Rose, pp.151–164.

York, G.K. 2002. Motor testing in neurology: An historical overview. In Louis 2002, pp.367–374.

York, G.K. 2015. Hughlings Jackson on joking. *Brain 138*:1435–1439.

York, G.K., Koehler, P.J. 2000. Jacksonian epilepsy. In Koehler et al., pp.94–99.

York, G.K., Steinberg, D.A. 1993. Hughlings Jackson's rejection of the unconscious. *JHN 2*:65–78.

York, G.K., Steinberg, D.A. 1994. Hughlings Jackson's theory of cerebral localization. *JHN 3*:153–168.

York, G.K., Steinberg, D.A. 1995. Hughlings Jackson's theory of recovery. *Neurology 45*:834–838.

York, G.K., Steinberg, D.A. 2002. The philosophy of Hughlings Jackson. *Journal of the Royal Society of Medicine 95*:314–318.

York, G.K., Steinberg, D.A. 2006. *An Introduction to the Life and Work of John Hughlings Jackson with a Catalogue Raissoné of his Writings: Medical History, Supplement 26*. London: Wellcome Trust Centre for the History of Medicine at UCL.

York, G.K., Steinberg, D.A. 2009. Broadbent's Law and cerebral localization in the nineteenth century. *JHN 18*:134–135

Youmans, E.L., ed. 1869. *The Correlation and Conservation of Forces: A Series of Expositions*. New York: D. Appleton.

Young, G.M. 1953. *Victorian England. Portrait of an Age*. 2 ed. Oxford: Oxford University Press. Reprinted in paperback 1989.

Young, R.M. 1970. *Mind, Brain and Adaptation in the Nineteenth Century. Cerebral Localization and its Biological Context from Gall to Ferrier*. Oxford: Oxford University Press. Reprinted 1990 with a new Preface.

Young, R.M. 1970a. The impact of Darwin on conventional thought. In Symondson, pp.13–35.

Young, R.M. 1985. *Darwin's Metaphor. Nature's Place in Victorian Culture*. Cambridge: Cambridge University Press.

Zifkin, B.G., Avanzini, G. 2009. Clinical neurophysiology with special reference to the electro-encephalogram. *Epilepsia 50*(Suppl.3):30–38.

Index

Footnotes are indicated by an 'n' after the page number. Boxes, Figures, and Tables are indicated by italics *b*, *f, and t*, following the page numbers.